Applications of Clinical Pharmacology in Drug Development

Applications of Clinical Pharmacology in Drug Development

Edited by **Mark Avis**

SYRAWOOD
PUBLISHING HOUSE

New York

Published by Syrawood Publishing House,
750 Third Avenue, 9th Floor,
New York, NY 10017, USA
www.syrawoodpublishinghouse.com

Applications of Clinical Pharmacology in Drug Development
Edited by Mark Avis

International Standard Book Number: 978-1-68286-198-1 (Hardback)

Contents

Preface

The main aim of this book is to educate learners and enhance their research focus by presenting diverse topics covering this vast field. This is an advanced book which compiles significant studies by distinguished experts. This book addresses successive solutions to the challenges arising in the area of application, along with it; the book provides scope for future developments.

Clinical pharmacology plays a vital role in drug development to ascertain how the drug affects the human subject. The aim of this book is to discuss some essential researches and advancements in this field through concepts like drug toxicity, therapeutic drugs, clinical trials, pharmacokinetics, etc. In this book, using various studies and examples, constant effort has been made to make the understanding of the different applications of clinical pharmacology in drug development as easy and informative as possible, for the readers.

It was a great honour to edit this book, though there were challenges, as it involved a lot of communication and networking between me and the editorial team. However, the end result was this all-inclusive book covering diverse themes in the field.

Finally, it is important to acknowledge the efforts of the contributors for their excellent chapters, through which a wide variety of issues have been addressed. I would also like to thank my colleagues for their valuable feedback during the making of this book.

Editor

Hit identification of IKKβ natural product inhibitor

Chung-Hang Leung[1]*, Daniel Shiu-Hin Chan[2], Ying-Wei Li[3], Wang-Fun Fong[3] and Dik-Lung Ma[2]*

Abstract

Background: The nuclear factor-κB (NF-κB) proteins are a small group of heterodimeric transcription factors that play an important role in regulating the inflammatory, immune, and apoptotic responses. NF-κB activity is suppressed by association with the inhibitor IκB. Aberrant NF-κB signaling activity has been associated with the development of cancer, chronic inflammatory diseases and auto-immune diseases. The IKK protein complex is comprised of IKKα, IKKβ and NEMO subunits, with IKKβ thought to play the dominant role in modulating NF-κB activity. Therefore, the discovery of new IKKβ inhibitors may offer new therapeutic options for the treatment of cancer and inflammatory diseases.

Results: A structure-based molecular docking approach has been employed to discover novel IKKβ inhibitors from a natural product library of over 90,000 compounds. Preliminary screening of the 12 highest-scoring compounds using a luciferase reporter assay identified 4 promising candidates for further biological study. Among these, the benzoic acid derivative (**1**) showed the most promising activity at inhibiting IKKβ phosphorylation and TNF-α-induced NF-κB signaling *in vitro*.

Conclusions: In this study, we have successfully identified a benzoic acid derivative (**1**) as a novel IKKβ inhibitor via high-throughput molecular docking. Compound **1** was able to inhibit IKKβ phosphorylation activity *in vitro*, and block IκBα protein degradation and subsequent NF-κB activation in human cells. Further *in silico* optimization of the compound is currently being conducted in order to generate more potent analogues for biological tests.

Background

The nuclear factor-κB (NF-κB) proteins are a small group of heterodimeric transcription factors that play an important role in regulating inflammatory, immune, and apoptotic responses [1-3]. NF-κB is ubiquitously present in the cytoplasm and its activity is normally suppressed by association with inhibitor IκB [4]. The intracellular NF-κB signaling cascade is initiated by a variety of inducers including proinflammatory cytokines TNF-α, IL-1 or endotoxins [5,6]. The aberrant activity to the NF-κB signaling pathway has been implicated in the development of a number of human diseases including cancer, auto-immune and chronic inflammatory conditions [3,7,8]. Therefore, inhibitors of the NF-κB signaling pathway could offer potential therapeutic value for the treatment of such diseases [9,10].

The IκB kinase is a multi-component complex composed of two catalytic subunits, IKKα and IKKβ and a regulatory unit NF-κB essential modulator (NEMO) [11-13]. Although both catalytic units are able to phosphorylate IκB, IKKβ has been shown to play the dominant role in activating NF-κB signaling in response to inflammatory stimuli [14,15]. Phosphorylated IκB is subsequently tagged by the E1 ubiquitin enzyme and degraded by the proteasome to liberate active NF-κB. Free NF-κB then translocates into the nucleus, where it binds to its cognate DNA site and enhances the expression of a number of genes related to the immune response, cell proliferation and survival [16,17]. Consequently, IKKβ represents an attractive target in the NF-κB pathway for the development of anti-inflammatory or anti-cancer therapeutics.

Virtual screening (VS) has emerged as a powerful tool in drug discovery complementing the vast array of popular but relatively costly high-throughput screening technologies [18,19]. Using virtual screening, the number of compounds to be evaluated *in vitro* could be dramatically decreased, which could greatly reduce the time and resource costs of drug discovery efforts. Meanwhile, natural products (NPs) have long provided a valuable source of inspiration to

* Correspondence: duncanleung@umac.mo; edmondma@hkbu.edu.hk
[1]State Key Laboratory of Quality Research in Chinese Medicine, Institute of Chinese Medical Sciences, University of Macau, Macao, China
[2]Department of Chemistry, Hong Kong Baptist University, Kowloon Tong, Hong Kong
Full list of author information is available at the end of the article

medicinal chemists due to the diversity of their molecular scaffolds, favourable biocompatibility and evolutionarily validated bioactive substructures [20,21]. Combining these two ideas, our group has previously identified natural product or small molecule inhibitors antagonizing cancer or inflammation-related targets using virtual screening [22-28]. For example, we have successfully identified natural product or natural product-like compounds targeting the c-*myc* oncogene G-quadruplex, tumor necrosis factor-alpha (TNF-α) and NEDD8-activating enzyme (NAE) [29-34].

In recent years, many small molecule inhibitors of IKKβ have been identified using pharmacophore-based or high-throughput screening approaches [32-39]. However, the recent publication of the IKKβ X-ray crystal structure with its inhibitor [40] enables the use of powerful structure-based *in silico* methods for the discovery of novel IKKβ inhibitors. We thus set out to identify interesting molecular scaffolds for the development of future IKKβ inhibitors from a large natural product library using high-throughput structure-based virtual screening. The X-ray co-crystal structure of the IKKβ with the reference inhibitor ((4-{[4-4-chlorophenyl) pyrimidin-2-yl]amino}phenyl[4-(2-hydroxyethyl)piperazin-1-yl]methanone (PDB: 3RZF) was used for our molecular modeling investigations (Figure 1) [40]. To our knowledge, this work is the first example of an IKKβ inhibitor identified using high-throughput molecular docking of a natural product database against the IKKβ X-ray co-crystal structure.

Results and Discussion
High-throughput virtual screening
The workflow of this virtual screening (VS) campaign is outlined in Scheme 1. The molecular model of IKKβ for VS was built using the recently reported X-ray co-crystal structure of IKKβ with its inhibitor. The binding site of IKKβ was defined to be within 3Å of the bound

inhibitor, which is situated at the hinge loop connecting the N and C lobes of the IKKβ KD domain. Over 90,000 structures from a chemical library of natural products and natural product-like compounds were screened *in silico* against the binding pocket of IKKβ [31]. The flexible ligands were docked to a grid representation of the receptor and assigned a score reflecting the quality of the complex according to the Internal Coordinate Mechanics (ICM) method [ICM-Pro 3.6-1d molecular docking software (Molsoft)]. Compounds with ICM docking scores of under -30 kcal/mol were shortlisted. Based on visual inspection and availability from the commercial sources, 12 compounds containing distinctive chemical scaffolds were chosen (Additional file 1: Figure S1). These compounds were purchased and were subjected to a preliminary luciferase assay (Additional file 1: Figure S2). The results showed that 4 out of the 12 compounds were able to inhibit NF-κB transcription activity by 20% or more compared to the untreated control at a concentration of 20 μM. The benzoic acid derivative (**1**) (Figure 1) inhibited NF-κB activity by over 40% relative to the untreated control, while compounds **3**, **9** and **10** exhibited weaker inhibitory activities of 20–30%. Compounds containing the benzoic acid moiety are known to display a variety of pharmacological effects and a number of benzoic acid derivatives possessing anti-inflammatory properties have been isolated from natural sources. For example, (*E*)-3-acetyl-6-(3,7-dimethylocta-2,6-dienyloxy)-2,4-dihydroxybenzoic acid isolated from *M. semecarpifolia* has been reported to suppress fmet-Leu-Phe (fMLP)-induced superoxide anion generation and elastase release by human neutrophils (Additional file 1: Table S1) [41]. In addition, the natural benzenoid antrocamphin A extracted from the fruiting body of *A. camphorata* was found to downregulate iNOS and COX-2 expression at both transcriptional and translational levels *via* suppression of NF-κB nuclear translocation [42]. A synthetic benzoic acid-derived compound GS143 reported by Furuichi, Shimbara and co-workers blocked NF-κB translocation through inhibition of IκBα ubiquitination and subsequent IκBα degradation [43]. To our knowledge, no biological activity of **1** has been reported in the literature. The identification of this natural product-derived benzoic acid scaffold as an IKKβ inhibitor could contribute to an understanding of the molecular mechanisms of the anti-inflammatory properties of this class of compounds. Furthermore, we envisage that this natural product derivative could serve as a valuable scaffold for the development of future IKKβ inhibitors.

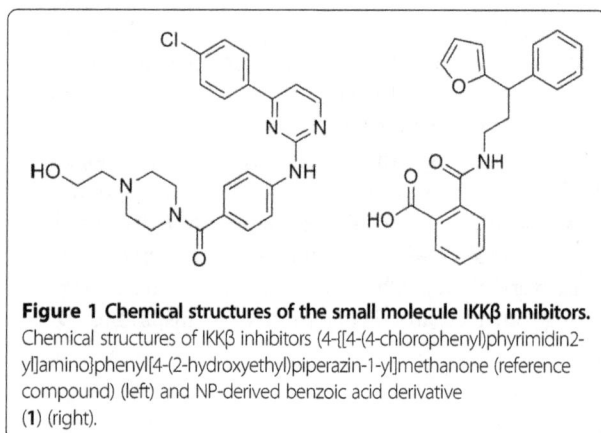

Figure 1 Chemical structures of the small molecule IKKβ inhibitors. Chemical structures of IKKβ inhibitors (4-{[4-(4-chlorophenyl)phyrimidin2-yl]amino}phenyl[4-(2-hydroxyethyl)piperazin-1-yl]methanone (reference compound) (left) and NP-derived benzoic acid derivative (**1**) (right).

Molecular modeling analysis
The ATP binding site of kinases generally consists of a narrow and hydrophobic region located between the N-lobe and C-lobe of the kinase domain (KD), with the

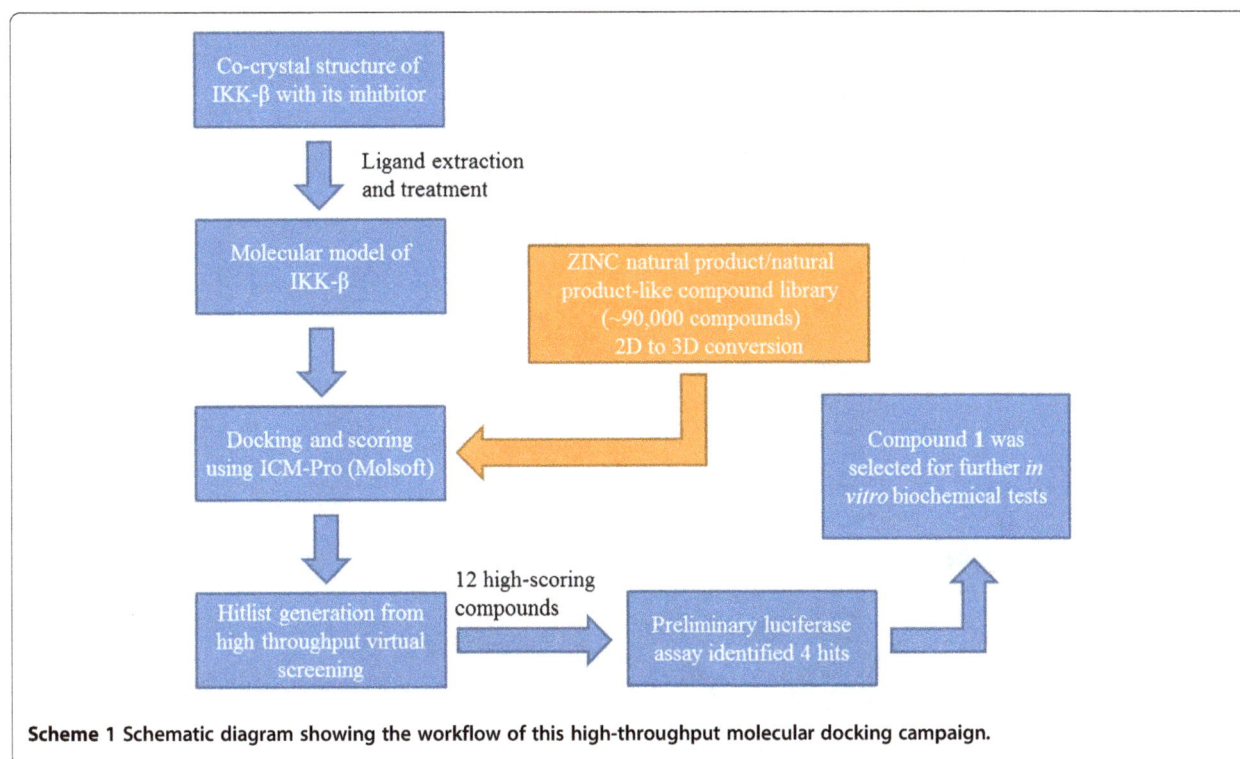

Scheme 1 Schematic diagram showing the workflow of this high-throughput molecular docking campaign.

two lobes linked together by a hinge region consisting of hydrogen bond donor and acceptor residues from the protein backbone [44]. The most important receptor residue in determining kinase inhibitor specificity is the "gatekeeper" residue, which controls the access of the inhibitor to the hydrophobic pocket. In the crystal structure of IKKβ, the gatekeeper residue is Met96, while Glu97, Tyr98 and Cys99 form the hinge region of the KD of IKKβ. The backbone groups of Glu97 and Cys99 are able to provide hydrogen bonding interactions with the inhibitor. In addition, the ATP binding site of IKKβ is partly covered by an activation loop comprised of serine, threonine and tyrosine residues in the unphosphorylated state. In particular, the N-terminal side of the activation loop contains the Asp166, Leu167 and Gly168 DLG triad which is involved in catalytic transfer of the γ-phosphate group in most kinase ATP binding sites (Figure 2a) [40].

Our molecular docking analysis revealed that the top-scoring binding mode of the natural product derivative **1** to the IKKβ complex is similar to that of the reference compound. The bound inhibitor in the co-crystal structure of IKKβ interacts with the ATP binding pocket in shape-driven manner [40]. While the structure of the reference compound contains the anilinopyrimidine motif that is found in other kinase inhibitors such as imatinib [45], no detectable hydrogen bonds between the hinge region of IKKβ and the anilinopyrimidine

moiety of the reference compound were recorded. The aromatic rings of the reference compound span the hinge loop while its terminal chlorine atom points towards the gatekeeper residue Met96 (Figure 2b).

By comparison, the benzoic acid moiety of **1** is situated at the end of the hinge loop with predicted hydrogen bonding interactions between the carboxyl oxygen and amide oxygen atoms of **1** with the phenolic hydrogen atom of Tyr98 and the backbone amino group of Gly102, respectively (Figure 2c). The pendant side chain of **1** is predicted to be situated in a hydrophobic binding pocket also occupied by the reference compound. We envisage that **1** could act as a reversible inhibitor of IKKβ by blocking the nucleotide recognition domain that binds ATP [40]. The binding score for **1** with the IKKβ complex was calculated to be -35.28 kcal/mol, reflecting a strong interaction between the compound and the IKKβ binding site.

The other eleven compounds were also predicted to situate in the hinge region of the binding pockets in the docking analysis. Most of the compounds could form hydrogen bonds with the hinge residues including Glu97, Cys99 and Glu100. Furthermore, several of the compounds formed additional hydrogen bonds with the residues in the solvent accessible region (Arg31 and Lys106). The lowest energy binding pose of the other compounds are summarized in Additional file 1: Table S2.

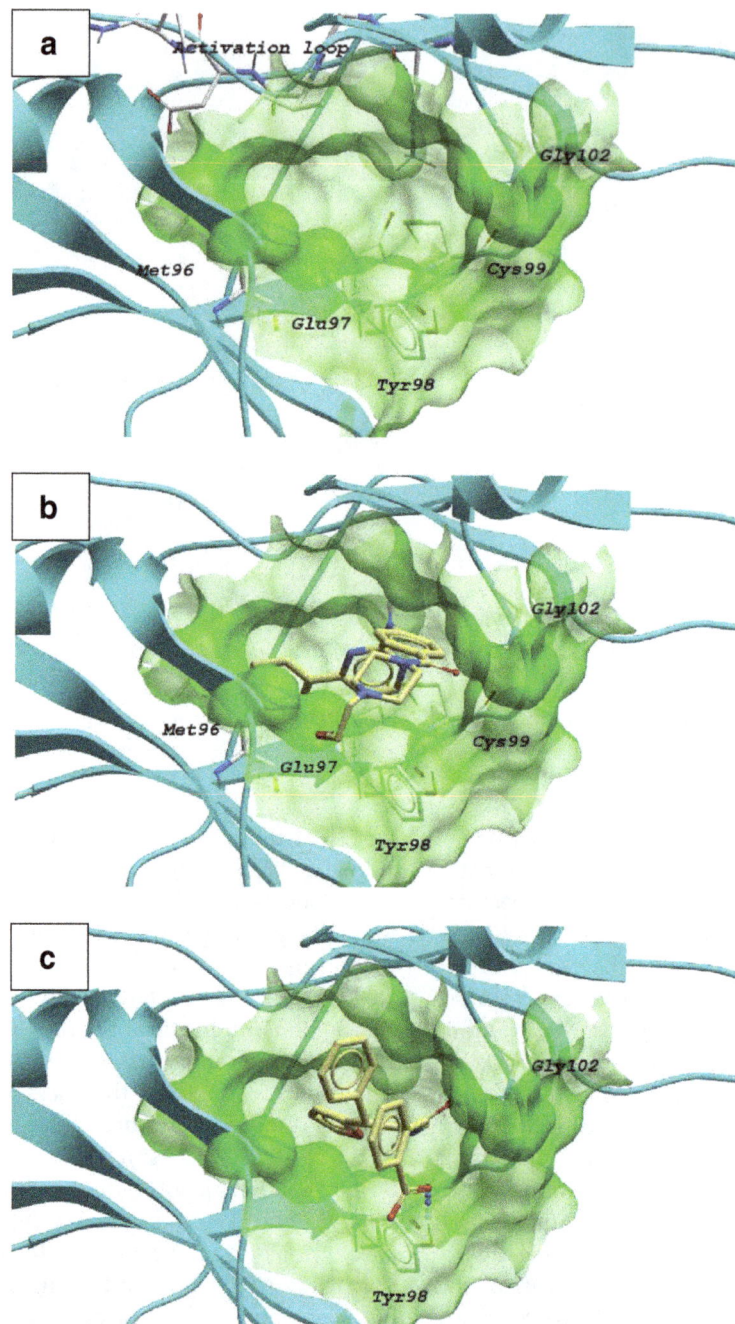

Figure 2 Molecular docking analysis of reference compound and 1 to the IKKβ protein complex. a) The KD domain of IKKβ is displayed in the ribbon form. The activation loop, gatekeeper residue (Met 96), hinge region (Glu97-Cys99) are visualized. Low-energy binding conformations of **b**) **1** and **c**) reference compound to IKKβ protein complex were generated by virtual ligand docking. Small molecules inhibitor **1** and reference compound is depicted as a ball-and-stick model showing carbon (yellow), hydrogen (grey), oxygen (red) and nitrogen (blue) atoms. H-bonds are indicated as dotted lines. The binding pocket of the IKKβ is represented as a translucent green surface.

We also investigated the selectivity of compound **1** for IKKβ over four other kinases (PKCα, PAK4, CaMK2α and JAK2) using molecular modeling. While compound **1** was predicted to bind at the ATP binding sites of the four other kinases, the ICM docking energies of the **1**-kinase complexes were significantly less negative than that for IKKβ (Additional file 1: Table S3). Molecules exhibiting such weak binding energies would be expected to be inactive *in vitro*.

1 inhibits IκBα phosphorylation *in vitro*

Encouraged by the molecular docking results and the preliminary luciferase screening experiment, we investigated the effect of compound **1** on IKKβ phosphorylation activity. Inhibition of IKKβ phosphorylation activity would be expected to lead to a decrease in GST-IκBα substrate phosphorylation level. Encouragingly, a dose-dependent reduction in IKKβ activity was observed upon the incubation with **1**, with an estimated IC_{50} value of *ca.* 50 μM (Figure 3).

1 inhibits TNF-α induced NF-κB signaling in a HepG2 cell line

We sought to investigate the ability of compound **1** to inhibit NF-κB signaling in human cells using a luciferase assay. A stably-transfected HepG2 cell line carrying the luciferase reporter gene driven by a promoter containing multiple copies of the NF-κB response element was used in this study. The transcriptional activity of NF-κB was

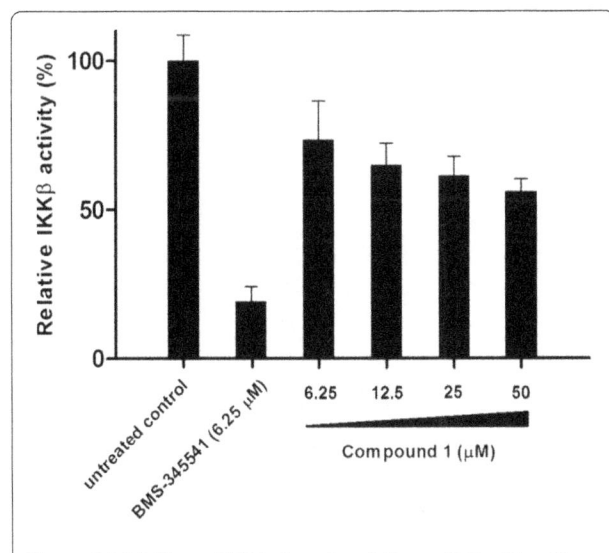

Figure 3 Inhibition of IKKβ phosphorylation activity. Microtiter plates with GST-IκBα were incubated with IKKβ together with **1** at the indicated concentrations. GST-IκBα phosphorylated level was detected using an anti-phospho IκBα (Ser32/Ser36) antibody and horseradish peroxidase conjugated secondary antibody. Approximate IC_{50} value of **1** = 50 μM. Error bars represent the standard deviations of the results from three independent experiments.

determined by measuring the luciferase activity of the cell lysates using a luminometer. We performed a dose response analysis of compound **1** and three other hit compounds in attenuating TNF-α-induced NF-κB signaling (Figure 4). Compound **1** inhibited TNF-α-induced luciferase activity in a dose-dependent manner with an estimated IC_{50} value of *ca.* 10 μM. While the three other compounds also inhibited TNF-α-induced luciferase activity, their inhibition potencies were around 10-fold lower compared to compound **1**.

Based on the results of the IKKβ assay and the molecular modeling analysis, we envisage that the inhibition of TNF-α-induced NF-κB signaling by **1** could be attributed, at least in part, to the inhibition of IKKβ activity *in vitro*, thus preventing the degradation of the NF-κB repressor IκBα. The slightly higher potency of **1** in the cell-based luciferase assay compared to the enzyme assay is possibly due to a multi-target effect of **1**, suggesting that this compound could potentially influence other steps involved in NF-κB activation.

Conclusions

In conclusion, we have discovered a new small molecule IKKβ inhibitor from a large natural product library of 90,000 compounds using high-throughput structure-based molecular docking. The benzoic acid derivative **1** is able to inhibit IKKβ activity in both cell-free and system with micromolar potency. Furthermore, compound **1** could inhibit IKKβ-mediated NF-κB signaling pathway in human cancer cells. We envisage that compound **1** attenuates the *in cellulo* transcriptional activity of NF-κB, at least in part, by abrogating the activity of IKKβ. The discovery of this natural product-like derivative provides medicinal chemists with a structurally interesting scaffold, facilitating further chemical modifications in order to sample greater regions of the chemical space of potential IKKβ inhibitors. We are currently investigating the effects of **1** on the proteins involved in NF-κB signaling and conducting *in silico* lead optimization to generate more potent analogues of **1** for *in vitro* biological testing.

Methods

Materials and cell lines

The NP/NP-like compound collection, which includes compound **1** and the other tested compounds, was obtained from InterBioScreen (Moscow, RUS). The K-LISA™ IKKβ Inhibitor Screening Kit was obtained from Calbiochem (Darmstadt, Germany). Passive lysis buffer and luciferase assay reagent were obtained from Promega Corporation (Madison, WI, USA). HepG2 and HepG2-NF-κB-Luc cells were provided by Prof. Y.C. Cheng (Department of Pharmacology, Yale University School of Medicine, USA). Cells cultured in Minimum

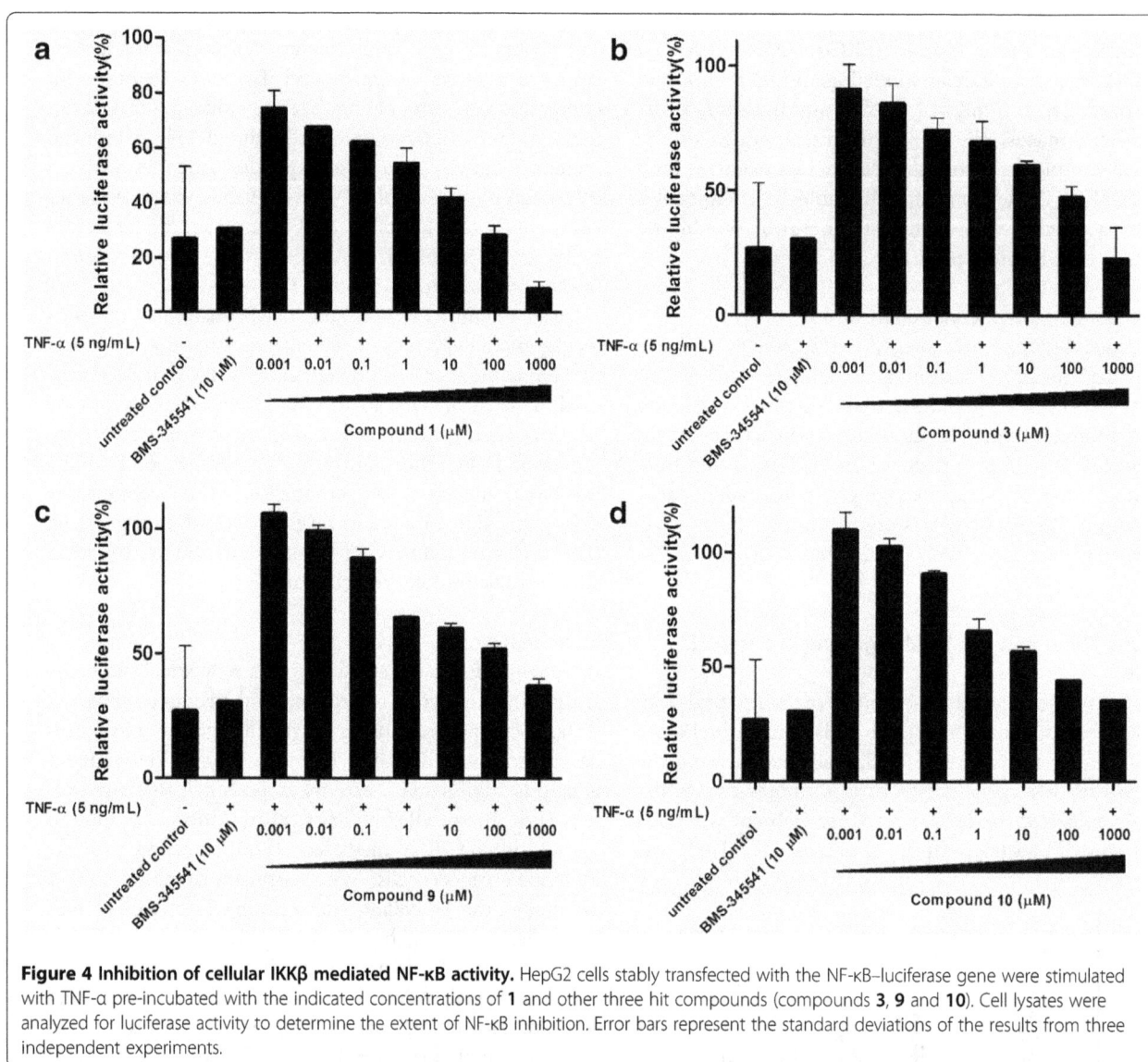

Figure 4 Inhibition of cellular IKKβ mediated NF-κB activity. HepG2 cells stably transfected with the NF-κB–luciferase gene were stimulated with TNF-α pre-incubated with the indicated concentrations of **1** and other three hit compounds (compounds **3**, **9** and **10**). Cell lysates were analyzed for luciferase activity to determine the extent of NF-κB inhibition. Error bars represent the standard deviations of the results from three independent experiments.

Essential Media containing 10% fetal bovine serum were incubated at 37°C/5% CO_2 and passaged three times a week.

IKKβ enzymatic activity

IKKβ activity was determined using the ELISA-based (K-LISA™) IKKβ Inhibitor Screening Kit according to the manufacturer's instructions. The GST-IκBα 50-amino acid peptide that includes the Ser32 and Ser36 IKKβ phosphorylation sites was used as a substrate and was incubated for 30 min at 30°C with human recombinant IKKβ in the presence of DMSO vehicle or different concentrations of **1** in a glutathione-coated 96-well plate. The phosphorylated GST-IκBα substrate was subsequently detected using anti-phospho-IκBα (Ser32/Ser36) antibody and a horseradish peroxidase-conjugated secondary antibody. The samples were finally incubated with TMB solution, and the color development was monitored at 450 nm on a plate reader (Bio-Rad).

NF-κB transactivation activity

Exponentially growing HepG2-NF-κB-Luc cells were seeded overnight at 1×10^4 cells/well in a 48-well plate. On the next day, the cells were pre-incubated with the indicated concentrations of **1** for 1 h before stimulation by 5 ng/mL of TNF-α for an additional 3 h. Passive lysis buffer (50 μL) was added to each well and the plate was incubated for 15 min with shaking. A 20 μL aliquot from each well was mixed with 70 μL luciferase assay reagent in a 96-well white plate. The transcriptional activity was determined by measuring the activity of firefly luciferase in a multi-well plate luminometer (Fusion α-FP, Perkin-Elmer).

Molecular modeling

A natural product or natural product-like chemical library containing over 90,000 compounds was screened *in silico*. Molecular docking was performed by using the ICM-Pro 3.6-1d program (Molsoft). According to the ICM method, the molecular system was described by using internal coordinates as variables. Energy calculations were based on the ECEPP/3 force field with a distance-dependent dielectric constant. The biased probability Monte Carlo (BPMC) minimization procedure was used for global energy optimization. The BPMC global-energy-optimization method consists of 1) a random conformation change of the free variables according to a predefined continuous probability distribution; 2) local-energy minimization of analytical differentiable terms; 3) calculation of the complete energy including nondifferentiable terms such as entropy and solvation energy; 4) acceptance or rejection of the total energy based on the Metropolis criterion and return to step (1). The binding between the small molecules and NAE-NEDD8 were evaluated with a full-atom ICM ligand binding score from a multireceptor screening benchmark as a compromise between approximated Gibbs free energy of binding and numerical errors. The score was calculated by:

$$S_{bind} = E_{int} + T\Delta S_{Tor} + E_{vw} + \alpha_1 E_{el} + \alpha_2 E_{hb} + \alpha_3 E_{hp} + \alpha_4 E_{sf}$$

where E_{vw}, E_{el}, E_{hb}, E_{hp}, and E_{sf} are Van der Waals, electrostatic, hydrogen bonding, and nonpolar and polar atom solvation energy differences between bound and unbound states, respectively. E_{int} is the ligand internal strain, ΔS_{Tor} is its conformational entropy loss upon binding, and $T = 300$ K, and α_i are ligand- and receptor independent constants. The initial model of IKKβ was built from the X-ray crystal structure of the Inhibitor of kappaB kinase beta (PDB: 3RZF) according to a previously reported procedure. Hydrogen and missing heavy atoms were added to the receptor structure followed by local minimization by using the conjugate gradient algorithm and analytical derivatives in the internal coordinates. In the docking analysis, the binding site was assigned across the entire structure of the protein complex. Each compound was assigned the MMFF force field atom types and charges and was then subjected to Cartesian minimization. The ICM docking was performed to find the most favorable orientation. The resulting trajectories of the complex between the small molecules and protein complex were energy minimized, and the interaction energies were computed. Each compound was docked three times and the minimum of the three scores was used. The 12 highest scoring compounds were utilized for biological testing without

further selection. The crystal structures of PAK4 (4APP), PKCα (3IW4), CAMK2α (2VZ6) and JAK2 (3IOK) were also prepared and compound **1** was docked to these molecular models individually using the aforementioned procedures.

Additional file

Additional file 1: Figure S1. Chemical structures of the 11 other high-scoring compounds selected for preliminary biological evaluation. **Figure S2.** Preliminary experimental screening of the 12 compounds on inhibition of cellular IKKβ mediated NF-κB activity. **Table S1.** Chemical name and structures of benzoic acid derivatives reported to target the NF-κB signaling pathway. **Table S2.** Lowest-energy binding pose of the 11 other compounds with the ATP binding site in the KD domain of IKKβ. **Table S3.** Binding poses and ICM docking energies of compound 1 to other four kinases. The reference compounds are displayed in cyan.

Competing interests
The authors declare that they have no competing interests.

Authors' contributions
C.-H. Leung and D.-L. Ma conceived the study, designed the experiments and performed the *in silico* high-throughput screening. Y.-W. Li and D. S.-H. Chan analyzed the experimental results, performed the experiments and wrote the manuscript. C.-H. Leung, D.-L. Ma and W.-F. Fong analyzed the experimental results and edited the manuscript. All authors have read and approved the final manuscript.

Acknowledgements
This work is supported by Hong Kong Baptist University (FRG2/11-12/009), Centre for Cancer and Inflammation Research, School of Chinese Medicine (CCIR-SCM, HKBU), the Health and Medical Research Fund (HMRF/11101212), the Research Grants Council (HKBU/201811 and HKBU/204612), the Science and Technology Development Fund, Macao SAR (001/2012/A) and the University of Macau MYRG091(Y1-L2)-ICMS12-LCH and MYRG121(Y1-L2)-ICMS12-LCH).

Author details
[1]State Key Laboratory of Quality Research in Chinese Medicine, Institute of Chinese Medical Sciences, University of Macau, Macao, China. [2]Department of Chemistry, Hong Kong Baptist University, Kowloon Tong, Hong Kong. [3]Centre for Cancer and Inflammation Research, School of Chinese Medicine, Hong Kong Baptist University, Kowloon Tong, Hong Kong.

References
1. Hayden MS, Ghosh S: **Shared Principles in NF-κB Signaling.** *Cell* 2008, **132**:344–362.
2. Vallabhapurapu S, Karin M: **Regulation and Function of NF-κB Transcription Factors in the Immune System.** *Annu Rev Immunol* 2009, **27**:693–733.
3. Karin M: **Nuclear factor-κB in cancer development and progression.** *Nature* 2006, **441**:431–436.
4. Baldwin AS: **The NF-κB AND IκB Proteins: New Discoveries and Insights.** *Annu Rev Immunol* 1996, **14**:649–681.
5. Hideshima T, Chauhan D, Richardson P, Mitsiades C, Mitsiades N, Hayashi T, Munshi N, Dang L, Castro A, Palombella V, *et al*: **NF-κB as a Therapeutic Target in Multiple Myeloma.** *J Biol Chem* 2002, **277**:16639–16647.
6. Schmid JA, Birbach A: **IκB kinase β (IKKβ/IKK2/IKBKB)—A key molecule in signaling to the transcription factor NF-κB.** *Cytokine Growth Factor Rev* 2008, **19**:157–165.
7. Lee CH, Jeon Y-T, Kim S-H, Song Y-S: **NF-κB as a potential molecular target for cancer therapy.** *Biofactors* 2007, **29**:19–35.
8. Karin M, Cao Y, Greten FR, Li Z-W: **NF-κB in cancer: from innocent bystander to major culprit.** *Nat Rev Cancer* 2002, **2**:301–310.

9. Kim HJ, Hawke N, Baldwin AS: NF-κB and IKK as therapeutic targets in cancer. *Cell Death Differ* 2006, 13:738–747.

10. Senftleben U: Anti-inflammatory interventions of NF-κB signaling: Potential applications and risks. *Biochem Pharmacol* 2008, 75:1567–1579.

11. Gilmore TD: Introduction to NF-κB: players, pathways, perspectives. *Oncogene* 2005, 25:6680–6684.

12. Perkins ND: Integrating cell-signaling pathways with NF-[kappa]B and IKK function. *Nat Rev Mol Cell Biol* 2007, 8:49–62.

13. Karin M, Ben-Neriah Y: Phosphorylation Meets Ubiquitination: The Control of NF-κB Activity. *Annu Rev Immunol* 2000, 18:621–663.

14. Karin M: How NF-κB is activated: the role of the IκB kinase (IKK) complex. *Oncogene* 1999, 18:6867–6874.

15. Strnad J, Burke JR: IκB kinase inhibitors for treating autoimmune and inflammatory disorders: potential and challenges. *Trends Pharmacol Sci* 2007, 28:142–148.

16. Karin M, Yamamoto Y, Wang QM: The IKK NF-κB system: a treasure trove for drug development. *Nat Rev Drug Discov* 2004, 3:17–26.

17. Gilmore TD: The Rel/NF-B signal transduction pathway: introduction. *Oncogene* 1999, 18:6842–6844.

18. Bajorath J: Integration of virtual and high-throughput screening. *Nat Rev Drug Discov* 2002, 1:882–894.

19. Shoichet BK: Virtual screening of chemical libraries. *Nature* 2004, 432:862–865.

20. Breinbauer R, Vetter IR, Waldmann H: From Protein Domains to Drug Candidates—Natural Products as Guiding Principles in the Design and Synthesis of Compound Libraries. *Angew Chem Int Ed* 2002, 41:2878–2890.

21. Ertl P, Roggo S, Schuffenhauer A: Natural Product-likeness Score and Its Application for Prioritization of Compound Libraries. *J Chem Inf Model* 2007, 48:68–74.

22. Leung C-H: Chan DS-H, Kwan MH-T, Cheng Z, Wong C-Y, Zhu G-Y, Fong W-F, Ma D-L: Structure-Based Repurposing of FDA-Approved Drugs as TNF-α Inhibitors. *ChemMedChem* 2011, 6:765–768.

23. Chan DS-H, Yang H, Kwan MH-T, Cheng Z, Lee P, Bai L-P, Jiang Z-H, Wong C-Y, Fong W-F, Leung C-H, Ma D-L: Structure-based optimization of FDA-approved drug methylene blue as a c-myc G-quadruplex DNA stabilizer. *Biochimie* 2011, 93:1055–1064.

24. Yang H, Zhong H-J, Leung K-H, Chan DS-H, Ma VP-Y, Fu W-C, Nanjunda R, Wilson WD, Ma D-L, Leung C-H: Structure-based design of flavone derivatives as c-myc oncogene down-regulators. *Eur J Pharm Sci* 2013, 48:130–141.

25. Ma D-L: Chan DS-H, Leung C-H: Molecular docking for virtual screening of natural product databases. *Chem. Sci.* 2011, 2:1656–1665.

26. Ma D-L: Chan DS-H, Lee P, Kwan MH-T, Leung C-H: Molecular modeling of drug–DNA interactions: Virtual screening to structure-based design. *Biochimie* 2011, 93:1252–1266.

27. Ma D-L: Ma VP-Y, Chan DS-H, Leung K-H, Zhong H-J, Leung C-H: In silico screening of quadruplex-binding ligands. *Methods* 2012, 57:106–114.

28. Ma D-L, Chan DS-H, Leung C-H: Drug repositioning by structure-based virtual screening. *Chem Soc Rev*, .

29. Leung C-H, Chan DS-H, Yang H, Abagyan R, Lee SM-Y, Zhu G-Y, Fong W-F, Ma D-L: A natural product-like inhibitor of NEDD8-activating enzyme. *Chem Commun* 2011, 47:2511–2513.

30. Ma D-L, Lai T-S, Chan F-Y, Chung W-H, Abagyan R, Leung Y-C, Wong K-Y: Discovery of a Drug-Like G-Quadruplex Binding Ligand by High-Throughput Docking. *ChemMedChem* 2008, 3:881–884.

31. Chan DS-H, Lee H-M, Yang F, Che C-M, Wong CCL, Abagyan R, Leung C-H, Ma D-L: Structure-Based Discovery of Natural-Product-like TNF-α Inhibitors. *Angew Chem Int Ed* 2010, 49:2860–2864.

32. Lee H-M: Chan DS-H, Yang F, Lam H-Y, Yan S-C, Che C-M, Ma D-L, Leung C-H: Identification of natural product Fonsecin B as a stabilizing ligand of c-myc G-quadruplex DNA by high-throughput virtual screening. *Chem Commun* 2010, 46:4680–4682.

33. Zhong H-J: Ma VP-Y, Cheng Z, Chan DS-H, He H-Z, Leung K-H, Ma D-L, Leung C-H: Discovery of a natural product inhibitor targeting protein neddylation by structure-based virtual screening. *Biochimie* 2012, 94:2457–2460.

34. Ma D-L, Chan DS-H, Fu W-C, He H-Z, Yang H, Yan S-C, Leung C-H: Discovery of a Natural Product-Like c-myc G-Quadruplex DNA Groove-Binder by Molecular Docking. *PLoS One* 2012, 7:e43278.

35. Miller DD, Bamborough P, Christopher JA, Baldwin IR, Champigny AC, Cutler GJ, Kerns JK, Longstaff T, Mellor GW, Morey JV, *et al*: 3,5-Disubstituted-indole-7-carboxamides: The discovery of a novel series of potent, selective inhibitors of IKK-β. *Bioorg Med Chem Lett* 2011, 21:2255–2258.

36. Crombie AL, Sum F-W, Powell DW, Hopper DW, Torres N, Berger DM, Zhang Y, Gavriil M, Sadler TM, Arndt K: Synthesis and biological evaluation of tricyclic anilinopyrimidines as IKKβ inhibitors. *Bioorg Med Chem Lett* 2010, 20:3821–3825.

37. Kempson J, Spergel SH, Guo J, Quesnelle C, Gill P, Belanger D, Dyckman AJ, Li T, Watterson SH, Langevine CM, *et al*: Novel Tricyclic Inhibitors of IκB Kinase. *J Med Chem* 2009, 52:1994–2005.

38. Kempson J, Guo J, Das J, Moquin RV, Spergel SH, Watterson SH, Langevine CM, Dyckman AJ, Pattoli M, Burke JR, *et al*: Synthesis, initial SAR and biological evaluation of 1,6-dihydroimidazo[4,5-d]pyrrolo[2,3-b]pyridin-4-amine derived inhibitors of IκB kinase. *Bioorg Med Chem Lett* 2009, 19:2646–2649.

39. Christopher JA, Bamborough P, Alder C, Campbell A, Cutler GJ, Down K, Hamadi AM, Jolly AM, Kerns JK, Lucas FS, *et al*: Discovery of 6-Aryl-7-alkoxyisoquinoline Inhibitors of IκB Kinase-β (IKK-β). *J Med Chem* 2009, 52:3098–3102.

40. Xu G, Lo Y-C, Li Q, Napolitano G, Wu X, Jiang X, Dreano M, Karin M, Wu H: Crystal structure of inhibitor of κB kinase β. *Nature* 2011, 472:325–330.

41. Chen J-J, Cho J-Y, Hwang T-L, Chen I-S: Benzoic Acid Derivatives, Acetophenones, and Anti-inflammatory Constituents from Melicope semecarpifolia. *J Nat Prod* 2007, 71:71–75.

42. Hsieh Y-H, Chu F-H, Wang Y-S, Chien S-C, Chang S-T, Shaw J-F, Chen C-Y, Hsiao W-W, Kuo Y-H, Wang S-Y: Antrocamphin A, an Anti-inflammatory Principal from the Fruiting Body of Taiwanofungus camphoratus, and Its Mechanisms. *J Agric Food Chem* 2010, 58:3153–3158.

43. Nakajima H, Fujiwara H, Furuichi Y, Tanaka K, Shimbara N: A novel small-molecule inhibitor of NF-κB signaling. *Biochem Biophys Res Commun* 2008, 368:1007–1013.

44. Ghose AK, Herbertz T, Pippin DA, Salvino JM, Mallamo JP: Knowledge Based Prediction of Ligand Binding Modes and Rational Inhibitor Design for Kinase Drug Discovery. *J Med Chem* 2008, 51:5149–5171.

45. Cowan-Jacob SW, Fendrich G, Manley PW, Jahnke W, Fabbro D, Liebetanz J, Meyer T: The Crystal Structure of a c-Src Complex in an Active Conformation Suggests Possible Steps in c-Src Activation. *Structure* 2005, 13:861–871.

2

Safety, tolerability, pharmacokinetics and pharmacodynamics of GSK2239633, a CC-chemokine receptor 4 antagonist, in healthy male subjects: results from an open-label and from a randomised study

Anthony Cahn[1*], Simon Hodgson[1], Robert Wilson[1], Jonathan Robertson[1], Joanna Watson[2], Misba Beerahee[1], Steve C Hughes[3], Graeme Young[3], Rebecca Graves[1], David Hall[1], Sjoerd van Marle[4] and Roberto Solari[1]

Abstract

Background: The CC-chemokine receptor 4 (CCR4) is thought potentially to play a critical role in asthma pathogenesis due to its ability to recruit type 2 T-helper lymphocytes to the inflamed airways. Therefore, CCR4 provides an excellent target for anti-inflammatory therapy.

Methods: The safety, tolerability, pharmacokinetics and pharmacodynamics of the CCR4 antagonist GSK2239633, N-(3-((3-(5-chlorothiophene-2-sulfonamido)-4-methoxy-1H-indazol-1-yl)methyl)benzyl)-2-hydroxy-2-methylpropanamide, were examined in healthy males. Two studies were performed: 1) an open-label, study in which six subjects received a single intravenous infusion of [^{14}C]-GSK2239633 100 μg (10 kBq) (NCT01086462), and 2) a randomised, double-blind, placebo-controlled, cross-over, ascending dose study in which 24 subjects received single oral doses of GSK2239633 150–1500 mg (NCT01371812).

Results: Following intravenous dosing, plasma GSK2239633 displayed rapid, bi-phasic distribution and slow terminal elimination ($t_{1/2}$: 13.5 hours), suggesting that GSK2239633 was a low to moderate clearance drug. Following oral dosing, blood levels of GSK2239633 reached C_{max} rapidly (median t_{max}: 1.0–1.5 hours). Estimated GSK2239633 bioavailability was low with a maximum value determined of only 16%. Food increased GSK2239633 systemic exposure (as assessed by AUC and C_{max}). Increases in AUC and C_{max} were less than dose proportional. Adverse events were reported by three subjects (50%) following intravenous administration, and by 19 subjects (79%) following oral administration; most (46/47; 98%) events were mild/moderate in intensity. GSK2239633 1500 mg inhibited thymus- and activation-regulated chemokine-induced (TARC) actin polymerisation reaching a mean CCR4 occupancy of 74%.

Conclusion: In conclusion, GSK2239633 was well-tolerated and capable of inhibiting TARC from activating the CCR4 receptor.

Keywords: GSK2239633, CCR4, Microdose, Healthy

* Correspondence: tony.x.cahn@gsk.com
[1]Medicines Discovery and Development, Gunnels Wood Road, Stevenage Herts SG1 2NY, UK
Full list of author information is available at the end of the article

Background

Allergic asthma is characterised by chronic inflammation of the airways, commonly triggered by environmental aeroallergens. This inflammatory process in asthma is characterised by inflammatory cell recruitment, increased mucus production, periodic airway smooth muscle contraction and vascular vasodilation [1-4]. Subsequently, Type 2 T helper (Th2) lymphocytes, and other cell types, are recruited from peripheral blood into the inflamed tissue where they produce cytokines that induce eosinophil recruitment, stimulate the production of allergen-specific immunoglobulin E by B-cells and increase the permeability of the endothelium to allow further recruitment of inflammatory cells [5-7].

One mode of Th2 lymphocyte recruitment to inflamed airways [8-11] is through the specific binding of the chemokines thymus- and activation-regulated chemokine (TARC) and monocyte-derived chemokine (MDC) to the CC-chemokine receptor 4 (CCR4) expressed on the surface of a subset of Th2 cells [12-17]. High levels of TARC and MDC have been detected in the lungs of patients with asthma following an allergen challenge [18,19], and high numbers of Th2 cells recovered in bronchial biopsies from patients with asthma have been found to be CCR4 positive [20-22]. As chemokine receptors play a key role in inflammatory processes, they provide excellent targets for anti-inflammatory therapy [23-26]. The targeting of CCR4 is believed to be a safe strategy as initial clinical studies with mogamulizumab, a humanised anti-CCR4 monoclonal antibody, have given no indication of an increase in the number of infections or any degree of immunosuppression related to mogamulizumab [27]. Further, there was no evidence of any CCR4-specific adverse clinical effects in patients with T-cell lymphomas treated with mogamulizumab [27].

GSK2239633 N-(3-((3-(5-chlorothiophene-2-sulfonamido)-4-methoxy-1H-indazol-1-yl)methyl)benzyl)-2-hydroxy-2-methylpropanamide, compound 7r in [28], is an allosteric antagonist of human CCR4 [29]. *In vitro*, GSK2239633 inhibited the binding of $[^{125}I]$-TARC to human CCR4 with a pIC_{50} of 7.96 ± 0.11 and also inhibited TARC-induced increases in the F-actin content of isolated human $CD4^+$ $CCR4^+$ T-cells with a pA_2 of 7.11 ± 0.29 [unpublished observations]. Conflicting pharmacokinetic profiles for GSK2239633 were obtained in the rat and dog, leading to variable predictions of the human pharmacokinetic profile. Therefore, before oral GSK2239633 was administered to humans for the first time, a Microdose Intravenous Study using a radio-labelled dose [30] of GSK2239633 was conducted in healthy subjects. This Microdose Intravenous Study revealed that plasma clearance of GSK2239633 was low to moderate or approximately 40% of liver blood flow when plasma clearance was converted to blood clearance. To obtain information at a potentially clinically relevant dose level, a study using single ascending oral doses of GSK2239633 was conducted in healthy subjects. Here we report the results obtained in both of these clinical studies.

Methods

Study population

All subjects provided signed and dated informed consent prior to screening. Local Ethics Review Committees provided approval for both studies (Microdose Intravenous Study: Independent Ethics Committee of the Foundation "Evaluation of the Ethics of Biomedical Research", Assen, The Netherlands; Single Oral Dose Study: Medische Ethische ToetsingsCommissie, Stichting Beoordeling Ethik Biomedisch Onderzoek, Assen, The Netherlands) and they were conducted in accordance with Good Clinical Practice and the guiding principles of the 2008 Declaration of Helsinki [31].

Microdose intravenous study

Healthy subjects aged 18–50 years with a body mass index of 18.5–29.9 kg/m^2 were eligible. Subjects had to be non-smokers or ex-smokers for a minimum of 6 months prior to screening and with a smoking history of <5 pack years. Exclusion criteria included positive testing for hepatitis B surface antigen, hepatitis C antibody and human immunodeficiency virus. Subjects unwilling to abstain from red wine, Seville oranges, grapefruit or grapefruit products 7 days prior to dosing were also ineligible.

Single oral dose study

Healthy subjects aged 18–65 years with a body mass index of 18.5–29.9 kg/m^2 and a smoking history as described for the Microdose Intravenous Study were eligible. Key exclusion criteria were as for the Microdose Intravenous Study.

Study design

Microdose intravenous study

This was an open-label, single-dose study conducted from 21 January 2010 to 18 February 2010 at PRA International, Zuidlaren, The Netherlands (GlaxoSmithKline protocol: CC4114041; Clinicaltrials.gov identifier: NCT01086462). Subjects received a single intravenous infusion of approximately 10 kBq $[^{14}C]$-GSK2239633 100 μg over 15 minutes. Subjects attended a screening visit within 30 days prior to receiving the first dose of study medication. Subjects were admitted to the clinical unit on Day −1 and remained there until 48 hours post-dose. As this was the first time GSK2239633 100 μg had been administered to humans, dosing was staggered so that only one subject received the study medication on Day 1. As the study medication was well-tolerated, the remaining subjects were dosed the following day in a staggered dosing schedule (20-minute interval between dosing of the subjects). Subjects received a follow-up telephone call 4–10 days after the last dose of study medication.

Single oral dose study

This was a randomised, double-blind, placebo-controlled, cross-over, single ascending-dose study conducted from 29 March 2011 to 1 July 2011 at PRA International, Zuidlaren, the Netherlands (GlaxoSmithKline protocol: CC4114660; Clinicaltrials.gov identifier: NCT01371812). Subjects completed a screening visit within 28 days prior to receiving the first dose of study medication. Subjects were admitted to the clinical unit the day before each dosing session for baseline assessments that included a physical examination and clinical laboratory tests. Single ascending oral doses of GSK2239633 or placebo were administered to two interlocking and alternating cohorts (Additional file 1: Figure S1) (Cohort 1 and Cohort 2), each of which consisted of 12 male subjects randomised to receive either active or placebo (eight active: four placebo). The randomisation schedule was generated prior to the start of the study using validated internal software. Subjects from Cohort 1 underwent four dosing sessions; the starting dose of GSK2239633 was 150 mg, followed by 600 mg, 1200 mg and 1200 mg after eating the standard United States Food and Drug Administration (FDA) high fat/high caloric meal to assess any food effect. Subjects from Cohort 2 underwent three dosing sessions; the starting dose of GSK2239633 was 300 mg, followed by 900 mg and 1500 mg. As this was a first-time-in-human study, dosing was staggered over 2 days so that on Day 1 one subject received GSK2239633 and one subject received placebo at each dosing session in both cohorts (with the exception of the food effect dosing session for Cohort 1). On Day 2, the remaining subjects were dosed provided GSK2239633 was well-tolerated on Day 1. Subjects fasted for 10 hours before each dosing session, except those in last period of Cohort 1 who ate 30 minutes prior to administration of GSK2239633 1200 mg. For both cohorts, no food was permitted up to 4 hours after administration of study medication. During a 2-hour period (1 hour pre-dose until 1 hour post-dose), no water was allowed with the exception of that taken with the study medication (240–300 mL). After receiving randomised treatment, subjects underwent a period of observation and assessments for 3 days. They returned to the clinical unit, following a washout period of approximately 14 days, to receive their next randomised dose of study medication, with additional 3-day inpatient assessments. Subjects returned for a follow-up visit 10–14 days after their last dose of study medication.

Dosing and sample collection

Microdose intravenous study

Subjects were dosed over 15 minutes with: 10 μg/mL GSK2239633 (^{14}C-labelled) in a saline solution for infusion (0.9% w/v sodium chloride solution) containing 10% w/v (2-hydroxypropyl)-beta-cyclodextrin.

Blood samples for pharmacokinetic analysis of plasma total radioactivity and GSK2239633 were collected at screening, Day –1, pre-dose and at 5, 10, 15, 20, 30, 45 minutes and 1, 1.5, 1.75, 2.25, 3.25, 4.25, 6.25, 8.25, 12.25, 16.25, 18.25, 24.25, 30.25, 36.25 and 48.25 hours from start of the infusion. Urine samples were collected prior to dosing and then until 24 hours after the infusion ended.

Single oral dose study

Subjects were dosed with GSK2239633 as a capsule formulation (Swedish orange coloured opaque hard gelatin capsules) with a unit dosage strength of 150 mg. Subjects received between one and 10 capsules (depending on the dose level), which were swallowed with 240 mL of water (or up to 300 mL of water in total for the higher number of capsules). Subjects randomised to placebo in each dosing session received the same number of capsules as those randomised to active treatment for the same dosing session.

Blood samples were drawn for pharmacokinetic analysis pre-dose and at 5, 15 and 30 minutes and 1, 2, 3, 4, 8, 10, 24 and 48 hours post-dose. For pharmacodynamic analysis, blood was collected pre-dose and at 1, 4 and 24 hours post-dose. The pharmacodynamic analysis was only conducted for subjects in the fasted condition; no analysis was performed for the fed cohort. An aliquot of urine was collected pre-dose; after dosing, all urine was collected and pooled during a 24-hour interval.

Pharmacokinetic analysis

Microdose intravenous study

The primary endpoints were maximum observed concentration (C_{max}), area under the concentration-time curve from time 0 to last measurable concentration (AUC_{0-t}), AUC from time 0 extrapolated to infinity ($AUC_{0-\infty}$) and terminal half-life ($t_{1/2}$) of GSK2239633 and [^{14}C]-radioactivity, apparent clearance (CL) and volume of distribution at steady state (V_{ss}) of GSK2239633 and cumulative urinary excretion of total radioactivity for 24 hours post-dose. Total radioactivity was measured directly by accelerator mass spectrometry. Plasma GSK2239633 concentrations were determined using an internally validated analytical method by accelerator mass spectrometry (further details provided as Additional file 1 material).

Urine radioactivity levels were measured by liquid scintillation counting with an external standardisation method. The lower limit of quantification (LLQ) was

0.98 pg/mL for the plasma assay and 10 pg GSK2239633 equiv/mL for the total plasma radioactivity assay. The LLQ for GSK2239633 in urine was 5 μg GSK2239633 equiv. Pharmacokinetic parameters for each subject were derived from plasma GSK2239633 concentration-time profiles by non-compartmental analysis using Win-Nonlin Professional Edition Version 5.2 or above (Pharsight Corporation, Mountain View, USA). Maximum observed concentration, time to C_{max} (t_{max}), AUC from time 0 to 48 hours post-dose (AUC_{0-48}), AUC_{0-t}, $AUC_{0-\infty}$, CL, $t_{1/2}$, volume of distribution during terminal elimination phase (Vd) and V_{ss} were determined.

Single oral dose study

Blood concentrations of GSK2239633 were determined by an internally validated analytical method based on extraction from a dried blood spot disc by addition of methanol, followed by high performance liquid chromatography/tandem mass spectrometry. The LLQ of the assay was 10 ng/mL (further details provided as Additional file 1 material). Analysis and derivation of pharmacokinetic parameters were conducted as for the Microdose Intravenous Study.

Safety and tolerability assessments
Microdose and single dose studies

The primary endpoints of the Single Oral Dose Study were adverse events and clinically relevant changes in safety parameters. Adverse events were recorded throughout both studies. For each event, the potential causal relationship with the study drug was assessed by the investigator. Other safety assessments in both studies included clinical laboratory tests (chemistry, haematology, urinalysis), vital signs, 12-lead electrocardiogram (ECG) and continuous cardiac telemetry.

Pharmacodynamic analysis
Single oral dose study

Blood samples (9 volumes) were collected into a 3.8% sodium citrate solution (1 volume) and incubated for 15 minutes at room temperature with saturating concentrations of fluorescein isothiocyanate (FITC)-conjugated mouse anti-human CD4 antibody and non-inactivating phycoerythrin (PE)-conjugated mouse anti-human CCR4 antibody (BD Biosciences, Oxford, United Kingdom), or appropriate isotype control antibodies. The samples were then incubated for 30 minutes at 37°C. For preclinical studies, antagonists or vehicle were added at the beginning of this incubation. Following this, the blood cells were incubated for 15 seconds with varying concentrations of TARC (PeproTech EC, London, United Kingdom) before addition of 10 volumes of fluorescence-activated cell sorting (FACS) lysing solution (BD Biosciences, Oxford, United Kingdom). After 30 minutes, the blood cell suspension was centrifuged ($500\,g$ for 5 minutes)

and resuspended in fresh FACS lysing solution for further 10 minutes to ensure complete red blood cell lysis. The cell suspensions were centrifuged ($500\,g$ for 5 minutes) again and washed twice by resuspending in phosphate buffered saline (PBS) solution and centrifuging at $500\,g$ for 5 minutes. After incubating the cell suspensions for 15 minutes with lysophosphatidylcholine (100 μg/mL) and Alexa fluor 647 phalloidin (0.075 units/mL), the cells were recovered by centrifugation at $500\,g$ for 5 minutes and resuspended in PBS. The F-actin content of the $CD4^+$ $CCR4^+$ lymphocytes in each sample was determined on a FACSCantoII flow cytometer by measuring the mean Alexa fluor 647 fluorescence intensity of 1,000 cells. This was expressed as a fraction of the Alexa fluor 647 fluorescence intensity of the $CCR4^-$ lymphocytes in the same sample. The fractional occupancy of CCR4 (Ro) was then estimated by determining the dose-ratio (DR) from the change in effective concentration giving 50% of the maximal response (EC_{50}) of the TARC concentration-response curve before and after dosing with GSK2239633 and using the formula Ro = (DR − 1)/DR [32].

Statistical analysis
Microdose intravenous study

No formal sample size estimation was performed. As this was an exploratory study, no formal statistical hypotheses for safety, tolerability or pharmacokinetics were tested.

Single oral dose study

No statistical analysis was done to determine the sample size. There was no statistical analysis of safety parameters.

Dose proportionality was primarily evaluated based on C_{max}, AUC_{0-10} and AUC_{0-t} using the power model. Each parameter was log_e-transformed prior to analysis. Additionally, a mixed model was fitted to the dose-normalised pharmacokinetic parameters to compare each dose with the reference dose (GSK2239633 150 mg). The data were log_e-transformed prior to analysis and the results were then back-transformed to calculate ratios between the doses. Food effect was assessed by performing a statistical analysis of C_{max}, AUC_{0-10} and AUC_{0-t} after log_e-transformation of the data. An analysis of variance (ANOVA) model was fitted along with 90% confidence intervals (CIs) by a mixed effects model, with fed/fasted condition as a fixed effect and subject as a random effect. Using data obtained in the Microdose Intravenous Study it was possible to make an estimation of GSK2239633 bioavailability following oral administration. For that, AUC_{0-10} was used as a comparison.

For the pharmacodynamic analysis, population estimates of the parameters, such as EC_{50}, were derived using non-linear mixed effects models in NonMEM Version 7 (ICON Development Solutions, PA, USA) for all profiles generated. Analysis of the entire individual pharmacodynamic and pharmacokinetic datasets was conducted to derive mean EC_{50} estimates pre-dose and in the presence of GSK2239633 (each subject acted as their own control as their pre-dose data was compared with their post-dose data). Although not a direct method for formal calculation of Ro, this DR was used to give an estimate of Ro as described above.

Results

Subject disposition and demographics

Microdose intravenous study

Six male subjects were enrolled and completed the study. The population mean [range] age was 22.7 [20.0–26.0] years and mean [range] body mass index was 22.1 [19.3–24.6] kg/m^2 (Table 1). All subjects were Caucasian.

Single oral dose study

Twenty-four male subjects were enrolled and completed the study. The population mean [range] age was 37.2 [20.0–65.0] years and mean [range] body mass index was 24.9 [19.8–29.1] kg/m^2 (Table 1). Twenty (83%) subjects were of Caucasian/European heritage, one (4%) subject was of Central/South Asian heritage, one (4%) subject was of South East Asian heritage and two (8%) subjects were of Arabic/North Africa heritage.

Pharmacokinetics

Microdose intravenous study

Following infusion, the plasma pharmacokinetics of GSK2239633 and total plasma radioactivity showed a rapid bi-exponential distribution phase followed by a slow terminal elimination phase. Terminal elimination $t_{1/2}$ values were 13.5 hours (95% CI: 9.6, 18.8) for

GSK2239633 and 31.6 hours (95% CI: 25.4, 39.3) for total plasma radioactivity (Table 2). Values of AUC for GSK2239633 were half those obtained for total plasma radioactivity (AUC$_{0–48}$: GSK2239633, 4.420 ng.hour/mL; total plasma radioactivity: 8.840 ng GSK2239633 equiv. hour/mL). The intrinsic plasma clearance (CL: 21.9 L/hour) was low to moderate. The observed Vss and Vd values of 119 L (95% CI: 78.4, 182.0) and 424 L (95% CI: 275.0, 654.0), respectively, for GSK2239633 were relatively high suggesting good distribution of GSK2239633 from the plasma compartment into tissues. However, a degree of caution should be taken when interpreting the apparent high distribution since there was evidence in several subjects of secondary peaks in the concentration-time profiles although data were sparse. The amount of radioactive drug-related material recovered in the urine accounted for approximately 20% of the administered dose.

Single oral dose study

Absorption of GSK2239633 was rapid with C_{max} at 1.0–1.5-hours across the dose range (Table 3). Values of $t_{1/2}$ could only be calculated for one subject after the 150 mg and the 1200 mg (fed) doses, and two subjects after the 1200 mg (fed) dose as blood concentrations of GSK2239633 were too erratic and low during the terminal phase for other subjects; for these three subjects, $t_{1/2}$ values ranged from 2.9 to 28.3 hours. Generally, both AUC (Additional file 1: Figure S2A) and C_{max} (Additional file 1: Figure S2B) increased with GSK2239633 dose. Results from the power model analysis indicated a less than dose proportional increase for AUC$_{0–10}$ (adjusted mean slope: 0.61; 90% CI: 0.54, 0.68) and C_{max} (adjusted mean slope: 0.76; 90% CI: 0.63, 0.89) as the 90% CIs did not contain unity (Additional file 1: Table S1). Dose proportionality

Table 1 Summary of subjects demographic characteristics

Demographics	Microdose intravenous study (n = 6)	Single oral dose study (n = 24)
Age, years; Mean [range]	22.7 [20.0–26.0]	37.2 [20.0–65.0]
Sex; n (%)		
Male	6 (100%)	24 (100%)
Height, cm; Mean [range]	180.0 [172.0–187.0]	180.5 [163.0–197.0])
Weight, kg; Mean [range]	71.8 [60.1–85.5]	81.0 [65.7–106.0]
Body mass index, kg/m^2; Mean [range]	22.1 [19.3–24.6]	24.9 [19.8–29.1]
Ethnicity; n (%)		
Hispanic or Latino	0	1 (4%)
Not Hispanic or Latino	6 (100%)	23 (96%)
Race; n (%)[a]		
White-White/Caucasian/European heritage	6 (100%)	20 (83%)
White-Arabic/North African heritage	0	1 (4%)
Asian-Central/South Asian heritage	0	1 (4%)
Asian-South East Asian heritage	0	2 (8%)

Table 2 Summary of derived plasma GSK2239633 pharmacokinetic parameters in the microdose intravenous study

	[^{14}C]-GSK2239633 (n = 6)	Total plasma drug-related radioactivity (n = 6)
Parameters	Geometric mean (95% CI)	Geometric mean (95% CI)*
C_{max} (ng/mL)	7.451 (6.114, 9.079)	8.380 (7.503, 9.359)
AUC_{0-48} (ng.hour/mL)	4.420 (3.515, 5.556)	8.840 (7.538, 10.368)
$AUC_{0-\infty}$ (ng.hour/mL)	4.577 (3.606, 5.810)	11.418 (9.004, 14.480)
$t_{1/2}$ (hour)[1]	13.5 [8.0–21.2]	31.6 [25.1–43.0]
CL (L/hour)	21.9 (17.2, 27.7)	8.8 (6.9, 11.1)
V_{ss} (L)	119.0 (78.4, 182.0)	249.0 (200.0, 309.0)
Vd (L)	424.0 (275.0, 654.0)	399.0 (322.0, 494.0)

* Concentrations are in ng GSK2239633 equiv/mL and ng GSK2239633 equiv.hour/mL for C_{max} and AUC, respectively.
[1] Median [range].
CI: confidence interval; C_{max}: maximum observed concentration; AUC_{0-48}: area under the concentration-time curve from time 0 to 48 hours post-dose; $AUC_{0-\infty}$: area under the concentration-time curve from time 0 extrapolated to infinity; $t_{1/2}$: half-life; CL: apparent clearance; V_{ss}: volume of distribution at steady state; Vd: volume of distribution during terminal elimination phase.

results were supported by mixed model analysis as assessed by comparison with the GSK2239633 150 mg dose level. Mean C_{max} and AUC_{0-t} for GSK2239633 following a dose of 1200 mg were 695 ng/mL and 2330 ng. hour/mL, respectively; these increased to 1410 ng/mL and 6520 ng.hour/mL when the study medication was administered after a standard FDA high fat/high caloric meal. The analysis of the food effect for GSK2239633 showed an increase of 208% in AUC_{0-10}, 180% in AUC_{0-t} and 103% in C_{max} (GSK2239633 1200 mg fed:fasted) in the fed state; all these differences achieved statistical significance (Supplemental Table S2). In addition to the increases observed for C_{max} and AUC parameters, absorption of GSK2239633 was more protracted in the fed condition with a median t_{max} of 3.0 hours. GSK2239633 bioavailability in the fasted state ranged from 12–14% for the two lowest doses studied (GSK2239633 150 mg and 300 mg). For GSK2239633 600 mg and above, estimated bioavailability decreased ranging from 5–9%. In the fed state,

GSK2239633 estimated bioavailability increased to approximately 16%.

Safety and tolerability
Microdose intravenous study
Adverse events were reported by three of the six (50%) study subjects. The events reported were abdominal discomfort (n = 1), diarrhoea (n = 1), rhinitis (n = 1) and headache (n = 1); all were mild, transient and had resolved at follow-up. The episode of diarrhoea was the only event judged to be possibly drug-related by the investigator. There were no clinically significant abnormalities in clinical laboratory results, physical exam, vital signs, 12-lead ECG parameters or continuous cardiac telemetry.

Single oral dose study
Nineteen of the 24 (79%) subjects reported adverse events (Table 4). There was no dose response in the

Table 3 Summary of derived blood GSK2239633 pharmacokinetic parameters in the single oral dose study (geometric mean, 95% confidence interval)

Parameter	GSK2239633 Dose						
	150 mg (n = 8)	300 mg (n = 8)	600 mg (n = 8)	900 mg (n = 8)	1200 mg (n = 8)	1500 mg (n = 8)	1200 mg (Fed) (n = 8)
AUC_{0-10} (ng.hour/mL)	534 (430, 663)	923 (695, 1227)	1210 (1055, 1393)	2060 (1552, 2741)	1520 (1175, 1963)	2560 (2026, 3234)	4670 (3783, 5769)
AUC_{0-t} (ng.hour/mL)	718 (518, 995)	1560 (971, 2511)	1970 (1563, 2492)	3110 (2242, 4324)	2330 (1499, 3611)	4150 (3121, 5528)	6520 (4264, 9980)
$AUC_{0-\infty}$ (ng.hour/mL)	420	ND	ND	ND	ND	ND	5180 (3101, 8654)
%AUCex (%)	13.7	ND	ND	ND	ND	ND	9.4 (3.6, 24.8)
C_{max} (ng/mL)	178 (124, 256)	353 (237, 526)	538 (391, 739)	869 (622, 1215)	695 (476, 1016)	1210 (778, 1889)	1410 (1127, 1761)
t_{max} (hour)[1]	1.5 [1.0–3.0]	1.0 [1.0–3.0]	1.0 [0.5–2.0]	1.5 [0.5–3.0]	1.0 [0.5–3.0]	1.0 [0.5–4.0]	3.0 [0.6–4.0]

[1] Median [range].
AUC_{0-10}: area under the concentration-time curve from time 0 to 10 hours post-dose; AUC_{0-t}: AUC from time 0 to last measurable concentration; $AUC_{0-\infty}$: AUC from time 0 extrapolated to infinity; ND: not determined; %AUCex: percentage of $AUC_{0-\infty}$ obtained by extrapolation; C_{max}: maximum observed concentration; t_{max}: time to C_{max}.

Table 4 Summary of the adverse events reported by two or more subjects in the single oral dose study

| | Placebo (n = 24) n (%) | GSK2239633 | | | | | | 1200 mg (Fed) (n = 8) n (%) | Placebo (Fed) (n = 4) n (%) | Total (n = 24) n (%) |
		150 mg (n = 8) n (%)	300 mg (n = 8) n (%)	600 mg (n = 8) n (%)	900 mg (n = 8) n (%)	1200 mg (n = 8) n (%)	1500 mg (n = 8) n (%)			
Any event	9 (38)	4 (50)	5 (63)	5 (63)	1 (13)	2 (25)	3 (38)	2 (25)	1 (25)	19 (79)
Headache	3 (13)	2 (25)	0	0	1 (13)	1 (13)	1 (13)	0	0	5 (21)
Diarrhoea	2 (8)	0	2 (25)	1 (13)	1 (13)	0	2 (25)	0	0	4 (17)
Rhinitis	1 (4)	1 (13)	0	0	0	0	1 (13)	0	0	2 (8)
Abdominal pain	0	0	0	0	0	0	1 (13)	0	0	1 (4)

incidence of adverse events across dose and treatment groups. Forty-six of the 47 (98%) events were graded as mild or moderate; none was graded as severe. One subject had a skin mole at screening that was subsequently excised and found to be a malignant melanoma. This was reported as an adverse event. The most frequently reported adverse events were headache and diarrhoea. Six subjects experienced events judged to be drug-related by the investigator, the most frequent of which was diarrhoea reported by three (13%) subjects (GSK2239633 600 mg: one; GSK2239633 1500 mg: two; placebo: one). Other events judged to be drug-related were abdominal pain, chest discomfort, headache, oral herpes and somnolence (one subject each). All adverse events resolved by the end of the study except for one episode of joint injury and one episode of folliculitis. No trends were detected in changes from baseline for clinical laboratory test values. The investigator judged there to be no clinically significant abnormalities in vital sign, 12-lead ECG parameters or continuous cardiac telemetry.

Pharmacodynamics

Single oral dose study

Dose–response curves for the relative increase in filamentous actin (F-actin) content of $CD4^+$ $CCR4^+$ cells in response to TARC showed that, although highly variable, CCR4 inhibition was evident from GSK2239633 150 mg to 1500 mg (Figure 1). For comparison, the results from in vitro studies assessing the effect of GSK2239633 (1–10 μM) on TARC-induced increases in F-actin content of $CD4^+$ $CCR4^+$ T-cells are also presented (Figure 2). At the GSK2239633 1500 mg dose, the calculated mean level of CCR4 inhibition equated to a predicted Ro of approximately 74% at 1 hour after dosing. Predicted Ro levels decreased over time following the blood pharmacokinetic profile, which showed an initial rapid peak in blood GSK2239633 exposure followed by a rapid decline to much lower levels 4–8 hours post-dose. The Ro estimates for each dose group at 1 and 4 hours post-dose are presented in Table 5. Receptor occupancy estimates at 4 hours post-dose were more variable than those at 1 hour post-

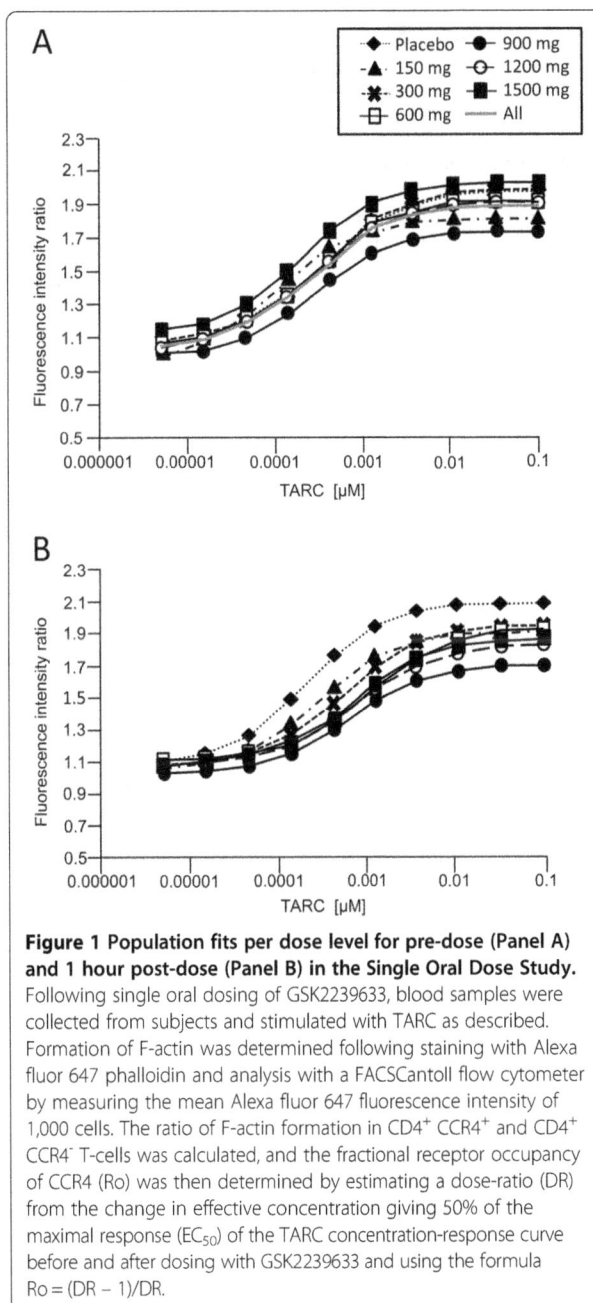

Figure 1 Population fits per dose level for pre-dose (Panel A) and 1 hour post-dose (Panel B) in the Single Oral Dose Study. Following single oral dosing of GSK2239633, blood samples were collected from subjects and stimulated with TARC as described. Formation of F-actin was determined following staining with Alexa fluor 647 phalloidin and analysis with a FACSCantoll flow cytometer by measuring the mean Alexa fluor 647 fluorescence intensity of 1,000 cells. The ratio of F-actin formation in $CD4^+$ $CCR4^+$ and $CD4^+$ $CCR4^-$ T-cells was calculated, and the fractional receptor occupancy of CCR4 (Ro) was then determined by estimating a dose-ratio (DR) from the change in effective concentration giving 50% of the maximal response (EC_{50}) of the TARC concentration-response curve before and after dosing with GSK2239633 and using the formula $Ro = (DR - 1)/DR$.

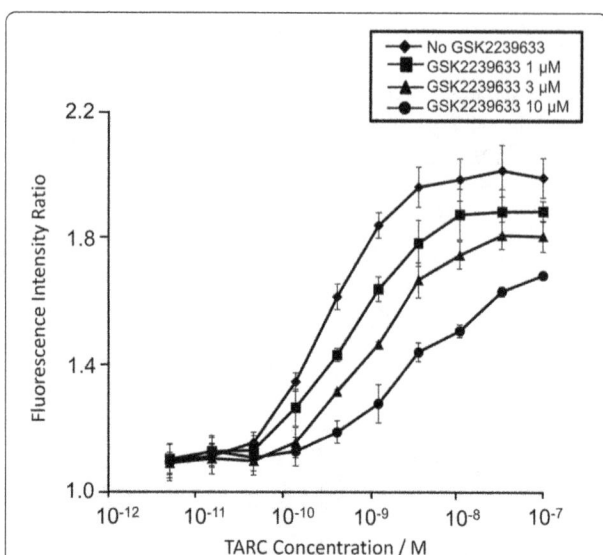

Figure 2 Thymus- and activation-regulated chemokine-induced increases in F-actin content of CD4+ CCR4+ T-cells in whole human blood in the absence or presence of GSK2239633 at 1 μM, 3 μM or 10 μM. The data presented are the mean of independent determinations in three donors. Error bars represent standard error of the mean.

dose and therefore, difficult to interpret. Although, this was not unexpected given the low blood exposure of GSK2239633 at the 4 hours post-dose time-point. Blood from placebo subjects, analysed in the same way and at the same time-points, did not show any shifts in the response curves, which would indicate CCR4 inhibition, when the post-dose curves were compared with the pre-dose curves. The placebo data also revealed the inherent variability in the technique as shown by the approximately 3-fold range in variability for the derived EC_{50} of TARC (pre-dose = 0.34 nM; all data = 0.1–0.34 nM).

Table 5 Changes in estimated receptor occupancy in the presence of GSK2239633 in the single oral dose study

GSK22939633 dose	Parameter[1,2]	Post-dose time point	
		1 hour	4 hours**
150 mg	Ro (95% CI) (%)	63 (NC)	53 (NC)
300 mg	Ro (95% CI) (%)	37 (29, 54)	9 (0, 45)
600 mg	Ro (95% CI) (%)	72 (71, 75)	14 (13, 14)
900 mg	Ro (95% CI) (%)	55 (50, 58)	42 (0, 56)
1200 mg	Ro (95% CI) (%)	64 (60, 67)	0 (0, 1)
1500 mg	Ro (95% CI) (%)	74 (62, 79)	61 (52, 67)

[1] Ro: CCR4 occupancy by GSK2239633 derived from the EC_{50} ratio (DR) for each dose group divided by the pre-dose EC_{50} and converted to an estimate of CCR4 occupancy (DR-1/DR).
[2] 95% CI: calculated from the 95% confidence interval (when available) of the modelled EC_{50}.
** Data generated at 4 hours post-dose with GSK2239633 was highly variable. Ro: receptor occupancy; CI: confidence interval; NC: not calculated, insufficient data to generate a measure of variability.

Discussion

In the Microdose Intravenous Study, the clearance of GSK2239633 was low to moderate (approximately 40% of liver blood flow) with a proportion of the drug appearing to be well distributed based on the long terminal elimination rate observed, albeit at relatively low levels and with signs of secondary input. Prior to the conduct of the Single Oral Dose Study, the systemic bioavailability of GSK2239633 in humans was predicted to be, at best, approximately 70%, based on results of the Microdose Intravenous Study and those obtained in the pre-clinical studies. This assumed that bioavailability was limited only by first pass extraction equivalent to the systemic clearance measured in the Microdose Intravenous Study. However, findings in the Single Oral Dose Study showed that this was an overestimate (see below). Unchanged GSK2239633 accounted for only 50% of the total plasma radioactivity following intravenous administration with the remaining circulating drug-related material comprised of one or more metabolites. A glucuronide conjugate was identified as a major component of the metabolised fraction through a pooled plasma analysis.

The blood exposure of GSK2239633 achieved in the Single Oral Dose Study was substantially lower than that expected based on the high oral bioavailability obtained in several pre-clinical species; however, it may be consistent with the physicochemical properties of the molecule, high molecular weight (549) and low solubility (0.02 mg/mL), and could explain the limited absorption window observed in humans. Gastric motility and the presence of food in the stomach could influence the systemic exposure profile of GSK2239633 in the manner observed in this first in man oral study. The food effect analysis supports this hypothesis and administration of GSK2239633 1200 mg in the fed state led to statistically significant increases in C_{max} (103%) and AUC parameters (AUC_{0-10}: 208%; AUC_{0-t}: 180%) compared with the fasted state. However, other factors, such as solubility, cannot be excluded. In addition, in the fed state, t_{max} was delayed by approximately 1.5 hours compared with the fasted state. The estimated bioavailability of GSK2239633 was considerably lower than predicted, achieving a maximum of only approximately 16% (either fasted or fed). Therefore, GSK2239633 exposure in the blood was notably lower than that required to explore a full pharmacodynamic response, which was reflected in the low estimated Ro observed for the actin polymerisation pharmacodynamic endpoint.

In these early studies, GSK2239633 had a satisfactory safety and tolerability profile in healthy subjects. No dose-limiting toxicity or maximum tolerated dose was identified. There was no relationship in the frequency or severity of adverse events with increasing doses of GSK2239633. The anti-CCR4 antibody, mogamulizumab, has been tested in clinical studies, although the study population for this was patients with relapsed CCR4+ adult T-cell lymphomas and other peripheral T-cell lymphomas [27]. Mogamulizumab has thus far been shown to be well-tolerated in that study population and none of the adverse events reported were specific to inhibition of CCR4 [27].

Pharmacodynamic analysis in the Single Oral Dose Study revealed that GSK2239633 inhibited TARC-induced increases in the F-actin content of CCR4+ T cells in human whole blood. Although, even at the highest dose (1500 mg), the magnitude of inhibition was low (the potency of TARC decreased only 4-fold indicating that the mean estimated receptor occupancy was 74% at 1 hour post-dose) and relatively short-acting (reflecting the rapid reduction of drug concentration and inhibition in the blood at 4 hours post-dose). GSK2239633 failed to achieve the minimum target level of CCR4 inhibition in the blood ($\geq$90% at peak and 50% at trough), and there was no indication of an extended duration of action (prolonged pharmacodynamic response in the absence of pharmacokinetic exposure) in whole blood ex vivo. In this study, we were unable to obtain systemic exposure of GSK2239633 high enough to inhibit CCR4 by more than 80% as measured in the whole blood CCR4 pharmacodynamic assay. This would substantially limit the degree to which we would be able to assess the blockade of CCR4 for clinical benefit in further studies.

CC-Chemokine receptor 4 is potentially involved in the pathogenesis of allergic diseases due to its involvement in the pathways leading to the recruitment of Th2 cells to the sites of allergen exposure [22,33]. A number of small-molecule CCR4 antagonists have shown promising results in various animal models of inflammation, such as reduction in ovalbumin-induced ear swelling in mice [34], inhibition of ovalbumin-induced airway inflammation in guinea pigs [35] and a reduction in the recruitment of Th2 cells to the lungs in a mouse model of ovalbumin-induced airway allergy [36]. However, no small molecules have progressed to clinical studies thus far [2,26], which may be due, in part, to poor oral exposure noted in pre-clinical animal models with some of the small molecules reported. A further general challenge with chemokines often speculated upon is the potential for redundancy within the chemokine system and alteration of function during evolution [2,37]. Results from some studies [38-40] indicate that chemokine receptors are also a good target for adjuvant discovery, in particular CCR4, as this receptor is expressed by regulatory T cells, a subset of T cells which normally functions in the down-regulation of immune responses induced by dendritic cells [41]. One of these studies identified CCR4 antagonists acting as adjuvants for both cellular and humoral immune responses.

Conclusions

Results obtained from these early studies conducted in healthy subjects, indicate that GSK2239633 was generally safe and well tolerated. GSK2239633 exhibited low and saturable systemic exposures and at the highest dose level of 1500 mg the peak inhibition of CCR4 by GSK2239633 in the blood (at 1 hour) was below 80% and less than 50% by 4 hours post-dose. Based on the low exposure and target engagement in blood, this molecule is not considered suitable for further development for an asthma indication at this time.

Additional file

Additional file 1: Safety, tolerability, pharmacokinetics and pharmacodynamics of GSK2239633, a CC-chemokine receptor 4 antagonist, in healthy male subjects. Detailed information of the pharmacokinetic assays, 2 Tables, 2 Figures and figure legends.

Abbreviations

ANOVA: Analysis of variance; AUC_{0-48}: Area under the concentration-time curve from time 0 to 48 hours post-dose; AUC_{0-t}: AUC from time 0 to last measurable concentration; $AUC_{0-\infty}$: AUC from time 0 extrapolated to infinity; CCR4: CC-chemokine receptor 4; CI: Confidence Intervals; CL: Apparent clearance; C_{max}: Maximum observed concentration; DR: Dose-Ratio; EC_{50}: Effective concentration giving 50% of the maximal response; FACS: Fluorescence-activated cell sorting; FDA: United states food and drug administration; FITC: Fluorescein isothiocyanate; LLQ: Lower limit of quantification; MDC: Monocyte-derived chemokine; PBS: Phosphate buffered saline; PE: Phycoerythrin; Ro: Fractional occupancy; TARC: Thymus- and activation-regulated chemokine; $t_{1/2}$: Terminal half-life; t_{max}: Time to C_{max}; Th2: Type 2 T helper; Vd: Volume of distribution during terminal elimination phase; V_{ss}: Volume of distribution at steady state.

Competing interests

Anthony Cahn, Simon Hodgson, Robert Wilson, Jonathan Robertson, Joanna Watson, Misba Beerahee, Steve C. Hughes, Graeme Young, Rebecca Graves, David Hall and Roberto Solari are GlaxoSmithKline employees. Sjoerd van Marle has no competing interests.

Authors' contributions

AC, RW, JR and MB participated in the conception and design of the study, and in the analysis and interpretation of the data. JW and SCH participated in the conception and design of the study, and in the acquisition, analysis and interpretation of the data. SH, DH and SVM took part in the acquisition, analysis and interpretation of the data. GY, RG and RS contributed in the analysis and interpretation of the data. All authors have made critical revisions of draft versions of the manuscript and approved the final manuscript.

Acknowledgements

The authors would like to thank the subjects and staff who participated in the studies. All listed authors meet the criteria for authorship set forth by the International Committee for Medical Journal Editors. Medical writing and editorial support to prepare the manuscript were provided by Dr Justin Cook and Dr Severina Moreira of Niche Science and Technology Ltd (Richmond-upon-Thames, United Kingdom), who were paid by GlaxoSmithKline for these services. These studies (NCT01086462 and NCT01371812) were funded by GlaxoSmithKline.

Author details

[1]Medicines Discovery and Development, Gunnels Wood Road, Stevenage Herts SG1 2NY, UK. [2]GlaxoSmithKline, Stockley Park West, Uxbridge, Middlesex UB11 1BT, UK. [3]GlaxoSmithKline, Park Road, Ware SG12 0DP, UK. [4]PRA International, Stationsweg 163, Zuidlaren 9741 GP, the Netherlands.

References

1. Finiasz M, Otero C, Bezrodnik L, Fink S: The role of cytokines in atopic asthma. *Curr Med Chem* 2011, 18:1476–1487.
2. Pease JE: Targeting Chemokine receptors in allergic disease. *Biochem J* 2011, 434:11–24.
3. Azzawi M, Bradley B, Jeffery PK, Frew AJ, Wardlaw AJ, Knowles G, Assoufi B, Collins JV, Durham S, Kay AB: Identification of activated T lymphocytes and eosinophils in bronchial biopsies in stable atopic asthma. *Am Rev Respir Dis* 1990, 142:1407–1413.
4. Fanta CH: Asthma. *N Engl J Med* 2009, 360:1002–1014.
5. Hamid Q, Tulic M: Immunobiology of asthma. *Annu Rev Physiol* 2009, 71:489–507.
6. Long AA: Immunomodulators in the treatment of asthma. *Allergy Asthma Proc* 2009, 30:109–119.
7. Minai-Fleminger Y, Levi-Schaffer F: Mast cells and eosinophils: the two key effector cells in allergic inflammation. *Inflamm Res* 2009, 58:631–638.
8. Vestergaard C, Yoneyama H, Murai M, Nakamura K, Tamaki K, Terashima Y, Imai T, Yoshie O, Irimura T, Mizutani H, Matsushima K: Overproduction of Th2-specific Chemokines in NC/Nga mice exhibiting atopic dermatitis-like lesions. *J Clin Invest* 1999, 104:1097–1157.
9. Vestergaard C, Bang K, Gesser B, Yoneyama H, Matsushima K, Larsen CG: A Th2 Chemokine, TARC, produced by keratinocytes may recruit CLA + CCR4+ lymphocytes into lesional atopic dermatitis skin. *J Invest Dermatol* 2000, 115:640–646.
10. Sekiya T, Miyamasu M, Imanishi M, Yamada H, Nakajima T, Yamaguchi M, Fujisawa T, Pawankar R, Sano Y, Ohta K, Ishii A, Morita Y, Yamamoto K, Matsushima K, Yoshie O, Hirai K: Inducible expression of a Th2-type CC Chemokine thymus- and activation-regulated Chemokine by human bronchial epithelial cells. *J Immunol* 2000, 165:2205–2213.
11. Zheng X, Nakamura K, Furukawa H, Nishibu A, Takahashi M, Tojo M, Kaneko F, Kakinuma T, Tamaki K: Demonstration of TARC and CCR4 mRNA expression and distribution using in situ RT-PCR in the lesional skin of atopic dermatitis. *J Dermatol* 2003, 30:26–32.
12. Liu YJ: Thymic stromal lymphopoietin: master switch for allergic inflammation. *J Exp Med* 2006, 203:269–273.
13. Imai T, Baba M, Nishimura M, Kakizaki M, Takagi S, Yoshie O: The T cell-directed CC Chemokine TARC is a highly specific biological ligand for CC Chemokine receptor 4. *J Biol Chem* 1997, 272:15036–15042.
14. Imai T, Chantry D, Raport CJ, Wood CL, Nishimura M, Godiska R, Yoshie O, Gray PW: Macrophage-derived Chemokine is a functional ligand for the CC Chemokine receptor 4. *J Biol Chem* 1998, 273:1764–1768.
15. Imai T, Nagira M, Takagi S, Kakizaki M, Nishimura M, Wang J, Gray PW, Matsushima K, Yoshie O: Selective recruitment of CCR4-bearing Th2 cells toward antigen-presenting cells by the CC Chemokines thymus and activation-regulated Chemokine and macrophage-derived Chemokine. *Int Immunol* 1999, 11:81–88.
16. Sallusto F, Lenig D, Mackay CR, Lanzavecchia A: Flexible programs of Chemokine receptor expression on human polarized T helper 1 and 2 lymphocytes. *J Exp Med* 1998, 187:875–883.
17. D'Ambrosio D, Iellem A, Bonecchi R, Mazzeo D, Sozzani S, Mantovani A, Sinigaglia F: Selective up-regulation of Chemokine receptors CCR4 and CCR8 upon activation of polarized human type 2 Th cells. *J Immunol* 1998, 161:5111–5115.
18. Bochner BS, Hudson SA, Xiao HQ, Liu MC: Release of both CCR4-active and CXCR3-active Chemokines during human allergic pulmonary late-phase reactions. *J Allergy Clin Immunol* 2003, 112:930–934.
19. Pilette C, Francis JN, Till SJ, Durham SR: CCR4 Ligands are up-regulated in the airways of atopic asthmatics after segmental allergen challenge. *Eur Respir J* 2004, 23:876–884.
20. Panina-Bordignon P, Papi A, Mariani M, Di Lucia P, Casoni G, Bellettato C, Buonsanti C, Miotto D, Mapp C, Villa A, Arrigoni G, Fabbri LM, Sinigaglia F: The C-C Chemokine receptors CCR4 and CCR8 identify airway T cells of allergen-challenged atopic asthmatics. *J Clin Invest* 2001, 107:1357–1364.
21. Morgan AJ, Symon FA, Berry MA, Pavord ID, Corrigan CJ, Wardlaw AJ: IL-4-expressing bronchoalveolar T cells from asthmatic and healthy subjects

preferentially express CCR 3 and CCR 4. *J Allergy Clin Immunol* 2005, 116:594–600.
22. Vijayanand P, Durkin K, Hartmann G, Morjaria J, Seumois G, Staples KJ, Hall D, Bessant C, Bartholomew M, Howarth PH, Friedmann PS, Djukanovic R: Chemokine receptor 4 plays a key role in T cell recruitment into the airways of asthmatic patients. *J Immunol* 2010, 184:4568–4574.
23. Barnes PJ: Immunology of asthma and chronic obstructive pulmonary disease. *Nat Rev Immunol* 2008, 8:183–192.
24. Barnes PJ: The cytokine network in asthma and chronic obstructive pulmonary disease. *J Clin Invest* 2008, 118:3546–3556.
25. Donnelly LE, Barnes PJ: Chemokine receptors as therapeutic targets in chronic obstructive pulmonary disease. *Trends Pharmacol Sci* 2006, 27:546–553.
26. Hall D, Ford A, Hodgson S: Therapeutic potential of CCR4 antagonists. In *New drugs and targets for asthma and COPD. Volume 39.* Karger: Prog Respir Res Basel; 2010:161–165.
27. Yamamoto K, Utsunomiya A, Tobinai K, Tsukasaki K, Uike N, Uozumi K, Yamaguchi K, Yamada Y, Hanada S, Tamura K, Nakamura S, Inagaki H, Ohshima K, Kiyoi H, Ishida T, Matsushima K, Akinaga S, Ogura M, Tomonaga M, Ueda R: Phase I study of KW-0761, a defucosylated humanized anti-CCR4 antibody, in relapsed patients with adult T-cell leukemia-lymphoma and peripheral T-cell lymphoma. *J Clin Oncol* 2010, 28:1591–1598.
28. Procopiou PA, Ford AJ, Graves RH, Hall DA, Hodgson ST, Lacroix YM, Needham D, Slack RJ: Lead optimisation of the N1 substituent of a novel series of indazole arylsulfonamides as CCR4 antagonists and identification of a candidate for clinical investigation. *Bioorg Med Chem Lett* 2012, 22:2730–2733.
29. Hodgson ST, Lacroix YML, Procopiou PA: *US patent 2010216860A1.* 2010. http://www.google.co.uk/patents?hl=en&lr=&vid=USPATAPP12711283&id=5OrUAAAAEBAJ&oi=fnd&dq=hodgson+patent+ccr4&printsec=abstract#v=onepage&q=hodgson%20patent%20ccr4&f=false.
30. *ICH M3 (R2) - guideline on nonclinical safety studies for the conduct of human clinical trials and marketing authorization for pharmaceuticals.* http://www.ema.europa.eu/docs/en_GB/document_library/Scientific_guideline/2009/09/WC500002941.pdf.
31. World Medical Association: *Declaration of Helsinki - ethical principles for medical research involving human subjects.* http://www.wma.net/en/30publications/10policies/b3.
32. Paton WDM: A theory of drug action based on the rate of drug-receptor combination. *Proc R Soc Lond B* 1961, 154:21–69.
33. Banfield G, Watanabe H, Scadding G, Jacobson MR, Till SJ, Hall DA, Robinson DS, Lloyd CM, Nouri-Aria KT, Durham SR: CC Chemokine receptor 4 (CCR4) in human allergen-induced late nasal responses. *Allergy* 2010, 65:1126–1133.
34. Nakagami Y, Kawashima K, Yonekubo K, Etori M, Jojima T, Miyazaki S, Sawamura R, Hirahara K, Nara F, Yamashita M: Novel CC Chemokine receptor 4 antagonist RS-1154 inhibits ovalbumin-induced ear swelling in mice. *Eur J Pharmacol* 2009, 624:38–44.
35. Nakagami Y, Kawase Y, Yonekubo K, Nosaka E, Etori M, Takahashi S, Takagi N, Fukuda T, Kuribayashi T, Nara F, Yamashita M: RS-1748, a novel CC Chemokine receptor 4 antagonist, inhibits ovalbumin-induced airway inflammation in guinea pigs. *Biol Pharm Bull* 2010, 33:1067–1079.
36. Sato T, Komai M, Iwase M, Kobayashi K, Tahara H, Ohshima E, Arai H, Miki I: Inhibitory effect of the new orally active CCR4 antagonist K327 on CCR4 + CD4+ T cell migration into the lung of mice with ovalbumin-induced lung allergic inflammation. *Pharmacology* 2009, 84:171–182.
37. Catley MC, Coote J, Bari M, Tomlinson KL: Monoclonal antibodies for the treatment of asthma. *Pharmacol Ther* 2011, 132:333–351.
38. Bayry J, Tchilian EZ, Davies MN, Forbes EK, Draper SJ, Kaveri SV, Hill AV, Kazatchkine MD, Beverley PC, Flower DR, Tough DF: In silico identified CCR4 antagonists target regulatory T cells and exert adjuvant activity in vaccination. *Proc Natl Acad Sci USA* 2008, 105:10221–10226.
39. Davies MN, Bayry J, Tchilian EZ, Vani J, Shaila MS, Forbes EK, Draper SJ, Beverley PC, Tough DF, Flower DR: Toward the discovery of vaccine adjuvants: coupling in silico screening and *in vitro* analysis of antagonist binding to human and mouse CCR4 receptors. *PLoS One* 2009, 4:e8084.
40. Pere H, Montier Y, Bayry J, Quintin-Colonna F, Merillon N, Dransart E,

Badoual C, Gey A, Ravel P, Marcheteau E, Batteux F, Sandoval F, Adotevi O, Chiu C, Garcia S, Tanchot C, Lone YC, Ferreira LC, Nelson BH, Hanahan D, Fridman WH, Johannes L, Tartour E: **A CCR4 antagonist combined with vaccines induces antigen-specific CD8+ T cells and tumor immunity against self antigens.** *Blood* 2011, **118**:4853–4862.

41. Miyara M, Sakaguchi S: **Natural regulatory T cells: mechanisms of suppression.** *Trends Mol Med* 2007, **13**:108–116.

3

Quantitation of small intestinal permeability during normal human drug absorption

David G Levitt

Abstract

Background: Understanding the quantitative relationship between a drug's physical chemical properties and its rate of intestinal absorption (QSAR) is critical for selecting candidate drugs. Because of limited experimental human small intestinal permeability data, approximate surrogates such as the fraction absorbed or Caco-2 permeability are used, both of which have limitations.

Methods: Given the blood concentration following an oral and intravenous dose, the time course of intestinal absorption in humans was determined by deconvolution and related to the intestinal permeability by the use of a new 3 parameter model function ("Averaged Model" (AM)). The theoretical validity of this AM model was evaluated by comparing it to the standard diffusion-convection model (DC). This analysis was applied to 90 drugs using previously published data. Only drugs that were administered in oral solution form to fasting subjects were considered so that the rate of gastric emptying was approximately known. All the calculations are carried out using the freely available routine PKQuest Java (www.pkquest.com) which has an easy to use, simple interface.

Results: Theoretically, the AM permeability provides an accurate estimate of the intestinal DC permeability for solutes whose absorption ranges from 1% to 99%. The experimental human AM permeabilities determined by deconvolution are similar to those determined by direct human jejunal perfusion. The small intestinal pH varies with position and the results are interpreted in terms of the pH dependent octanol partition. The permeability versus partition relations are presented separately for the uncharged, basic, acidic and charged solutes. The small uncharged solutes caffeine, acetaminophen and antipyrine have very high permeabilities (about 20×10^{-4} cm/sec) corresponding to an unstirred layer of only 45 μm. The weak acid aspirin also has a large AM permeability despite its low octanol partition at pH 7.4, suggesting that it is nearly completely absorbed in the first part of the intestine where the pH is about 5.4.

Conclusions: The AM deconvolution method provides an accurate estimate of the human intestinal permeability. The results for these 90 drugs should provide a useful benchmark for evaluating QSAR models.

Background

Despite the multitude of publications describing the different factors that affect the rate of intestinal absorption of drugs, there is only limited experimental data for the human small intestinal permeability of the thousands of drugs that are orally absorbed. The quantitative structure activity relationship (QSAR) between a drug's physical chemical properties and its rate of intestinal absorption is obviously of great importance in selecting candidate drugs. The standard approach is to relate some property of the drug (e.g. octanol/water partition, Caco-2 cell permeability, etc.) to the fraction absorbed in humans [1,2]. Although the fraction absorbed is a useful clinical parameter [3], it is a crude measure of permeability. Since most successful drugs are nearly 100% absorbed, they cannot provide any quantitative data about their relative permeability. Furthermore, the fraction absorbed may be influenced in uncertain ways by factors such as intestinal metabolism or large intestinal absorption.

More recently, there have been direct measurements of human small intestinal permeability using the regional perfusion technique. In a recent communication, Dahan,

Correspondence: levit001@umn.edu
Department of Integrative Biology and Physiology, University of Minnesota, 6-125 Jackson Hall, 321 Church St. S. E, Minneapolis, MN 55455, USA

Lennernas and Amidon [4] discuss the various reasons why these measurement of "...jejunal permeability (alone) may not always adequately predict" the fraction absorbed. This includes small intestinal heterogeneity (such as variations in pH and membrane transport systems) and large intestinal absorption. In addition, the regional perfusion conditions used in these measurements may differ from the normal physiological conditions. For example, the high pressure and volume in the perfusion system may increase access to the intervillous space allowing increased paracellular transport of PEG markers [5].

This paper describes a new approach to measuring human intestinal permeability during normal drug absorption. It is well recognized that the time course of intestinal absorption can be determined from deconvolution of the plasma concentrations following oral and intravenous input in the same subject. There are a variety of mathematical approaches to this deconvolution [6]. Some care is required in this procedure because random errors in the plasma concentration data can lead to non-physiological fluctuations or negative values in the predicted absorption rate. The simplest procedures assume that the absorption can be described by some simple function (e.g. 3 parameter gamma [6] or Hill function [7]) which is then adjusted to give the best fit to the oral plasma absorption curve. More sophisticated approaches use generalized functions with varying numbers of parameters [8,9]. This absorption function must then be interpreted in terms of the intestinal permeability. This is difficult because intestinal transit, dispersion and absorption is complicated and poorly understood. The most widely used quantitative model of intestinal absorption is the "compartmental absorption and transit" (CAT) model which has been incorporated into the commercial program GastroPlus™ [10,11]. This CAT model describes the small intestine in terms of 7 sequential well mixed compartments with passive absorption (determined by the permeability) and one way transport in the aboral direction. Because the solution of this model's equations requires numerical calculations and does not have an analytical solution, it cannot be easily adapted for the deconvolution approach.

In this paper a new 3 parameter function ("Averaged Model" (AM)) that accurately mimics the transit, dispersion and absorption of the small intestine is used to determine the intestinal permeability by deconvolution. The range of validity of this AM model is evaluated by comparing it with the more exact diffusion convection model (DC). This AM procedure is then applied to published data to determine the human intestinal permeability of 90 drugs. The main criterion for the selection of drugs for this analysis is that they were administered as an oral solution in order to eliminate the ambiguity and variability in the rate of gastric emptying.

Methods

Numerical solution of the Diffusion-Convection (DC) model equations

Ni et. al. [12] have described a model of intestinal transit which combines convection, dispersion and absorption (DC model). The main assumption is that there is an equal volume flow into and out of each intestinal region so that the cross-sectional area (radius = r) and the convective flow (F) remains constant as the solute spreads along the intestine by convection and dispersion. The differential equation describing this DC model is:

$$\pi r^2 \frac{\partial c}{\partial t} = \pi r^2 D \frac{\partial^2 c}{\partial x^2} - F \frac{\partial c}{\partial x} - 2\pi r P c \qquad (1)$$

The left hand side is the time dependent change in the concentration c(x,t) (where x is the distance from the pyloric sphincter). The first term on the right is the dispersive mixing, the second is the convective flow and the third is the absorption term where r is the intestinal radius (cm), D is the dispersion coefficient (cm^2/sec), F is the volume flow (cm^3/sec) and P is the permeability (cm/sec).

Ni et. al. [12] derived an exact analytical solution to Equation (1) that assumes as a boundary condition an exponential concentration at x = 0. This condition is not physiological because it implies that, in addition to the convective flux out of the stomach, there is also a non-physiological dispersive flux both out of and into the stomach (and out of and into the large intestine). For this reason the analytical solution will not be used here and, instead, a finite difference numerical approximation to Equation (1) will be used in which there is only a convective flux from the stomach to the small intestine and from the small intestine to the large intestine. (Also, the numerical solution is computationally much faster than the analytical solution). The small intestine is divided into N equal sections with the following difference equations:

$$i = 1 : \quad \Delta V \frac{dc[1]}{dt} = I_G(t) - (F + \Delta P + De)\,c[1] + De\,c[2]$$

$$0 < i < N : \quad \Delta V \frac{dc[i]}{dt} = (F + De)\,c[i-1] - (F + \Delta P + 2De)\,c[i] + De\,c[i+1]$$

$$i = N : \quad \Delta V \frac{dc[N]}{dt} = (F + De)\,c[N-1] - (F + De + \Delta P)\,c[N]$$

$$(2)$$

where c[i] is the concentration in the ith compartment at time t, $I_G(t)$ is the rate of gastric emptying into the intestine, r = intestinal radius, L = intestinal length, S = surface area = $2\pi r L$, V = volume = $\pi r^2 L$, $\Delta P = PS/N$, ΔV = V/N and De = $\pi r^2 DN/L$. The rate $E_{DC}(t)$ that the unabsorbed solute exits the small intestine and passes into the large intestine is:

$$E_{DC}(t) = F c[N] \tag{3}$$

The cumulative amount $A_{DC}(t_i)$ that has entered the large intestine at time $t_i = i \, \Delta t$ is:

$$A_{DC}(t_i) = \sum_{j=1}^{i} E_{DC}(t_j) \, \Delta t \tag{4}$$

The absorption rate $R_{DC}(t)$ at time t_i is:

$$R_{DC}(t_i) = \Delta P \sum_{i=1}^{N} c[i] \tag{5}$$

Gastric emptying in humans of non-caloric fluids is approximately exponential with a half time of about 15 minutes [13,14] and it will be assumed that $I_G(t)$ is exponential:

$$I_G(t) = FC_0 \exp(-t/T_G) \tag{6}$$

where T_G is the time constant for gastric emptying, C_0 is the gastric concentration at $t = 0$ and $FC_0 = Dose/T_G$. In addition, the parameters D, F and P will be described in terms of 3 other time constants:

$$T_P = r/(2P) \qquad T_F = V/F \qquad T_D = L^2/(2D) \tag{7}$$

Equation (2) is solved numerically using N = 50 and the Rosenbrock method as implemented in Maple (Maplesoft™). Some of the figures shown here are Maple plots.

Derivation and description of the "Averaged Model (AM)"

The DC equation (Equation (1)) has the interesting property that, if the drug is completely absorbed in the small intestine and the amount entering the large intestine can be neglected, it has the same kinetics as a well stirred compartment. This can be seen by integrating Equation (1) over x from 0 (pyloric sphincter) to x = L (the ileocecal junction):

$$\pi r^2 L \frac{dC}{dt} = I_0(t) - I_L(t) - 2\pi r L P C$$
$$C = (1/L)\int_0^L c(x,t)dx \quad I_0(t) = -\pi r^2 D \frac{dc(0,t)}{dx} + Fc(0,t) \tag{8}$$
$$I_L(t) = -\pi r^2 D \frac{dc(L,t)}{dx} + Fc(L,t)$$

where C is the average intestinal concentration and $I_0(t)$ and $I_L(t)$ are the inflow and outflow rates. If the outflow term $I_L(t)$ is negligible, then this equation reduces to:

$$V \frac{dC}{dt} = I_0(t) - PSC \tag{9}$$

This is identical to the case of a well mixed compartment of volume V with arbitrary input $I_0(t)$. Assuming that $I_0(t) = I_G(t)$ (Equation (6)) and solving the

differential Equation (9) one obtains the "averaged model" (AM) equation for the case of 100% absorption:

$$C(t) = (Dose/V) \, T_P [\exp(-t/T_G) - \exp(-t/T_P)]/(T_G - T_P) \tag{10}$$

where T_P and T_G are the permeability and gastric emptying time constants (Equation (6) and (7)). The rate of absorption (R(t)) from the small intestine is:

$$R(t) = PSC(t) = Dose \, [\exp(-t/T_G) - \exp(-t/T_P)]/(T_G - T_P) \tag{11}$$

This AM R(t) is identical to the absorption rate for the DC model for the case where all the solute is absorbed ($I_L(t) = 0$, Equation (8)). It should be emphasized that although Equation (9) is similar to the well-mixed equation it is not physically equivalent because C is the average concentration and it is not assumed that the intestine is well mixed. For example, it would be erroneous to assume that the rate of solute flow into the large intestine was equal to F*C.

As discussed above, Equation (11) is a rigorously accurate description of the intestinal absorption for the DC model only for the case where all of the solute is absorbed in the small intestine. This result can be generalized to the arbitrary permeability case where only a fraction F_A of the total Dose is absorbed in the small intestine:

$$R_M(t) = M \, [\exp(-t/T_G) - \exp(-t/T_P)]/(T_G - T_P)$$
$$M = F_A \, Dose \tag{12}$$

where M is the total amount absorbed. In addition, the relationship between T_P and P must be modified for this general case. The C in Equation (8) is based on the assumption of 100% absorption. If, for example, only 50% were absorbed the actual concentration would be twice this value of C and the value of P would be reduced by half. Thus, the general relationship between T_P and the averaged model intestinal permeability (P_M) is:

$$P_M = F_A P = F_A r/(2T_P) \tag{13}$$

The amount absorbed ($A_M(t)$) as a function of time is:

$$A_M(t) = \int_0^t R_M(\tau)dt = M\{1 + [T_P \exp(-t/T_P) \tag{14}$$
$$- T_G \exp(-t/T_G)]/(T_G - T_P)\}$$

These AM model expressions for the intestinal absorption rate $R_M(t)$ and P_M are only approximations to the exact DC model for this general case where not all the solute is absorbed. The range of validity of this approximation will be evaluated by comparing it to the DC model for a range of experimental parameters (see Results, Comparison of DC and AM models).

R_M and M represent the rate and total amount absorbed across the small intestinal epithelial luminal membrane. Assuming a linear system, the rate of solute entering the systemic circulation (R_{SM}) is:

$$R_{SM}(t) = M_S \left[\exp(-t/T_G) - \exp(-t/T_P) \right]/(T_G - T_P)$$
$$M_S = F_A(1 - E_H)(1 - E_I) Dose \qquad (15)$$

where E_H and E_I are the hepatic and intestinal extraction ratios [15]. The hepatic extraction (E_H) can be estimated from the liver blood flow (Q_H) [15] and the whole blood liver clearance (Cl_H):

$$E_H = Cl_H/Q_H \qquad (16)$$

The liver clearance (Cl_H) was estimated by correcting the whole blood clearance following the IV infusion for the fractional renal clearance using data obtained in the same subjects that were used for the permeability estimates.

Equation (15) is a simple 3 parameter function whose parameters (M_S, T_G and T_P) can be determined experimentally by deconvolution (see below for details) of the blood concentration time course following IV and oral doses. The fraction absorbed (F_A) can be determined from M_S and estimates of E_H and E_I (Equation (15)). Finally, the AM model intestinal permeability (P_M) can be determined from F_A and T_P (Equation (13)).

Equation (15) is symmetrical in T_G and T_P so that there is an ambiguity in distinguishing the gastric emptying time constant T_G from the permeability time constant T_P. Most of the applications described here will be based on data obtained using oral solutions (not tablets) given to fasting subjects and the time constant that is closest to 10 to 15 minutes will be assumed to be T_G.

The theoretical accuracy of the AM model absorption rate RM (Equation 12) was evaluated by comparing it with the exact DC model R_{DC} (Equation 5). A set of the 7 DC parameters (Dose, T_G, T_P, T_B, T_D, r, L) were selected and the DC model intestinal absorption rate and fraction absorbed was determined. Then, the AM model parameters (M, T_G, T_P, Equation (12)) that provided the best fit to the DC absorption rate were determined by minimizing the following error function using the optimization routine in Maple (Maplesoft™):

$$Error = (1/N) \sum_{i=1}^{N} (R_{DC}[i] - R_M(t_i))^2 \qquad (17)$$

where $t_i = i \, \Delta t$ and comparing the AM model parameters (F_A, T_P and T_G) with the actual input DC parameters.

Experimental determination of the averaged model (AM) parameters by deconvolution

The determination of the 3 AM model parameters (M_S, T_G and T_P) is based on standard procedures that have been described previously [6]. First, the 2 or 3 exponential systemic bolus response function r(t) is determined from the experimental blood concentration time course following the known IV infusion. The blood concentration $C_{oral}(t)$ following the oral dose is equal to the convolution of r(t) and the AM model systemic absorption rate $R_{SM}(t)$ (Equation (15)):

$$C_{oral}(t) = \int_0^t r(t-\tau) R_{SM}(\tau) \, d\tau \qquad (18)$$

The 3 AM model parameters (M_S, T_G and T_P) are then estimated by finding the parameter set that minimizes the error function:

$$Err = \sum_k \frac{|C_{oral}(t_k) - C_k|}{C_k + noise} \qquad (19)$$

where C_k is the experimental blood concentration at time t_k following the oral dose. The "noise" determines the relative weighting of each data point and can be arbitrarily adjusted but is usually set to 10% of the average blood value. The optimized set of parameters is determined by a non-linear Powell minimization routine [16]. Most of the drugs were administered as oral solutions in fasting subjects and T_G was forced to be in the range of 10 to 20 minutes (the normal range for non-caloric fluids [13,14]) and only the two parameters T_P and M_S were freely adjusted. For a few solutes that were administered as capsules or tablets, all 3 parameters were adjusted.

These procedures have been implemented in PKQuest Java, a freely distributed software program that has been used previously for pharmacokinetic analysis of more than 30 different solutes in a series of publications [7]. The implementation is designed to be user friendly and simple to use. The user only needs to enter 1) the dose and duration of the constant IV infusion; 2) the experimental blood concentration for the IV dose (which can be copied and pasted from a standard Excel file); and 3) the experimental blood concentration following the oral dose. The program then finds the optimum set of AM parameters. It also outputs 4 plots that are useful for evaluating the results: 1) A comparison of the experimental blood concentration for the IV dose versus the blood concentration predicted by bolus response function (there is usually nearly perfect agreement). 2) The AM model absorption rate as a function of time; 3) AM total absorption as a function of time; and 4) a comparison of the experimental blood concentration following the oral dose versus the AM model prediction (Equation (18)). This last plot is especially useful because it provides the best measure of the quality of the AM model. See Figures 1, 2, 3 and 4 for examples of these plots. PKQuest Java and a detailed tutorial can be freely downloaded from www.pkquest.com. Also available for download are the complete data sets for the 90 solutes

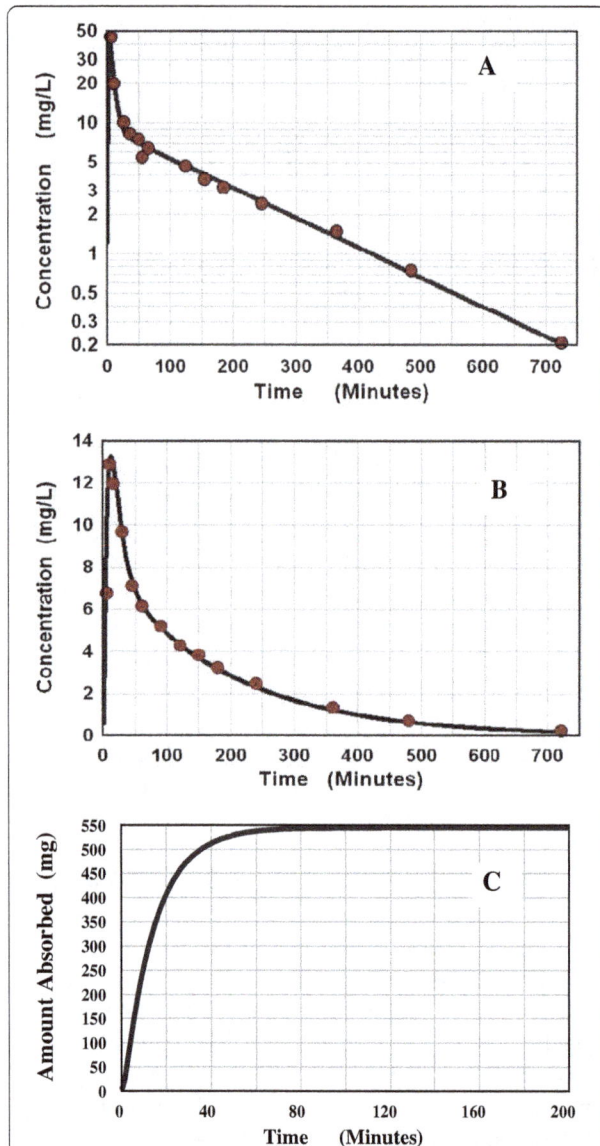

Figure 1 AM model deconvolution solution for intestinal absorption of acetaminophen. Figure 1**A** shows a comparison of the experimental blood concentration data points (red circles) following an IV input versus the theoretical blood concentration determined from the 2 exponential systemic response function (line). Figure 1**B** shows a comparison of the experimental blood concentration data points (red circles) following an oral input with the theoretical blood concentration prediction determined from the deconvolution solution of the AM absorption rate function. Figure 1**C** shows the cumulative AM absorption amount as a function of time.

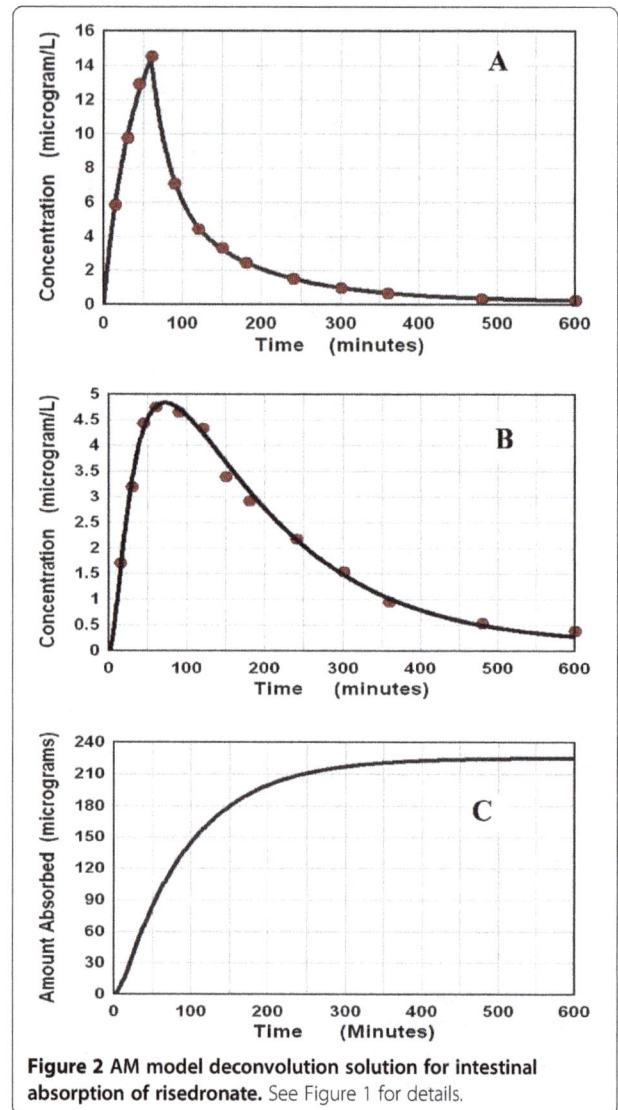

Figure 2 AM model deconvolution solution for intestinal absorption of risedronate. See Figure 1 for details.

discussed in this paper. This allows the user to reproduce all of the results.

Experimental intestinal absorption data

In order to be a candidate for determination of intestinal permeability it was required that the solute met the following 4 conditions: 1) intravenous and oral dose pharmacokinetics in the same subject; 2) the oral dose was in the form of a solution (not tablet) to fasting subjects; 3) the drug's pharmacokinetics are linear, at least in the concentration range that is investigated; 4) the drug is soluble at the concentrations used in the absorption study. These conditions severely limit the number of experimental results that can be used. Condition #1 is satisfied in only a small fraction of permeability studies. Condition #2 also severely restricts the number of possible candidates because tablets or capsules are used in most oral drug studies. A thorough search of the published

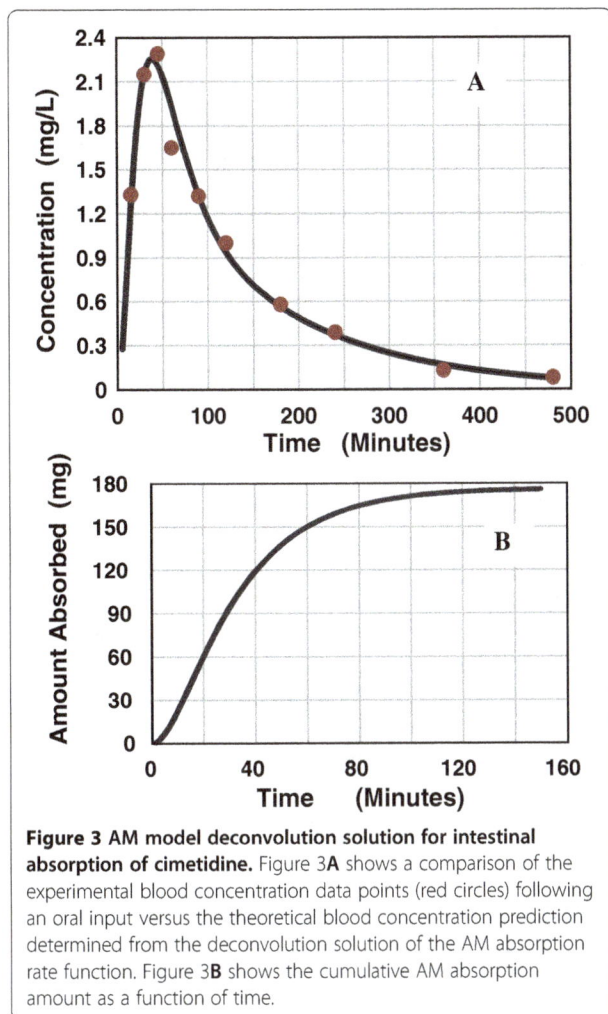

Figure 3 AM model deconvolution solution for intestinal absorption of cimetidine. Figure 3**A** shows a comparison of the experimental blood concentration data points (red circles) following an oral input versus the theoretical blood concentration prediction determined from the deconvolution solution of the AM absorption rate function. Figure 3**B** shows the cumulative AM absorption amount as a function of time.

using the following relations (this assumes that only the neutral solute has a finite octanol partition) [17]:

$$Mono\,protic\,base:\quad logPow_2 = logPow_1 + log\big(1 + 10^{(pKa-pH1)}\big)$$
$$- log\big(1 + 10^{(pka-pH2)}\big)$$
$$Mono\,protic\,acid:\quad logPow_2 = logPow_1 + log\big(1 + 10^{(pH1-pKa)}\big)$$
$$- log\big(1 + 10^{(pH2-pKa)}\big)$$

$$(20)$$

The experimental perfused human jejunum permeability [18] and the Caco-2 permeability are also listed in Additional file 1: Table 2 if they were available. The form of the oral dose (solution, tablet, capsule) is listed and solutes which may have solubility limitations are marked in the table. If there is suggestive evidence that the intestinal absorption is protein mediated (either influx or efflux), this is also indicated. The experimental data points

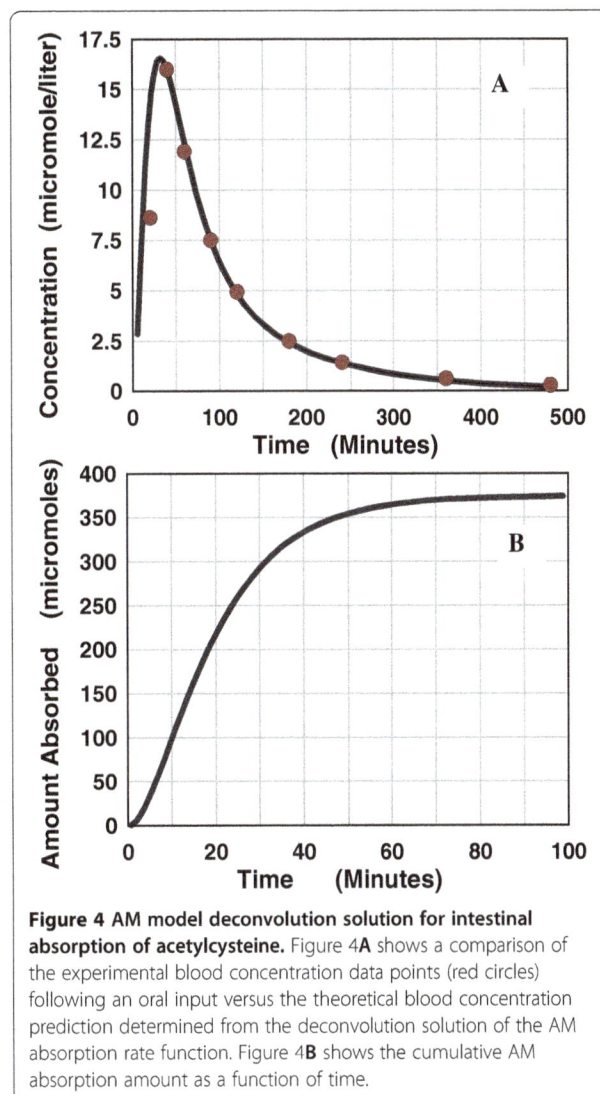

Figure 4 AM model deconvolution solution for intestinal absorption of acetylcysteine. Figure 4**A** shows a comparison of the experimental blood concentration data points (red circles) following an oral input versus the theoretical blood concentration prediction determined from the deconvolution solution of the AM absorption rate function. Figure 4**B** shows the cumulative AM absorption amount as a function of time.

literature returned 90 drugs that met these conditions. A few drugs that were administered as tablets have been included if the drug had a high water solubility so that the tablet would be rapidly dissolved and a low permeability (long T_P) that could not be confused with the T_G. The results and analyses are summarized in the Excel file that is included in the Additional file 1: "Table 2". Additional file 1: Table 2 lists the solute, a link to the reference publication, the AM model parameters, a subjective measure of the quality of the AM fit to the data and the calculated permeability. The table includes the ionization behavior of the solute (weak acid, base, neutral or always ionized) in the pH range of 4 to 8 and the pKa if it is a weak base or acid. Also listed is an estimate of the experimental log(octanol/water) partition coefficient at pH 7.4 (log D). For most solutes there are multiple reported values of log D that can vary by as much a log unit. For those solutes which are available on the LOGKOW site maintained by James Sangster, the value listed is an approximate average of the listed values. When necessary, the log Pow values were converted from pH1 to a different pH2

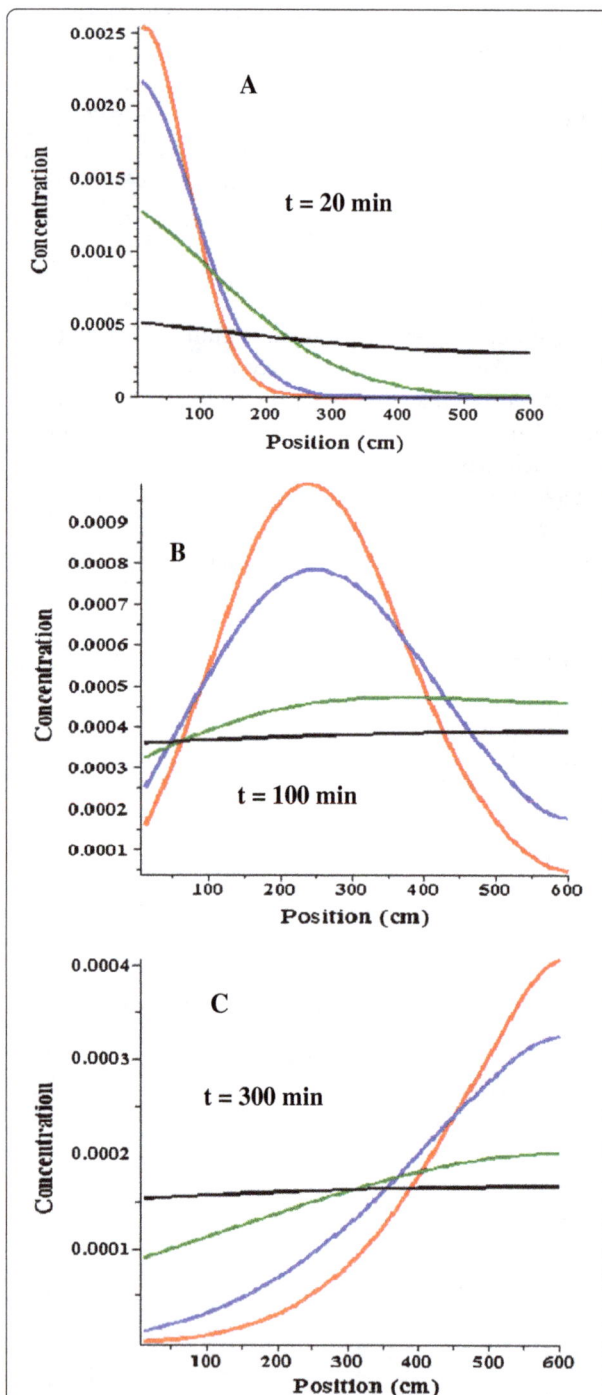

Figure 5 Diffusion convection concentration profile. The diffusion convection model concentration as a function of distance from the pyloric sphincter is shown at 20 (Figure 5**A**), 100 (**B**) and 300 minutes (**C**) after administering the oral dose as a bolus to the stomach for an impermeable (P = 0) solute. The profile is shown for 4 different values of the dispersion time constant (T_D): 2000 (red); 1000 (blue); 200 (green); and 20 minutes (black). For all profiles T_F = 200 minutes; T_G = 15 minutes; r = 1 cm; L = 600 cm and Dose = 1.

were read from the published figures using UN-SCAN-IT (Silk Scientific Corporation).

Results

Solution and parameter study of the Diffusion-Convection (DC) model

The DC model differential equation (Equation (2)) was solved numerically. Figure 5A, B and C show the DC concentration profile for a non-permeable ($\Delta P = 0$) solute at time = 20, 100 and 300 minutes after the oral dose with T_D (dispersive transit time) values of 2000 (red curve), 1000 (blue), 200 (green) and 20 (black) minutes. Unless otherwise stated, all of the plots described here have T_G = 15 minutes (gastric emptying time constant), T_F = 240 minutes (convective small intestinal transit time), N = 50 (there is no significant change in the results for greater N), Δt = 1 minute, Dose = 1.0, r = 1 cm and L = 600 cm. Since the concentration profile has a strong dependence on T_D, these plots could be used to estimate the value of T_D (and T_F) in the human if experimental measurements of the concentration profile along the small intestine for impermeable solutes were available. Unfortunately, no such measurements have been reported for humans or other large mammals (they have been made in rats [19]).

The experimental measurement in humans that can be used to estimate T_D is the distribution of small intestinal transit times determined from the appearance of some non-permeable label in the large intestine [20]. Figure 6 shows the DC cumulative amount entering the large intestine as a function of time (Equation (4)) for T_D = 2000 (red), 1000

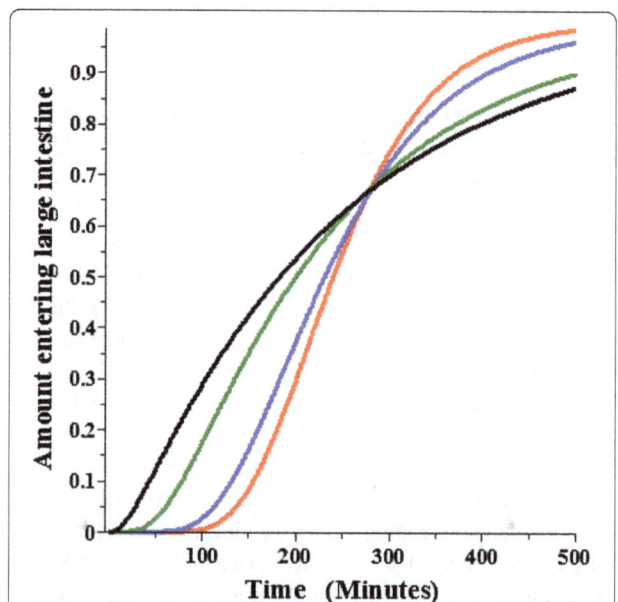

Figure 6 Diffusion convection small intestinal transit time. The diffusion convection amount leaving the small intestine and entering the large intestine as a function of time for an impermeable solute. Same conditions as for Figure 5.

(blue), 200 (green) and 20 (black) minutes for the same conditions as in Figure 5. The shape of the curves can be roughly characterized by the time of first appearance of solute and the half time. Caride et. al. [21] reported the time of arrival (time at which a "sustained" increase in breath hydrogen or [99m]technetium-diethylenetriaminepentaacetic acid was first detected) of about 73 minutes. Based on an extensive literature review, Davis et. al. [22] found an average small intestinal half time of about 240 minutes. From Figure 6, a T_D of about 200 minutes provides the best fit to these experimental measurements in humans.

In the next section, the DC model will be used to evaluate the accuracy of the AM model approximation. The plots in Figures 5 and 6 are for non-permeable solutes. Figure 7 shows a plot of the DC fraction absorbed versus the permeability (10^{-4} cm/sec) for $T_D = 1000$ (blue) and 200 (green) minutes. It can be seen that for the high permeability solutes the fraction absorbed increases by about 5% as T_D increases 5 fold (i.e. as the dispersion rate decreases). This produces a small dependence of the error in the AM absorption rate on T_D (see below) which is quantitated in the next section.

Comparison of DC and AM models – theoretical evaluation of accuracy of AM model approximation

The procedure that will be used to measure the experimental permeability is to fit the AM absorption rate Equation (15) to the systemic absorption rate determined by deconvolution. The accuracy of this procedure will be theoretically tested here by fitting Equation 15 to the general DC model absorption rate and comparing the AM permeability to the permeability that is used to generate the DC absorption data. Figure 8A and B compare the absorption rate as a function of time for the DC model (red) versus the best fit AM model (blue) for the case where the DC $T_D = 200$ minutes and $T_F = 240$ minutes (and $T_G =$

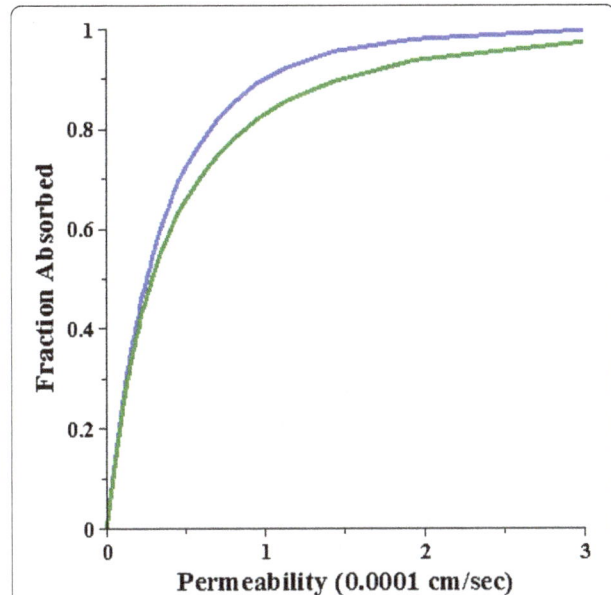

Figure 7 Permeability dependence of the diffusion convection intestinal absorption. The fractional absorption of the diffusion convection model as a function of the permeability in units of 10^{-4} cm/sec for a dispersion time constant (T_D) of 1000 (blue) or 200 minutes (green). The rest of the conditions are the same as in Figure 5.

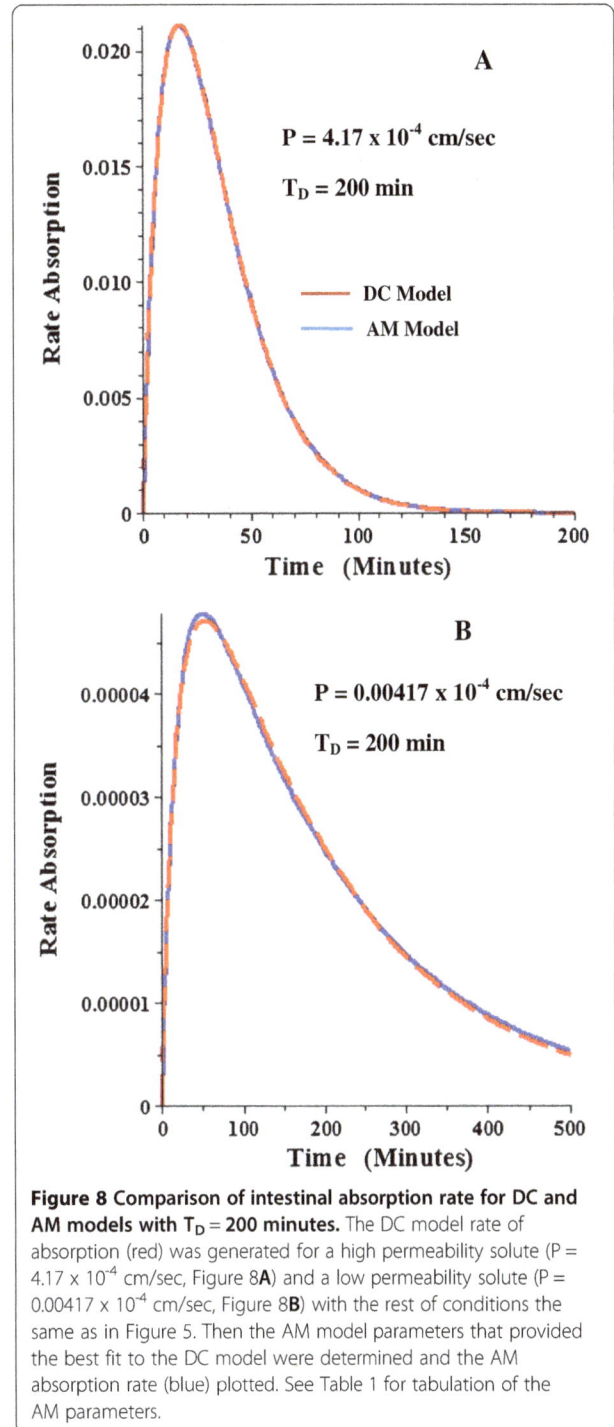

Figure 8 Comparison of intestinal absorption rate for DC and AM models with $T_D = 200$ minutes. The DC model rate of absorption (red) was generated for a high permeability solute (P = 4.17 x 10^{-4} cm/sec, Figure 8**A**) and a low permeability solute (P = 0.00417 x 10^{-4} cm/sec, Figure 8**B**) with the rest of conditions the same as in Figure 5. Then the AM model parameters that provided the best fit to the DC model were determined and the AM absorption rate (blue) plotted. See Table 1 for tabulation of the AM parameters.

15 min, r = 1 cm, L = 700 cm). Figure 8A shows that the AM model provides a nearly perfect fit to the DC absorption rate for the case of a relatively high permeability solute (T_P = 200 min, corresponding to P = 4.167 × 10^{-4} cm/sec). This is expected because only 1% of the solute passes from the small to large intestine for this high permeability and, as shown above, the AM and DC models are theoretically identical if all the solute is absorbed. More surprisingly, the DC and AM models are nearly identical (Figure 8B) even for solutes with a very low permeability (P = 0.004167 × 10^{-4} cm/sec) where only 1% of the solute is absorbed. If the dispersion time constant (T_D) is increased to 1000 minutes, the AM model provides a poorer approximation to the DC absorption rate for solutes with a low permeability (Figure 9B).

The quantitative comparison between the DC parameters used to generate the absorption rate and the AM parameters (T_G, T_P and F_A) that provide an optimal fit to this DC absorption rate are listed in Table 1 for a large range of values of the DC parameters. For T_D = 200 min, the AM permeability is within 20% of the DC permeability for a thousand fold permeability range (total absorption varying from 1% to 99%). For T_D =1000 min, the AM permeability can reach values 60% greater than the DC permeability for very low permeability solutes. Since the normal human T_D is about 200 minutes (Results, previous section), these results show that the AM model provides a good approximation to the exact DC model for a wide range of permeabilities.

AM model estimates of the human intestinal permeability of 90 solutes

The Excel Table in the Additional file 1: Table 2 lists the values of the intestinal permeability for 90 solutes determined using the AM model and deconvolution. As discussed in the Methods there are two time constants in the AM model. For most of the solutes in this table, an oral solution was administered to fasting subjects so that the value of T in the range of 10 to 20 minutes can be assumed to be T_G. For the few solutes in the table in which a tablet or capsule was administered, the solute had such a low permeability that it was clear that the longer T must correspond to T_P.

In order to determine the permeability it is essential to relate the rate of solute absorption into the systemic circulation determined by deconvolution to the rate of intestinal absorption and this requires estimates of the liver and intestinal first pass extraction (Equation (15)). The liver extraction was determined from the estimated liver blood flow and the liver clearance (Equation (16)). The liver clearance is equal to the total systemic clearance (determined from the IV input blood data) corrected for the fractional renal clearance. These values are listed in Additional file 1: Table 2 for each solute. The value for the liver flow is just an estimate and for some drugs, e.g. β-blockers, the value is reduced. The intestinal extraction is more uncertain. Although certain drug classes are known to have significant intestinal metabolism, there is no quantitative data available in humans [23]. In Additional file 1: Table 2 the column labeled "Est Fraction Absorbed" represents the final estimate taking account of the best guess for intestinal extraction.

Three representative examples of AM model deconvolution calculations will be described in detail. Acetaminophen is the classic example of a high permeability drug. Its intestinal absorption rate is usually assumed to be so fast that its absorption rate is a measure of the rate limiting gastric emptying [24-26]. The deconvolution

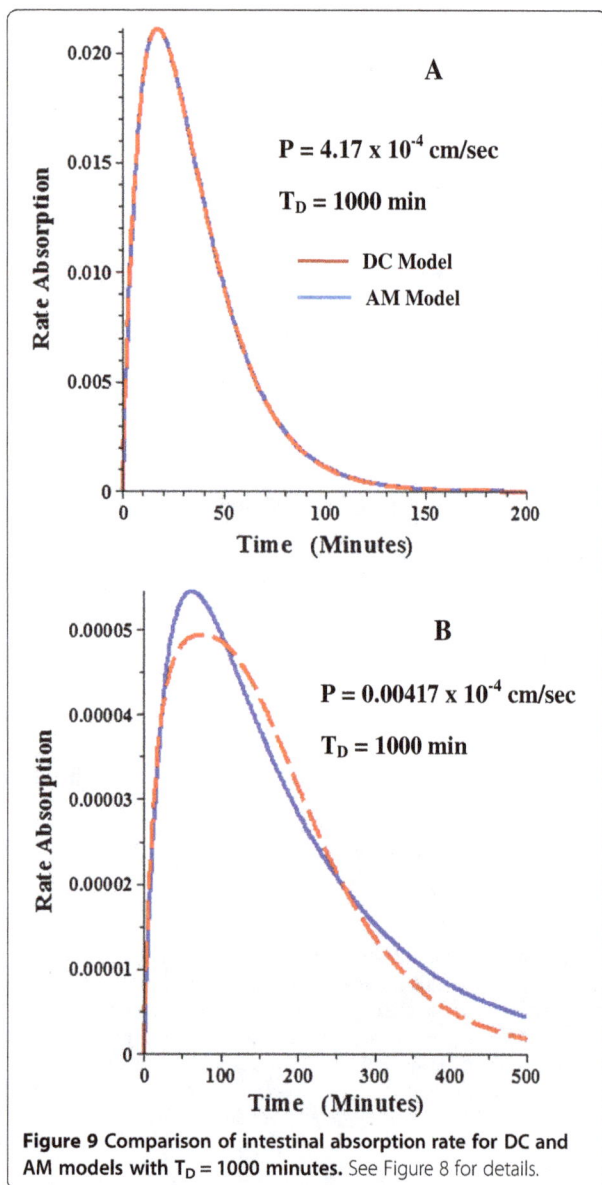

Figure 9 Comparison of intestinal absorption rate for DC and AM models with T_D = 1000 minutes. See Figure 8 for details.

Table 1 Comparison of "averaged" (AM) and dispersion convection (DC) absorption rates

DC Model				AM Model		
P_{DC} (10^{-4} cm/sec)	T_D (min)	T_G (min)	Fr. Absorb	P_{AM} (10^{-4} cm/sec)	T_G (min)	Fr. Absorb
4.167	200	15	.987	4.77	17.2	.989
0.4167	200	15	0.600	0.493	18.56	0.604
0.04167	200	15	0.109	0.0514	19.76	0.111
0.004167	200	15	0.0119	0.00517	19.9	.012
4.167	1000	15	0.999	4.167	15	0.999
0.4167	1000	15	0.658	0.522	20.8	0.690
0.04167	1000	15	0.111	0.0645	29	0.121
0.004167	1000	15	0.0119	0.0067	30	0.0129
4.167	200	60	0.997	4.155	60.0	0.997
0.04167	200	60	0.109	0.062	86	0.107
4.167	1000	60	0.999	4.167	60.0	0.999
0.04167	1000	60	0.112	0.0879	114.5	0.121

The theoretical time dependent absorption rate was generated for the DC parameters listed in the table (P_{DC} = permeability, T_D and T_G = the dispersion and gastric emptying time constants). For all results, T_F = 240 min, r = 1 cm, L = 700 cm. The DC "Fr. Absorb" is the resultant cumulative fraction absorbed. The AM parameters (permeability (P_{AM}), T_G and Fr. Absorb) were then adjusted to obtain the optimum fit to the DC absorption rate, similar to the procedure used to determine the experimental human small intestinal permeability by deconvolution.

results shown in Figure 1 are based on the data of Ameer et. al. [27] for a 650 mg IV and oral (elixir) dose (data for one "representative" subject). Figure 1A shows the 2 exponential response function fit to the IV input data. Figure 1B compares the AM model prediction of the blood concentration with the experimental data for the oral dose, and Figure 1C shows the cumulative predicted absorption rate. The AM parameters are M = 545 mg, and the two time constants are 2 and 14 minutes. As discussed above, it is assumed that the time constant closest to 15 minutes is T_G, and therefore T_P = 2 minutes. Correcting M for the liver extraction (Equation (16)) yields a fraction absorbed of 1.07; i.e. 100% absorption which is expected given the fact that the amount absorbed reaches its maximum by 50 minutes (Figure 1C), well before one would expect a significant amount to pass into the large intestine. From Equation (13), assuming an r of 1 cm, the acetaminophen permeability P_M is 41.7×10^{-4} cm/sec. There are two other published sets of acetaminophen data that can be used to estimate the permeability by deconvolution. The data of Divoll et. al. [28] (650 mg oral elixir data for representative "elderly" subject) has a P_M of 54×10^{-4} and that of Eandi et. al. [29] (averaged data (n = 9) for 1 gm oral "drops") has a P_M of 12.6×10^{-4} cm/sec.

Risedronate is a pyridinyl bisphosphonate with a very low intestinal permeability (bioavailability < 1%). Despite this low permeability, the plasma pharmacokinetics described by Mitchell et. al. [30] after an oral (30 mg solution) and IV infusion (0.3 mg) can be used to determine the time course of intestinal absorption by deconvolution (Figure 2). The AM model provides an excellent fit to the oral plasma data (Figure 2B) with M = 220 mg

(= 0.73% of 30 mg oral dose), T_G = 14 and T_P = 79.4 minutes. Using the fraction absorbed of 0.0073 in Equation (13), $P_M = 0.008 \times 10^{-4}$ cm/sec. (Since risedronate is not metabolized [30], there is no significant first pass metabolism.) The absorption is complete by 300 minutes (Figure 2C) presumably because this is the time required for complete emptying into the large intestine. This result also suggests that there is no significant absorption from the large intestine.

First pass intestinal extraction cannot be quantitatively measured in humans. In Additional file 1: Table 2 the assumed intestinal metabolism is indicated by the difference between the estimated total absorption (the column labeled "Est Fract Abs Small Intestine") and the systemic absorption corrected for the liver extraction (column labeled "Fract Abs Corrected for Liver Clearance"). For example, cimetidine has a highly variable bioavailability of about 65% that has been attributed to either low intestinal permeability or intestinal metabolism [31]. The AM model provides a good fit (Figure 3A) to the blood concentration following a 300 mg oral solution dose [32]. The AM parameters are M = 175 mg, T_G = 10 and T_P = 25 minutes. Correcting for liver extraction raises the amount absorbed to 203 mg (68% of the oral dose). From the AM model time course of the amount absorbed (Figure 3B) it can be seen that the absorption is complete by about 100 minutes. This is short compared to the presumed small intestinal transit time of about 300 minutes, suggesting that permeability is not limiting and that intestinal metabolism is responsible for the incomplete absorption. This approach of assuming that permeability is not rate limiting if the absorption is completed in, e.g.,

150 minutes can be used as a general criteria for determining if intestinal metabolism is important. (Note: this criteria is not applicable to acidic drugs, see Discussion). The extreme example of this for the drugs in Additional file 1: Table 2 is domperidone for which as much as 63% may be cleared by intestinal metabolism [33]. Cimetidine and domperidone are exceptions and for most of the drugs in Additional file 1: Table 2 intestinal metabolism is not significant.

Discussion

As shown above (Results, Comparison of DC and AM models), the 3 parameter averaged model (AM) provides a good estimate of the small intestinal permeability if the following 2 conditions are met: 1) gastric emptying can be described by a single exponential process; and 2) the assumptions underlying the diffusion-convection (DC) model are valid. In addition, to convert the AM value of T_P to an absolute permeability requires an assumption about the small intestinal radius (r, Equation (13), assumed = 1 cm). The analysis listed in the Additional file 1: "Table 2" is limited primarily to drugs that were administered as oral solutions to fasting subjects, conditions for which the exponential emptying should be a good approximation [14]. The basic assumption of the DC model is that the small intestine can be described by a uniform volume cylinder with convective flow into each segment exactly balanced by flow out, combined with a mixing dispersion term, with all properties uniform for its entire length. This is, at best, an approximate description of the small intestine. Little is known about the details of small intestinal volume, mixing and dispersion in a fasting human subject that has swallowed the small volume of water (about 200 ml) that is usually administered in these oral solution dose studies.

Probably the most severe limitation of the DC model is the assumption that the parameters do not vary over the length of the intestine. The luminal pH definitely varies with position and, since the permeability of weak acids and bases depends critically on pH, this implies that their permeability will also vary with position. There have been a number of measurements of the pH position dependence of the human intestine. In a review of the older literature, Gray and Dressman [34] reported pH values of 4.9 in proximal duodenum, 5.3 in terminal duodenum, 4.4-6.5 in proximal jejunum, 6.6 in mid and terminal jejunum and varying from 6.5 in proximal ileum to 7.4 in terminal ileum. Using in situ pH microelectrodes Ovesen et. al. [35] simultaneously measured a fasting pH of 2.05 in stomach, 3.03 in duodenal bulb, 4.9 in mid duodenum and 4.92 in proximal jejunum. Using radiotelemetry capsules swallowed "with a small quantity of water", Evans et. al. [36] reported pH values of 6.63 in jejunum, 7.41 in mid small bowel, 7.49 in ileum and

from 6.37 to 7.04 in colon. Using the "smart pill", Lalezari [37] recently reported pH values varying from 5.6, 6.2, 6.68, 6.9 for proximal to terminal small intestinal quartiles. Thus, the small intestinal pH can be assumed to start at about 4.4 in an initial short segment of the duodenum, increasing to 5.4 in the first part of the jejunum, to 6.4 in mid intestine and to 7.4 in the terminal ileum.

The results in Additional file 1: Table 2 will be discussed in terms of the classical pH partition assumption that the permeability is proportional to the concentration of the neutral moiety, using the octanol/water partition (log D) as representative of the epithelial membrane partition and the pKa to estimate the neutral concentration [38]. Since the small intestinal pH varies from about 4.4 to 7.4, this pH partition hypothesis implies that the intestinal permeability can vary by as much as 1000 fold over its entire length. Although more complicated approaches that combine log D with estimates of polar surface area and hydrogen bond donors can improve permeability estimates [39], log D captures the main features and will be focused on here. It is hoped that the data set in Additional file 1: Table 2 will be used in future evaluations of these advanced models.

Since the permeability of the 18 uncharged solutes in Additional file 1: Table 2 should not be affected by this pH heterogeneity, one would predict that the AM permeability for these solutes should be a good approximation to the true permeability. Figure 10 shows a plot of the log D versus the log of the permeability (cm/sec). The 5 colored points indicate solutes for which there is strong evidence of protein mediated transport. The 3 green points have P-glycloprotein mediated efflux (digoxin and β-methyl digoxon [40] and colchicine [41]) which should reduce their permeability. The blue point is lamivudine which is a substrate for the organic cation transporters [42] and the red point is xylose which has a carrier mediated transport (probably the glucose transport system) [43-45], both of which will increase the "permeability". The black line is the least squares regression fit to the black (non-protein mediated) points. There is only a weak correlation between permeability and log D. Presumably other factors besides simple octanol partition are important. The 4 points with the highest permeability (caffeine, acetaminophen, antipyrine and cotinine) are all low molecular weight (< 200) solutes. The 2 points with log D < −1.5 (acyclovir and ganciclovir) may have significant paracellular transport.

One would predict that the small intestinal pH heterogeneity should significantly influence the apparent AM "permeability" of the basic solutes listed in Additional file 1: Table 2. Since the basic solutes have a higher uncharged concentration at the higher pH, they will tend to be absorbed in the terminal small intestine – delaying

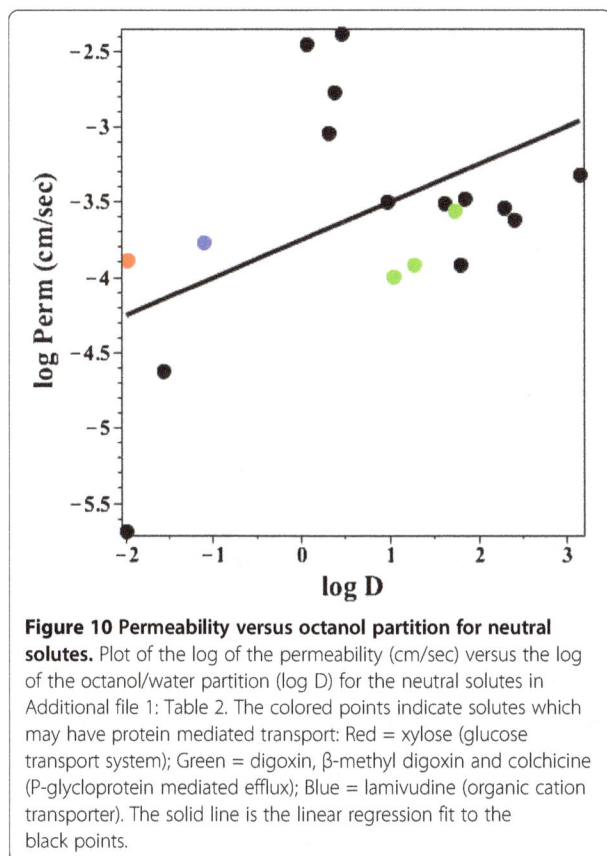

Figure 10 Permeability versus octanol partition for neutral solutes. Plot of the log of the permeability (cm/sec) versus the log of the octanol/water partition (log D) for the neutral solutes in Additional file 1: Table 2. The colored points indicate solutes which may have protein mediated transport: Red = xylose (glucose transport system); Green = digoxin, β-methyl digoxin and colchicine (P-glycloprotein mediated efflux); Blue = lamivudine (organic cation transporter). The solid line is the linear regression fit to the black points.

their absorption and decreasing the calculated permeability. This delay should have a complicated dependence on log D. Solutes with a relatively high log D at pH 6.5 will be absorbed in the first part of the intestine and have a correspondingly higher apparent permeability then solutes with a low log D whose absorption will be delayed until they reach the pH of 7.4 in the ileum. Figure 11 shows a plot of log D versus log permeability for the basic solutes in Additional file 1: Table 2 for a log D determined at pH 7.4 (Figure 11A), pH 6.4 (Figure 11B) and pH 5.4 (Figure 11C) using Equation (20) to convert the log D to the different pHs. The orange point is midodrine which is a known substrate for the peptide transport system [46]. The solid line is the linear regression fit to the black points and the dashed line is the regression for the neutral solutes (Figure 10). The pH 6.4 plot provides the best fit to the neutral solute permeability data (which should not be pH dependent), suggesting that pH 6.4 is the best average approximation for basic solutes. This is consistent with the current recommendation to use a pH of 6.8 for studies of "simulated" intestinal fluid [34]. As predicted, the AM permeability of the basic solutes with low log D at pH 6.4 or 7.4 is less than that of the neutral solutes (dashed line) because their absorption should be delayed until they reach the ileum. This comparison

between the neutral and basic solutes is only suggestive because of the small number of neutral solutes in Additional file 1: Table 2 and their poor correlation with log D (Figure 10).

The opposite effect should occur for the acidic solutes which should be absorbed in the proximal (acidic) section of the intestine. The classic example is aspirin, which has a pKa of 3.49 and a log D of about −1.8 (average from LOGKOW) at pH 7.4. From the plots in Figures 10 or 11, one would predict that a solute with this log D should have a low permeability of about 0.4×10^{-4} cm/sec, about 25 times smaller than the experimental AM aspirin permeabilities (Additional file 1: Table 2) of 6.69×10-4 cm/sec (Rowland et al. [47] for one subject) or 20.8×10^{-4} cm/sec (Bochner et al. [48], average of 6 subjects). The explanation of this high permeability has been controversial. Hogben et al. [49] used this rapid absorption of aspirin to infer that there must be a pH of about 5.3 at the luminal surface of the epithelial cell maintained by some unknown mechanism combined with a large unstirred luminal fluid layer. However, the recognition that the unstirred layer in humans is only about 35 μm [50] makes this idea untenable and direct measurements in guinea pig jejunum do not find evidence for this acidic mircroclimate [51]. An alternative explanation is that the salicylates are transported by a monocarboxylic acid carrier system [52,53]. However, Takagi et al. [54] suggested this result is an artifact and that pure phospholipid liposomes show the same apparent "carrier" behavior. The most likely explanation is simply that aspirin is absorbed in the duodenum and proximal jejunum where the pH varies from 4.4 to 5.4. At a pH of 5.4, the log D of aspirin is about 0.19 (Equation (20)) and small neutral solutes with this log D (e.g. caffeine, see Figure 10) have high AM permeabilities, equal to or greater than are observed for aspirin. The aspirin permeability at pH 5.4 is presumably high enough that it can be nearly completely absorbed in this short proximal region.

A dramatic illustration of the effect of this pH heterogeneity on the absorption of weak acids is provided by acetylcysteine which has a pKa of 3.25 and a very low log D of −2.5 at pH 7.4 with a corresponding log D of −1.5 at pH 6.4 and −0.6 at pH 5.4. The AM fit to the blood concentration following the oral dose and the time course of the intestinal absorption is shown in Figure 4. Even though the permeability time constant T_P is very fast (6.95 minutes), only about 12% of the 3676 μm oral dose is absorbed and the absorption stops after about 50 minutes (Figure 4B). This suggests that the absorption occurred only in the low pH proximal small intestine and this region was cleared by about 50 minutes after 12% was absorbed and that there was no significant absorption in the rest of the intestine.

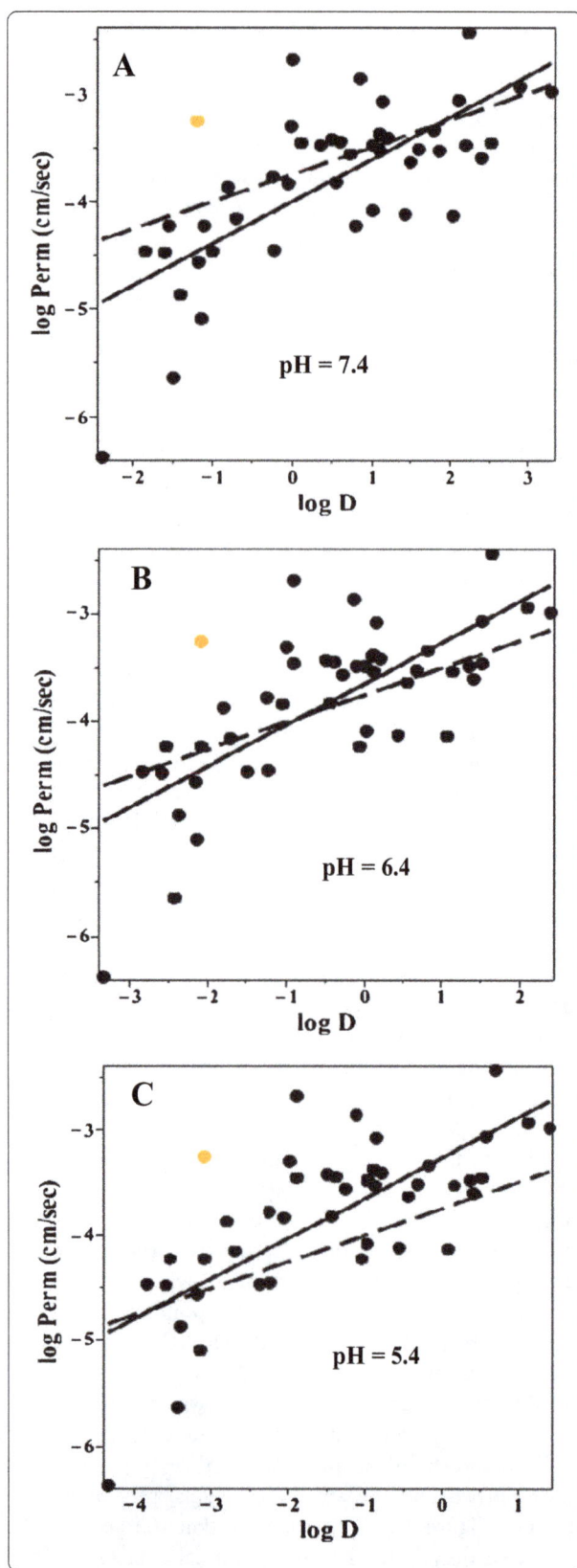

Figure 11 Permeability versus octanol partition for basic solutes. Plot of the log of the permeability (cm/sec) versus the log of the octanol/water partition (log D) for the basic solutes in Additional file 1: Table 2. The log D was determined at pH = 7.4 (Figure 11**A**), 6.4 (Figure 11**B**) and 5.4 (Figure 11**C**). The solid line is the linear regression fit to the black points and the dashed line is the linear regression fit to the neutral solutes (Figure 10). The orange point is midodrine which is a substrate for the peptide transport system.

Figure 12 shows a plot of the log permeability versus the log D at pH 7.4 (Figure 12A), 6.4 (Figure 12B) and 5.4 (Figure 12C) for the 10 acidic solutes in Additional file 1: Table 2. The solid line is the linear regression fit to the black points and the dashed line is the regression for the neutral solutes (Figure 10). There is no significant correlation between log D and the permeability. This is probably because most of these solutes are relatively rapidly and nearly completely absorbed in the proximal intestine and the log D varies over a smaller range than the basic solutes (Figure 11).

Figure 13 shows a plot of the log permeability versus the log D for the 7 solutes in Additional file 1: Table 2 that are charged over the entire pH range 5.4 to 7.4. The 2 green points indicate solutes that may be substrates for the peptide transport system. All the solutes have low permeabilities that are less than are predicted by the neutral solute plot (dashed line). These solutes are probably absorbed primarily by paracellular transport.

The best currently available measurements of human small intestinal permeability are the single-pass jejunal perfusion results of Lennernas and colleagues. Currently, they have published the jejunal permeability for 28 drugs [18]. Figure 14 shows a log-log plot of the AM versus the perfused jejnunal permeability for the 8 drugs that were studied by both methods. The dashed line is the line of identity. The black and red points are weak bases and acids, respectively, and the green point is the uncharged solute antipyrine. It can be seen that for most solutes the AM permeability is in good absolute agreement with the direct perfusion permeability - a surprising result considering the marked differences in experimental approaches and assumptions for the two methods. The major exception is the weak acid furosemide (red point) whose AM permeability (1.54×10^{-4} cm/sec) is 30 times greater than the perfusion permeability, presumably because furosemide is absorbed primarily in the proximal jejunum that has a pH significantly more acid than the pH of 6.5 used in the perfusion studies.

One can use the AM permeability of the highest permeability solutes to estimate a lower bound for the unstirred aqueous layer. For the passively absorbed high lipid solubility drugs, the permeability (P) should be approximately equal to that of the total fluid

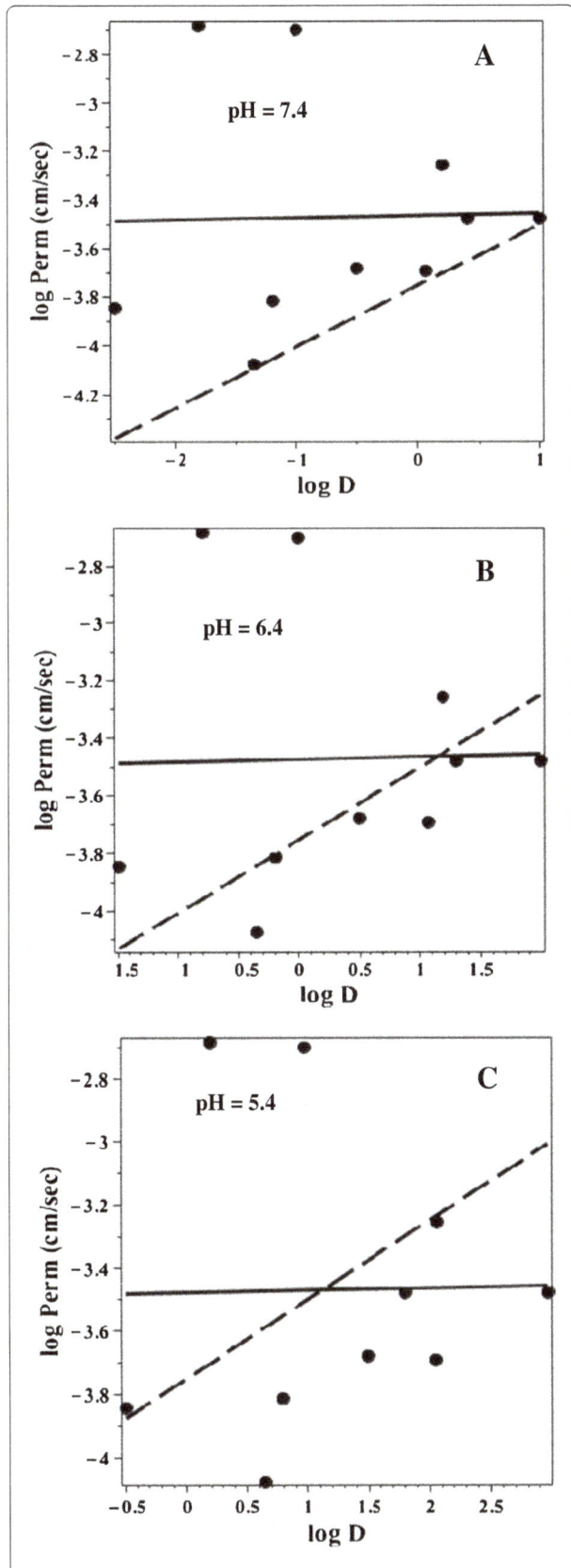

Figure 12 Permeability versus octanol partition for acidic solutes. Plot of the log of the permeability (cm/sec) versus the log of the octanol/water partition (log D) for the acidic solutes in Additional file 1: Table 2. The log D was determined at pH = 7.4 (Figure 12A), 6.4 (Figure 12B) and 5.4 (Figure 12C). The solid line is the linear regression fit to the black points and the dashed line is the linear regression fit to the neutral solutes (Figure 10).

layer separating the intestinal capillaries from the well stirred lumen:

$$P = D_{US}/L_{US} \qquad (21)$$

where L_{US} is the thickness and D_{US} is the average diffusion coefficient for this fluid layer. The small uncharged solutes (e.g. caffeine, acetaminophen and antipyrine) have the highest AM permeabilities of about 20×10^{-4} cm/sec (Additional file 1: Table 2). Assuming a D of 9.1×10^{-6} cm^2/sec for, e.g., antipyrine in water at 37°C [55], L = 45 μm. Since the epithelial cell thickness is about 25 μm [56], this corresponds to an unstirred luminal layer of only about 20 μm, similar to the value of 35 μm found by Levitt et al. [50] for human jejunum. This AM antipyrine permeability value is about 3 times larger than the value found by Fagerholm and Lennernas [55] at the highest rates of jejunal perfusion. The perfusion at a pressure of about 20 mm Hg [57] produces an unphysiological distended

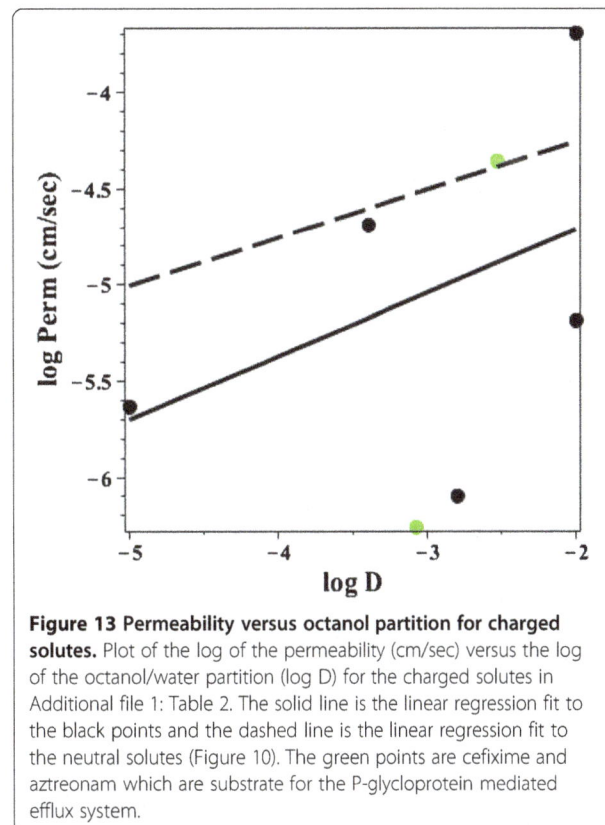

Figure 13 Permeability versus octanol partition for charged solutes. Plot of the log of the permeability (cm/sec) versus the log of the octanol/water partition (log D) for the charged solutes in Additional file 1: Table 2. The solid line is the linear regression fit to the black points and the dashed line is the linear regression fit to the neutral solutes (Figure 10). The green points are cefixime and aztreonam which are substrate for the P-glycloprotein mediated efflux system.

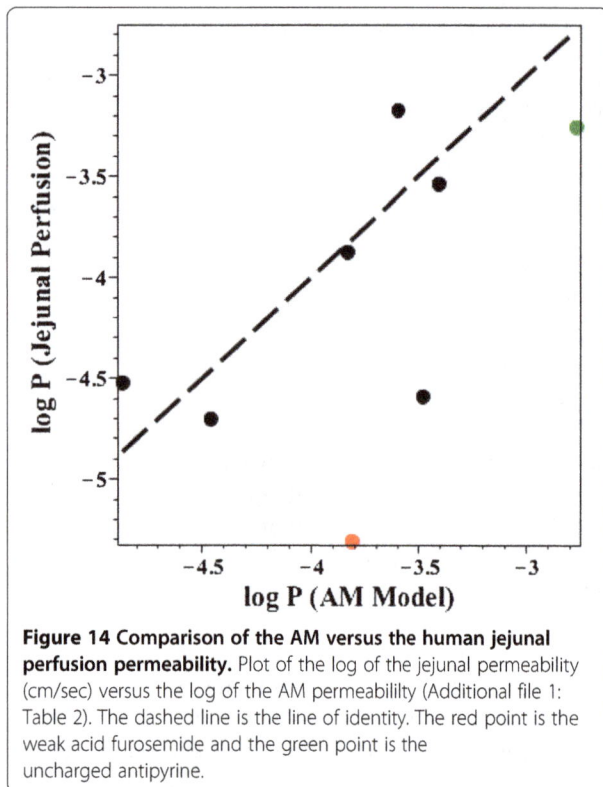

Figure 14 Comparison of the AM versus the human jejunal perfusion permeability. Plot of the log of the jejunal permeability (cm/sec) versus the log of the AM permeabililty (Additional file 1: Table 2). The dashed line is the line of identity. The red point is the weak acid furosemide and the green point is the uncharged antipyrine.

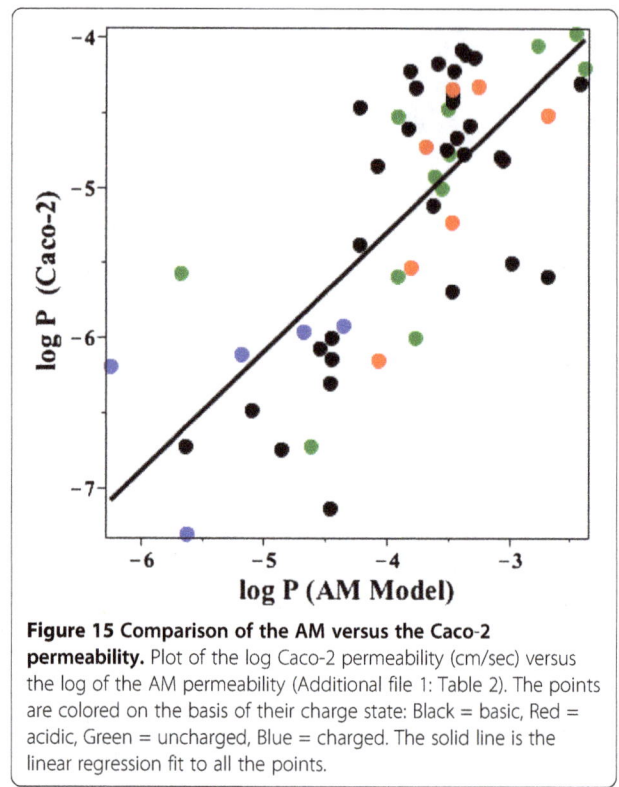

Figure 15 Comparison of the AM versus the Caco-2 permeability. Plot of the log Caco-2 permeability (cm/sec) versus the log of the AM permeability (Additional file 1: Table 2). The points are colored on the basis of their charge state: Black = basic, Red = acidic, Green = uncharged, Blue = charged. The solid line is the linear regression fit to all the points.

jejunum (radius of 1.61 cm) [58] and one might expect greater unstirred layers than during the nearly fasting conditions used for the AM studies.

The standard procedure for screening for the intestinal permeability of drugs is the Caco-2 cell culture system. Comparison of the AM permeability with the Caco-2 permeability is inexact because of the variety of techniques that have been used for reported Caco-2 values, with results differing by as much as 10 fold between different labs [1]. Larregieu and Benet [59] recently reviewed some of the problems in using Caco-2 as a surrogate for human permeability measurements. Thomas et al. [60] recently published a compilation of results for 120 drugs determined in their lab by the same method and these values were compared with the AM values for the drugs studied by both methods (Additional file 1: Table 2). In addition, Additional file 1: Table 2 was filled in with Caco-2 results from other labs. When more than one value was available, usually the larger permeability was used. Figure 15 shows a log-log plot of the AM versus Caco-2 permeability. The solid line is the linear regression fit. At the high permeability end of the regression, the AM permeability is about 40 times greater than the Caco-2 permeability. This is consistent with a Caco-2 unstirred layer that varies, depending on the stirring rate, from 564 to 2500 μm [61], which is 12 to 55 times

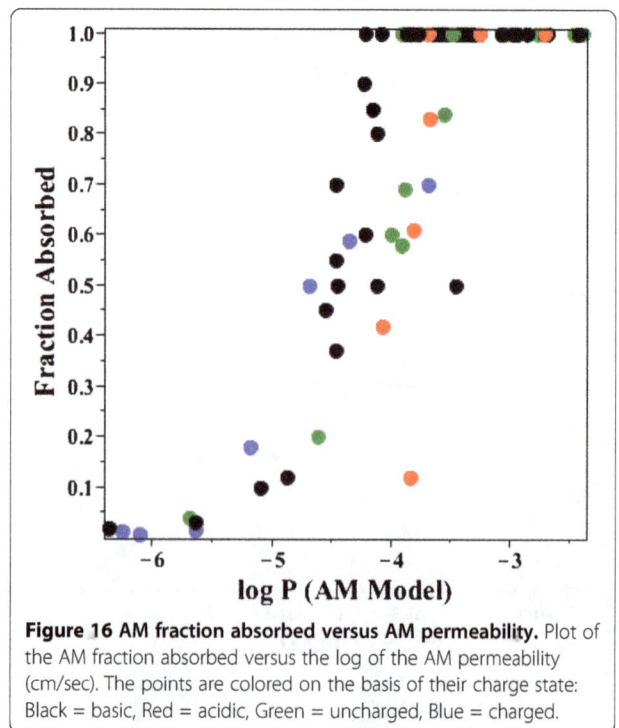

Figure 16 AM fraction absorbed versus AM permeability. Plot of the AM fraction absorbed versus the log of the AM permeability (cm/sec). The points are colored on the basis of their charge state: Black = basic, Red = acidic, Green = uncharged, Blue = charged.

greater than the AM value. At the low permeability end where the unstirred layer is not limiting, the AM permeability is 6.8 times greater than the Caco-2 permeability.

As discussed in the Background section, the standard approach for evaluating QSAR predictions of intestinal drug permeability is to use the human fraction absorbed as a surrogate for the permeability. Although the limitations of this approach are well recognized [1], it is the only available correlate of absorption for most drugs. The plot of the fraction absorbed versus the log of the AM permeability for the drugs in Additional file 1: Table 2 (Figure 16) dramatically illustrates this limitation. For values of the AM P greater than about 10^{-4} cm/sec, the drugs are 100% absorbed and, for P less than about 10^{-5}, absorption drops to 10% or less. Thus, although the permeability varies over a 10,000 fold range, the fraction absorbed varies from 0.1 to 1 over just a 10 fold permeability range. Although the fraction absorbed is the clinically most important prediction, it would clearly be useful to be able predict the permeability over a wider range. The data in Additional file 1: Table 2 should provide a useful benchmark for QSAR analysis.

Conclusions

The "averaged model" (AM) model accurately describes intestinal absorption if the assumptions of the diffusion convection (DC) model are satisfied. This new simple 3 parameter function (Equation (15)) can be used to determine by deconvolution the human intestinal permeability during the normal human drug absorption process. The AM permeability is similar to the values measured using direct jejunal perfusion. Its main limitation results from the heterogeneity in the small intestinal permeability of weak acids and bases produced by the variation in intestinal pH. Weak acids will tend to be absorbed in the proximal intestine and weak bases in the terminal intestine and this will be represented in the "permeability" determined by this method. The permeability data for the 90 drugs described in the Additional file 1: "Table 2" provides a large data base that should be useful in drug development and QSAR analysis.

Additional file

Additional file 1: Table 2. Summary of averaged model (AM) deconvolution analysis of human intestinal absorption. Tabulated summary of all the permeability data used in the paper "Quantitation of small intestinal permeability during normal human drug absorption", D. G. Levitt.

Abbreviations

AM: Averaged model; DC: Diffusion convection model; D: Dispersion coefficient; D_{US}: average unstirred layer diffusion coefficient; L_{US}: Unstirred layer thickness; F: Intestinal convective flow; P: Permeability for DC model; P_M: AM permeability for case where F_A of dose is absorbed; R: Intestinal radius; L: Intestinal length; S: Surface area = $2\pi rL$; V: Volume = $\pi r^2 L$; N: Number of finite segments in numerical solution; ΔP: PS/N; ΔV: V/N;

De: $\pi r^2 DN/L$; Dose: Total oral dose; F_A: Fraction of dose absorbed; $I_G(t)$: Convective solute input from stomach; E_{DC}: DC flux from small to large intestine; $A_{DC}(t)$: DC cumulative amount leaving small intestine; A_M: AM cumulative amount absorbed for case where F_A of dose is absorbed; E_H: Fractional liver extraction; E_I: Fractional intestinal mucosal extraction; Cl_H: Liver clearance; Q_H: Liver blood flow; M: Amount absorbed = F_A Dose; M_S: AM amount entering the systemic circulation; R_{DC}: DC rate of intestinal absorption; R: AM rate of intestinal absorption for case where 100% absorbed in small intestine; R_M: AM rate of absorption for case where F_A of dose is absorbed; R_{SM}: AM rate of absorption corrected for intestinal and liver extraction; c(x,t): DC concentration at position x at time t; C(t): "averaged" AM concentration; C_{oral}: Experimental blood concentration following an oral dose; T_F: DC convective time constant; T_D: DC dispersion time constant; T_p: Intestinal permeability time constant; T_G: Gastric emptying time constant; pKa: Acid dissociation constant; P_{ow}: Octanol/water partition; log D: log P_{ow} at pH = 7.4.

Competing interests
The author declares that he has no competing interests.

Authors' contributions
DGL is the sole contributor to this work.

References

1. Egan WJ, Lauri G: **Prediction of intestinal permeability.** *Adv Drug Deliv Rev* 2002, **54**(3):273–289.
2. Zhao YH, Le J, Abraham MH, Hersey A, Eddershaw PJ, Luscombe CN, Butina D, Beck G, Sherborne B, Cooper I, *et al*: **Evaluation of human intestinal absorption data and subsequent derivation of a quantitative structure-activity relationship (QSAR) with the Abraham descriptors.** *J Pharm Sci* 2001, **90**(6):749–784.
3. Amidon KS, Langguth P, Lennernas H, Yu L, Amidon GL: **Bioequivalence of oral products and the biopharmaceutics classification system: science, regulation, and public policy.** *Clin Pharmacol Ther* 2011, **90**(3):467–470.
4. Dahan A, Lennernas H, Amidon GL: **The fraction dose absorbed, in humans, and high jejunal human permeability relationship.** *Molecular pharmaceutics* 2012, **9**(6):1847–1851.
5. Soderholm JD, Olaison G, Kald A, Tagesson C, Sjodahl R: **Absorption profiles for polyethylene glycols after regional jejunal perfusion and oral load in healthy humans.** *Dig Dis Sci* 1997, **42**(4):853–857.
6. Levitt DG: **The use of a physiologically based pharmacokinetic model to evaluate deconvolution measurements of systemic absorption.** *BMC Clin Pharmacol* 2003, **3**:1.
7. Levitt DG: **PKQuest_Java: free, interactive physiologically based pharmacokinetic software package and tutorial.** *BMC research notes* 2009, **2**:158.
8. Sparacino G, Pillonetto G, Capello M, De Nicolao G, Cobelli C: **WINSTODEC: a stochastic deconvolution interactive program for physiological and pharmacokinetic systems.** *Comput Methods Programs Biomed* 2002, **67**(1):67–77.
9. Verotta D: **Estimation and model selection in constrained deconvolution.** *Ann Biomed Eng* 1993, **21**(6):605–620.
10. Agoram B, Woltosz WS, Bolger MB: **Predicting the impact of physiological and biochemical processes on oral drug bioavailability.** *Adv Drug Deliv Rev* 2001, **50**(Suppl 1):S41–S67.
11. Yu LX, Amidon GL: **A compartmental absorption and transit model for estimating oral drug absorption.** *Int J Pharm* 1999, **186**(2):119–125.
12. Ni PF HONFH, Fox JL, Leuenberger H, Higuchi HI: **Theoretical model studies of intestinal drug absorption V. Non-steady-state fluid flow and absorption.** *Int J Pharm* 1980, **5**:33–47.
13. Collins PJ, Horowitz M, Cook DJ, Harding PE, Shearman DJ: **Gastric emptying in normal subjects–a reproducible technique using a single scintillation camera and computer system.** *Gut* 1983, **24**(12):1117–1125.
14. George JD: **New clinical method for measuring the rate of gastric emptying: the double sampling test meal.** *Gut* 1968, **9**(2):237–242.
15. Wu CY, Benet LZ, Hebert MF, Gupta SK, Rowland M, Gomez DY, Wacher VJ: **Differentiation of absorption and first-pass gut and hepatic metabolism in humans: studies with cyclosporine.** *Clin Pharmacol Ther* 1995, **58**(5):492–497.
16. Press WH, Teukolsky SA, Vetterling WT, Flannery BP: *Numerical Recipes in C.* 2nd edition. Cambridge: Cambridge University Press; 1992.

17. Poulin P, Schoenlein K, Theil FP: **Prediction of adipose tissue: plasma partition coefficients for structurally unrelated drugs.** *J Pharm Sci* 2001, **90**(4):436–447.

18. Lennernas H: **Intestinal permeability and its relevance for absorption and elimination.** *Xenobiotica* 2007, **37**(10–11):1015–1051.

19. Miller MS, Galligan JJ, Burks TF: **Accurate measurement of intestinal transit in the rat.** *J Pharmacol Methods* 1981, **6**(3):211–217.

20. Yu LX, Amidon GL: **Characterization of small intestinal transit time distribution in humans.** *Int J Pharm* 1998, **171**(2):157–163.

21. Caride VJ, Prokop EK, Troncale FJ, Buddoura W, Winchenbach K, McCallum RW: **Scintigraphic determination of small intestinal transit time: comparison with the hydrogen breath technique.** *Gastroenterology* 1984, **86**(4):714–720.

22. Davis SS, Hardy JG, Fara JW: **Transit of pharmaceutical dosage forms through the small intestine.** *Gut* 1986, **27**(8):886–892.

23. Yang J, Jamei M, Yeo KR, Tucker GT, Rostami-Hodjegan A: **Prediction of intestinal first-pass drug metabolism.** *Curr Drug Metab* 2007, **8**(7):676–684.

24. Clements JA, Heading RC, Nimmo WS, Prescott LF: **Kinetics of acetaminophen absorption and gastric emptying in man.** *Clin Pharmacol Ther* 1978, **24**(4):420–431.

25. Heading RC, Nimmo J, Prescott LF, Tothill P: **The dependence of paracetamol absorption on the rate of gastric emptying.** *Br J Pharmacol* 1973, **47**(2):415–421.

26. Ogungbenro K, Vasist L, Maclaren R, Dukes G, Young M, Aarons L: **A semi-mechanistic gastric emptying model for the population pharmacokinetic analysis of orally administered acetaminophen in critically ill patients.** *Pharm Res* 2011, **28**(2):394–404.

27. Ameer B, Divoll M, Abernethy DR, Greenblatt DJ, Shargel L: **Absolute and relative bioavailability of oral acetaminophen preparations.** *J Pharm Sci* 1983, **72**(8):955–958.

28. Divoll M, Ameer B, Abernethy DR, Greenblatt DJ: **Age does not alter acetaminophen absorption.** *J Am Geriatr Soc* 1982, **30**(4):240–244.

29. Eandi M, Viano I, Ricci Gamalero S: **Absolute bioavailability of paracetamol after oral or rectal administration in healthy volunteers.** *Arzneimittelforschung* 1984, **34**(8):903–907.

30. Mitchell DY, Barr WH, Eusebio RA, Stevens KA, Duke FP, Russell DA, Nesbitt JD, Powell JH, Thompson GA: **Risedronate pharmacokinetics and intra- and inter-subject variability upon single-dose intravenous and oral administration.** *Pharm Res* 2001, **18**(2):166–170.

31. Hui YF, Kolars J, Hu Z, Fleisher D: **Intestinal clearance of H2-antagonists.** *Biochem Pharmacol* 1994, **48**(2):229–231.

32. Walkenstein SS, Dubb JW, Randolph WC, Westlake WJ, Stote RM, Intoccia AP: **Bioavailability of cimetidine in man.** *Gastroenterology* 1978, **74**(2 Pt 2):360–365.

33. Heykants J, Hendriks R, Meuldermans W, Michiels M, Scheygrond H, Reyntjens H: **On the pharmacokinetics of domperidone in animals and man. IV. The pharmacokinetics of intravenous domperidone and its bioavailability in man following intramuscular, oral and rectal administration.** *Eur J Drug Metab Pharmacokinet* 1981, **6**(1):61–70.

34. Gray VA, Dressman JB: **Change of pH requirement for simulated intestinal fluid TS.** *Pharmacopeial Forum* 1996, **22**(1):1943–1945.

35. Ovesen L, Bendtsen F, Tage-Jensen U, Pedersen NT, Gram BR, Rune SJ: **Intraluminal pH in the stomach, duodenum, and proximal jejunum in normal subjects and patients with exocrine pancreatic insufficiency.** *Gastroenterology* 1986, **90**(4):958–962.

36. Evans DF, Pye G, Bramley R, Clark AG, Dyson TJ, Hardcastle JD: **Measurement of gastrointestinal pH profiles in normal ambulant human subjects.** *Gut* 1988, **29**(8):1035–1041.

37. Lalezari D: **Gastrointestinal pH profile in subjects with irritible syndrome.** *Ann Gastroenterol* 2012, **25**(4):1–5.

38. Avdeef A: *Absorption and drug development. Solubility, permeability and charge state.* Hoboken, New Jersey: John Wiley and Sons,Inc; 2003.

39. Kramer SD: **Absorption prediction from physicochemical parameters.** *Pharm Sci Technology Today* 1999, **2**(9):373–380.

40. Pauli-Magnus C, Murdter T, Godel A, Mettang T, Eichelbaum M, Klotz U, Fromm MF: **P-glycoprotein-mediated transport of digitoxin, alpha-methyldigoxin and beta-acetyldigoxin.** *Naunyn Schmiedebergs Arch Pharmacol* 2001, **363**(3):337–343.

41. Dahan A, Amidon GL: **Grapefruit juice and its constituents augment colchicine intestinal absorption: potential hazardous interaction and the role of p-glycoprotein.** *Pharm Res* 2009, **26**(4):883–892.

42. Jung N, Lehmann C, Rubbert A, Knispel M, Hartmann P, van Lunzen J, Stellbrink HJ, Faetkenheuer G, Taubert D: **Relevance of the organic cation transporters 1 and 2 for antiretroviral drug therapy in human immunodeficiency virus infection.** *Drug Metab Dispos* 2008, **36**(8):1616–1623.

43. Levitt DG, Hakim AA, Lifson N: **Evaluation of components of transport of sugars by dog jejunum in vivo.** *Am J Physiol* 1969, **217**(3):777–783.

44. Rolston DD, Mathan VI: **Xylose transport in the human jejunum.** *Dig Dis Sci* 1989, **34**(4):553–558.

45. Csaky TZ, Ho PM, Csaky TZ, Ho PM: **Intestinal transport of D-xylose.** *Proceedings of the Society for Experimental Biology and Medicine Society for Experimental Biology and Medicine (New York, NY)* 1965, **120**(2):403–408.

46. Tsuda M, Terada T, Irie M, Katsura T, Niida A, Tomita K, Fujii N, Inui K: **Transport characteristics of a novel peptide transporter 1 substrate, antihypotensive drug midodrine, and its amino acid derivatives.** *J Pharmacol Exp Ther* 2006, **318**(1):455–460.

47. Rowland M: **Influence of route of administration on drug availability.** *J Pharm Sci* 1972, **61**(1):70–74.

48. Bochner F, Williams DB, Morris PM, Siebert DM, Lloyd JV: **Pharmacokinetics of low-dose oral modified release, soluble and intravenous aspirin in man, and effects on platelet function.** *Eur J Clin Pharmacol* 1988, **35**(3):287–294.

49. Hogben CA, Tocco DJ, Brodie BB, Schanker LS: **On the mechanism of intestinal absorption of drugs.** *J Pharmacol Exp Ther* 1959, **125**(4):275–282.

50. Levitt MD, Strocchi A, Levitt DG: **Human jejunal unstirred layer: evidence for extremely efficient luminal stirring.** *Am J Physiol* 1992, **262**(3 Pt 1): G593–G596.

51. Rechkemmer G, Wahl M, Kuschinsky W, von Engelhardt W: **pH-microclimate at the luminal surface of the intestinal mucosa of guinea pig and rat.** *Pflugers Arch* 1986, **407**(1):33–40.

52. Takanaga H, Tamai I, Tsuji A: **pH-dependent and carrier-mediated transport of salicylic acid across Caco-2 cells.** *J Pharm Pharmacol* 1994, **46**(7):567–570.

53. Tamai I, Takanaga H, Maeda H, Yabuuchi H, Sai Y, Suzuki Y, Tsuji A: **Intestinal brush-border membrane transport of monocarboxylic acids mediated by proton-coupled transport and anion antiport mechanisms.** *J Pharm Pharmacol* 1997, **49**(1):108–112.

54. Takagi M, Taki Y, Sakane T, Nadai T, Sezaki H, Oku N, Yamashita S: **A new interpretation of salicylic acid transport across the lipid bilayer: implications of pH-dependent but not carrier-mediated absorption from the gastrointestinal tract.** *J Pharmacol Exp Ther* 1998, **285**(3):1175–1180.

55. Fagerholm U, Lennernas H: **Experimental estimation of the effective unstirred water layer thickness in the human jejunum, and it importance in oral drug absorption.** *Eur J Pharm Sci* 1995, **3**:247–253.

56. Mackenzie NM: **Comparison of the metabolic activities of enterocytes isolated from different regions of the small intestine of the neonate.** *Biol Neonate* 1985, **48**(5):257–268.

57. Lennernas H: **Human intestinal permeability.** *J Pharm Sci* 1998, **87**(4):403–410.

58. Knutson T, Fridblom P, Ahlstrom H, Magnusson A, Tannergren C, Lennernas H: **Increased understanding of intestinal drug permeability determined by the LOC-I-GUT approach using multislice computed tomography.** *Mol Pharm* 2009, **6**(1):2–10.

59. Larregieu CA, Benet LZ: **Drug discovery and regulatory considerations for improving in silico and in vitro predictions that use caco-2 as a surrogate for human intestinal permeability measurements.** *AAPS J* 2013, **15**(2):483–497.

60. Thomas S, Brightman F, Gill H, Lee S, Pufong B: **Simulation modelling of human intestinal absorption using Caco-2 permeability and kinetic solubility data for early drug discovery.** *J Pharm Sci* 2008, **97**(10):4557–4574.

61. Hidalgo IJ, Hillgren KM, Grass GM, Borchardt RT: **Characterization of the unstirred water layer in Caco-2 cell monolayers using a novel diffusion apparatus.** *Pharm Res* 1991, **8**(2):222–227.

4

Empiric guideline-recommended weight-based vancomycin dosing and nephrotoxicity rates in patients with methicillin-resistant *Staphylococcus aureus* bacteremia: a retrospective cohort study

Ronald G Hall II[1,2]*, Kathleen A Hazlewood[1,7], Sara D Brouse[1,8], Christopher A Giuliano[3,9], Krystal K Haase[3], Chistopher R Frei[4], Nicolas A Forcade[4,10], Todd Bell[5], Roger J Bedimo[6] and Carlos A Alvarez[1,2]

Abstract

Background: Previous studies have established a correlation between vancomycin troughs and nephrotoxicity. However, data are currently lacking regarding the effect of guideline-recommended weight-based dosing on nephrotoxicity in methicillin-resistant *Staphylococcus aureus* bacteremia (MRSAB).

Methods: Adults who were at least 18 years of age with methicillin-resistant *Staphylococcus aureus* bacteremia and received of empiric vancomycin therapy for at least 48 hours (01/07/2002 and 30/06/2008) were included in this multicenter, retrospective cohort study. The association between guideline-recommended, weight-based vancomycin dosing (at least 15 mg/kg/dose) and nephrotoxicity (increase in serum creatinine (SCr) by more than 0.5 mg/dl or at least a 50% increase from baseline on at least two consecutive laboratory tests) was evaluated. Potential independent associations were evaluated using a multivariable general linear mixed-effect model.

Results: Overall, 23% of patients developed nephrotoxicity. Thirty-four percent of the 337 patients who met study criteria received weight-based dosing. The cohort was composed of 69% males with a median age of 55 years. The most common sources of MRSAB included skin/soft tissue (32%), catheter-related bloodstream bacteremia (20%), pulmonary (18%). Eighty-six percent of patients received twice daily dosing. Similar rates of nephrotoxicity were observed regardless of the receipt of guideline-recommended dosing (22% vs. 24%, OR 0.91 [95% CI 0.53-1.56]). This finding was confirmed in the multivariable analysis (OR 1.52 [95% CI 0.75-3.08]). Independent predictors of nephrotoxicity were (OR, 95% CI) vancomycin duration of greater than 15 days (3.36, 1.79-6.34), weight over 100 kg (2.74, 1.27-5.91), Pitt bacteremia score of 4 or greater (2.73, 1.29-5.79), vancomycin trough higher than 20 mcg/ml (2.36, 1.07-5.20), and age over 52 years (2.10, 1.08-4.08).

Conclusions: Over one out of five patients in this study developed nephrotoxicity while receiving vancomycin for MRSAB. The receipt of guideline-recommended, weight-based vancomycin was not an independent risk factor for the development of nephrotoxicity.

Keywords: Adverse events, Nephrotoxicity, Vancomycin, Dosing, Weight, Obesity, MRSA

* Correspondence: ronald.hall@ttuhsc.edu
[1]Department of Pharmacy Practice, Texas Tech University Health Sciences
Center, School of Pharmacy, Dallas, USA
[2]Department of Clinical Sciences, University of Texas Southwestern, Dallas,
USA
Full list of author information is available at the end of the article

Background

Decreased vancomycin efficacy has been reported by several investigators for methicillin-resistant *Staphylococcus aureus* (MRSA) isolates with a vancomycin MIC of 1 µg/ml or higher [1-3]. This has been accompanied by a trend of increased vancomycin minimum inhibitory concentrations (MIC) in MRSA isolates [4]. Experts in the field have responded in two ways. First, the Clinical and Laboratory Standards Institute lowered the susceptibility breakpoint for vancomycin versus *S. aureus* [5]. Second, several influential organizations endorsed a consensus review recommending higher vancomycin trough concentrations [6]. Weight-based dosing was recommended to achieve these new target vancomycin trough concentrations. The impact of these two changes on the safety profile of vancomycin is unknown. Recent studies suggest increased vancomycin trough concentrations are a risk factor for increased rates of nephrotoxicity [1,7-10]. However, no studies have yet evaluated the effect of guideline-recommended, weight-based vancomycin dosing on nephrotoxicity. We performed a multi-center retrospective cohort study to assess the risk of nephrotoxicity associated with guideline-recommended, weight-based vancomycin dosing.

Methods

Design

We conducted a multi-center, retrospective cohort study at three hospitals between July 2002 and June 2008. This retrospective cohort evaluated the association between the receipt of weight-based vancomycin dosing as recommended in the 2009 guideline and the development of nephrotoxicity in patients with MRSA bacteremia [6]. The development of nephrotoxicity during vancomycin therapy was the primary outcome of interest. All data were collected from the patient's medical record at each study institution. The results of our evaluation of guideline-recommended, weight-based dosing and mortality can be found elsewhere [11].

Setting

The three study hospitals were a 400 bed tertiary hospital, a 350 bed Veteran Affairs hospital, and a 600 bed university hospital. The requirement for informed consent was waived by each of the institutional review boards (IRBs) that approved the study (North Texas Veterans Health Care System, Texas Tech University Health Sciences Center, and University of Texas Health Science Center, San Antonio) due to the retrospective nature of the study and being deemed as minimal risk.

Patients

All adults (18 years or older) admitted with MRSA bacteremia (identified by microbiological records) who received parenteral vancomycin for at least 48 hours were evaluated for study inclusion. Patients were excluded if at the time of the first vancomycin dose they were pregnant, had moderate-to-severe renal dysfunction (defined as a creatinine clearance (CrCl) $\leq$ 30 ml/min or receipt of dialysis), received vancomycin within the same hospital stay, or had a culture-proven MRSA infection within six months [12]. Patients with a CrCl $\leq$ 30 ml/min were excluded because these patients were considered more likely to require a dosing frequency adjustment to less than once daily dosing and the measure of vancomycin dosing intensity used was mg/kg/day. Prior MRSA infections were excluded due to the likely prior receipt of vancomycin.

Definitions

The study team agreed upon the following definitions while designing this study. Nephrotoxicity was defined as an increase in serum creatinine (SCr) by greater than a 0.5 mg/dl or 50% increase from baseline on at least two consecutive laboratory tests during the period from initiation of vancomycin to completion of therapy [6]. We compared the nephrotoxicity rates among patients treated with guideline-recommended vancomycin doses (at least 30 mg/kg/day; at least 15 mg/kg/day for CrCl 30-50 ml/min) to those treated with lower vancomycin doses (less than 30 mg/kg/day; less than 15 mg/kg/day for CrCl 30-50 ml/min). Vancomycin trough concentrations were determined by the assay used for routine patient care at each institution. All concentrations labeled as "trough" were utilized. Only the first/initial vancomycin trough concentration was utilized in the analysis. All study hospitals did not have a mandatory therapeutic drug monitoring service and therefore vancomycin trough concentrations were only obtained as clinically indicated by the prescribing physician. Pitt bacteremia score and Charlson comorbidity index were used to quantify severity of illness and comorbid conditions. Both of these indices have been described in detail elsewhere [13-15].

Statistical analysis

All analyses were performed using SAS 9.2 (Cary, North Carolina) and RTREE (Available at: http://c2s2.yale.edu/software/rtree/). It was determined that seven to eight variables would likely be evaluated in the multivariable model. In order to prevent overfitting, a total of 70-80 events would be required. Assuming a nephrotoxicity rate of 25% based on prior literature, 280-320 patients would be required for the multivariable analysis [1,7]. Candidate variables selected for consideration in the multivariable model were identified *a priori*. Univariable associations were explored using either Chi-square or Fisher's Exact tests. Dichotomization of continuous variables was achieved by recursive partitioning to determine significant cut-points [16]. A Pitt bacteremia score ≥ 4 was used based on previous literature [17]. A vancomycin trough greater than 20 mcg/ml was based on previous observations of increased rates of nephrotoxicity compared with troughs of 15-20 mcg/ml [10]. The univariable analysis included the following candidate variables: receipt of guideline-recommended, weight-based vancomycin dosing, vancomycin trough greater than 20 mcg/ml, duration of vancomycin treatment greater than 15 days, gender, age greater than 52 years, weight greater than 100 kg, Pitt bacteremia score of 4 or higher, intensive care unit (ICU) residence, use of concomitant nephrotoxins (e.g. contrast dye, aminoglycosides, vasopressors), baseline serum creatinine, and Charlson comorbidity index score of 5 or higher.

Consideration for inclusion in the multivariable model was based on our conceptual model as well as significant associations observed in the univariable analysis (p<0.1). Independent predictors of nephrotoxicity were determined using a multivariable generalized linear mixed-effect model. Hospital site was treated as a random effect whereas other covariates were treated as fixed effects. A p value of <0.05 was considered statistically significant for the multivariable model. The analysis also included an extensive evaluation of effect measure modification and biologic interaction.

Results

Of the 798 patients with MRSA bacteremia, 337 were included in the cohort (Hospital A = 156, Hospital B = 100, Hospital C = 81). Reasons for patient exclusion were not collected by the automated screening process.

The baseline characteristics of the cohort are shown in Table 1. The cohort was predominantly male (79.2%) and was comprised of Caucasians (65%), African-Americans (14%), and Hispanics (17%). Data regarding race/ethnicity were missing for 5 patients and documented as other in seven patients. Vancomycin was dosed according to 2009 guidelines in 33.6% percent of patients. Patients weighing ≥ 100 kg received similar doses per day to those weighing < 100 kg (1941 mg vs. 1919 mg, p = 0.72). Patients receiving guideline-recommended, weight-based vancomycin dosing had a median daily dose of 32.0 mg/kg/day (interquartile range 29.0, 36.0), while those receiving lower doses received 21.3 mg/kg/day (interquartile range 17.0, 26.0) (p < 0.001). As expected, vancomycin trough concentrations were higher in patients receiving guideline-recommended, weight-based dosing (12.3 mcg/ml, IQR 8.3, 17.5) compared to patients who received lower doses (10.1 mcg/ml, IQR 7.1, 14.9), p = 0.03. The most common dosing frequencies administered were once (11.3%) or twice daily (86.3%). Other dosing frequencies included thrice daily (2.1%) or every other day (0.3%). The most common sources of infection for patients receiving weight-based vancomycin dosing according to the 2009 guideline were bloodstream catheter-related (16.6%), central nervous system (0.4%), gastrointestinal (0.9%), genitourinary (6.7%), osteomyelitis (1.3%), pulmonary (19.3%), skin/soft tissue (37.7%), and other (0.5%). The source of infection was undocumented for 16.6% of patients. For patients receiving lower doses, the sources of infection were bloodstream catheter-related (27.4%), genitourinary (10.6%), osteomyelitis (0.9%), pulmonary (15%), skin/soft tissue (20.4%). The source of infection was undocumented in 25.7% of patients receiving lower dosing.

Table 1 Baseline characteristics of the cohort[A]

Characteristic	Guideline-recommended dosing (n = 113)[*]	Lower dosing (n = 223)[+]	p-value
Male gender (%)	76%	81%	0.97
Age (years)	57 (46, 71)	54 (44, 63)	0.03
Height (cm)	172 (163, 178)	175 (168, 183)	<0.001
Weight (kg)	63 (57, 68)	88 (75, 104)	<0.001
Serum creatinine (mg/dl)	0.9 (0.7, 1.3)	0.9 (0.7, 1.2)	0.70
Creatinine clearance (ml/min)	71 (47, 104)	86 (66, 124)	<0.001
Charlson comorbidity index > 5	20%	13%	0.06
Length of hospital stay (days)	17 (9, 37)	18 (9, 32)	0.60
Intensive care unit resident	41%	41%	0.99
Pitt bacteremia ≥ 4	21%	22%	0.80
Concomitant nephrotoxin	50%	49%	0.85
Nephrotoxicity	22%	24%	0.74
Initial Vancomycin Dose (mg/kg/day)	32 (29, 36)	21 (17, 26)	<0.001

A = Results are presented as median (interquartile range) unless otherwise noted.
* = Vancomycin ≥ 30 mg/kg/day, ≥ 15 mg/kg/day for creatinine clearance of 30-50 ml/min.
+ = Vancomycin < 30 mg/kg/day, < 15 mg/kg/day for creatinine clearance of 30-50 ml/min.

Nephrotoxicity occurred in 78 patients (23%), occurring in 56%, 11%, and 33% of patients at Hospitals A, B, and C, respectively. The median (interquartile range) increase from baseline to peak serum creatinine was 0.0 mg/dL (0.0, 0.2) for patients who did not develop nephrotoxicity versus 1.0 mg/dL (0.6, 2.1) for patients who developed nephrotoxicity. Fifteen percent of patients had a vancomycin trough concentration greater than 20 mcg/ml. Concurrent nephrotoxins included contrast dye (34%), aminoglycosides (19%), and vasopressors (12%). Concomitant antimicrobials active against MRSA were used in 23% of patients.

In the univariable analysis (Table 2), nephrotoxicity was similar between patients that received guideline-recommended, weight-based vancomycin dosing versus lower dosing (22% vs. 24%). Factors associated with increased risk for nephrotoxicity included duration of vancomycin treatment greater than 15 days, weight greater than 100 kg, Pitt bacteremia score of 4 or higher, vancomycin trough greater than 20 mcg/ml, age greater than 52 years, ICU residence, and concomitant nephrotoxin. In the multivariable analysis there was not a statistically significant association between vancomycin dosing and nephrotoxicity (Table 3). Independent predictors of nephrotoxicity in the multivariable model were duration of vancomycin treatment greater than 15 days, weight greater than 100 kg, Pitt bacteremia score of 4 or higher, vancomycin trough greater than 20 mcg/ml, and age greater than 52 years.

Discussion

We did not observe a statistically significant relationship between the receipt of guideline-recommended, weight-based dosing of vancomycin and the development of nephrotoxicity in patients in our cohort. This finding is

Table 2 Univariable analysis of risk factors for nephrotoxicity

Variable	Odds ratio	95% confidence interval
Guideline-recommended vancomycin dosing	0.91	0.53-1.56
Vancomycin duration > 15 days	3.65	2.16-6.17
Weight greater than 100 kilograms	2.08	1.18-3.67
Pitt Bacteremia Score of four or greater	3.80	2.17-6.63
Vancomycin trough greater than 20 mcg/ml	2.51	1.28-4.92
Age greater than 52 years	2.40	1.38-4.15
Intensive care unit resident	3.64	2.15-6.18
Concomitant nephrotoxin	2.08	1.24-3.49
Male gender	1.04	0.56-1.57
Charlson comorbidity index 5 or greater	1.14	0.57-2.27
Baseline serum creatinine greater than 1.0 mg/dL	0.94	0.56-1.57

Table 3 Multivariable analysis of independent risk factors for nephrotoxicity

Variable	Odds ratio	95% confidence interval
Guideline-Recommended Vancomycin Dosing	1.52	0.75-3.08
Vancomycin duration greater than 15 days	3.36	1.79-6.34
Weight greater than 100 kilograms	2.74	1.27-5.91
Pitt Bacteremia Score of four or greater	2.73	1.29-5.79
Vancomycin trough greater than 20 mcg/ml	2.36	1.07-5.20
Age greater than 52 years	2.10	1.08-4.08
Intensive care unit residence	1.90	0.95-3.80
Concomitant nephrotoxin	1.64	0.87-3.11

clinically important because weight-based vancomycin dosing is now recommended by the vancomycin guidelines [6].

The impact of vancomycin on the development of nephrotoxicity has been debated for decades. Multiple prospective clinical trials suggest that traditional vancomycin doses (1 gram IV every 12 hours) cause nephrotoxicity 5% of the time, or less, when concomitant nephrotoxins are not used [18-21]. A 7-35% rate of nephrotoxicity was reported with the concomitant use of nephrotoxins [22,23].

The controversy surrounding vancomycin-associated nephrotoxicity has resurfaced in parallel with the increased utilization of higher vancomycin doses to achieve higher target trough concentrations in response to rising vancomycin MIC values. The nephrotoxicity rate in our study (23%) is consistent with recent data utilizing a standard definition of nephrotoxicity (11-42%) [1,7-10].

Our study also agreed with other studies that have identified an association between vancomycin trough concentrations and nephrotoxicity [1,7-10]. These studies, and our own, are unable to determine whether this association is causative in nature. Our observation of an association between duration of vancomycin treatment and nephrotoxicity is also consistent with previous work [1,7,9]. Whether vancomycin duration is a causative factor in nephrotoxicity is also unclear.

The factors significantly associated with the development of nephrotoxicity in our study are clinically reasonable. We found that a Pitt bacteremia score of 4 or greater was predictive of nephrotoxicity in our study. This is consistent with other studies that have observed a significant association between nephrotoxicity and ICU residence upon antibiotic initiation or increased APACHE II scores [7,8,24]. We observed that greater patient weight was significantly associated with the development of nephrotoxicity, which is also consistent with previous investigations [8,24].

The application of our study is limited by its retrospective nature and the potential lack of external validity in patients being treated with vancomycin for conditions other than MRSA bacteremia. The lack of information regarding reasons for exclusion may also limit how other institutions are able to use these findings for their patient population. Retrospective studies may have differences between the comparison groups in regards to measured and unmeasured confounders. To address potential confounding, a stratified analysis was conducted on variables considered to potentially affect the primary outcome. Biologically plausible factors that demonstrated confounding were included in the multivariable model. A multivariable mixed-effects model using hospital site as the random effect was utilized to minimize the impact of the differences in measured confounders as well as the risk of clustering. One major difference between the institutions is the much longer length of stay at Hosptial A due to two long-term care wings in the facility compared to none for the Hospitals B and C. Therefore, the higher nephrotoxicity rate at Hospital A may be in part due to an observation bias due to patients on vancomycin remaining in the hospital longer than patients at the other institutions.

The fact that we did not observe an association between concomitant nephrotoxins and nephrotoxicity may have been due to the lack of recording the dose and duration of concomitatnt nephrotoxin use. Our results may have also been subject to a selection bias since patients weighing greater than 70 kilograms were less likely to receive weight-based vancomycin dosing as recommended by the 2009 guideline. This selection bias could have reduced our ability to detect guideline-recommended, weight-based dosing as an independent risk factor for nephrotoxicity. The utilization of all vancomycin concentrations labeled as "troughs" could have biased our results. The potential for each institution to use different vancomycin assays could have also biased our results. However, our study found that vancomycin troughs greater than 20 mcg/ml is associated with nephrotoxicity mirroring those of previous studies. This lack of effect is common for most non-differential misclassification biases. If any effect were to occur to this bias, it would have been to lessen the ability to determine that vancomycin trough concentrations are a risk factor for nephrotoxicity. The exclusion of patients with missing vancomycin trough concentrations from the multivariable model may have also biased the results. This exclusion may have created a selection bias that decreased the ability to detect severity of illness or length of vancomycin therapy as patients without therapeutic drug monitoring tend to be less severely ill patients who do not require long durations of therapy. The fact that both of these characteristics remained independent predictors of nephrotoxicity in spite of this selection bias reinforces the strength of these associations. Last, our study evaluated dosing practices prior to the publication of the 2009 guidelines. However, this standard measure created two distinct groups supported by the 2009 guideline regardless of how often weight-based vancomycin was utilized during the study period.

Furthermore, the implications of loading doses and therapeutic drug monitoring programs on nephrotoxicity need further evaluation since none of our institutions utilized loading doses or formal therapeutic drug monitoring services (e.g. automatic pharmacy consultation for vancomycin management). Each study institution employs clinical pharmacists who monitor vancomycin trough concentrations and provide recommendations for the physician to clinically evaluate.

Conclusions

In this multi-center study, more than one in five patients developed nephrotoxicity. We did not observe a significant relationship between weight-based guideline-recommended dosing and nephrotoxicity. If this finding is confirmed by others, clinicians should be able to utilize weight-based, guideline-recommended dosing. Careful management of patients with MRSAB is needed to avoid vancomycin trough concentrations associated with nephrotoxicity.

Competing interests
Grant funding from AstraZeneca, Ortho-McNeil Janssen, and Pfizer: CRF. Scientific Advisory Board for Tibotec Therapeutics and Gilead Sciences: RJB. None: RGH, CAA, CAG, KKH, KAH, NAF, SDB, TB.

Author contributions
RGH, CAG, KKH, KAH, SDB, RJB were involved in the study concept and design. RGH, CAG, CAA, CRF were involved in the data analysis and interpretation. RGH, CAG, KKH, KAH, CAA, CRF, NAF, SDB, TB, RJB were involved in the drafting of the manuscript for important intellectual content and had final approval of the manuscript.

Acknowledgements
Drs. CA and RH were supported by Grant Number KL2RR024983, titled, "North and Central Texas Clinical and Translational Science Initiative" (Milton Packer, M.D., PI) from the National Center for Research Resources (NCRR), a component of the National Institutes of Health (NIH), and NIH Roadmap for Medical Research, and its contents are solely the responsibility of the authors and do not necessarily represent the official views of the NCRR or NIH. Information on NCRR is available at http://www.nih.gov/about/almanac/archive/2003/organization/NCRR.htm. Information on Re-engineering the Clinical Research Enterprise can be obtained from http://or.org/pdf/NIH_Roadmap-ClinicalResearch.pdf. Dr. CF was supported by National Institutes of Health grant KL2RR025766.
Presented in part at the 2010 Society of Critical Care Medicine's 39th Critical Care Congress (Abstract #956) and at the Infectious Diseases Society of America 2010 Annual Meeting (Abstract #288).

Author details
[1]Department of Pharmacy Practice, Texas Tech University Health Sciences Center, School of Pharmacy, Dallas, USA. [2]Department of Clinical Sciences, University of Texas Southwestern, Dallas, USA. [3]Department of Pharmacy Practice, Texas Tech University Health Sciences Center, School of Pharmacy, Amarillo, USA. [4]Division of Pharmacotherapy, University of Texas, Austin, USA. [5]Department of Internal Medicine, Texas Tech University Health Sciences Center, School of Medicine, Amarillo, USA. [6]Department of Internal Medicine, University of Texas Southwestern, Dallas, USA. [7]Current affiliation: University of Wyoming School of Pharmacy, Swedish Family Medicine Residency Program, Englewood, USA. [8]Current affiliation: University of Kentucky

Healthcare, Lexington, USA. [9]Current affiliation: Wayne State University Eugene Applebaum College of Pharmacy and Health Sciences, Detroit, USA. [10]Current affiliation: Mission Regional Medical Center, Mission, USA.

References

1. Hidayat LK, Hsu DI, Quist R, Shriner KA, Wong-Beringer A: High-dose vancomycin therapy for methicillin-resistant *Staphylococcus aureus* infections: efficacy and toxicity. *Arch Intern Med* 2006, 166:2138–2144.

2. Lodise TP, Graves J, Evans A, et al: Relationship between vancomycin MIC and failure among patients with methicillin-resistant *Staphylococcus aureus* bacteremia treated with vancomycin. *Antimicrob Agents Chemother* 2008, 52:3315–3320.

3. Sakoulas G, Moise-Broder PA, Schentag J, Forrest A, Moellering RC Jr, Eliopoulos GM: Relationship of MIC and bactericidal activity to efficacy of vancomycin for treatment of methicillin-resistant *Staphylococcus aureus* bacteremia. *J Clin Microbiol* 2004, 42:2398–2402.

4. Wang G, Hindler JF, Ward KW, Bruckner DA: Increased vancomycin MICs for *Staphylococcus aureus* clinical isolates from a university hospital during a 5-year period. *J Clin Microbiol* 2006, 44:3883–3886.

5. Tenover FC, Moellering RC Jr: The rationale for revising the clinical and laboratory standards institute vancomycin minimal inhibitory concentration interpretive criteria for *staphylococcus aureus*. *Clin Infect Dis* 2007, 44:1208–1215.

6. Rybak M, Lomaestro B, Rotschafer JC, et al: Therapeutic monitoring of vancomycin in adult patients: a consensus review of the American Society of Health-System Pharmacists, the Infectious Diseases Society of America, and the Society of Infectious Diseases Pharmacists. *Am J Health Syst Pharm* 2009, 66:82–98.

7. Jeffres MN, Isakow W, Doherty JA, Micek ST, Kollef MH: A retrospective analysis of possible renal toxicity associated with vancomycin in patients with health care-associated methicillin-resistant *Staphylococcus aureus* pneumonia. *Clin Ther* 2007, 29:1107–1115.

8. Lodise TP, Patel N, Lomaestro BM, Rodvold KA, Drusano GL: Relationship between initial vancomycin concentration-time profile and nephrotoxicity among hospitalized patients. *Clin Infect Dis* 2009, 49:507–514.

9. Pritchard L, Baker C, Leggett J, Sehdev P, Brown A, Bayley KB: Increasing vancomycin serum trough concentrations and incidence of nephrotoxicity. *Am J Med* 2010, 123:1143–1149.

10. Kullar R, Davis SL, Levine DP, Rybak MJ: Impact of vancomycin exposure on outcomes in patients with methicillin-resistant staphylococcus aureus bacteremia: support for consensus guidelines suggested targets. *Clin Infect Dis* 2011, 52:975–981.

11. Hall RG, Giuliano CA, Haase KK, et al: Empiric guideline-recommended weight based dosing and mortality in methcillin-resistant *Staphylococcus aureus* bacteremia: a retrospective cohort study. *BMC Infect Dis* 2012, 12:104.

12. Cockcroft DW, Gault MH: Prediction of creatinine clearance from serum creatinine. *Nephron* 1976, 16:31–41.

13. Charlson ME, Pompei P, Ales KL, MacKenzie CR: A new method of classifying prognostic comorbidity in longitudinal studies: development and validation. *J Chronic Dis* 1987, 40:373–383.

14. Chow JW, Fine MJ, Shlaes DM, et al: Enterobacter bacteremia: clinical features and emergence of antibiotic resistance during therapy. *Ann Intern Med* 1991, 115:585–590.

15. Chow JW, Yu VL: Combination antibiotic therapy versus monotherapy for gram-negative bacteraemia: a commentary. *Int J Antimicrob Agents* 1999, 11:7–12.

16. Zhang H, Singer B: *Recursive partitioning in the health sciences*. New York: Springer; 1999.

17. Rhee JY, Kwon KT, Ki HK, et al: Scoring systems for prediction of mortality in patients with intensive care unit-acquired sepsis: a comparison of the Pitt bacteremia score and the Acute Physiology and Chronic Health Evaluation II scoring systems. *Shock* 2009, 31:146–150.

18. Arbeit RD, Maki D, Tally FP, Campanaro E, Eisenstein BI: The safety and efficacy of daptomycin for the treatment of complicated skin and skin-structure infections. *Clin Infect Dis* 2004, 38:1673–1681.

19. Ellis-Grosse EJ, Babinchak T, Dartois N, Rose G, Loh E: The efficacy and safety of tigecycline in the treatment of skin and skin-structure infections: results of 2 double-blind phase 3 comparison studies with vancomycin-aztreonam. *Clin Infect Dis* 2005, 41:S341–S353.

20. Weigelt J, Itani K, Stevens D, Lau W, Dryden M, Knirsch C: Linezolid versus vancomycin in treatment of complicated skin and soft tissue infections. *Antimicrob Agents Chemother* 2005, 49:2260–2266.

21. Wilcox MH, Tack KJ, Bouza E, et al: Complicated skin and skin-structure infections and catheter-related bloodstream infections: noninferiority of linezolid in a phase 3 study. *Clin Infect Dis* 2009, 48:203–212.

22. Downs NJ, Neihart RE, Dolezal JM, Hodges GR: Mild nephrotoxicity associated with vancomycin use. *Arch Intern Med* 1989, 149:1777–1781.

23. Sorrell TC, Collignon PJ: A prospective study of adverse reactions associated with vancomycin therapy. *J Antimicrob Chemother* 1985, 16:235–241.

24. Lodise TP, Lomaestro B, Graves J, Drusano GL: Larger vancomycin doses (at least four grams per day) are associated with an increased incidence of nephrotoxicity. *Antimicrob Agents Chemother* 2008, 52:1330–1336.

5

Hypersensitivity to oxaliplatin: clinical features and risk factors

Marie Parel[1†], Florence Ranchon[2†], Audrey Nosbaum[3], Benoit You[4], Nicolas Vantard[1], Vérane Schwiertz[1], Chloé Gourc[1], Noémie Gauthier[1], Marie-Gabrielle Guedat[1], Sophie He[1], Eléna Kiouris[1], Céline Alloux[1], Thierry Vial[5], Véronique Trillet-Lenoir[4], Gilles Freyer[4], Frédéric Berard[3†] and Catherine Rioufol[2*†]

Abstract

Background: Oxaliplatin-based regimens induce a potential risk of hypersensitivity reaction (HSR), with incidence varying from 10% to 25% and lack of clearly identified risk factors. The present study aimed to assess incidence and risk factors in HSR.

Methods: All patients treated with oxaliplatin in the Medical Oncology Department of the Lyon Sud University Hospital (Hospices Civils de Lyon, France) from October 2004 to January 2011 were enrolled. Incidence and severity of HSR were analyzed retrospectively and the potential clinicopathological covariates were tested on univariate and multivariate analysis.

Results: A total of 1,221 doses of oxaliplatin were administered for 191 patients, 8.9% of whom experienced an HSR. Seventeen HSRs were observed, with 1.6% grade 3 and no grade 4 events. The first reaction appeared after a median of 3 oxaliplatin infusions. Using univariate analysis, HSR was associated with younger age (mean age, 56.2 years; p = 0.04), female gender (p = 0.01) and prior exposure to platinum salts (p = 0.02). No increased risk was associated with mean dose or with presence of atopic background. Multivariate analysis confirmed that women were at higher risk of oxaliplatin HSR than men (p < 0.05). Reintroduction of oxaliplatin was effective in 64.7% of hypersensitive patients using an appropriate premedication strategy. Patients who experienced a grade 3 HSR were not rechallenged.

Conclusion: The risk of developing oxaliplatin HSR should not be underestimated (8.9% of patients). The medical team's vigilance should be increased with women, younger patients and patients with prior exposure to platinum salts.

Keywords: Oxaliplatin, Hypersensitivity, Risk factors, Platinum salts, Desensitization

Background

Chemotherapy agents can induce hypersensitivity reaction (HSR), reducing the use of critical drugs in fragile patients for fear of inducing severe reaction and possibly death. However, with improved outcomes in cancer care, longer patient survival and extended treatment courses, patients are exposed to drugs more frequently and for longer periods, increasing the risk of sensitization and of HSR. Prevention and management of acute infusion

reactions in oncology remain essential [1], particularly with platinum agents (carboplatin, cisplatin and oxaliplatin) [2]. HSR should be an important concern, due to its potential life-threatening risk and the subsequent treatment withdrawal [3].

Oxaliplatin, a third-generation platinum agent, has been approved for the treatment of metastatic colorectal cancer and for adjuvant treatment in stage-III colon cancer [4]. It is also used worldwide in other malignancies, such as ovarian cancer [5]. As colorectal cancer is the third most common cancer in the world and the second leading cause of cancer death in western countries, its treatment is currently a public health priority and oxaliplatin represents a key chemotherapeutic agent [6].

* Correspondence: catherine.rioufol@chu-lyon.fr
†Equal contributors
2Hospices Civils de Lyon, Clinical Oncology Pharmacy Department, Pierre-Bénite - Université Lyon 1, EMR 3738, Lyon, France
Full list of author information is available at the end of the article

HSR to oxaliplatin has been less frequently described than to cisplatin and carboplatin. However the increasing use of oxaliplatin in clinical practice shows significant incidence, varying from 10% to 23.8% [3,7-13]. Identifying patients with high risk of oxaliplatin-HSR is a major clinical issue and several studies assessed risk factors, although with heterogeneous results [3,7,9,10,14]. Moreover, Asian populations were mostly investigated [3,7,8,10,12-15], but only some studies evaluated the risk factors using multivariate analysis [3,7,9,12].

The aim of this retrospective cohort study was to investigate the clinical features and the risk factors of oxaliplatin-HSR.

Methods

Source of data

All patients who received at least one dose of oxaliplatin in the Medical Oncology Department of the Lyon Sud University Hospital (Hospices Civils de Lyon, France) over a 6-year period from October 2004 to January 2011 were identified using the pharmaceutical software dedicated to antineoplastic preparation. Routine premedication before oxaliplatin infusion included 120 mg of methylprednisolone given intravenously and antiemetic prophylaxis.

The following clinical data were collected from medical files: sex, age, history of allergy, oxaliplatin HSR, type of cancer, previous exposure to platinum agents, and oxaliplatin exposure during the study period (total number of courses, doses and cumulative dose), and treatment line number.

Data from patients who experienced oxaliplatin-associated HSR were compared to that of controls patients who received oxaliplatin without experiencing HSR.

For the purposes of the present study, HSR was defined as any unexpected adverse manifestation including non-allergic drug hypersensitivity and drug allergy reactions like the typical symptoms of IgE-mediated reactions, including cutaneous symptoms such as palmar or facial flushing, respiratory symptoms such as shortness of breath, and cardiovascular symptoms such as any alteration in pulse or blood pressure [16]. Expected side-effects, such as chemotherapy-induced nausea or vomiting and diarrhea, were excluded. Severity was graded according to the Ring and Messmer's classification [17] and the National Cancer Institute Common Terminology Criteria for Adverse Events (NCI-CTCAE v 4) because of its frequent use by medical oncologists worldwide (Table 1). The outcome data was also recorded for each patient.

Statistical analysis

Clinicopathological variables potentially associated with oxaliplatin HSR were subjected to univariate analysis. Statistical analysis was carried out using Wilcoxon's test to determine whether age or mean dose were associated with hypersensitivity. The other factors (sex, prior platinum exposure and atopic background) were evaluated using Fisher's exact test.

For multivariate analysis, a logistic regression model was applied. All variables with a p-value ≤ 0.1 on univariate analysis were considered candidates for multiple logistic regression. Two-sided p values exceeding 0.05 were considered statistically significant. Statistical analysis used SAS software, version 8.

Since data were collected retrospectively and that patients' management was not modified, according to the French law (n°2004-806, 9th august 2004), this study did not need to be approved by a research ethics committee [18]. It was conducted in accordance with the law on data protection (n°2004-801, 6th august 2004).

Results

A total of 191 patients treated with oxaliplatin were included. Patient characteristics are listed in Table 2.

Table 1 Clinical severity scale of immediate reactions

	According to ring and messmer [17]	According to NCI-CTCAE
Grade	Clinical signs	
1	Cutaneous-mucous signs	Mild transient reaction with no infusion interruption
2	Cutaneous-mucous signs	Therapy or infusion interruption indicated but responds promptly to symptomatic treatment (antihistamines, corticosteroids, narcotics, IV fluids)
	Cardiovascular signs (tachycardia, hypotension)	
	Respiratory signs	
3	Cardiovascular collapse	Prolonged reaction not rapidly responsive to symptomatic medication and/or brief interruption of infusion.
	Bronchospam	Recurrence of symptoms following initial improvement
		Hospitalization indicated for clinical sequelae
4	Cardiac arrest	Life-threatening consequences with urgent intervention indicated
5	-	Death

NCI-CTCAE: National Cancer Institute Common Terminology Criteria for Adverse Events.

Table 2 Patient characteristics

Patient characteristics (n = 191)	Mean (range)	n (%)
Age (years)	62.4 (23–84)	
Sex, male		78 (41)
Atopic diseases		32 (17)
Diagnosis		
Colon		86 (45)
Stomach		10 (5)
Ovary		35 (18)
Pancreas		9 (5)
Peritoneum		8 (4)
Rectum		25 (13)
Other[1]		18 (10)
Prior platinum exposure, yes		45 (24)
Treament regimen		
FOLFOX4 (oxaliplatin, 5-fluorouracil and leucovorin)		101 (53)
FOLFOX4-bevacizumab		10 (5)
FOLFOX4-cetuximab		4 (2)
GEMOX (oxaliplatin and gemcitabine)		47 (25)
Oxaliplatin alone		5 (3)
TOMOX(oxaliplatin and raltitrexed)		12 (6)
Other[2]		12 (6)
Total infusion courses	6.4 (1–18)	
Oxaliplatin dose (mg/m[2])	85.3 (42–160)	

[1]Includes: appendix (2), gallbladder (4), liver (2), mouth (1), oesophagus (2), endometrium (1) and unknown primary (6).
[2]Includes: 2 ELOGEM (combination of oxaliplatin and gemcitabine), 2 EOX (combination of oxaliplatin, epirubicin and capecitabine), 2 FOLFIRINOX (combination of oxaliplatin, irinotecan, 5-fluorouracil and leucovorin), 1 FOLFOX6 (combination of oxaliplatin, 5-fluorouracil and leucovorin), 2 FOLFOX7 (combination of oxaliplatin, 5-fluorouracil and leucovorin), 1 patient treated with oxaliplatin and epirubicine, 1 oxaliplatin with cetuximab and 1 XELOX (combination of oxaliplatin and capecitabine).

Table 3 Hypersensitivity reactions to oxaliplatin

	Hypersensitivity reactions to oxaliplatin
Hypersensitivity reactions	17 (8.9%)
Severity according to Ring and Messmer [17]	
Grade 1 events	12 (6.3%)
Grade 2 events	2 (1.0%)
Grade 3 events	3 (1.6%)
Grade 4 events	0
Severity according to to NCI-CTCAE	
Grade 1 events	5 (2.9%)
Grade 2 events	9 (4.7%)
Grade 3 events	3 (1.6%)
Grade 4 events	0
Grade 5 events	0
Cycle number at event	
Median (range)	3 (1–13)

NCI-CTCAE: National Cancer Institute Common Terminology Criteria for Adverse Events.

without bronchospasm. Severity of HSRs according to the Ring and Messmer's classification and the National Cancer Institute Common Terminology Criteria for Adverse Events (NCI-CTCAE v 4) was similar (Table 3). Most reactions were moderate but three patients presented grade 3 HSRs with hypotension, hypothermia and symptomatic larynx spasm (1 patient), acute hypertension, symptomatic larynx spasm and dyspnea (1 patient), and hypotension, bradycardia, hypothermia and fainting (1 patient). There was no grade 4 event (heart failure or respiratory arrest which required urgent intervention) and no death. Nine patients responded promptly to symptomatic treatments (antihistamines, corticosteroids, narcotics or IV fluids) and 3 patients had a more prolonged reaction not rapidly responsive to symptomatic medications and/or brief interruption of infusion.

After their first HSR episode, 13 patients (76%) were rechallenged with a mean 4.8 further cycles of oxaliplatin, associated in most cases with strengthened premedication including antihistamines and higher-dose corticosteroids. Patients who experienced a grade 3 HSR were not rechallenged. Four (30.8%) experienced another HSR at the following course: 1 second reaction in 3 patients and 2 in another patient, which 1 required definitive withdrawn of oxaliplatin. A total 22 HSRs occurred in 17 patients and required definitive withdrawn of oxaliplatin in 2 patients. Clinical signs and severity were generally similar in first and repeat episodes. Three clinicopathological parameters emerged as potential risk factors for oxaliplatin HSR using univariate analysis (Tables 4 and 5). Patients from the HSR group were younger (mean age, 56.2 years) than controls (mean age, 62.6 years; $p < 0.05$). The rate of

About 59% had colorectal cancer, 70% of whom were treated with a FOLFOX4 regimen (combination of oxaliplatin, 5-fluorouracil and leucovorin). During the 6-year follow-up, 17 patients experienced an HSR to oxaliplatin, representing an incidence of 8.9% of all treated patients (Table 3). A total of 1,221 doses of oxaliplatin were administered, with 1.8% overall frequency of HSR. Patients received median of 4.7 infusions, with a mean 85.3 mg/m[2] oxaliplatin per infusion. First HSR appeared after median of 3 infusions, and before the 7th course in most patients (80%). Among the 7 patients who developed a first HSR at the 1st or 2nd course, 3 have already been exposed to platinum agents. Sixteen of the 17 patients with HSR were women (94%) and 2 of them were treated for ovarian cancer.

During the first reaction, the most common effects were flushing (10 patients), urticaria (4 patients) and fever (4 patients). Two patients experienced dyspnea

Table 4 Results of univariate analysis (n = 191)

	Patients (n)	HSR (n)	HSR (%)	p value[1]
Sex				
Female	113	16	14.2	0,0147
Male	78	1	1.3	
Prior exposure to platinum salts				
Yes	45	8	17.8	0,0220
No	146	9	6.2	
Atopic background				
Yes	32	4	12.5	0,4367
No	159	13	8.2	

[1]Fischer exact test.

oxaliplatin HSR was higher in women than men ($p < 0.05$), with 14.2% of all women treated with oxaliplatin having reactions compared to only 1.3% of all men. Thirdly, HSR was more frequent in patients previously treated with platinum salts ($p < 0.05$). Mean oxaliplatin dose and presence of atopic background were not significantly associated with HSR. Using multivariate analysis, sex was the only remaining significant covariate, thereby confirming that women are at higher risk of oxaliplatin than men ($p < 0.05$).

Discussion

Hypersensitivity reactions to antineoplastic agents are commonly overlooked. However, for some drugs, particularly L-asparaginase, taxanes and platinum salts, hypersensitivity may lead to the withdrawal of the chemotherapy, thereby reducing the number of therapeutic options. The incidence of oxaliplatin HSR is rising as a consequence of its increased clinical use. Given the limited number of active agents in colorectal malignancy, it is now necessary to understand this kind of reactions and ways of prevent them [19]. The present retrospective study of 191 French patients aimed at bringing new insights to the clinical features of oxaliplatin HSR and its risk factors.

Incidence of oxaliplatin HSR and number of previous cycles appeared to differ from other reports, with lower incidence (8.9%) and earlier onset (before the 6th course), compared to 10–23.8% incidence [3,7-11,13,20] and onset mostly after 6–10 courses [3,10,14,20-22]. As previously described, age and female gender were identified as risk factors [7,9,13]. Interestingly, we showed that 94% of hypersensitive patients were women, finding which was not reported yet. The reasons for this increased risk amongst females are not known. However, it is well

established that, for unknown reasons, anaphylaxis is more frequent in women. Kim *et al.* suggest that an association between female gender and younger age may be explained by a possible role of hormonal influences [9]. Another hypothesis could be the important proportion of women (89%) among patients with a previous exposure to platinum agents which is a risk factor of oxaliplatin HSR in univariate analysis in this study. We also investigated the influence of prior exposure to platinum salts. Previous infusions appeared as a risk factor for oxaliplatin HSR. The effect of the platinum-free interval on the incidence and severity of HSR to platinum-containing agents is still a matter of discussion [7]. The impact of concomitant drugs on the risk of HSR is still an issue. In the present study, among 5 patients received oxaliplatin concomitantly with cetuximab, known to induce reaction at the time of administration, 1 patient developed an HSR. Our patients were treated with 14 different regimens which prevent us to assess the involvement of associated treatment due to a lack of power. The efficiency of premedication on HSR is naturally expected. A recent study demonstrated a significant improvement of tolerance with increased doses of dexamethasone and antihistamine [23]. Our patients were systematically treated with 120 mg methylprednisolone before oxaliplatin infusion, leading to a lower incidence of HSR. Several studies assessed the effect of re-exposure to oxaliplatin with or without premedication. In most cases, steroids plus antihistamines and prolongation of oxaliplatin infusion were helpful. A secondary prevention regimen comprising 40 mg famotidine, 20 mg dexamethasone plus 50 mg diphenhydramine was investigated before re-exposure to oxaliplatin in 30 patients with prior HSR: oxaliplatin was well tolerated in 19 of 30 patients (63.3%) for at least 2 cycles [20].

Management of patients with oxaliplatin HSR remains the question of importance in terms of possible therapeutic options. In the present study, 13 of the 17 hypersensitive patients were re-exposed to oxaliplatin; only 4 developed further reactions. Nevertheless, patients who experienced a grade 3 HSR were not rechallenged. Consistently with previous reports, reintroduction of oxaliplatin is generally possible in grade 1/2 hypersensitive patients using an appropriate premedication strategy: i.e. anti-histamine and/or steroids, and reduced infusion flow [24-26]. But uniform approach to prevent oxaliplatin HSR has not been established and reintroduction remains associated with recurrence of HSR, which requires permanent withdrawal of oxaliplatin infusion with obvious harmful

Table 5 Results of univariate analysis (n = 191)

	Patients with HSR (n = 17)	Patients without HSR (n = 174)	p value[2]
Mean age (years)	56.2 ±10.5	62.6 ±12	0.0405
Mean oxaliplatin dose (mg/m²)	88.5 ±15.2	87.4 ±13.1	0.7473

[2]Wilcoxom's test.

consequences for the patient. Efforts strengthening prevention are needed. Consistently with our results, reinforced premedication could be assessed after 3 courses of oxaliplatin (median of our study) for example or for women with prior exposure to platinum salts. Moreover, when oxaliplatin treatment is considered fundamental for the patient after severe HSR, desensitization should be performed. The need to offer first-line therapy has urged the clinical development of rapid desensitization, which allows hypersensitive patients to be re-treated with medications. Such protocols are safe and effective and allow patients to continue with the treatment that initially caused an HSR [27,28].

Finally, another therapeutic option is the switch for carboplatin or cisplatin, in case of gynecological malignancies for example. Successful replacement of carboplatin by cisplatin has been demonstrated but cases of severe reactions have also been reported [29]. The incidence of cross reaction with oxaliplatin is not known and less described. Some authors suggested to perform skin tests to exclude cross-reactivity before substituting one platinum analog for another [30,31]. Skin tests have been reported to predict oxaliplatin allergic HSR [32], but are rarely used in daily practice. Indeed there are time-consuming, uncomfortable for the patient and only available in some drug allergy care centers. Nonetheless, skin tests and the basophile activation test contribute to identifying the mechanism of HSR which remains unclear. Because of HSR usually occurs after multiple infusions, platinum agents are thought to induce a type I response mediated by IgE, followed by the release of histamine and cytokines. Recent studies have suggested the involvement of type II and III reactions [33]. Further analysis of the mechanism may lead to the development of effective therapeutic strategies.

Several limitations of this study should be noted. As this was a retrospective study, hypersensitivity symptoms were not actively pursued. Some medical records were insufficient and the incidence of HSR was probably underestimated. The number of study subjects is small, so data presented should be interpreted with caution.

Conclusions

Given the frequency and potential severity of oxaliplatin HSR, identification of risk factors could be of therapeutic benefit. In the present analysis, women, younger patients (mean age, 56.2 years) and patients who had experienced a prior exposure to platinum salts presented increased risk. Reintroduction of oxaliplatin is generally possible in grade 1/2 hypersensitive patients using an appropriate premedication strategy but uniform approach to prevent oxaliplatin HSR has not been established and reintroduction remains associated with recurrence of HSR, which requires permanent withdrawal of oxaliplatin infusion.

The risk of developing HSR during oxaliplatin treatment should not be underestimated. Patients need to be informed about clinical manifestations, so they can be handled early by physicians and nursing staff. These findings underline that a close monitoring should be systematic during oxaliplatin infusion, especially if risk factors are identified.

Competing interests
No conflict of interests.
No direct funding was received for this study. The authors were personally salaried by their institutions during the period of writing, although no specific salary was set aside or given for writing the paper.

Authors' contributions
MP, FR, AN, BY, TV, VTL, GF, FB, CR have made substantial contributions to conception and design, or acquisition of data, or analysis and interpretation of data; 2) have been involved in drafting the manuscript or revising it critically for important intellectual content; and 3) have given final approval of the version to be published. All authors have been involved in drafting the manuscript or revising it critically for important intellectual content; and 3) have given final approval of the version to be published. All authors have read and approved the manuscript.

Acknowledgements
We would like to acknowledge the medical, pharmaceutical, and nursing teams at the Centre Hospitalier Lyon Sud, Hospices Civils de Lyon, France.

Author details
[1]Hospices Civils de Lyon, Clinical Oncology Pharmacy Department, Pierre-Bénite, France. [2]Hospices Civils de Lyon, Clinical Oncology Pharmacy Department, Pierre-Bénite - Université Lyon 1, EMR 3738, Lyon, France. [3]Hospices Civils de Lyon, Allergy and Clinical Immunology Department, Pierre-Bénite, France. [4]Oncologie Médicale, Centre d'Investigation des Thérapeutiques en Oncologie et Hématologie de Lyon (CITOHL), Centre Hospitalier Lyon-Sud, Hospices Civils de Lyon, Lyon - Université Lyon 1, EMR 3738, Lyon, France. [5]Centre Régional de pharmacovigilance de Lyon, France.

References
1. Joerger M: Prevention and handling of acute allergic and infusion reactions in oncology. *Ann Oncol* 2012, 23(10):x313–319.
2. Makrilia N, Syrigou E, Kaklamanos I, Manolopoulos L, Saif MW: Hypersensitivity reactions associated with platinum antineoplastic agents: a systematic review. *Met Based Drugs* 2010, 2010:1–11.
3. Shao YY, Hu FC, Liang JT, Chiu WT, Cheng AL, Yang CH: Characteristics and risk factors of oxaliplatin-related hypersensitivity reactions. *J Formos Med Assoc* 2010, 109(5):362–368.
4. Grothey A, Goldberg RM: A review of oxaliplatin and its clinical use in colorectal cancer. *Expert Opin Pharmacother* 2004, 5(10):2159–2170.
5. Ray-Coquard I, Weber B, Cretin J, Haddad-Guichard Z, Levy E, Hardy-Bessard AC, Gouttebel MC, Geay JF, Aleba A, Orfeuvre H, *et al*: Gemcitabine-oxaliplatin combination for ovarian cancer resistant to taxane-platinum treatment: a phase II study from the GINECO group. *Br J Cancer* 2009, 100(4):601–607.
6. American Cancer Society: *Cancer facts and figures*. Atlanta: American Cancer Society; 2009.
7. Mori Y, Nishimura T, Kitano T, Yoshimura K, Matsumoto S, Kanai M, Hazama M, Ishiguro H, Nagayama S, Yanagihara K, *et al*: Oxaliplatin-free interval as a risk factor for hypersensitivity reaction among colorectal cancer patients treated with FOLFOX. *Oncology* 2010, 79(1–2):136–143.
8. Ichikawa Y, Goto A, Hirokawa S, Kijima M, Ishikawa T, Chishima T, Suwa H, Yamamoto H, Yamagishi S, Osada S, *et al*: Allergic reactions to oxaliplatin in a single institute in Japan. *Jpn J Clin Oncol* 2009, 39(9):616–620.
9. Kim BH, Bradley T, Tai J, Budman DR: Hypersensitivity to oxaliplatin: an investigation of incidence and risk factors, and literature review. *Oncology* 2009, 76(4):231–238.

10. Siu SW, Chan RT, Au GK: Hypersensitivity reactions to oxaliplatin: experience in a single institute. *Ann Oncol* 2006, 17(2):259–261.

11. Andre T, Boni C, Mounedji-Boudiaf L, Navarro M, Tabernero J, Hickish T, Topham C, Zaninelli M, Clingan P, Bridgewater J, et al: Multicenter international study of oxaliplatin/5-fluorouracil/leucovorin in the adjuvant treatment of colon cancer (MOSAIC) investigators. *N Engl J Med* 2004, 350(23):2406–2408.

12. Mi-Yeong K, Sung-Yoon K, Suh-Young K, Min-Suk Y, Min-Hye K, Woo-Jung S, Sae-Hoon K, You Jung K, Keun-Wook L, Sang-Heon C, et al: Hypersensitivity reactions to oxaliplatin: clinical features and risk factors in Koreans. *Asian Pacific J Cancer Prev* 2012, 13:1213–1215.

13. Seki K, Senzaki K, Tsuduki Y, Ioroi T, Fujii M, Yamauchi H, Shiraishi Y, Nakata I, Nishiguchi K, Matsubayashi T, et al: Risk factors for oxaliplatin-induced hypersensitivity reactions in Japanese patients with advanced colorectal cancer. *Int J Med Sci* 2011, 8(3):210–215.

14. Shibata Y, Ariyama H, Baba E, Takii Y, Esaki T, Mitsugi K, Tsuchiya T, Kusaba H, Akashi K, Nakano S: Oxaliplatin-induced allergic reaction in patients with colorectal cancer in Japan. *Int J Clin Oncol* 2009, 14(5):397–401.

15. Zhao Y, An X, Xiang XJ, Feng F, Wang FH, Wang ZQ, Xu RH, He YJ, Li YH: Clinical features of hypersensitivity reactions to oxaliplatin among Chinese colorectal cancer patients. *Chin J Cancer* 2010, 29(1):102–105.

16. Johansson SG, Bieber T, Dahl R, Friedmann PS, Lanier BQ, Lockey RF, Motala C, Ortega Martell JA, Platts-Mills TA, Ring J, et al: Revised nomenclature for allergy for global use: report of the nomenclature review committee of the world allergy organization, october 2003. *J Allergy Clin Immunol* 2004, 113(5):832–836.

17. Ring J, Messmer K: Incidence and severity of anaphylactoid reactions to colloid volume substitutes. *Lancet* 1977, 1(8009):466–469.

18. Claudot F, Alla F, Fresson J, Calvez T, Coudane H, Bonaiti-Pellie C: Ethics and observational studies in medical research: various rules in a common framework. *Int J Epidemiol* 2009, 38(4):1104–1108.

19. Shepherd GM: Hypersensitivity reactions to chemotherapeutic drugs. *Clin Rev Allergy Immunol* 2003, 24(3):253–262.

20. Suenaga M, Mizunuma N, Shinozaki E, Matsusaka S, Chin K, Muto T, Konishi F, Hatake K: Management of allergic reactions to oxaliplatin in colorectal cancer patients. *J Support Oncol* 2008, 6(8):373–378.

21. Brandi G, Pantaleo MA, Galli C, Falcone A, Antonuzzo A, Mordenti P, Di Marco MC, Biasco G: Hypersensitivity reactions related to oxaliplatin (OHP). *Br J Cancer* 2003, 89(3):477–481.

22. Polyzos A, Tsavaris N, Gogas H, Souglakos J, Vambakas L, Vardakas N, Polyzos K, Tsigris C, Mantas D, Papachristodoulou A, et al: Clinical features of hypersensitivity reactions to oxaliplatin: a 10-year experience. *Oncology* 2009, 76(1):36–41.

23. Kidera Y, Satoh T, Ueda S, Okamoto W, Okamoto I, Fumita S, Yonesaka K, Hayashi H, Makimura C, Okamoto K, et al: High-dose dexamethasone plus antihistamine prevents colorectal cancer patients treated with modified FOLFOX6 from hypersensitivity reactions induced by oxaliplatin. *Int J Clin Oncol* 2011, 16(3):244–249.

24. Giacchetti S, Perpoint B, Zidani R, Le Bail N, Faggiuolo R, Focan C, Chollet P, Llory JF, Letourneau Y, Coudert B, et al: Phase III multicenter randomized trial of oxaliplatin added to chronomodulated fluorouracil-leucovorin as first-line treatment of metastatic colorectal cancer. *J Clin Oncol* 2000, 18(1):136–147.

25. Levi FA, Zidani R, Vannetzel JM, Perpoint B, Focan C, Faggiuolo R, Chollet P, Garufi C, Itzhaki M, Dogliotti L, et al: Chronomodulated versus fixed-infusion-rate delivery of ambulatory chemotherapy with oxaliplatin, fluorouracil, and folinic acid (leucovorin) in patients with colorectal cancer metastases: a randomized multi-institutional trial. *J Natl Cancer Inst* 1994, 86(21):1608–1617.

26. Yanai T, Iwasa S, Hashimoto H, Kato K, Hamaguchi T, Yamada Y, Shimada Y, Yamamoto H: Successful rechallenge for oxaliplatin hypersensitivity reactions in patients with metastatic colorectal cancer. *Anticancer Res* 2012, 32(12):5521–5526.

27. Castells M, Sancho-Serra Mdel C, Simarro M: Hypersensitivity to antineoplastic agents: mechanisms and treatment with rapid desensitization. *Cancer Immunol Immunother* 2012, 61(9):1575–1584.

28. Cortijo-Cascajares S, Nacle-Lopez I, Garcia-Escobar I, Aguilella-Vizcaino MJ, Herreros-de-Tejada A, Cortes-Funes Castro H, Calleja-Hernandez MA: Effectiveness of oxaliplatin desensitization protocols. *Clin Transl Oncol* 2013, 15(3):219–225.

29. Couraud S, Planus C, Rioufol C, Mornex F: Platinum salts hypersensitivity. *Rev Pneumol Clin* 2008, 64(1):20–26.

30. Elligers KT, Davies M, Sanchis D, Ferencz T, Saif MW: Rechallenge with cisplatin in a patient with pancreatic cancer who developed a hypersensitivity reaction to oxaliplatin. Is skin test useful in this setting? *JOP* 2008, 9(2):197–202.

31. Meyer L, Zuberbier T, Worm M, Oettle H, Riess H: Hypersensitivity reactions to oxaliplatin: cross-reactivity to carboplatin and the introduction of a desensitization schedule. *J Clin Oncol* 2002, 20(4):1146–1147.

32. Pagani M, Bonadonna P, Senna GE, Antico A: Standardization of skin tests for diagnosis and prevention of hypersensitivity reactions to oxaliplatin. *Int Arch Allergy Immunol* 2008, 145(1):54–57.

33. Syrigou E, Syrigos K, Saif MW: Hypersensitivity reactions to oxaliplatin and other antineoplastic agents. *Curr Allergy Asthma Rep* 2008, 8(1):56–62.

6

The favorable kinetics and balance of nebivolol-stimulated nitric oxide and peroxynitrite release in human endothelial cells

R Preston Mason[1,2], Robert F Jacob[2], J Jose Corbalan[3], Damian Szczesny[3], Kinga Matysiak[3] and Tadeusz Malinski[3*]

Abstract

Background: Nebivolol is a third-generation beta-blocker used to treat hypertension. The vasodilation properties of nebivolol have been attributed to nitric oxide (NO) release. However, the kinetics and mechanism of nebivolol-stimulated bioavailable NO are not fully understood.

Methods: Using amperometric NO and peroxynitrite ($ONOO^-$) nanosensors, β_3-receptor (agonist: L-755,507; antagonists: SR59230A and L-748,337), ATP efflux (the mechanosensitive ATP channel blocker, gadolinium) and P2Y-receptor (agonists: ATP and 2-MeSATP; antagonist: suramin) modulators, superoxide dismutase and a NADPH oxidase inhibitor (VAS2870), we evaluated the kinetics and balance of NO and $ONOO^-$ stimulated by nebivolol in human umbilical vein endothelial cells (HUVECs). NO and $ONOO^-$ were measured with nanosensors (diameter ~ 300 nm) placed 5 ± 2 μm from the cell membrane and ATP levels were determined with a bioluminescent method. The kinetics and balance of nebivolol-stimulated NO and $ONOO^-$ were compared with those of ATP, 2-MeSATP, and L-755,507.

Results: Nebivolol stimulates endothelial NO release through β_3-receptor and ATP-dependent, P2Y-receptor activation with relatively slow kinetics (75 ± 5 nM/s) as compared to the kinetics of ATP (194 ± 10 nM/s), L-755,507 (108 ± 6 nM/s), and 2-MeSATP (105 ± 5 nM/s). The balance between cytoprotective NO and cytotoxic $ONOO^-$ was expressed as the ratio of [NO]/[$ONOO^-$] concentrations. This ratio for nebivolol was 1.80 ± 0.10 and significantly higher than that for ATP (0.80 ± 0.08), L-755,507 (1.08 ± 0.08), and 2-MeSATP (1.09 ± 0.09). Nebivolol induced ATP release in a concentration-dependent manner.

Conclusion: The two major pathways (ATP efflux/P2Y receptors and β_3 receptors) and several steps of nebivolol-induced NO and $ONOO^-$ stimulation are mainly responsible for the slow kinetics of NO release and low $ONOO^-$. The net effect of this slow kinetics of NO is reflected by a favorable high ratio of [NO]/[$ONOO^-$] which may explain the beneficial effects of nebivolol in the treatment of endothelial dysfunction, hypertension, heart failure, and angiogenesis.

Keywords: Nevibolol, Nitric oxide, Peroxynitrite, ATP, β_3-adrenergic receptors, P2Y-purinergic receptors

Background

Arterial endothelial cells modulate vascular tone through release of nitric oxide (NO), a potent vasodilator that regulates regional blood flow [1,2]. Beyond vasodilation, NO has various vascular benefits that reduce the risk for cardiovascular disease. NO inhibits smooth muscle cell proliferation and migration, adhesion of leukocytes to the vascular endothelium, and platelet aggregation [3].

An uncoupling of endothelial nitric oxide synthase (eNOS) along with reduced endothelial-dependent NO release and generation of peroxynitrite ($ONOO^-$) has been linked to atherogenesis and its clinical manifestations [4,5]. Agents that enhance NO bioavailability have been shown to reduce cardiovascular events, as well as central arterial blood pressure, in patients with hypertension [4,5]. NO generation in the endothelium is accompanied by the production of $ONOO^-$. Peroxynitrite, a major component of nitroxidative stress, is cytotoxic and can trigger a cascade of events leading to vasoconstriction, dysfunction of the endothelium, and apoptosis

* Correspondence: malinski@ohio.edu
[3]Department of Chemistry and Biochemistry, Ohio University, 45701 Athens, OH, USA
Full list of author information is available at the end of the article

[6]. Therefore, a change in the balance between NO and ONOO⁻ generated by the endothelium can significantly affect the endothelial function, and as a result, lead to the dysfunction of the cardiovascular system.

ATP, which widely regulates cell and tissue function through autocrine or paracrine stimulation of purinergic (P2Y) receptors, has also been shown to be an important mediator of endothelial-dependent NO [7]. The vascular effect of ATP was first characterized in aortic segments from spontaneously hypertensive rats, as well as normotensive Wistar-Kyoto rats, in which direct application of ATP caused NO-mediated relaxation [8]. Similar effects were observed in hepatic arterial tissue isolated from New Zealand White rabbits and shown to be dependent on endothelial P2Y receptors [9]. In renal tissue, isolated from Wistar-Kyoto rats, ATP was further shown to induce relaxation of the glomerular microvasculature by activating P2Y receptors, followed by eNOS and guanylate cyclase pathway activation [10].

Nebivolol is a third-generation, β_1-adrenergic receptor antagonist with vasodilatory properties that appear to be independent of its β_1-receptor interactions [11-13]. Its mechanism of action is attributed to eNOS activation since its vasodilatory effects can be reversed with specific eNOS inhibitors such as N^G-monomethyl-L-arginine (L-NMMA) and N_ω-nitro-L-arginine methyl ester (L-NAME) [14-16]. In a number of independent studies, nebivolol-induced NO release has also been linked to β_3-receptor interactions as well as ATP-dependent, P2Y-mediated eNOS activation [17-20]. Nebivolol has also been reported to reverse eNOS uncoupling and interfere with oxidative stress processes, by reducing NADPH oxidase activity or by directly scavenging oxygen-derived free radicals [13,20-23].

We conducted this study to evaluate simultaneously the kinetics of nebivolol-stimulated NO and ONOO⁻ production and the role of ATP efflux along with P2Y- and β_3-receptor activation in human endothelial cells. We hypothesized that the slow kinetics of NO release in the endothelium, through integrated cellular mechanism that include both the ATP autocrine and/or paracrine pathway and these specific receptors, may be at least partially responsible for favorable balance between bioavailable NO and cytotoxic ONOO⁻. The high level of NO and low ONOO⁻ generated by nebivolol may explain its pleiotropic and therapeutic effects on the restoration of endothelial function in the cardiovascular system.

Methods
Materials
Nebivolol HCl (in powder form) was provided by Forest Research Institute (Commack, NY). The β_3-agonist, L-755,507, and β_3-antagonists, SR59230A and L-748,337, were purchased from Tocris Bioscience (Ellisville, MO).

ATP, 2-MeSATP, and the non-selective P2Y receptor antagonist, suramin, were purchased from Sigma-Aldrich (St. Louis, MO). Gadolinium (Gd^{3+}), a mechanosensitive, ATP-release channel blocker, superoxide dismutase (PEG-SOD) and the NADPH oxidase inhibitor, VAS2870, were also purchased from Sigma-Aldrich.

Cell culture
Primary human umbilical vein endothelial cells (HUVECs) were purchased from Lonza Inc. (Walkersville, MD). Cells were cultured in the recommended complete endothelial cell growth medium and maintained at 37°C in a 95% air / 5% CO_2 humidified incubator. As recommended by the supplier, cells were supplied with fresh medium every other day and propagated by an enzymatic (trypsin) procedure for a maximum of 16 population doublings. Our studies were performed in accordance with the guidelines established by the Ohio University Office of Institutional Research Compliance. These guidelines conform with the principles of the World Medical Association Declaration of Helsinki.

NO and ONOO⁻ measurement
Endothelial NO and ONOO⁻ release was measured using amperometric nanosensors as previously described [21,24]. Briefly, each of the sensors was made by depositing a sensing material on the tip of a carbon fiber (length 4-5 μm; diameter 200-300 nm), i.e., a conductive film of polymeric nickel(II)tetrakis(3-methoxy-4-hydroxyphenyl)porphyrin for the NO sensor and a conductive film of polymeric manganese(III)-[2]paracyclophenylporphyrin for the ONOO⁻ sensor. The fiber was sealed with a nonconductive epoxy and connected to copper electrical wires with a conductive silver epoxy. Confluent HUVECs were rinsed with endothelial basal medium (EBM; Lonza Inc., Walkersville, MD) and the tandem of nanosensors was gently lowered to within 5 ± 2 μm from the surface of an endothelial cell using a remote-controlled micromanipulator (Sensapex, Finland). Amperometric measurements were performed using a Gamry Reference 600™ dual potentiostat (Gamry instruments, Warminster, PA). Basal NO and ONOO⁻ levels were measured by differential pulse voltammetry (DPV) in separate experiments. The DPV current at the peak potential characteristic for NO and ONOO⁻ is directly proportional to the local concentration of NO and ONOO⁻ in the immediate vicinity of the sensor. The nanosensors were calibrated before measurements in cells using a linear calibration curve (current versus concentration) constructed from standard NO or ONOO⁻ solutions ranging from 50 nM to 700 nM. The sensors response and calibration was tested again after measurements in cells, using the standard addition method. The detection limit of the sensors was 10^{-9} M.

Changes in current, proportional to the concentration of NO or ONOO⁻, were observed after the injection of nebivolol and other agents used in this study, including modulators of the ATP pathway and both agonists and antagonists of the β_3-receptor. To test their direct effects, the compounds were administered acutely by a nanoinjector prior to measurements of NO and ONOO⁻ release from the cells. For combination studies, cells were treated with various β_3-receptor and ATP pathway modulators, VAS2870 or PEG-SOD for 30 minutes prior to treatment with nebivolol.

ATP measurement

Extracellular ATP was quantified using a luciferin-luciferase assay kit (BioAssay Systems, Hayward, CA). The ATP measurement was performed following the supplier's recommendations. Briefly, confluent HUVECs were rinsed and incubated at 37°C in EBM medium for 5 minutes in the absence or presence of the various test agents. Aliquots (100 µL) of each sample supernatant were then transferred to a white opaque 96-well plate, along with luciferin and luciferase, and then luminescence was measured on a luminometer (BioTek, Winooski, VT). The ATP concentration was obtained using a standard calibration, prepared as recommended in the kit.

Calculations and statistical analysis

All data are presented as mean ± standard deviation (SD) of the mean of n > 3. Statistical analysis of the mean difference between multiple groups was performed using one-way analysis of variance (ANOVA) with Student-Newman-Keuls multiple comparisons post hoc analysis; and between two groups, using Student's t-test. The alpha level for all the tests was 0.05. A P value <0.05 was considered to be statistically significant. All statistical analyses were performed using Origin (v 6.1 for Windows; OriginLab, Northampton, MA) and GraphPad Prism (v. 5.00 for Windows; GraphPad Software, San Diego, CA).

Results

Using nanonsensor technology, we measured *in situ*, near-real time NO and ONOO⁻ released from HUVECs following the acute administration of nebivolol, L-755, 507, 2-MeSATP or ATP over a range of concentrations. Representative amperograms (concentration/current vs. time) collected from endothelial cells treated with nebivolol, L-755,507, 2-MeSATP, and ATP are shown in the Figure 1. A distinctive difference between the slope and peak height of amperograms was observed for both NO and ONOO⁻ production. The slope of amperograms was used to calculate the rate of NO and ONOO⁻ generation by endothelial cells after stimulation with nebivolol, L-755,507, 2-MeSATP, and ATP (Figure 2). The kinetics of NO release was relatively slow for nebivolol, with a rate of

75 ± 4 nM/s, and significantly faster for L-755,507 (108 ± 6 nM/s) and 2-MeSATP (105 ± 5 nM/s); and very fast for ATP-stimulated NO release (194 ± 10 nM/s). The rates for ONOO⁻ followed this same pattern as NO – lowest rate for nebivolol and the highest for ATP.

As shown in the Figure 3, the maximal NO concentration of 225 ± 15 nM was observed after stimulation with nebivolol and was the highest among the four agents tested. Surprisingly, ONOO⁻ concentration was the lowest after nebivolol stimulation (125 ± 10 nM) and the highest after ATP stimulation (220 ± 13 nM). The maximal NO and ONOO⁻ concentrations were between that observed for nebivolol and ATP. We applied the ratio of [NO] and [ONOO⁻] concentrations to depict the chemical redox balance between these two molecules in the cellular milieu. A decrease in [NO]/[ONOO⁻] ratio indicates a decrease in the concentration of the cytoprotective NO and/or an increase in the level of highly oxidative, cytotoxic ONOO⁻. A ratio of [NO]/[ONOO⁻] below 1.0 is an indicator that the cellular environment is dominated by high oxidative/nitroxidative stress.

Nanosensors provide unique opportunities for the simultaneous measurement of NO and ONOO⁻ concentration in small volume ($\sim 10^{-15}$ L), at near real-time (10^{-5} s) in close proximity to the cell membrane (~ 5 µm). The ratios of [NO]/[ONOO⁻] are presented in the Figure 3B. There is a highly significant difference in the [NO]/[ONOO⁻] balance between nebivolol (1.80 ± 0.10) and ATP (0.80 ± 0.08). The ratio of [NO]/[ONOO⁻] for L-755,507 and 2-MeSATP are similar, 1.08 ± 0.08 and 1.09 ± 0.09 respectively. There is a 40-60% difference in the [NO]/[ONOO⁻] balance between nebivolol and 3 other agents tested here.

A very low ratio of [NO]/[ONOO⁻] (lower than one) was observed only after the stimulation of endothelial cells by ATP (Figure 3B). We validated this model of monitoring [NO]/[ONOO⁻] balance in endothelial cells by changing the level of superoxide (O_2^-), the precursor of ONOO⁻. In the presence of membrane permeable PEG-SOD (400 U/mL), a significant reduction in ONOO⁻ concentration with concomitant increase in the NO level was observed (Figure 4A). This effect was observed for both nebivolol and ATP. A similar effect of the increase in NO and proportional decrease in ONOO⁻ was noticed in the presence of NADPH oxidase inhibitor, VAS2870 (5 µM). The Inhibition of the NADPH oxidase increases NO concentration by 20-30% after stimulation with nebivolol or ATP. This indicates that about 20-30% of NO produced by the endothelium is consumed by O_2^- generated by NADPH oxidase. The source of the remaining 70-80% of O_2^- in nebivolol- or ATP-stimulated endothelium is most likely eNOS.

The decrease in O_2^- had a significant influence on the level of bioavailable NO and the concentration of ONOO⁻, as reflected by a significant increase in [NO]/

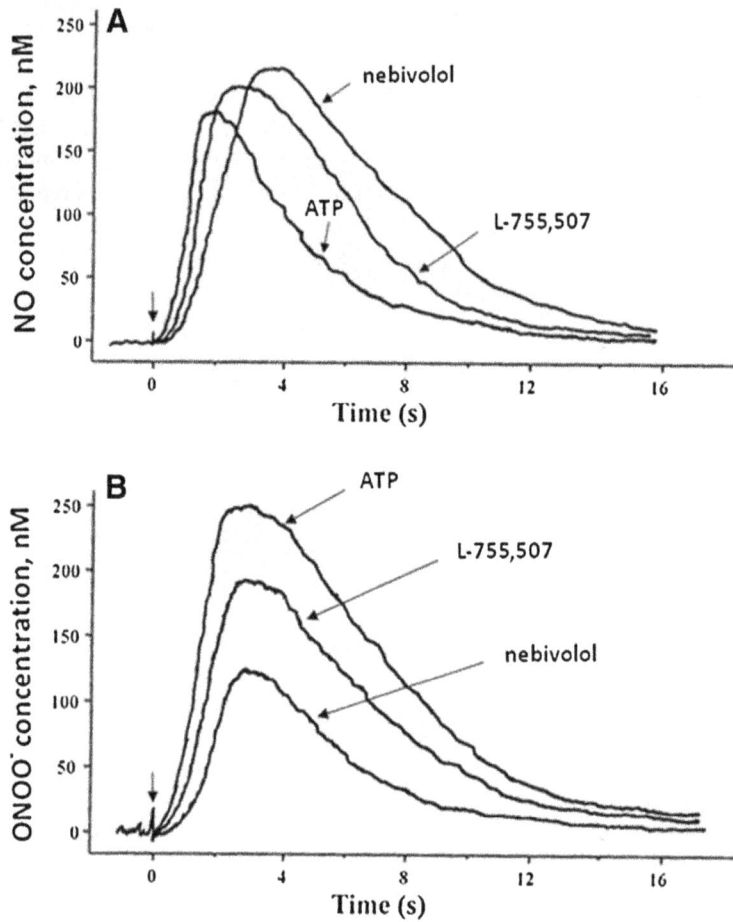

Figure 1 Representative amperograms showing endothelial NO and ONOO⁻ release stimulated with nebivolol, L-755,507, 2-MeSATP, and ATP. NO **(A)** and ONOO⁻ **(B)** release from HUVECs were stimulated with nebivolol, ATP, 2-MeSATP, or L-755,507 (each at 1 μM). The amperograms of the 2-MeSATP partially overlaps that of L-755,507 and are omitted. NO and ONOO⁻ release were measured with electrochemical nanosensors positioned 5 ± 2 μm from the surface of a single cell. Arrows indicate compound administration.

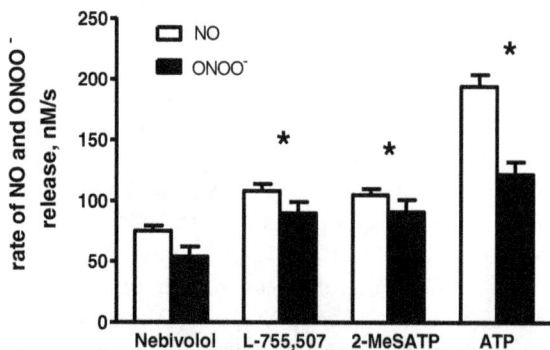

Figure 2 Rate of endothelial NO and ONOO⁻ release. NO and ONOO⁻ release from HUVECs were stimulated with nebivolol, L-755,507, 2-MeSATP, and ATP (each at 1 μM). Values are mean ± SD (n = 5). One-way ANOVA, Student-Newman-Keuls multiple comparison post-hoc test: *$P < 0.05$ compared with either the rate of NO or ONOO⁻ released by cells stimulated with nebivolol.

[ONOO⁻] ratio (Figure 4B). A favorable [NO]/[ONOO⁻] balance increased even further for nebivolol to 4.30 ± 0.21 in the presence of PEG-SOD. Also, in the presence of PEG-SOD, a favorable shift in the [NO]/[ONOO⁻] balance was observed for ATP.

Nebivolol increased endothelial NO release in a dose-dependent manner (Figure 5A). The effect of nebivolol on ATP concentration released from cells was significant and correlated well with a dose-dependent increase in NO production (Figure 5B). The ratio of [NO]/[ONOO⁻] decreased with the increase of nebivolol concentration (Figure 5C). This correlates well with a fast increase in nebivolol-stimulated ATP component in the overall stimulation process of NO release.

The relationship between NO bioavailability and ATP production was further tested using modulators of the ATP/purinergic pathway. Each of these agents significantly attenuated the effects of nebivolol on endothelial NO release (Figure 6A). At the specific concentrations

Figure 3 Maximal endothelial NO and ONOO⁻ concentrations, and [NO]/[ONOO⁻] ratio stimulated with nebivolol, L-755,507, 2-MeSATP, and ATP. (A) Maximal NO and ONOO⁻ concentration release from HUVECs stimulated with nebivolol, L-755,507, 2-MeSATP, and ATP (each at 1 µM). Values are mean ± SD (n = 5). One-way ANOVA, Student-Newman-Keuls multiple comparison post-hoc test: *P < 0.05 compared with either the maximal NO or ONOO⁻ concentration released by cells stimulated with nebivolol. (B) The [NO]/[ONOO⁻] ratio calculated from the maximal concentration in A. Values are mean ± SD (n = 5). One-way ANOVA, Student-Newman-Keuls multiple comparison post-hoc test: *P < 0.05 compared with [NO]/[ONOO⁻] ratio calculated for nebivolol.

Figure 4 Maximal endothelial NO and ONOO⁻ concentrations, and [NO]/[ONOO⁻] ratio stimulated with nebivolol and ATP following a PEG-SOD and VAS2870 incubation. (A) Maximal NO and ONOO⁻ concentrations stimulated with nebivolol and ATP (each at 1 µM) following a 30-minute incubation of HUVECs with PEG-SOD (400 U/mL) and VAS2870 (5 µM). Values are mean ± SD (n = 5). Student's t-test: *P < 0.05 compared with nebivolol. (B) The [NO]/[ONOO⁻] ratio calculated from the maximal concentration in A. Values are mean ± SD (n = 5). Student's t-test: *P < 0.05 compared with [NO]/[ONOO⁻] balance calculated for nebivolol.

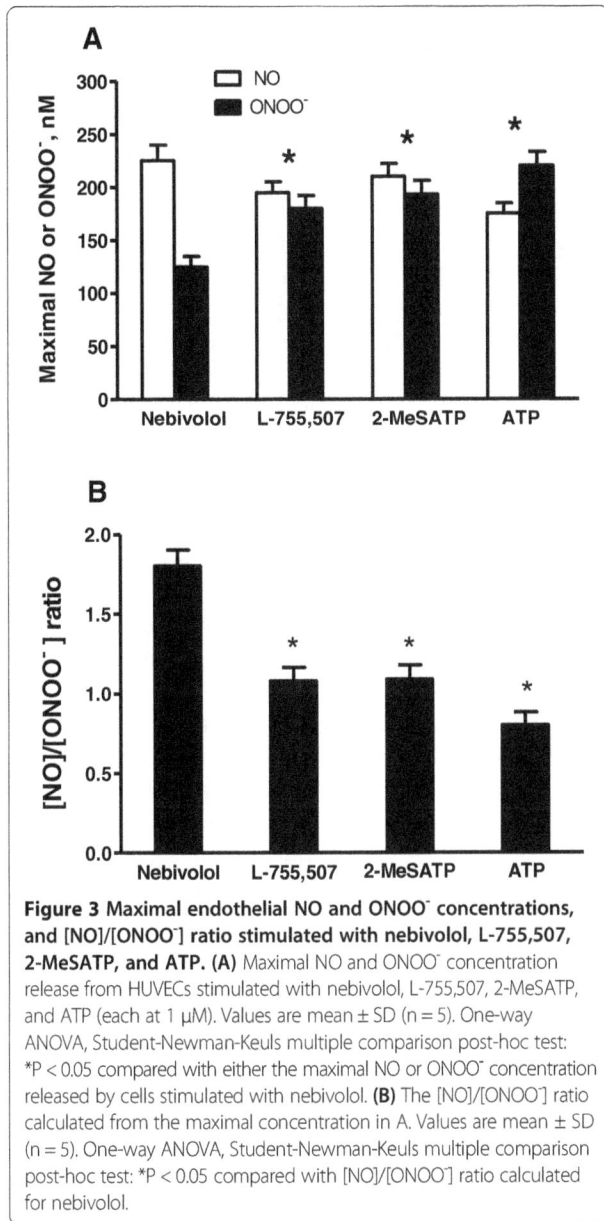

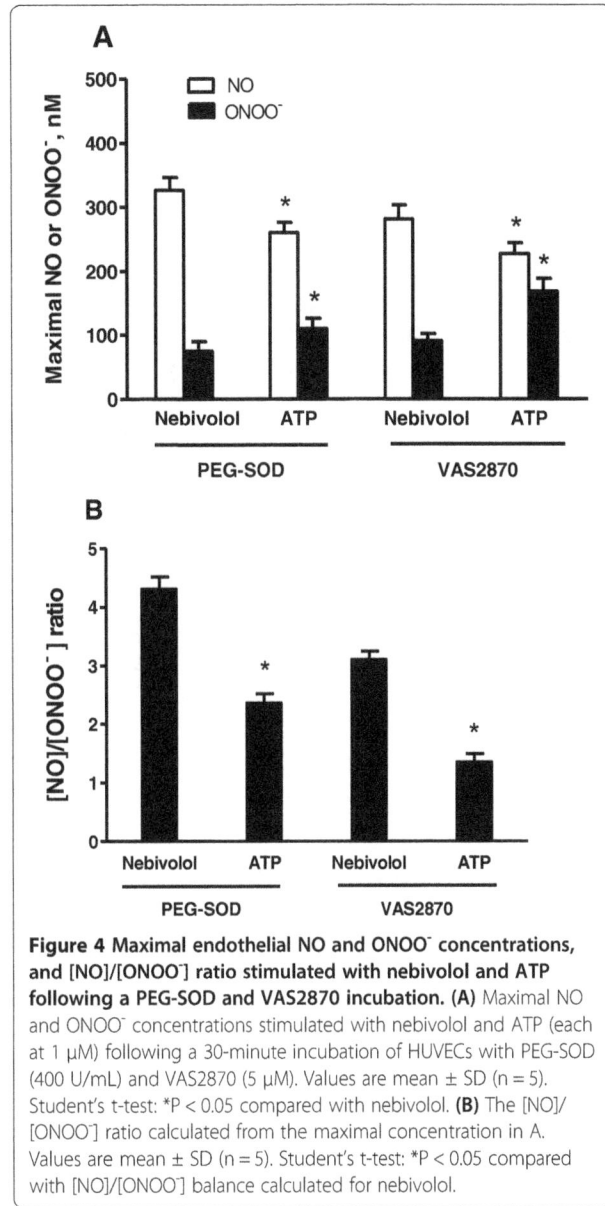

tested, suramin (10 µM) and Gd^{3+} (200 µM) inhibited nebivolol-induced NO release by 50 and 60%, respectively. These findings are consistent with the observation that the effects of nebivolol on endothelial-dependent NO release is casually associated with ATP production, especially at higher concentrations of nebivolol. We also measured the effects of nebivolol on endothelial NO release in the presence of β_3-receptor antagonists SR59230A (1 µM) or L-748,337 (3 µM). Both of these agents reduced the nebivolol-induced NO release by approximately 50% (Figure 6A). However, a combination of suramin and SR59230A reduced nebivolol stimulated NO by more than 90%.

Discussion

The key finding from this study is that nebivolol-stimulated NO release from human endothelial cells is multipathway and slow. This slow process preserves eNOS coupling and leads to a high production of bio-available NO and low production of ONOO⁻. The slow kinetics and dynamics of NO generation is a significant factor in the maintaining of the highly favorable balance between [NO] and [ONOO⁻] concentrations in the endothelium. The favorable kinetics of NO release, combined with O_2^- scavenging by nebivolol, may help to explain the pleiotropic effect of nebivolol on the cardiovascular system observed in clinical studies. The

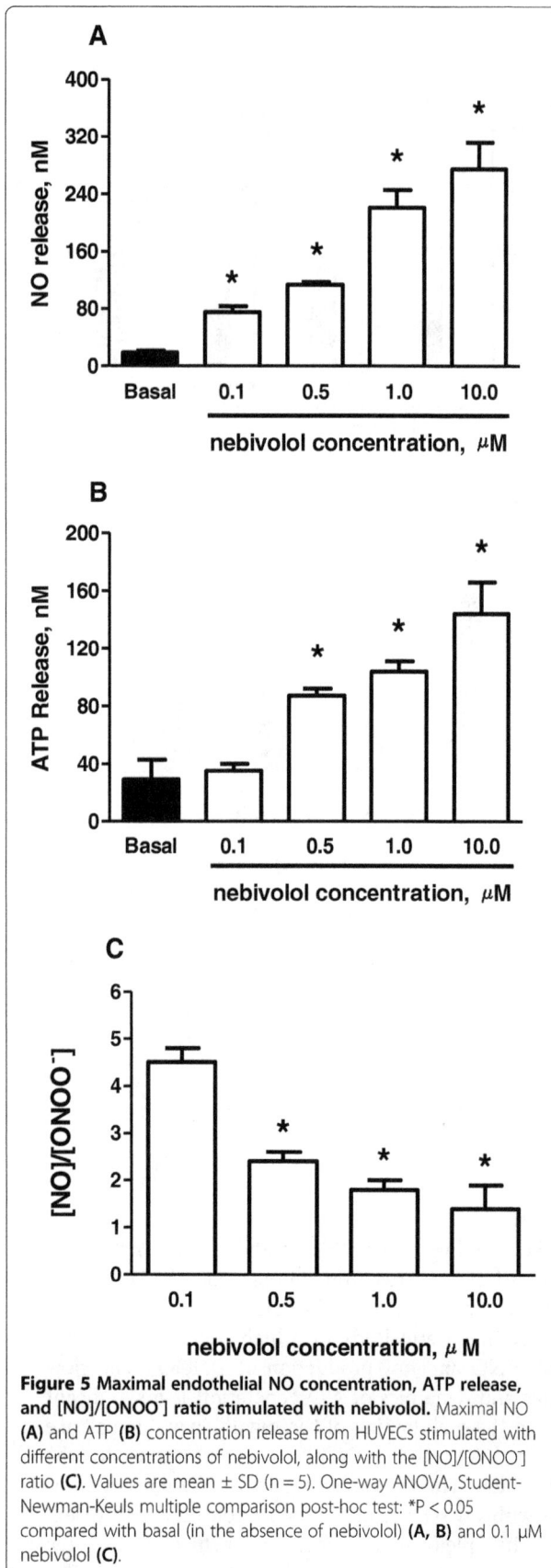

Figure 5 Maximal endothelial NO concentration, ATP release, and [NO]/[ONOO⁻] ratio stimulated with nebivolol. Maximal NO **(A)** and ATP **(B)** concentration release from HUVECs stimulated with different concentrations of nebivolol, along with the [NO]/[ONOO⁻] ratio **(C)**. Values are mean ± SD (n = 5). One-way ANOVA, Student-Newman-Keuls multiple comparison post-hoc test: *$P < 0.05$ compared with basal (in the absence of nebivolol) **(A, B)** and 0.1 μM nebivolol **(C)**.

rate of NO release by nebivolol is slower than that observed for the other three agents presented in this study (ATP, L-755,507, and 2-MeSATP). These three agents produced comparable NO concentrations with nebivolol, however, excessive and rapid NO production stimulated by these agents eventually leads to uncoupling of eNOS (rapid depletion of substrates and/or cofactors for NO production). The uncoupled eNOS is an efficient generator of O_2^- in one electron transfer reduction of oxygen. Therefore, uncoupled eNOS can produce, sequentially, both NO and O_2^-. NO and O_2^- generated in close proximity by eNOS can react rapidly in a diffusion controlled reaction to produce ONOO⁻. The studies with VAS2870 also elucidated that the second major source of O_2^- in the endothelium during the stimulation of NO release by nebivolol is NADPH oxidase. Our study shows that after the stimulation of endothelial cells with nebivolol, the contribution of NADPH oxidase to the pool of O_2^-, and subsequently the pool of ONOO⁻ is about 20-30%, while about 70-80% of O_2^- and ONOO⁻ comes from uncoupled eNOS. NADPH oxidase contribution to the pool of O_2^- and ONOO⁻ after stimulation with ATP is about 30-35% with eNOS contributing 65-70%. In addition to the favorable kinetics of NO release, nebivolol may also increase NO bioavailability through non-receptor-mediated mechanisms, such as conveying antioxidant benefits of the endothelium. Nebivolol has been shown to scavenge O_2^- independent of β_3-receptor blockade in animal and cell based models of cardiovascular diseases [13,17,20,21]. These effects are attributed to its specific interactions with plasma membrane and its efficiency as a chain-breaking antioxidant [13,25]. Nebivolol has also been shown to interact with enzymatic sources of oxygen radicals such as NADPH oxidase [21,22]. This correlates well with our data showing lower generation of O_2^-/ONOO⁻ by NADPH oxidase than eNOS after stimulation with nebivolol.

The scavenging properties of nebivolol cannot alone explain the low level of ONOO⁻ and slow kinetics of nebivolol stimulated NO production. The results of our study suggest that nebivolol increases NO release in the human endothelium through a complementary mechanism involving β3-receptor, ATP autocrine and/or paracrine, and P2Y-receptor activation. Two different β_3-receptor antagonists (SR59230A and L-748,337) were discovered to significantly reduce nebivolol-induced NO release in HUVECs. However, these β_3-receptor antagonists reduced NO production only by about 50%. A blockage with Gd^{3+} of mechanosensitive ATP channels of HUVECs reduced NO production by 60%, indicating a direct involvement of extracellular ATP in the stimulation process. Finally, in the presence of both antagonists of the P2Y-receptor, suramin, and β_3-receptor antagonist, SR59230A, NO concentration decreased by more than 90%.

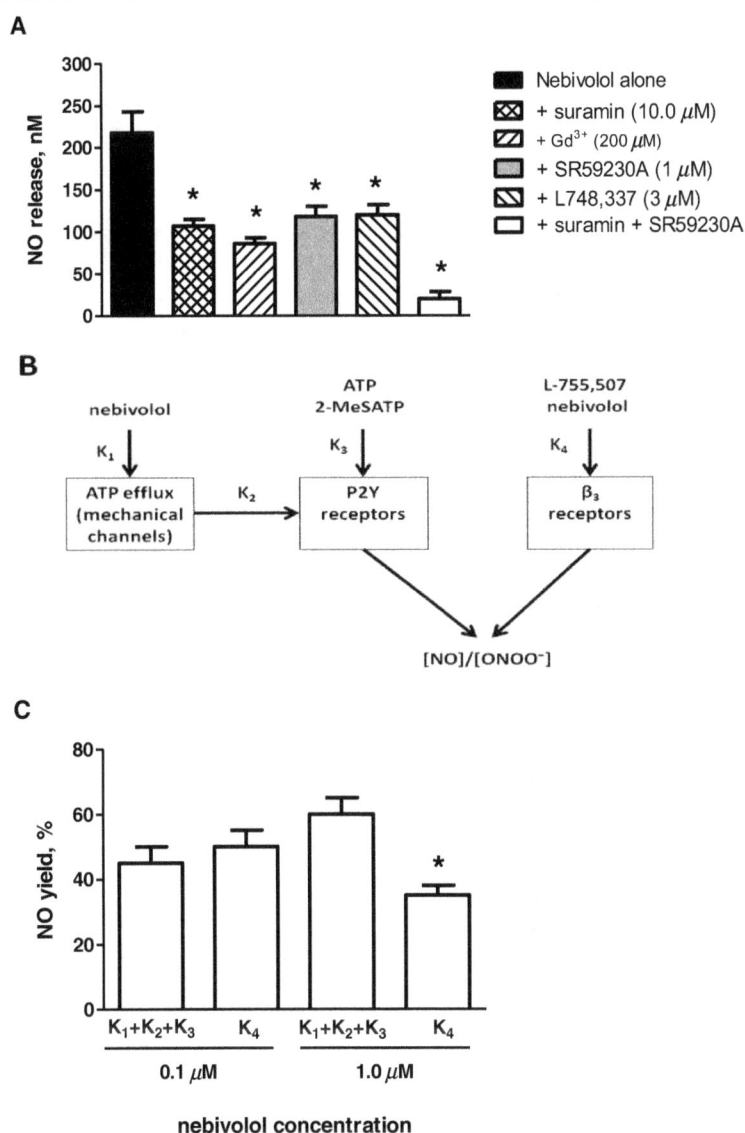

Figure 6 Major pathways involved in nebivolol-stimulated NO and ONOO⁻ generation, and maximal endothelial NO concentration stimulated with nebivolol alone or following an incubation with several modulators. (A) Maximal NO concentration release from HUVECs stimulated with nebivolol (1 µM). Cells were also incubated with suramin (10 µM), Gd^{3+} (200 µM), SR59230A (1 µM), L-748,337 (3 µM) and suramin + SR59230A for 30 minutes and NO release was stimulated with nebivolol (1 µM). Values are mean ± SD (n = 5). One-way ANOVA, Student-Newman-Keuls multiple comparison post-hoc test: *$P < 0.05$ compared with nebivolol alone. **(B)** Nebivolol-stimulated generation of NO and ONOO⁻ involves at least two major pathways and several steps. **(C)** At low nebivolol concentration, K_4 will be more determinant than at higher concentration. Values are mean ± SD (n = 5). Student's t-test: *$P < 0.05$ compared with $K_1 + K_2 + K_3$.

Our findings in this study argue for the involvement of β_3-receptors in eNOS activation and NO release in human endothelial cells stimulated by nebivolol. A role for β_3-receptors in nebivolol-induced NO release was previously demonstrated in human heart ventricular tissue and coronary microarteries [19]. Nebivolol was shown to activate cardiac β_3-receptors in a manner similar to that of the selective β_3-receptor agonist, BRL 37344, both of which resulted in a change in ventricular contraction attributed to NO release. The negative inotropic effects of nebivolol were modified by pretreatment with L-748, 337, but not with nadolol, a nonselective β_2/β_3-receptor antagonist [19]. These specific receptor-mediated effects of nebivolol on NO metabolism may contribute to favorable changes in vascular hemodynamic properties and calcium regulation given the relative distribution of β_1- and β_3-receptors in the failing heart. Clinical support for such potential benefit was demonstrated in a randomized trial of elderly patients with documented heart failure [26]. Nebivolol was also shown in another study to increase vasodilation in coronary microarteries essential for the regulation of coronary resistance and perfusion reserve [18]. Endothelial-dependent vasodilation was not reproduced with nebivolol in mice deficient for β_3-receptors [18]. Nebivolol also failed to induce neocapillary tube formation in animals deficient in either β_3-receptor or eNOS expression [18]. Another recent study showed that nebivolol increased levels of endothelial progenitor cells, promoted angiogenesis, and reversed left ventricular dysfunction in mice with extensive myocardial infarction [20]. The vasodilation effects of nebivolol could only be partially blocked with a specific β_3-adrenergic receptor antagonist [20]. The data presented in our work established an important connection between the cardioprotective effects of nebivolol and its β_3-mediated, ATP-mediated effects on eNOS function.

The results of this study also suggest a role for the ATP autocrine and/or paracrine pathway in the activation of eNOS. It was found that the mechanosensitive ATP channel blocker, Gd^{3+}, inhibited nebivolol-induced NO release by 60%. Moreover, the rate of NO stimulation with ATP is much faster than the stimulation with nebivolol. Therefore, we concluded that a rate determining factor in the kinetics of nebivolol-stimulated NO may be the ATP efflux from endothelial cells. The delivery of ATP from intracellular to extracellular space will require a buildup of the gradient of concentration, passage through mechanical channels and diffusion to receptors on the membrane surface. These delivery processes, based on efflux and diffusion, will be much slower than the direct high gradient diffusion of ATP to membrane receptors from an outer solution of ATP.

Extracellular ATP promotes vascular relaxation through the activation of P2Y receptors and the subsequent stimulation of eNOS and cytosolic guanylate cyclase [10]. Exogenous ATP has been shown to promote NO release from Wister-Kyoto rat glomerular endothelial cells with kinetic properties similar to those of nebivolol [17]. Inhibition of ATP efflux with Gd^{3+}, an inhibitor of stretch-activated channels, also reduced the effects of nebivolol [17]. We demonstrated that a pretreatment of cells with Gd^{3+} decreased the ability of nebivolol-induced endothelial NO release. This may suggest that nebivolol itself may be linked to opening of mechanosensitive ATP channels.

It appears from this study that the kinetics of NO production by eNOS is crucial in maintaining a favorable balance between [NO]/[ONOO⁻] concentrations. A rapid stimulation may produce high level of NO but also a high level of ONOO⁻. Therefore, the rapid generation of NO accompanied by high ONOO⁻ cancels the beneficial effect of NO and imposes a deleterious effect of ONOO⁻-induced nitroxidative stress with severe side effect for the endothelium. NO and ONOO⁻ stimulation by cerivastatin is a good example of this kind of "non-favorable kinetics"

of NO release [27]. A potentially excellent pleiotropic effect of cerivastatin was compromised by the negative effect of high ONOO⁻ generated by this drug. This negative side effect of cerivastatin on the cardiovascular system was the forced withdrawal of this otherwise excellent drug from the pharmaceutical market.

Limitations

HUVECs were used in this study as the sole source of endothelial cells. Further studies will be required to confirm these findings using other sources of endothelial cells.

Conclusions

We propose that nebivolol-stimulated generation of NO and ONOO⁻ involves at least two major pathways and several steps (Figure 6B). One of this pathways involves a stimulation of intracellular ATP efflux through mechanical channels (K_1), diffusion of extracellular ATP to P2Y receptors (K_2), and stimulation of P2Y receptors by ATP (K_3) followed by the release of NO and ONOO⁻. We propose that this pathway involving many steps is a rate determining factor in NO and ONOO⁻ production after stimulation with nebivolol. The other pathway, through β_3 receptors (K_4) is faster and the rate of NO and ONOO⁻ release comparable with that of K_3. Therefore, the yield of NO produced by each pathway will vary with the concentration of nebivolol. At low nebivolol concentration, K_4 pathway will be more determinant than at higher concentration (Figure 6C).

The results of this study provide additional insights into the cellular basis for nebivolol-induced NO release in human endothelial cells. The ability of nebivolol to stimulate NO release appears to be independent of its selective β_1-blockade properties and dependent on stimulation of β_3-receptors and ATP-mediated stimulation of P2Y-purinergic receptors. It seems to be also linked to direct opening of mechanosensitive ATP channels. A multistep stimulation of NO release is relatively slow and the production of NO does not significantly influence the supply of substrates or cofactors to eNOS, maintaining its relative high degree of coupling. The coupled eNOS can produce high NO concentration and low ONOO⁻ leading to a highly beneficial effect of nebivolol in the treatment of dysfunctional endothelium in cardiovascular diseases.

Competing interests

Dr Mason received an independent research grant in support of this study from Forest Laboratories. All other authors have no conflicts of interest to disclose.

Authors' contributions

RPM and TM designed the study. JJC, DS, and KM performed the experimental work. RPM, RFJ, JJC, and TM carried out the analyses, interpreted the data, drafted the manuscript and critically reviewed it. All authors read and approved the final manuscript.

Acknowledgements

Financial support was provided by the Marvin White Endowment Fund at Ohio University. A special thanks to Forest Laboratories for providing nebivolol, and to Collin Arocho and Paula Hale for their assistance in the preparation of this manuscript. This investigation was conducted in a facility constructed with support from Research Facilities Improvement Program Grant Number C06 RR-014575-01 from the National Center for Research Resources, National Institutes of Health.

Author details

[1]Cardiovascular Division, Department of Medicine, Brigham and Women's Hospital, Harvard Medical School, 02115 Boston, MA, USA. [2]Elucida Research LLC, 01915 Beverly, MA, USA. [3]Department of Chemistry and Biochemistry, Ohio University, 45701 Athens, OH, USA.

References

1. Ignarro LJ, Buga GM, Wood KS, Byrnes RE, Chaudhuri G: Endothelium-derived relaxing factor produced and released from artery and vein is nitric oxide. *Proc Natl Acad Sci U S A* 1987, **84**:9265–9269.
2. Rees DD, Palmer RM, Moncada S: The role of endothelium-derived nitric oxide in the regulation of blood pressure. *Proc Natl Acad Sci U S A* 1989, **86**:3375–3378.
3. Kojda G, Harrison DG: Interactions between NO and reactive oxygen species: pathophysiological importance in atherosclerosis, hypertension, diabetes and heart failure. *Cardiovas Res* 1999, **43**:562–571.
4. Mizuno Y, Jacob RF, Mason RP: Effects of calcium channel and renin-angiotensin system blockade on intravascular and neurohormonal mechanisms of hypertensive vascular disease. *Am J Hypertens* 2008, **21**:1076–1085.
5. Mizuno Y, Jacob RF, Mason RP: Advances in pharmacologic modulation of nitric oxide in hypertension. *Curr Cardiol Rep* 2010, **12**:472–480.
6. Mason RP, Jacob RF, Kubant R, Ciszewski A, Corbalan JJ, Malinski T: Dipeptidyl peptidase-4 inhibition with saxagliptin enhanced nitric oxide release and reduced blood pressure and sICAM-1 levels in hypertensive rats. *J Cardiovasc Pharmacol* 2012, **60**:467–473.
7. Corriden R, Insel PA: Basal release of ATP: an autocrine-paracrine mechanism for cell regulation. *Sci Signal* 2010, **3**:re1–re25.
8. Dominiczak AF, Quilley J, Bohr DF: Contraction and relaxation of rat aorta in response to ATP. *Am J Physiol* 1991, **261**:H243–H251.
9. Mathie RT, Ralevic V, Alexander B, Burnstock G: Nitric oxide is the mediator of ATP-induced dilatation of the rabbit hepatic arterial vascular bed. *Br J Pharmacol* 1991, **103**:1602–1606.
10. Jankowski M, Szczepanska-Konkel M, Kalinowski L, Angielski S: Cyclic GMP-dependent relaxation of isolated rat renal glomeruli induced by extracellular ATP. *J Physiol* 2001, **530**:123–130.
11. Bowman AJ, Chen CP, Ford GA: Nitric oxide mediated venodilator effects of nebivolol. *Br J Clin Pharmacol* 1994, **38**:199–204.
12. Ignarro LJ: Experimental evidences of nitric oxide-dependent vasodilatory activity of nebivolol, a third-generation beta-blocker. *Blood Press* 2004, **1**:2–16.
13. Mason RP, Kubant R, Jacob RF, Walter MF, Boychuk B, Malinski T: Effect of nebivolol on endothelial nitric oxide and peroxynitrite release in hypertensive animals: Role of antioxidant activity. *J Cardiovas Pharmacol* 2006, **48**:862–869.
14. Cockcroft JR: Exploring vascular benefits of endothleium-derived nitric oxide. *Am J Hypertens* 2005, **18**:177S–183S.
15. Georgescu A, Pluteanu F, Flonta ML, Badila E, Dorobantu M, Popov D: The cellular mechanisms involved in the vasodilator effect of nebivolol on the renal artery. *Eur J Pharmacol* 2005, **508**:159–166.
16. Tzemos N, Lim PO, MacDonald TM: Nebivolol reverses endothelial dysfunction in essential hypertension: A randomized, double-blind, crossover study. *Circulation* 2001, **104**:511–514.
17. Kalinowski L, Dobrucki LW, Szczepanska-Konkel M, Jankowski M, Martyniec L, Angilieski S, Malinski T: Third-generation b-blockers stimulate nitric oxide release from endothelial cells through ATP efflux: a novel mechanism for antihypertensive action. *Circulation* 2003, **107**:2747–2752.
18. Dessy C, Saliez J, Ghisdal P, Daneau G, Lobysheva II, Frerart F, Belge C, Jnaoui K, Noirhomme P, Feron O, Balligand JL: Endothelial beta3-adrenoreceptors mediate nitric oxide-dependent vasorelaxation of coronary microvessels in response to the third-generation beta-blocker nebivolol. *Circulation* 2005, **112**:1198–1205.
19. Rozec B, Erfanian M, Laurent K, Trochu JN, Gauthier C: Nebivolol, a vasodilating selective beta(1)-blocker, is a beta(3)-adrenoceptor agonist in the nonfailing transplanted human heart. *J Am Coll Cardiol* 2009, **53**:1532–1538.
20. Sorrentino SA, Doerries C, Manes C, Speer T, Dessy C, Lobysheva I, Mohmand W, Akbur R, Bahlmann F, Besler C, Schaefer A, Hilfiker-Kleiner D, Luscher TF, Balligand JL, Drexler H, Landmesser U: Nebivolol exerts beneficial effects on endothelial function, early endothelial progenitor cells, myocardial neovascularization, and left ventricular dysfunction early after myocardial infarction beyond conventional beta1-blockade. *J Am Coll Cardiol* 2011, **57**:601–611.
21. Mason RP, Kalinowski L, Jacob RF, Jacoby AM, Malinski T: Nebivolol reduces nitroxidative stress and restores nitric oxide bioavailability in endothelium of black Americans. *Circulation* 2005, **112**:3795–3801.
22. Mollnau H, Schulz E, Daiber A, Baldus S, Oelze M, August M, Wendt M, Walter U, Geiger C, Agrawal R, Kleschyov AL, Meinertz T, Munzel T: Nebivolol prevents vascular NOS III uncoupling in experimental hyperlipidemia and inhibits NADPH oxidase activity in inflammatory cells. *Arterioscler Thromb Vasc Biol* 2003, **23**:615–621.
23. Mason RP, Kubant R, Jacob RF, Malinski P, Huang X, Louka FR, Borowic J, Mizudo Y, Malinski T: Loss of arterial and renal nitric oxide bioavailability in hypertensive rats with diabetes. *Am J Hypertens* 2009, **22**:1160–1166.
24. Malinski T, Taha Z: Nitric oxide release from a single cell measured in situ by a porphyrinic-based microsensor. *Nature* 1992, **358**:676–678.
25. Janssen PM, Zeitz O, Hasenfuss G: Transient and sustained impacts of hydroxyl radicals on sarcoplasmic reticulum function: protective effect of nebivolol. *Eur J Pharmacol* 1999, **366**:223–323.
26. Flather MD, Shibata MC, Coats AJ, Van Veldhuisen DJ, Parkhomenko A, Borbola J, Cohen-Solal A, Dumitrascu D, Ferrari R, Lechat P, Soler-Soler J, Tavazzi L, Spinarova L, Toman J, Bohm M, Anker SD, Thompson SG, Poole-Wilson PA: Randomized trial to determine the effect of nebivolol on mortality and cardiovascular hospital admission in elderly patients with heart failure (SENIORS). *Eur Heart J* 2005, **26**:215–225.
27. Kalinowski L, Dobrucki LW, Brovkovych V, Malinski T: Increased nitric oxide bioavailability in endothelial cells contributes to the pleiotropic effect of cerivastatin. *Circulation* 2002, **105**:933–938.

7

Olanzapine in pregnancy and breastfeeding: a review of data from global safety surveillance

Elizabeth Brunner*†, Deborah M Falk†, Meghan Jones†, Debashish K Dey† and Chetan Chinmaya Shatapathy†

Abstract

Background: Olanzapine use has been reported during pregnancy and breastfeeding, but there are no controlled clinical trials assessing the safety of olanzapine exposure to infants and fetuses. The purpose of this report was to review and analyze prospective post-marketing cases of pregnancy and breastfeeding with olanzapine, in order to guide clinicians and women on the use of olanzapine therapy during pregnancy and/or breastfeeding.

Methods: A worldwide safety database maintained by Eli Lilly and Company was searched for all spontaneous-reported data regarding olanzapine use during pregnancy and/or breastfeeding. Cases reported prior to pregnancy outcome were considered to be prospective, and follow-up was pursued after the delivery date to assess outcome.

Results: Outcome data were available for 610 prospectively identified pregnancies during which olanzapine was used. The majority of women had normal births (66%), although premature births were reported in 9.8% and perinatal conditions in 8% of the pregnancies. A total of 102 pregnancies reported olanzapine treatment during breastfeeding. In these infants, the most commonly reported adverse events were somnolence (3.9%), irritability (2%), tremor (2%), and insomnia (2%), although the majority of pregnancies reported no adverse events (82.3%).

Conclusions: The frequency of fetal outcomes in these prospectively identified pregnancies exposed to olanzapine did not differ from rates of outcomes reported in the general population. These data may be useful to help guide clinicians and women decide to continue, or discontinue, olanzapine therapy during pregnancy and/or breastfeeding, but should be considered within the limitations associated with spontaneously reported data. Women should notify their clinicians if they become pregnant or intend to become pregnant while being treated with olanzapine. Because of limited experience in humans, olanzapine should be used in pregnancy only when potential benefit justifies potential risk to the fetus. Olanzapine should only be considered during breastfeeding when the potential benefit justifies the potential risk to the infant.

Keywords: Olanzapine, Breastfeeding, Pregnancy

Background

Women with psychiatric conditions may become pregnant, and motherhood is common in such women: in one sample, 63% of women with psychotic disorders were mothers [1]. Women with psychotic disorders who are pregnant or breastfeeding are often treated with antipsychotics [2]. Due to ethical constraints restricting inclusion of pregnant and breastfeeding women in clinical trials, there is a paucity of data available on the use of antipsychotic drugs in this population. The current literature on antipsychotic use during pregnancy and breastfeeding

stems from case reports and large, uncontrolled reports of prospective and retrospective data [3,4], making it difficult to draw conclusions concerning the safety of these medications for the mother and child. Adverse outcomes during pregnancy, delivery, post-natal care as well as birth defects, and perinatal complications have been reported in patients treated with antipsychotics [4].

Women with schizophrenia and bipolar disorder have a greater likelihood of complications, including placental abnormalities; hemorrhaging; fetal distress; congenital anomalies, such as cardiovascular defects; and neonatal complications [5]. Additionally, cessation of antipsychotic treatment for women with psychotic disorders may increase the risk of relapse, which in turn could lead to

* Correspondence: ebrunner@lilly.com
†Equal contributors
Eli Lilly and Company, Lilly Corporate Center, Indianapolis, Indiana 46285, USA

poor pre- and post-natal care as well as obstetric-related adverse events [4]. Therefore, clinicians and women must carefully weigh the benefits and the risks of remaining on or terminating antipsychotic treatment.

Olanzapine has been shown to be effective for treating the symptoms of schizophrenia and bipolar disorder in adults and schizophrenia and acute manic or mixed episodes associated with bipolar disorder in adolescents [6-10]. There have been reports about the safety of olanzapine in the fetus and infant, with some cases reporting normal births without complications and others reporting adverse outcomes, such as differences in birth weight [11] and neural development [2]. In preclinical trials, prenatal treatment with olanzapine did not disrupt spatial memory and short-term memory in rats, whereas other antipsychotics did [12].

In the absence of adequate and well-controlled clinical trials, spontaneous post-marketing adverse event data provides information on the safety of treatment with antipsychotic medications during pregnancy and breastfeeding. Spontaneous post-marketing data typically involve a much greater number of exposures to a much broader population of patients compared with data from clinical trials. This is particularly true in this population (women who are pregnant or breastfeeding), since pregnant women are excluded from clinical trials. However, this should be considered within the limitations associated with spontaneously reported data, which may sometimes under represent the true incidence of events, as not all patients or clinicians report pregnancies and their outcomes to Eli Lilly and Company. Here we present prospectively collected data from Eli Lilly and Company's safety database including spontaneous reports, clinical trial cases, and post-marketing observational study reports, regarding the use of olanzapine during pregnancy and/or breastfeeding.

Methods
Database
Eli Lilly and Company (Lilly) has maintained a worldwide safety database of all adverse events reported to Lilly relative to treatment with products marketed by Lilly since 1983. This database consists of all spontaneous adverse events—regardless of severity—reported in patients treated with olanzapine (including data from published literature and regulatory agency reports), and serious adverse event reports from clinical trials and post-marketing studies. Additionally, the database contains reports of olanzapine use during pregnancy and/or breastfeeding, even if no adverse outcome was reported. Cases are entered into the database regardless of the reporter type (e.g., healthcare provider, patient), concomitant medications or medical co-morbidities, or consideration of the potential relationship between olanzapine treatment and the outcome. In the cases that

were reported from clinical trials (the minority of cases), the institutional review boards approved the protocols for all these trials and studies were conducted in accordance with ethical principles of Good Clinical Practice and the Declaration of Helsinki and its guidelines. This review was a retrospective analysis of data from the Lilly Safety Database (the Lilly Safety Database is the global database application used for the collection, storage, and reporting of adverse events to regulatory agencies, investigators, and internal departments). The information that was prospectively collected is derived from spontaneously reported pregnancies. In all cases, the initial contact to Lilly is made by the reporter. Lilly then sends a letter and a questionnaire requesting additional information. When information is not provided directly by the patient, Lilly also requests the patient's consent for release of medical information. Authorizations were not possible to obtain from patients who did not provide any follow-up information. Since the population in this review consists of pregnancies with prospective follow-up data, subjects without any follow-up information were not included in this review. Ethical or Institutional Review Board approval is not mandated (as opposed to prospectively collected data for study purposes from clinical trial participants).

Reports of olanzapine exposure during pregnancy were categorized based on when the report was received relative to the report of the pregnancy outcome. For prospective pregnancy cases (in which the olanzapine exposure was reported before the report of the pregnancy outcome), each reporter was contacted after the expected delivery date for outcomes. Retrospective reports were not used to calculate frequency of pregnancy outcomes for comparison with the general population, since not all olanzapine exposures resulting in pregnancy, nor all outcomes of pregnancy, are reported.

Definitions
An event represents a clinical sign, symptom, or syndrome reported for a single reported outcome; therefore, more than one event may occur in a patient or the patient's child. Normal birth was defined as birth between 37 and 42 weeks of gestation, or at an undefined gestation time with no reported abnormalities; premature birth was defined as birth before 37 weeks of gestation; and post-term birth was defined as birth after 42 weeks of gestation.

As per the World Health Organization (WHO), 'Congenital anomalies, also known as birth defects, are structural or functional abnormalities, including metabolic disorders, which are present from birth. Congenital anomalies are a diverse group of disorders of prenatal origin which can be caused by single gene defects, chromosomal disorders, multifactorial inheritance, environmental teratogens and micronutrient deficiencies [13].

Perinatal condition was defined as an adverse event occurring within 7 days of birth, and post-perinatal condition was defined as an adverse event occurring any time after 7 days post-birth. Elective termination was defined as a planned abortion with no anomalies; therapeutic abortion as a planned abortion due to medical reasons; and a spontaneous abortion as a failure of embryonic development, fetal death in utero, or expulsion of any of all or part of the product of conception before the 20th week of gestation or a fetal weight of <500 grams. Stillbirth was defined as death of the fetus at any time after the 20th week of gestation, with no breathing or other evidence of life after birth, and may also be referred to as intrauterine death. Neonates born at 37 to 42 weeks' gestation, or at an unspecified gestation, with no reported adverse events were considered full term. Neonates born before 37 weeks' gestation were considered premature, while neonates born after 42 weeks of gestation were considered post-term.

After birth, neonates were classified as normal if there were no issues noted. A congenital anomaly was defined as a tissue malformation seen in a neonate, born at 37 to 42 weeks' gestation, or at an unspecified gestation, with a congenital anomaly noted at birth, or a report of a therapeutic abortion due to congenital anomalies in the fetus. A perinatal condition was defined as an adverse event (not considered to be a congenital anomaly) that occurred within 7 days of birth in neonates born at 37 to 42 weeks' gestation or at an unspecified gestation. A post-perinatal condition was defined as an adverse event (not considered to be a congenital anomaly) that occurred after 7 days of birth in neonates born at 37 to 42 weeks' gestation or at an unspecified gestation age.

Analysis

The safety database was searched for all reports of pregnancy and breastfeeding in temporal association with treatment with olanzapine occurring from first (10 September 1986) human dose in a clinical trial through 31 December 2010. Pregnancy outcomes, as well as trimester of olanzapine exposure, were analyzed through 31 December 2010. Qualitative comparisons were made between this dataset and historic reports from the general population on rates of outcomes of and during pregnancy, delivery, and fetal outcomes (see Table 1) [14-24].

Results

Pregnancy outcomes

Through 31 December 2010, there were 610 prospectively identified pregnancies with an available outcome reported and included in this analysis. In addition, 73 cases reported an elective termination without a fetal anomaly, and were not included in the analysis. Maternal oral olanzapine dose was reported in 535 of 610 (87.7%) pregnancies and oral olanzapine doses ranged from 0.6 mg/day to 35.0 mg/day,

with a mean dose of 10.3 mg/day. Intramuscular injections were reported in several cases (<1%) with reported maternal doses within the labeled dose range.

Of the 610 prospectively identified pregnancies exposed to olanzapine with an available outcome, there were 401 (66%) normal births, 60 (9.8%) premature births, 57 (9.3%) spontaneous abortions, 49 (8%) perinatal conditions, 27 (4.4%) congenital anomalies, and 16 (2.6%) other (post-perinatal condition, ectopic pregnancy, post-term birth, and stillbirth). There did not appear to be an increased risk of spontaneous abortion, ectopic pregnancy, stillbirth, premature or post-term birth, or congenital anomalies in pregnant women treated with olanzapine compared with historic control rates in the general population (Table 1). Given the well-known limitations of the data under review, the findings need to be interpreted with caution.

The timing of exposure to olanzapine during pregnancy was reported in 594 (97.4%) of the prospectively reported cases. Of these, the majority reported olanzapine exposure either during all three trimesters 263 (44.3%) or in the first trimester only 187 (31.5%). Approximately 47.1% (189/401) of women experiencing normal births were exposed to olanzapine during all three trimesters. The majority of women who experienced spontaneous abortions were exposed to olanzapine during the first trimester only (50/57, 87.7%). Approximately half of the women who experienced premature (27/60, 45%) or post-mature births (3/5, 60%) were treated with olanzapine throughout pregnancy. Among women who experienced perinatal conditions, 63.3% (31/49) were exposed to olanzapine for all three trimesters and 6.1% (3/49) were exposed to olanzapine during the third trimester only (Table 2). Forty-three percent of women reported continuation of treatment with olanzapine during all three trimesters of their pregnancy (Table 2). In patients who continued olanzapine treatment throughout all three trimesters, 71.9% had normal births. Exposure during only the first trimester of pregnancy was reported in 30.7% of pregnancies.

Of the prospectively identified pregnancies with an available reported outcome, 27 (4.4%) reported congenital anomalies; this risk did not appear to be greater in the population being treated with olanzapine compared with the general population (Table 1).

Breastfeeding

In women being treated with olanzapine while breastfeeding, from spontaneous reports, clinical trial cases, and post-marketing observational study reports, (N=102), 62 pregnancies included olanzapine dose information: doses ranged from 2.5 to 20.0 mg/day, with a mean dose of 7.4 mg/day. All reported an oral dose form. Duration of olanzapine exposure during breastfeeding was reported in

Table 1 Fetal outcomes in prospectively identified olanzapine-exposed pregnancies, compared to rates in the general population[†]

Fetal outcome	Outcome reported (%) (N=610)	Historic control rate in general population (%)
Spontaneous abortion	57 (9.3%)[g]	10% to 20% [19,20]
Ectopic pregnancy	3 (0.5%)	1.3% to 2.1% [21-23]
Normal birth[a]	401 (65.7%)	61% to 64% [24]
Premature[b]	60 (9.8%)	12.8% [25]
Post-term[c]	5 (0.8%)	5.6% [25]
Stillbirth	5 (0.8%)[h]	0.5% to 1.1%[i] [26,27]
Congenital anomaly[d]	27 (4.4%)	3.0% to 5.0% [28,29]
Perinatal condition[e]	49 (8.0%)	[j]
Post-perinatal condition[f]	3 (0.5%)	[j]

[a] Includes neonates born at 37–42 weeks' gestation, or at an unspecified gestation.
[b] Includes neonates born <37 weeks' gestation or reported as "premature."
[c] Includes neonates born >42 weeks or reported as "post-term."
[d] Includes neonates born at 37–42 weeks' gestation or at an unspecified gestation with a congenital abnormality (resulting from abnormal tissue formation) at birth, and reports of therapeutic abortions due to congenital abnormalities in the fetus.
[e] Includes neonates born at 37–42 weeks' gestation or at an unspecified gestation with adverse event ≤7 days of birth.
[f] Includes neonates born at 37–42 weeks' gestation or at an unspecified gestation with an adverse event >7 days after birth.
[g] Includes one report of a congenital anomaly in a 13-week aborted fetus.
[h] Includes one report of a normal fetus who died when the mother committed suicide at 8 months' gestation.
[i] Indicates range when stratified by race/ethnicity.
[j] Due to the specific definitions (gestation and adverse events in a timeframe after birth), historical population rates are not available.
[†] Clinical trial and spontaneous reports from the Lilly worldwide safety database (First human dose through 31 December 2010).

30 pregnancies, and ranged from 2 days to 13 months, with a mean exposure of 74 days, and a median exposure of 30 days. In a study in lactating, healthy women taking oral olanzapine, olanzapine was excreted in breast milk. Mean infant exposure (mg/kg) at steady state was estimated to be 1.8% of the maternal olanzapine dose (mg/kg) [25]. In the olanzapine safety database, there were no adverse events reported in the neonate/infant in the majority (82.3%) of pregnancies that reported breastfeeding during olanzapine treatment. A total of 15.6% of the pregnancies reported an adverse event in the neonate or infant in temporal association with breastfeeding. The most commonly reported adverse events included somnolence (3.9%), irritability (2%), tremor (2%), and insomnia (2%). Outcomes of these events noted in the neonate/infant were reported as recovered/recovering in 40% of the events, as not recovered in 24% of the events, and as unknown in 36% of the events.

Discussion

Through 31 December 2010, it is estimated that more than 33 million patients were treated with olanzapine. Based on the analysis of prospectively reported pregnancy where there was an outcome available, 66% of the outcomes of women treated with olanzapine at any time during pregnancy were normal. This rate of normal birth outcomes is comparable to that of the general population, which ranges from 61% to 64% [19]. Premature births (9.8%) and spontaneous abortion (9.3%) rates in this dataset were comparable to those of the

general population (12.8% [20] and 10% to 20% [14,15], respectively).

Prospective reports are subject to fewer reporting biases compared with retrospective reports [26]. Women whose children have major birth defects (abnormality that can affect the structure or function of an organ) are more likely to report the outcome, compared with women who have healthy babies [27]. Prospectively collected information provides more details about a case and helps to provide a risk estimate [28], whereas retrospective reports may be susceptible to systematic recall bias and underestimation of exposure to maternal psychiatric illness and non-psychotropic agents [29], and cannot be used in the calculation of outcome rates [30]. In addition, prospective cohorts are able to include specific variables, and the data can be collected with more reliability and accuracy [31], thus providing an opportunity to obtain follow-up information, and a more accurate ascertainment of exposure during pregnancy and in the perinatal period. Therefore, in this population, prospective reports were used to calculate frequency of pregnancy outcomes for comparison to the general population.

The risk of unfavorable outcomes in neonates and infants whose mothers were treated with olanzapine during pregnancy in this dataset did not appear to differ from that of the general population. This information is complementary to the findings of a previous prospective study of pregnancy outcomes in patients treated with atypical antipsychotics. The defects in the infant of the olanzapine-treated patient included the midline defects

Table 2 Trimester of olanzapine exposure in prospectively identified pregnancies by outcome from Lilly Worldwide Safety Database[†]

Pregnancy outcome	Outcomes reported by trimester(s) of exposure to Olanzapine (n)								
	1st only	2nd only	3rd only	1st & 2nd	1 & 3rd	2nd & 3rd	All	Unknown	Total
Normal birth[a]	109	14	18	37	7	21	189	6	**401**
Full-term	96	12	17	33	6	20	169	4	**357**
Unknown gestation	13	2	1	4	1	1	20	2	**44**
Spontaneous abortion[a]	50	1	0	4	0	0	0	2	**57[g]**
Ectopic pregnancy	3	0	0	0	0	0	0	0	**3**
Premature[b]	11	1	2	4	1	11	27	3	**60**
Normal	7	1	0	3	1	8	18	3	**41**
Congenital anomaly	2	0	0	0	0	0	2	0	**4**
Perinatal condition	2	0	2	1	0	3	7	0	**15**
Post-term[c]	0	0	2	0	0	0	3	0	**5**
Normal	0	0	2	0	0	0	1	0	**3**
Perinatal condition	0	0	0	0	0	0	2	0	**2**
Stillbirth	0	0	0	0	0	1	4	0	**5[h]**
Congenital anomaly[d]	3	1	2	4	0	7	8	2	**27**
Full-term	2	1	2	1	0	4	8	0	**18**
Unknown gestation	0	0	0	2	0	3	0	2	**7**
Therapeutic abortion	1	0	0	1	0	0	0	0	**2**
Perinatal condition[e]	9	0	3	2	0	1	31	3	**49**
Full-term	8	0	3	1	0	1	28	3	**44**
Unknown gestation	1	0	0	1	0	0	3	0	**5**
Post-perinatal condition[f]	2	0	0	0	0	0	1	0	**3**
Full-term	2	0	0	0	0	0	1	0	**3**
Totals	**187**	**17**	**27**	**51**	**8**	**41**	**263**	**16**	**610**

[a] Includes neonates born at 37–42 weeks' gestation, or at an unspecified gestation.
[b] Includes neonates born <37 weeks' gestation or reported as "premature."
[c] Includes neonates born >42 weeks' or reported as "post-term."
[d] Includes neonates born at 37–42 weeks' gestation or at an unspecified gestation with a congenital abnormality (resulting from abnormal tissue formation) at birth, and reports of therapeutic abortions due to congenital abnormalities in the fetus.
[e] Includes neonates born at 37–42 weeks' gestation or at an unspecified gestation with an adverse event ≤7 days after birth.
[f] Includes neonates born at 37–42 weeks' gestation or at an unspecified gestation with an adverse event >7 days after birth.
[g] Includes one report of a congenital anomaly in a 13-week aborted fetus.
[h] Includes one normal fetus who died when the mother committed suicide at 8 months' gestation.
[†] First Human Dose through 31 December 2010 (Data on file).

of cleft lip, encephalocele, and aqueductal stenosis. Yet all these events occurred in one child of an olanzapine-treated mother, compared with none in the other treatment groups [2]. Given the well-known limitations of the data under review, the findings need to be interpreted with caution.

Other congenital defects, including meningocele/ankyloblepharon [32], hip dysplasia [33], acheiria [34], and atrioventricular canal defect/unilateral clubfoot [35], have been reported in infants exposed to olanzapine in utero.

In a postmarketing safety database assessment of 68 prospective pregnancies, spontaneously reported with a known outcome in women who received risperidone [3], 37 pregnancies reported a normal outcome. Organ malformations were reported in 3.8% of the reports and

spontaneous abortions in 16.9% of the reports. The denominator used was subtracting the number of induced abortions (predominantly undertaken for nonmedical reasons) from the total 68 reports. In utero exposure to risperidone does not appear to increase the risk of spontaneous abortions, structural malformations, and fetal teratogenic risk above that of the general population.

In a prospective, controlled cohort study of 215 pregnancies in women exposed to haloperidol or penfluridol [36], rates of major abnormalities were compared to a control group of pregnancies (N=631) exposed to non-teratogenic agents reported to a European counseling center. Compared to the controlled group, the women treated with antipsychotics were older; and a significantly higher proportion smoked 5 or more cigarettes a day. No differences were noted in the number of previous miscarriages, number of pregnancies, history of elective terminations, or gestational age at first contact. No differences were observed between the antipsychotic-exposed group and the control group in the rates of major malformations (3.4% vs. 3.8% respectively) or in the rates of major malformations in live births with first trimester exposure (3.1% vs. 3.8% respectively). There were statistically significant differences observed between the antipsychotic-exposed group and the control group in the rates of delivery (81.9% vs. 90.3% respectively), elective termination of pregnancy (8.8% vs. 3.8% respectively), preterm birth (13.9% vs. 6.9% respectively), Cesarean section (25.5% vs. 16.3% respectively), and in the median gestational age [interquartile range] at delivery (40 [38-40] vs. 40 [39-41] weeks respectively), median birthweight [interquartile range] (3155 [2800–3500] vs. 3370 [3030–3700] g respectively), and median birthweight [interquartile range] of full-term infants (3250 [3000–3590] vs. 3415 [3140–3750] g respectively).

In this dataset, 66% of births were classified as normal births; premature births occurred in 9.8% of pregnancies. This is not consistent with the findings of Newham et al. [37], who found higher rates of premature births in infants whose mothers were treated with typical antipsychotics compared with a non-medicated reference group, although there was no significant difference between the atypical antipsychotic and the reference groups. This analysis, as ours, did not control for concomitant mediations or other potential confounders, which may have potentially affected gestational age.

Although this analysis did not examine birth weight, previous studies have found higher rates of low birth weight (31%) and neonatal intensive care unit admission (31%) reported in neonates whose mothers were treated with olanzapine during pregnancy compared with neonates of mothers who were treated with other atypical antipsychotics [11], although the differences were not statistically significant. Another study found that infants born to mothers who were treated with olanzapine or clozapine during pregnancy had significantly higher birth weights compared with infants of mothers who were treated with typical antipsychotics [37].

One study examining placental passage (defined as the ratio of umbilical cord to maternal plasma concentration) of antipsychotics found that olanzapine concentrations in the placenta were 72% of the mother's, which was significantly greater compared with concentrations of haloperidol, quetiapine, and risperidone [11]. However, another study reported the rate of placental passage of olanzapine to be much lower (17%) [38]. Potential fetal exposure to olanzapine should be taken into consideration when weighing the benefits and risks of remaining on olanzapine therapy.

Infant exposure to olanzapine via breast milk of olanzapine-treated mothers was lower than exposure in utero. Adverse events were reported in 15.6% of infants who were exposed to olanzapine through breast milk, and the most common events included somnolence, irritability, tremor, and insomnia. This differs from several studies of olanzapine in which either no adverse events were noted [39-43], or the types of adverse events (e.g., respiratory difficulties and hypotonia) were different [44]. The safety profile of olanzapine is based on exposures to the drug in adults and adolescents, the safety profile of exposure through uterus, during early and late developmental stages or via breast milk is likely to differ. Gilad et al. [44] found that the rate of adverse events in olanzapine-exposed breastfed infants were not statistically significantly different from infants not exposed to olanzapine.

The information reviewed in the current paper was voluntarily reported by (or on behalf of) the patient (spontaneous adverse event reports). There are several, well-known limitations to spontaneously reported data. Spontaneous reporting of adverse events may be highly variable [45]: clinicians may be less likely to report adverse events that are not serious or have been seen in the general population; this may skew the data toward more serious adverse events. Similarly, the information collected may lack details in particular key information, such as concurrent treatments, relevant medical history, and long-term follow-up of infant developmental outcomes. The data reported here included all reported cases regardless of concomitant medications, relevant medical co-morbidities, and potential causal relationship to olanzapine exposure. Since this is not a clinical trial, data are not collected like they typically are in a clinical trial or in a prospective observational study where there is a defined protocol. The follow-up rate cannot be calculated from spontaneously reported data as there is no pre-defined duration of follow-up for individual patient reports. Moreover, due to the nature of spontaneous reporting, and given the process of soliciting and obtaining follow-up information, a follow-up rate often does not provide an informative assessment of the completeness and accuracy of the follow-up. Although follow-up information may have been received, often the most relevant follow-up is the outcome of pregnancy/breastfeeding, which may not always be available. In addition, it is not possible to confirm the exact trimester in which the patients were exposed to olanzapine from spontaneously reported data. In summary, spontaneous data alone are not adequate to make definitive conclusions regarding the potential risk of adverse events following exposure to olanzapine.

Based on reports from the Adverse Event Reporting System (AERS), the Food and Drug Administration's (FDA) computerized information database designed to monitor for new adverse events and support post-marketing safety surveillance for approved drugs, various major regulatory agencies recently updated the prescribing information label language of all antipsychotics regarding use during pregnancy, informing of the potential risk of abnormal muscle movements (extrapyramidal signs) and/or withdrawal symptoms in neonates whose mothers were treated with antipsychotics during the third trimester of pregnancy [46]. It is important to assess the risks and benefits of treating women who are pregnant or breastfeeding with antipsychotics, and weigh these against possible risks of anomalies and developmental problems to the fetus and infant.

Conclusions

There are no controlled studies for the use of olanzapine therapy in pregnant women or in women who are breastfeeding. Given the well-known limitations of data under review, the findings need to be interpreted with caution. The relative risks and benefits of olanzapine treatment during pregnancy and/or breastfeeding should be carefully weighed by the clinician and the patient on a case-by-case basis. Because of limited experience in humans, olanzapine should be used in pregnancy only when potential benefit justifies potential risk to the fetus [25]. Olanzapine should only be considered during breastfeeding when the potential benefit justifies the potential risk to the infant. Women should be advised to notify their clinician if they become pregnant or intend to become pregnant during treatment with olanzapine. Presently, data are not sufficient to make definitive conclusions regarding the safety of olanzapine therapy during pregnancy and/or breastfeeding. However, acknowledging the limitations of the existing data, our review found that the frequency of fetal outcomes in prospectively identified pregnancies exposed to olanzapine did not differ from rates of outcomes reported in the general population. In the absence of data from clinical trials, the current analysis of post-marketing data attempts to provide greater information about the safety of olanzapine exposure during pregnancy and/or breastfeeding.

Competing interests
All authors are employees and stockholders of Eli Lilly and Company.

Authors' contributions
All authors (EB, DF, MJ, DD, and CS) have contributed to the conception and planning of the work that led to the manuscript, analysis and interpretation of the data, and drafting and critical revision of the manuscript for intellectual content. All authors read and approved the final manuscript.

Acknowledgements
We thank Deborah N. D'Souza, PhD who provided medical writing support on behalf of Eli Lilly and Company.

References

1. Howard LM, Kumar R, Thornicroft G: Psychosocial characteristics and needs of mothers with psychotic disorders. Br J Psychiatry 2001, 178:427–32.
2. McKenna K, Koren G, Tetelbaum M, Wilton L, Shakir S, Diav-Citrin O, Levinson A, Zipursky RB, Einarson A: Pregnancy outcome of women using atypical antipsychotic drugs: a prospective comparative study. J Clin Psychiatry 2005, 66:444–449.
3. Coppola D, Russo LJ, Kwarta RF Jr, Varughese R, Schmider J: Evaluating the postmarketing experience of risperidone use during pregnancy: pregnancy and neonatal outcomes. Drug Saf 2007, 30:247–264.
4. Gentile S: Antipsychotic therapy during early and late pregnancy. A systematic review. Schizophr Bull 2010, 36:518–544.
5. Jablensky AV, Morgan V, Zubrick SR, Bower C, Yellachich LA: Pregnancy delivery, and neonatal complications in a population cohort of women with schizophrenia and major affective disorders. Am J Psychiatry 2005, 162:79–91.
6. Beasley CM Jr, Sanger T, Satterlee W, Tollefson G, Tran P, Hamilton S: Olanzapine versus placebo: results of a double-blind, fixed-dose olanzapine trial. Psychopharmacology (Berl) 1996, 124:159–167.
7. Tohen M, Zhang F, Keck PE, Feldman PD, Risser RC, Tran PV, Breier A: Olanzapine versus haloperidol in schizoaffective disorder, bipolar type. J Affect Disord 2001, 67:133–140.
8. Tohen M, Kryzhanovskaya L, Carlson G, Delbello M, Wozniak J, Kowatch R, Wagner K, Findling R, Lin D, Robertson-Plouch C, Xu W, Dittmann RW, Biederman J: Olanzapine versus placebo in the treatment of adolescents with bipolar mania. Am J Psychiatry 2007, 164:1547–1556.
9. Kryzhanovskaya L, Schulz SC, McDougle C, Frazier J, Dittmann R, Robertson-Plouch C, Bauer T, Xu W, Wang W, Carlson J, Tohen M: Olanzapine versus placebo in adolescents with schizophrenia: a 6-week, randomized, double-blind, placebo-controlled trial. J Am Acad Child Adolesc Psychiatry 2009, 48:60–70.
10. Kryzhanovskaya LA, Robertson-Plouch CK, Xu W, Carlson JL, Merida KM, Dittmann RW: The safety of olanzapine in adolescents with schizophrenia or bipolar I disorder: a pooled analysis of 4 clinical trials. J Clin Psychiatry 2009, 70:247–258.
11. Newport DJ, Calamaras MR, DeVane CL, Donovan J, Beach AJ, Winn S, Knight BT, Gibson BB, Viguera AC, Owens MJ, Nemeroff CB, Stowe ZN: Atypical antipsychotic administration during late pregnancy: placental passage and obstetrical outcomes. Am J Psychiatry 2007, 164:1214–1220.
12. Rosengarten H, Quartermain D: Effect of prenatal administration of haloperidol, risperidone, quetiapine and olanzapine on spatial learning and retention in adult rats. Pharmacol Biochem Behav 2002, 72:575–579.
13. World Health Organization: Congenital anomalies. ; 2013. http://www.who.int/topics/congenital_anomalies/en/index.html.
14. American College of Obstetricians and Gynecologists: ACOG practice bulletin. Management of recurrent pregnancy loss. Number 24, February 2001. (Replaces Technical Bulletin Number 212, September 1995). American College of Obstetricians and Gynecologists. Int J Gynaecol Obstet 2002, 78:179–190.
15. Shields KE, Wiholm BE, Hostelley LS, Striano LF, Arena SR, Sharrar RG: Monitoring outcomes of pregnancy following drug exposure. Drug Saf 2004, 27:353–367.
16. Van Den Eeden SK, Shan J, Bruce C, Glasser M: Ectopic pregnancy rate and treatment utilization in a large managed care organization. Obstet Gynecol 2005, 105:1052–1057.
17. Farquhar CM: Ectopic pregnancy. Lancet 2005, 366:583–591.
18. Centers for Disease Control and Prevention (CDC): Ectopic pregnancy – United States, 1990 1992. MMWR Morb Mortal Wkly Rep 1995, 44:46–48.
19. Ventura SJ, Abma JC, Mosher WD, Henshaw SK: Estimated pregnancy rates by outcome for the United States, 1990–2004. Natl Vital Stat Rep 2008, 56:1–25. 28.
20. Heron M, Hoyert DL, Murphy SL, Xu J, Kochanek KD, Tejada-Vera B: Births: final data for 2006. Natl Vital Stat Rep 2009, 57:1–134.
21. MacDorman MF, Kirmeyer S: Fetal and perinatal mortality, United States, 2005. Natl Vital Stat Rep 2009, 57:1–19.
22. MacDorman MF, Kirmeyer S: The challenge of fetal mortality. NCHS Data Brief 2009, 16:1–8.

23. Centers for Disease Control: Update on overall prevalence of major birth defects – Atlanta, Georgia, 1978–2005. *MMWR Morb Mortal Wkly Rep* 2008, **57**:1–5.

24. Zhu JL, Basso O, Obel C, Bille C, Olsen J: Infertility, infertility treatment, and congenital malformations: Danish national birth cohort. *BMJ* 2006, **333**:679.

25. Eli Lilly and Company: *Zyprexa® (olanzapine) US prescribing information.* http://pi.lilly.com/us/zyprexa-pi.pdf.

26. Koren G, Pastuszak A, Ito S: Drugs in pregnancy. *N Engl J Med* 1998, **338**:1128–1137.

27. Bar-Oz B, Moretti ME, Mareels G, Van Tittelboom T, Koren G: Reporting bias in retrospective ascertainment of drug-induced embryopathy. *Lancet* 1999, **354**:1700–1701.

28. Rodriguez EM: *Guidance for industry establishing pregnancy registries. Pregnancy Registry Working Group Pregnancy Labeling Taskforce.* ; 2000. http://www.fda.gov/ohrms/dockets/ac/00/slides/3601s1e/sld001.htm.

29. Newport DJ, Brennan PA, Green P, Ilardi D, Whitfield TH, Morris N, Knight BT, Stowe ZN: Maternal depression and medication exposure during pregnancy: comparison of maternal retrospective recall to prospective documentation. *BJOG* 2008, **115**:681–688.

30. US Food and Drug Administration: *Reviewer Guidance: Evaluation of human pregnancy outcome data.* http://www.fda.gov/ohrms/dockets/98fr/991540gd.pdf.

31. Clark M: Retrospective versus prospective cohort study designs for evaluating treatment of pressure ulcers. A comparison of 2 studies. *J Wound Ostomy Continence Nurs* 2008, **35**:391–394.

32. Arora M, Praharaj SK: Meningocele and ankyloblepharon following in utero exposure to olanzapine. *Eur Psychiatry* 2006, **21**:345–346.

33. Spyropoulou AC, Zervas IM, Soldatos CR: Hip dysplasia following a case of olanzapine exposed pregnancy: a questionable association. *Arch Womens Ment Health* 2006, **9**:219–222.

34. Ramkisson R, Campbell M, Agius M: The clinical dilemma–prescribing in pregnancy. *Psychiatr Danub* 2008, **20**:88–90.

35. Yeshayahu Y: The use of olanzapine in pregnancy and congenital cardiac and musculoskeletal abnormalities. *Am J Psychiatry* 2007, **164**:1759–1760.

36. Diav-Citrin O, Schechtman S, Ornoy S, Arnon J, Schaefer C, Garbis H, Clementi M, Ornoy A: Safety of haloperidol and penfluridol in pregnancy: a multicenter, prospective, controlled study. *J Clin Psychiatry* 2005, **66**:317–322.

37. Newham JJ, Thomas SH, MacRitchie K, McElhatton PR, McAllister-Williams RH: Birth weight of infants after maternal exposure to typical and atypical antipsychotics: prospective comparison study. *Br J Psychiatry* 2008, **192**:333–337.

38. Schenker S, Yang Y, Mattiuz E, Tatum D, Lee M: Olanzapine transfer by human placenta. *Clin Exp Pharmacol Physiol* 1999, **26**:691–697.

39. Croke S, Buist A, Hackett LP, Ilett KF, Norman TR, Burrows GD: Olanzapine excretion in human breast milk: estimation of infant exposure. *Int J Neuropsychopharmacol* 2002, **5**:243–247.

40. Gardiner SJ, Kristensen JH, Begg EJ, Hackett LP, Wilson DA, Ilett KF, Kohan R, Rampono J: Transfer of olanzapine into breast milk, calculation of infant drug dose, and effect on breast-fed infants. *Am J Psychiatry* 2003, **160**:1428–1431.

41. Friedman SH, Rosenthal MB: Treatment of perinatal delusional disorder: a case report. *Int'l. J. Psychiatry in Medicine* 2003, **33**:391–394.

42. Lutz UC, Wiatr G, Orlikowsky T, Gaertner HJ, Bartels M: Olanzapine treatment during breast feeding: a case report. *Ther Drug Monit* 2008, **30**:399–401.

43. Whitworth A, Stuppaeck C, Yazdi K, Kralovec K, Geretsegger C, Zernig G, Alchhorn W: Olanzapine and breast-feeding: changes of plasma concentrations of olanzapine in a breast-fed infant over a period of 5 months. *J Psychopharmacol* 2010, **24**:121–123.

44. Gilad O, Merlob P, Stahl B, Klinger G: Outcome of infants exposed to olanzapine during breastfeeding. *Breastfeed Med* 2011, **6**:55–58.

45. Goldman SA: Limitations and strengths of spontaneous reports data. *Clin Ther* 1998, **20**(Suppl C):C40–C44.

46. US Food and Drug Administration: FDA Drug Safety Communication: *Antipsychotic drug labels updated on use during pregnancy and risk of abnormal muscle movements and withdrawal symptoms in newborns.* ; 2011. http://www.fda.gov/Drugs/DrugSafety/ucm243903.htm.

8

Polycomblike protein PHF1b: a transcriptional sensor for GABA receptor activity

Shamol Saha[1], Yinghui Hu[2†], Stella C Martin[1†], Sabita Bandyopadhyay[2], Shelley J Russek[2*] and David H Farb[1]

Abstract

Background: The γ-aminobutyric acid (GABA) type A receptor ($GABA_AR$) contains the recognition sites for a variety of agents used in the treatment of brain disorders, including anxiety and epilepsy. A better understanding of how receptor expression is regulated in individual neurons may provide novel opportunities for therapeutic intervention. Towards this goal we have studied transcription of a $GABA_AR$ subunit gene (*GABRB1*) whose activity is autologously regulated by GABA via a 10 base pair initiator-like element (β_1-INR).

Methods: By screening a human cDNA brain library with a yeast one-hybrid assay, the Polycomblike (PCL) gene product PHD finger protein transcript b (PHF1b) was identified as a β_1-INR associated protein. Promoter/reporter assays in primary rat cortical cells demonstrate that PHF1b is an activator at *GABRB1*, and chromatin immunoprecipitation assays reveal that presence of PHF1 at endogenous *Gabrb1* is regulated by $GABA_AR$ activation.

Results: PCL is a member of the Polycomb group required for correct spatial expression of homeotic genes in *Drosophila*. We now show that PHF1b recognition of β_1-INR is dependent on a plant homeodomain, an adjacent helix-loop-helix, and short glycine rich motif. In neurons, it co-immunoprecipitates with SUZ12, a key component of the Polycomb Repressive Complex 2 (PRC2) that regulates a number of important cellular processes, including gene silencing via histone H3 lysine 27 trimethylation (H3K27me3).

Conclusions: The observation that chronic exposure to GABA reduces PHF1 binding and H3K27 monomethylation, which is associated with transcriptional activation, strongly suggests that PHF1b may be a molecular transducer of $GABA_AR$ function and thus GABA-mediated neurotransmission in the central nervous system.

Background

The γ-aminobutyric acid (GABA) type A receptor ($GABA_AR$) plays a critical role in the pathophysiology of brain disorders such as anxiety and epilepsy, presenting an important therapeutic target for research. Of particular interest is the mechanism that underlies the expression of eight distinct $GABA_AR$ subunit classes whose collection of genes are differentially transcribed to form diverse receptor subtypes, with variable affinities for activation and modulation [1]. Variations in receptor subunit composition are also associated with different disease states. For instance, pilocarpine induces status epilepticus (SE) and spontaneous seizures in rats that are accompanied by a decrease in α_1 and β_1 subunit

mRNAs, and a marked increase in $\alpha4$ [2]. Recent reports using chromatin immunoprecipitation (ChIP) assays of primary neurons and slices of dentate gyrus from animals 24 hours after SE have shown that levels of these $GABA_A$ receptor subunits may be regulated by changes in transcription that are driven by activity-dependent transcription factors [3-6].

Most interesting to the study of $GABA_AR$ regulation is the fact that chronic activation leads to an associated decrease in the levels of particular $GABA_AR$ subunit mRNAs, their cognate proteins, and their promoter/reporter activity, as measured in primary cultured neurons and *in vivo*. While it is certainly well established that the majority of genes rely on upstream regulatory elements to control relevant levels of gene expression, our previous studies showed that an initiator (β_1 initiator element [INR]; a 10 base pair (bp) core sequence that contains the transcriptional start site of *GABRB1*) is critical for the expression of β_1 subunit mRNAs in neocortical and

* Correspondence: srussek@bu.edu

†Equal contributors

²Department of Pharmacology & Experimental Therapeutics, Laboratory of Translational Epilepsy, Boston University School of Medicine, 72 East Concord Street, Boston, MA 02118, USA

Full list of author information is available at the end of the article

hippocampal neurons [7]. In fact, sequential deletion of most of the *GABRB1* promoter (*GABRB1-p*) reveals that the initiator is indispensable for neuron-specific promoter activity that is autologously regulated (transcriptionally repressed after chronic GABA$_A$R activation). Replacing the core *GABRB1-p* with three concatenated copies of the β_1-INR reconstitutes full promoter/reporter activity that is both neural-specific and autologously regulated.

Transcriptional regulators function through DNA-protein or protein-protein interactions that regulate the recruitment and assembly of the pre-initiation complex (PIC), which contains RNA polymerase II and general transcription factors (GTFs), TFIID, B, A, E, F and H [8-11]. The TATA box is located nearly −30 nucleotides upstream of the transcription start site and directs the initiation of transcription and assembly of the general transcription apparatus [12]. The downstream INR contributes to start site selection and directs the transcriptional initiation of genes with non-canonical TATA boxes [13]. Although a number of INRs have been identified among mammalian genes, the initiator binding complex is poorly understood. RNA polymerase II recognizes core promoter sequences to influence start site selection at the core promoter [14,15]. TAF$_{II}$250 and TAF$_{II}$150 (TAFs 1 and 2) [16] contribute to the selective recognition of promoters containing INRs [17-21]. A number of transcriptional regulators such as TFII-I, E2F, YY1 and USF stimulate transcription by binding to sites that overlap core promoter sequences [12,22]. Specific INR-binding proteins like YY1 and TFII-I contain distinct motifs for DNA binding [23-25]. YY1 binds through two zinc finger (C2H2) domains [26] whereas TFII-I, a context-dependent DNA recognition protein, binds through multiple helix-loop-helix (HLH) motifs with the aid of a basic rich region [24].

Chromatin remodeling plays an important role in either facilitating or preventing RNA polymerase II access to promoter regions, targeting N-terminal histone tails for acetylation, methylation, phosphorylation and/or ubiquitination modification(s) [27-30]. Two groups of proteins are found to be involved in regulating the modification status of chromatin at promoter regions: Trithorax (trxG) and Polycomb-Group (PcG) proteins. Both protein groups maintain active and silent status of transcriptional activity, respectively [31,32]. PcG proteins are encoded by some 40 genes in *Drosophila*, which include Polycomb (PC), Polyhomeotic (PHO), Polycomblike (PCL) and Posterior sex comb (PSC). PcG proteins maintain promoters in an inactive state, whereas trxG proteins counteract silencing by stimulating transcription [28,32-34]. Recently, two main Polycomb groups of repressive complexes have been characterized: PRC1 and PRC2, which appear to form biochemically distinct repressive units. Four core components of PRC2 are EZH2, SUZ12, EED and RbAp46/48 [32] and

each protein in the complex has a distinct functional role in silencing transcriptional activity.

In this paper, we now show that PHF1b, a Polycomblike protein, binds to the β_1-INR to stimulate transcription. In addition, our results demonstrate that chronic GABA treatment reduces the presence of PHF and monomethylated histone H3 lysine 27 (H3K27) at endogenous rat *Gabrb1-p*, consistent with a role for PHF1b in remodeling the local chromatin environment of the core promoter region in response to neuronal signals.

Results

Isolation of a cDNA encoding an initiator-associated protein

To further understand neural-specific expression of *GABRB1-p* [7], we cloned the factor that associates with the β_1-INR. A one-hybrid screen was performed using a transformed *S. cerevisiae* strain (Figure 1A, top panel) that included two chromosomally integrated reporters and a human neonatal or adult brain cDNA library. Each reporter gene (*His3* and *LacZ*) was regulated by three tandem repeats of the β_1-INR, a configuration shown to reconstitute neuronal specificity and autologous regulation of *GABRB1* [7]. In a parallel experiment, nonselective media containing no aminotriazole was used to make sure that enough yeast transformants were obtained to cover the complexity of the cDNA library.

Five hundred yeast colonies carrying potential candidates were isolated from the *His3* screen. These yeast colonies were further tested for their ability to express the second reporter *LacZ*, which yielded 50 candidates that stimulated both reporters. Only four candidates (A4, A10, B33, B37) were positive upon retransformation of isolated clones. DNA sequencing and blast analysis revealed a perfect match of these four clones to a splice variant (b) of human Polycomblike protein PHF1. The full length PHF1b sequence in the database (ACC# BC008834) was compared to that of the isolated clones (see Figure 1, bottom panel). Candidates B33 and B37 are identical, whereas, candidate A10 is 10 amino acids longer than either B33 or B37. Candidate A4 lacks amino terminus of the PHF1b but contains two plant homeodomains (PHD) with the remainder of the carboxyl terminus. From the sizes of the clones and their amino terminus sequences, it was predicted that the zinc finger domain II with adjacent sequences is required for DNA recognition. This zinc finger is characterized by a C$_4$HC$_3$ motif and is found predominantly in proteins that are associated with chromatin remodeling [35]. The 120 amino acid carboxyl terminal region adjacent to the PHD finger II is predicted to form an HLH structure [36] whereas the carboxyl terminus showed no significant homology to any known structures. PHF1a, an alternatively spliced version of PHF1 [37], shares an identical amino terminus region comprising both finger

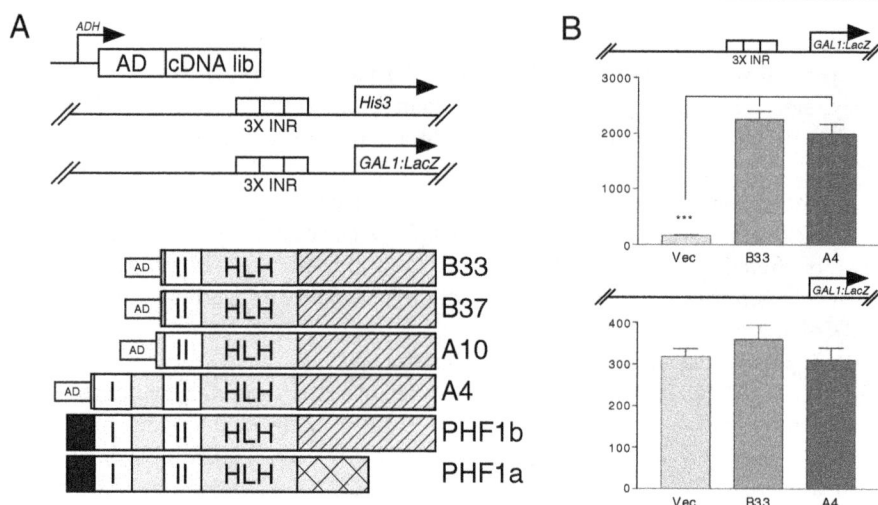

Figure 1 **Results of a yeast one-hybrid assay using expressed human brain cDNAs and β₁-INR sequences. A)** The NLY2 yeast strain was transformed to contain two integrated reporters (*His3* and *LacZ*) (top panel) under the control of three tandem β₁-INRs. This strain was used to screen a yeast expression library containing cDNAs derived from human adult or fetal brains. cDNAs were expressed from a yeast 2 micron based multi-copy plasmid with expression controlled by the *ADH* promoter. The libraries of expressed proteins contain a GAL4 activation domain (AD) fused to each cDNA in frame to facilitate one-hybrid screening in yeast. Transformed yeast colonies were screened for their ability to grow on selective solid media containing 10 mM 3-aminotriazole and lacking histidine. To confirm clone selection, expression of β-galactosidase was measured by plating yeast colonies on plates containing chromogenic dye (X-gal). Purified clones are shown in relation to the wild type and full length PHF1b (human Polycomblike protein) and PHF1a sequence. Two plant homeodomain (PHD) fingers are shown (I or II) with white boxes. Black box represents the amino terminus. Different carboxyl termini that result from alternative splicing are shown with hatched (PHF1b) and cross-hatched bars (PHF1a). A putative helix-loop-helix forming sequence is depicted by "HLH". **B)** Screened candidates require INR sequence for reporter gene activation. Top panel shows candidates A4 and B33 activates *β-galactosidase* reporter gene only when reporter promoter contains the INR sequence. A reporter without INR sequence (bottom panel) shows no activity from the candidates in comparison to the vector plasmid. Results are expressed as mean values ± SEM.

domains and the HLH, but differs in the carboxyl terminus due to a frame shift that gives rise to two unique ends of different sizes (Figure 1A, bottom panel). Surprisingly, none of the candidates isolated were PHF1a. A confirmatory experiment for INR site dependency demonstrated that candidates A4 and B33 require INR sequences for *β-galactosidase* reporter gene activity (Figure 1B, top panel). Absence of the INR sequence in this promoter/reporter construct does not support activity (Figure 1B, bottom panel).

PHD II and HLH are necessary for recognition of the β₁-INR

PHD fingers are protein domains consisting of two zinc ions coordinated by cysteine and histidine residues in a C4HC3 motif [38,39]. Thus far, no specific function for this motif has been identified, however, it has been proposed that proteins containing PHD fingers are involved in processes of chromatin remodeling [35].

To determine the minimum sequence of PHF1b necessary for INR recognition, a series of PHF1b truncation mutants were engineered (Figure 2). The GAL4 activation domain (AD) [40] was fused to zinc finger domains I, II, and to the predicted HLH part of the protein [36]. The DNA binding activity of these cDNA products was tested in yeast. A number of cDNAs containing

sequential deletions from the C-terminus were generated. Expression of cDNAs encoding either PHD I, II or HLH domains were not sufficient for DNA association as measured by growth on 10 mM 3-aminotriazole containing media and ability to activate the β-galactosidase reporter gene (Figure 2, rows 2, 3 and 4). A PHF1b fragment that terminated at the divergent sequence with PHF1a (Figure 2, row 8) [37] was also inactive. However, a longer version of PHF1b (Figure 2, row 14) that included an additional 40 amino acids beyond the putative HLH sequence was sufficient for growth support mediated by the β₁-INR. Further sequential deletions defined the PHD finger II, HLH, and a portion of the 40 amino acid domain (11 amino acid region) as being the required sequence for INR recognition (Figure 2, row 10). The importance of the 11 amino acids (SFPSGQGPGGG) (glycine-rich motif) was further tested in the context of either the PHD finger II or HLH domain. The 11 amino acid sequence was fused to the end of PHD finger II (Figure 2, row 6) and to the HLH domain where the 11 amino acid sequence was imbedded in a larger sequence (Figure 2, row 5). Both fusion proteins (rows 5 and 6) failed to support β₁-INR recognition as measured by the yeast one-hybrid assay. Similarly, the HLH alone was ineffective for INR recognition (Figure 2, row 4).

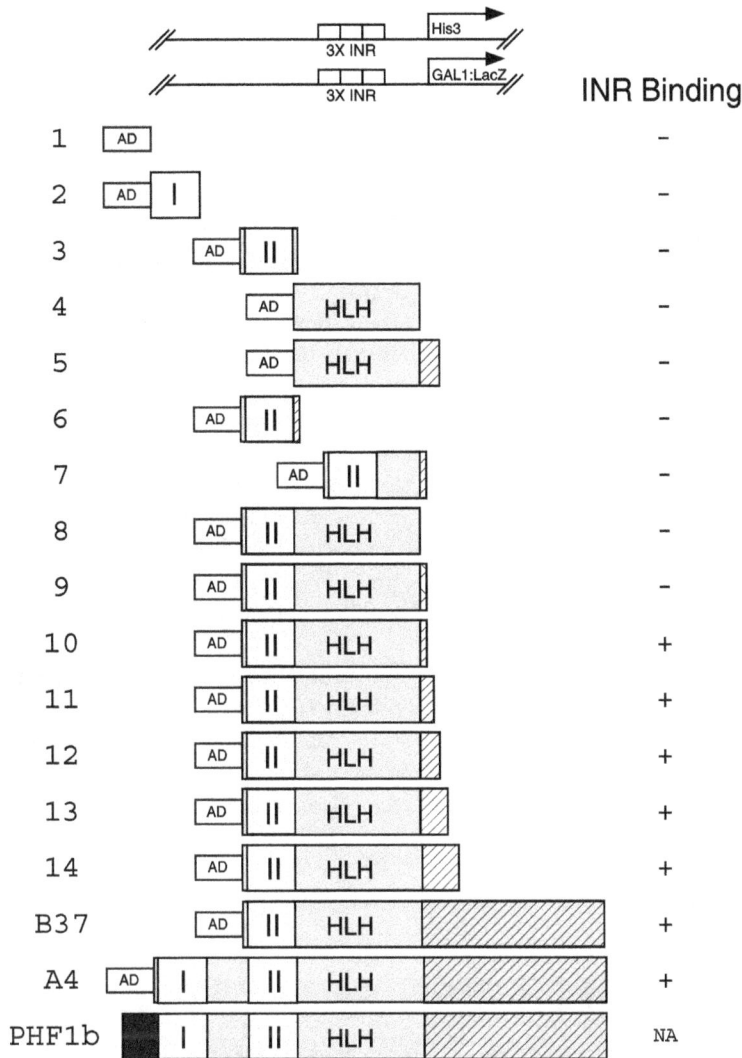

Figure 2 Mapping sequences that are required for PHF1b DNA recognition. Depicted is the yeast strain with chromosomally integrated reporters carrying three tandem β_1 initiator sites that was used for one-hybrid assays. Candidates identified by one-hybrid assays were used to construct a number of 5' and 3' sequential deletions of the PHF1b gene to define the minimal β_1-INR binding domain. The GAL4 AD was fused to all of the PHF1b fragments and tested for its ability to activate three tandem β_1-INR sites linked to either *His3* or *LacZ*. Full length PHF1b is shown for comparison to relate relative sizes of AD fused PHF1b fragments (#2-14 with the exception of #9, which is a derivative of PHF1a) and one-hybrid candidates B37 and A4. The DNA binding activities both positive (+) and negative (−) are as indicated. The criterion for DNA binding is measured by the ability of the constructs to activate both reporter genes (*His3* and *LacZ*) at levels comparable to B37 and A4 isolates. *His3* expression was measured by the survival of the yeast colonies that could grow on plates that contained 10 mM 3-aminotriazole and β-galactosidase activity from the second reporter, measured by β-galactosidase assays. The results from both assays were the same and are indicated by one column to the right.

It is apparent from the one-hybrid assays that finger II, HLH and the 11 amino acids beyond the frame shift point of PHF1 proteins are essential for DNA recognition. The significance of the glycine-rich 11 amino acid motif in the context of the HLH domain is not clear. The alternatively spliced version PHF1a does not contain the glycine-rich sequence and does not bind β_1-INR (Figure 2, row 9). The minimum PHF1b DNA binder requires 11 amino acids beyond the frame shift point of PHF1a (Figure 2, row 10). It is plausible that the 11 amino acids of PHF1b may not be essential for DNA binding but may be required for some structural stability of the protein.

PHF1 proteins are localized to the nucleus

The larger *Drosophila* homolog of PHF1/PCL1 proteins is localized in the nucleus [41], but the nuclear localization motif has not yet been identified. To determine the region of PHF1b that contains the nuclear localization signal, a number of truncated versions of PHF1b were constructed (Figure 3) and fused to the

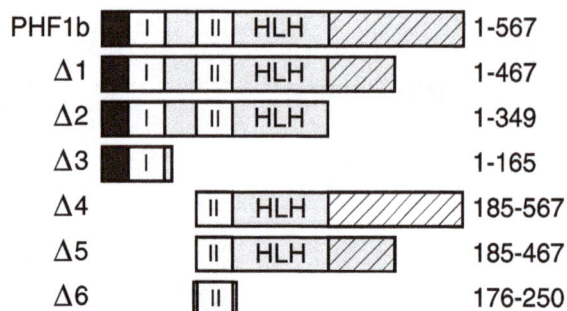

Figure 3 PHF1b deletion derivatives. PHF1b derivatives showing amino terminus and carboxyl terminus deletions. These deletions are used as GFP and GAL4(1–100) fusions to determine the nuclear localization and repressor domains of the protein. Numbers represent the amino acid positions that specify the sizes of the proteins.

green fluorescent protein (GFP) protein. Complementary DNAs coding for GFP-PHF1b fusion proteins were transfected into COS-7 cells that were fixed with paraformaldehyde. The transfected cells were viewed through a blue filter to detect the green fluorescence from the hybrid proteins. PHF1b Δ6 (Figure 4D) is sufficient for nuclear localization when compared with full length PHF1b (Figure 4A) or other PHF1b derivatives that contained amino terminus, PHD finger I and part of the carboxyl terminus of the protein (PHF1b Δ1 and Δ5) (Figure 4B and C). Taken together with the fact that the GFP fusion protein with the amino terminus and PHD

Finger I (PHF1b Δ3) (Figure 4E) did not localize to the nucleus, as compared with GFP alone (Figure 4F), the nuclear localization sequence (NLS) is most likely located within the PHD finger II region and facilitates an association with DNA by localizing the protein in the nucleus.

In addition to the COS-7 nuclear localization study, we also investigated the localization of the same GFP-PHF1b fusion proteins in primary rat neocortical neurons (Figure 5). Results of confocal microscopy using transfected neurons shows a similar pattern of PHF1b expression as was observed with COS-7 cells. Full length PHF1b (Figure 5D, PHF1b) is restricted to the nucleus. Location of the nucleus was visualized by co-transfection of cytomegalovirus (CMV)-DsRed-Nuclear (Figure 5E, H and K). The PHD finger II domain is sufficient for nuclear localization (Figure 5G, PHF1b Δ5). GFP alone (Figure 5A), PHF1b Δ3 (Figure 5J) and DsRed-Monomer (Figure 5B) are not restricted to the nucleus. As compared to COS-7, the GFP-PHF1b expression pattern is highly restricted within the larger neuronal nucleus (Figure 5D).

PHF1b stimulates *GABRB1* promoter activity in transfected primary cultured neurons

DNA alignment of the human, mouse, and rat β_1 promoters shows that the initiator sequence is identical and the region 192-bp upstream and downstream of the initiator is 94% similar (data not shown), suggesting that the key regulatory factors for the promoter are conserved across species. Considering the conserved nature of β_1

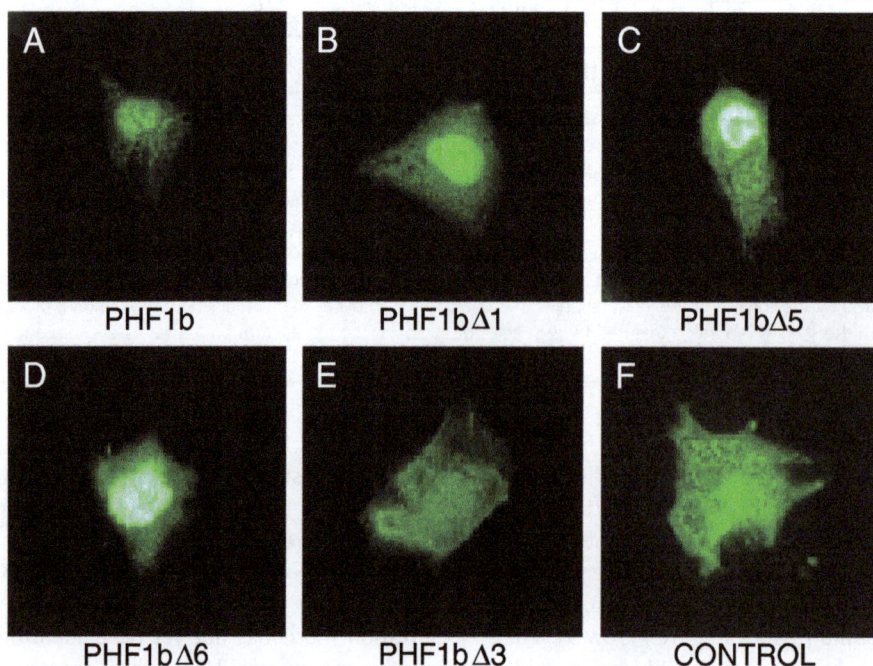

Figure 4 PHD domain II is necessary for the localization of PHF1b to COS cell nuclei. COS cells were transfected with GFP-PHF1b fusion constructs (see Figure 3 for PHF1b deletion derivatives). Control represents a vector expressing only GFP protein.

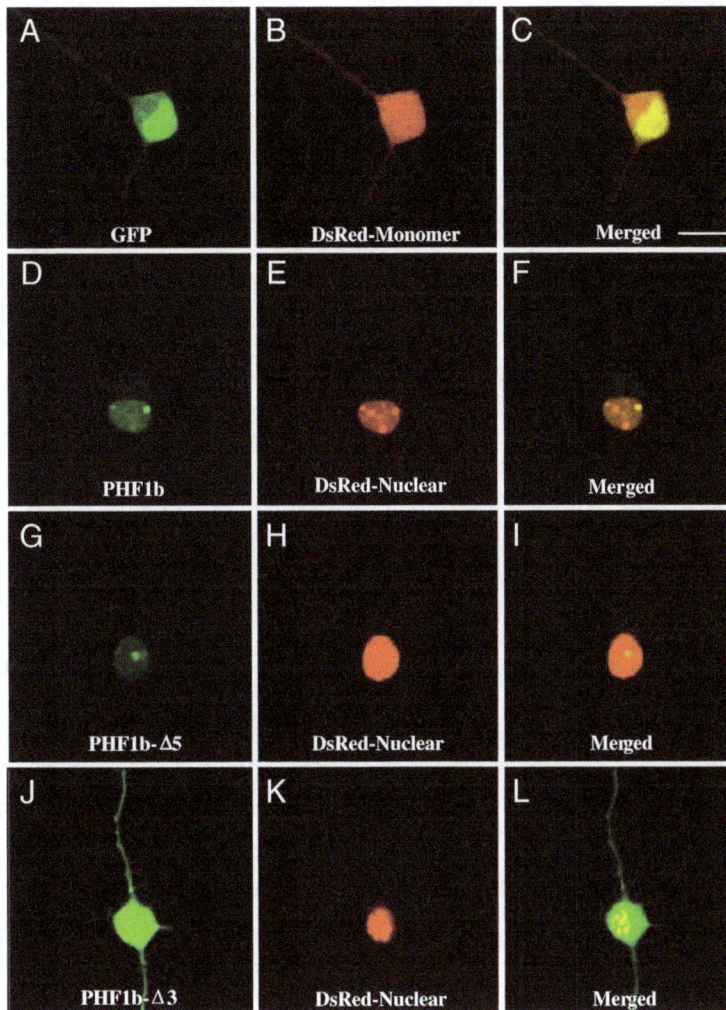

Figure 5 **PHF1b protein nuclear localization in rat neocortical neurons.** Primary rat neocortical neurons isolated from E18 brain and maintained one week *in vitro* were transfected with GFP-PHF1b fusion plasmids (CMV-GFP-PHF1b, CMV-GFP-PHF1b-Δ5, CMV-GFP-PHF1b-Δ3, see Figure 3) and examined 48 hours after transfection by confocal microscopy for nuclear localization relative to DsRed-Nuclear marker (CMV-DsRed-Nuclear), a red fluorescent protein that localizes to the nucleus. Control transfection of CMV-GFP **(A, C)** and CMV-DsRed-Monomer **(B, C)** construct expression is throughout cortical cells and expression is not restricted to the nucleus **(C)**. Both GFP-PHF1b **(D, F)** and GFP-PHF1b-Δ5 **(G, I)** fusion construct expression coincides with DsRed-Nuclear **(E, F and H, I)** indicating that both the PHF1b and the PHF1b-Δ5 protein contain a nuclear localization signal. In contrast, the GFP-PHF1b-Δ3 **(J, L)** fusion construct expression is not restricted to the nucleus **(DsRed-Nuclear, K, L)** suggesting that the nuclear localization signal of PHF1b is not localized at the N-terminus of the PHF1b protein. Scale bar is 10 μm.

promoters, the study of a human *GABRB1* promoter in rat primary neuronal cultures is quite likely to be relevant to gene regulation in humans. Towards this goal, an expression construct containing the human PHF1b cDNA under control of the CMV promoter was co-transfected into primary rat neocortical neurons to monitor the effects of such expression on human *GABRB1-p/*luciferase reporter activity. There is a 3-fold stimulation of *GABRB1* promoter activity observed upon PHF1b overexpression (Figure 6), suggesting that PHF1b may be an important regulatory factor of human *GABRB1* transcription.

Chronic GABA exposure regulates PHF1 binding to endogenous *Gabrb1*

ChIP was used to demonstrate that PHF1 proteins are bound to the endogenous rat *Gabrb1* core promoter of both hippocampal and neocortical neurons (Figure 7B) where high levels of endogenous β_1 subunit mRNAs have been reported [7]. Binding of PHF1 to *Gabrb1* is decreased after chronic treatment with GABA at a concentration reported to down-regulate β_1 mRNAs and subunit levels in cultured neocortical neurons (Figure 7C and D). Moreover, blockade of $GABA_A Rs$ by the antagonist

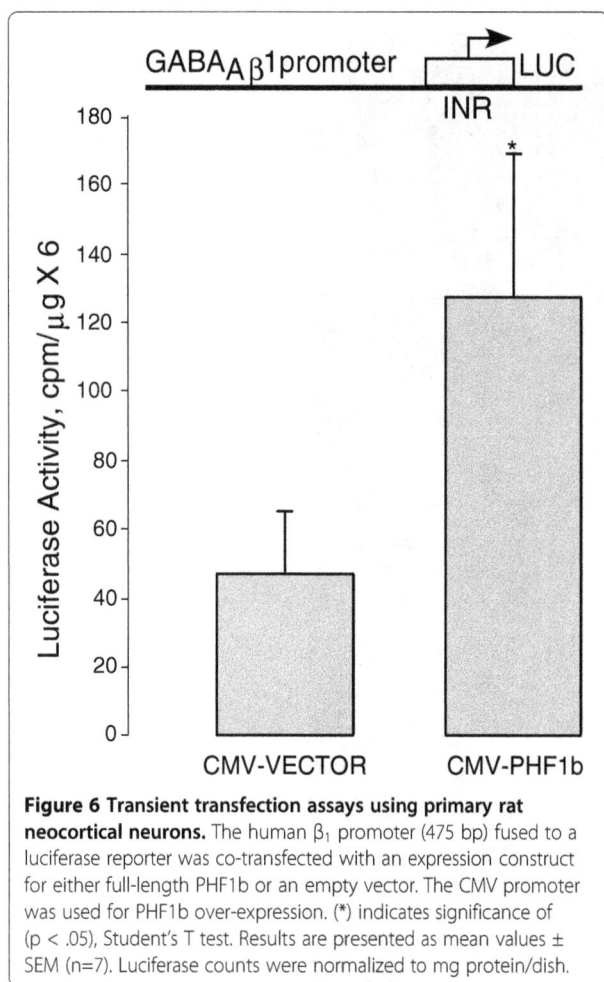

Figure 6 Transient transfection assays using primary rat neocortical neurons. The human β_1 promoter (475 bp) fused to a luciferase reporter was co-transfected with an expression construct for either full-length PHF1b or an empty vector. The CMV promoter was used for PHF1b over-expression. (*) indicates significance of (p < .05), Student's T test. Results are presented as mean values ± SEM (n=7). Luciferase counts were normalized to mg protein/dish.

bicuculline reverses GABA-induced removal of PHF1 from *Gabrb1* suggesting that the effects of GABA exposure are through the GABA$_A$ receptor.

A PRC2 complex protein EZH2 requires PHF1a (Pcl1) for efficient catalysis of (H3K27) trimethylation [42]. To determine if PHF1b functions in this regard at *Gabrb1*, we examined whether the trimethylation status of H3K27 is altered at the core promoter region after GABA treatment. No significant change in trimethylation at the H3K27 position was detected, however, there was a 26% decrease of monomethylation (n=6, p=0.0011) (Figure 8).

TAF1 and TAF2 as co-activators of PHF1b at the *GABRB1* promoter

TAF1 and TAF2 contribute to DNA binding and core promoter selectivity of RNA pol II [17]. It has been shown that the complex formed by TAF1 and TAF2 preferentially bind to INR-like DNA sequences compared to random DNA [21]. Independently, these two TAFs do not show DNA sequence specificity, but as a complex they recognize DNA and thereby recruit TFIID to TATA-less promoters [21]. Since β_1-INR shows

significant sequence similarity with the TdT-INR [13] (see Figure 9A), we tested whether TAF1 and TAF2, perhaps as a cofactor for PHF1b, would influence promoter activity that is dependent on the β_1-INR.

The transcriptional start site from β_1-INR was analyzed in the context of a synthetic GAL4 upstream activating sequence (UAS) (Figure 9B). Promoter activity of this construct (p5XG-β_1-INR-Luc construct) was significantly reduced in COS-7 cells when compared to a construct that contained the adenovirus E1B TATA instead of β_1-INR [43] (data not shown). This result is to be expected given the fact that the TATA-less promoters are in general weaker than TATA-containing promoters [12] and β_1-INR is derived from a neural specific gene.

In order to determine whether transcription initiated from the synthetic promoter through the β_1-INR, total RNA was prepared from COS-7 cells that had been co-transfected with the expression construct for the GAL4-VP16 activator and p5XG- β_1-INR-Luc. Primer extension analysis showed two major transcripts originating from use of the synthetic promoter (Figure 9C). The start sites we identified are different from those observed by Russek et al., [7], but both originate within the sequence of β_1-INR. This discrepancy of start sites is most likely due to the fact that the two promoters are structurally different from each other, one being in the original human *GABRB1* promoter, studied in neurons, and the other containing only the β_1-INR element in the context of GAL4 UAS, studied in COS-7 cells.

The p5XG-β_1-INR-Luc construct was also used in co-expression studies with either TAF1 or TAF2 and PHF1b to study the effect of TAF co-activator properties on promoter activation. Again, the GAL4-VP16 construct was used to express the common upstream activator that recognizes the GAL4 UAS for these experiments (Figure 9B and D). Over-expression of PHF1b shows enhancement of luciferase activity with greatest effect in the presence of either TAF1 or TAF2 (Figure 9D). PHF1b over-expression potentiates TAF co-activity two to three fold. Moreover, co-expression of TAF1 and TAF2 with PHF1b increases the activity of the p5XG-β_1-INR-Luc promoter as much as six fold compared to activation with the GAL4-VP16 activator alone.

PHF1b represses transcription from the TK promoter at a distance

In order to study transcriptional properties of various PHF1b domains the protein domains were individually fused to the GAL4 DNA binding domain and tested. A synthetic promoter containing the GAL4 UAS and the TK enhancer promoter was employed to test whether PHF1b could function as a repressor or activator from a distance. GAL4-PHF1b fusion constructs were co-transfected with the TK enhancer promoter construct

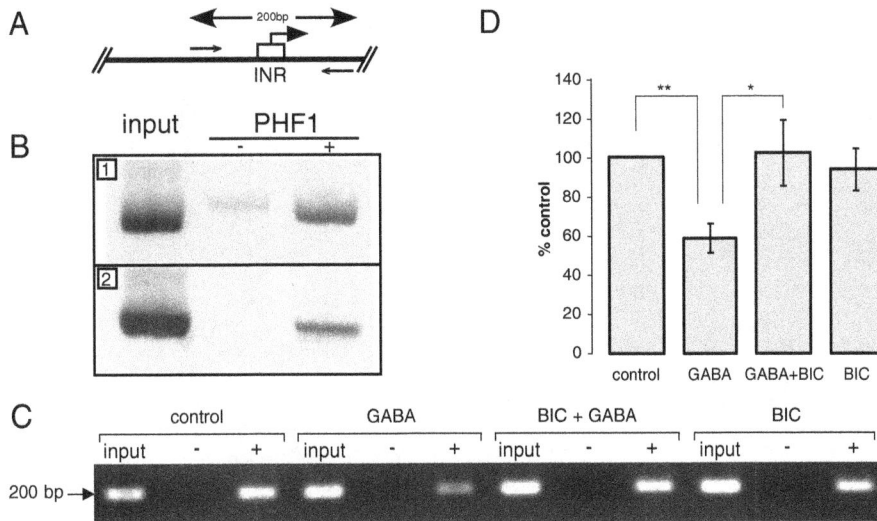

Figure 7 Association of PHF1 proteins with endogenous *Gabrb1* in neurons. ChIP assays were performed using a PHF1(a and b) specific antibody and precipitated genomic DNA was found to contain the core promoter region of *Gabrb1* in primary rat neocortical neurons. Detection of the endogenous *Gabrb1* promoter was accomplished by PCR as depicted in **(A)** using two primers (arrows) that flank the β_1-INR. The size of the PCR fragment is indicated above. Initiator position is depicted with a box and arrow showing the direction of transcription. **(B)** Bottom panel shows the presence or absence of *Gabrb1*-specific PCR products in fragments of genomic DNA that have been precipitated after addition of PHF1 antibodies. ChIP substrates are as indicated (1) primary neocortical neurons and (2) primary hippocampal neurons cultured for 7 days from E18 rat brains. **(C)** Representative data showing the presence or absence of *Gabrb1*-specific PCR products from ChIP performed with PHF1 antibody. Primary neocortical neurons were treated with either GABA (500 µM), GABA and the specific GABA$_A$R antagonist bicuculline (50 µM), bicuculline alone, or relevant vehicle for 48 h, as described in Russek et al [7]. Presence of IgG in reaction is represented as "-" and PHF1 antibody as "+". **(D)** Quantitation of ChIP data displayed in **(C)** is represented as mean ± SEM and expressed as percent increase from control (% control). (*=significantly different from control, $p < 0.05$). All samples were analyzed as ratios of PHF1 antibody/IgG after normalization to input.

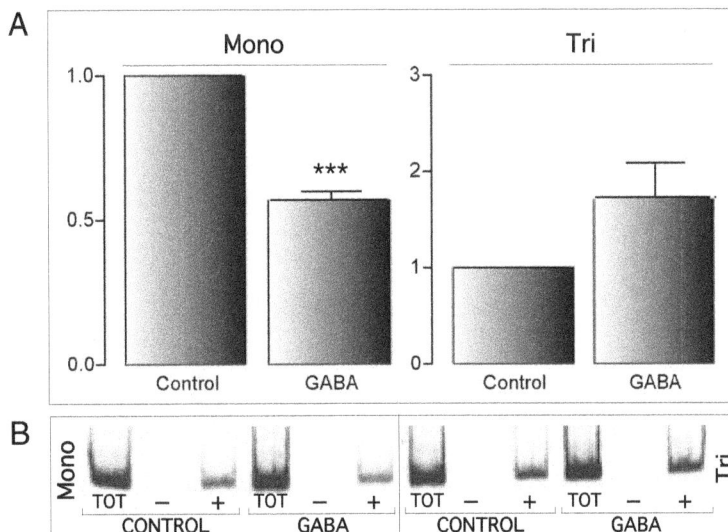

Figure 8 GABA decreases H3K27 mono methylation on the *Gabrb1* promoter. Real time PCR analysis of ChIP assays show a statistically significant (***) decrease (n=5) of H3K27 monomethylation at the core promoter region (P = 0.0001) **(A)** with no significant change in the status of trimethylation (n=5, p=0.1184). Y-axis represents relative signal of H3K27 (mono- or tri-) methylation as compared to vehicle control (set as 1). A Student's t-test was used to investigate the statistical significance of mono- and trimethylation. **(B)** Radiographic display showing amplified promoter fragments immunoprecipitated with H3K27me1 (mono) and H3K27me3 (tri) antibodies. Total input DNA and IgG lanes are marked by "TOT" and "-", respectively. Results are expressed as mean values ± SEM.

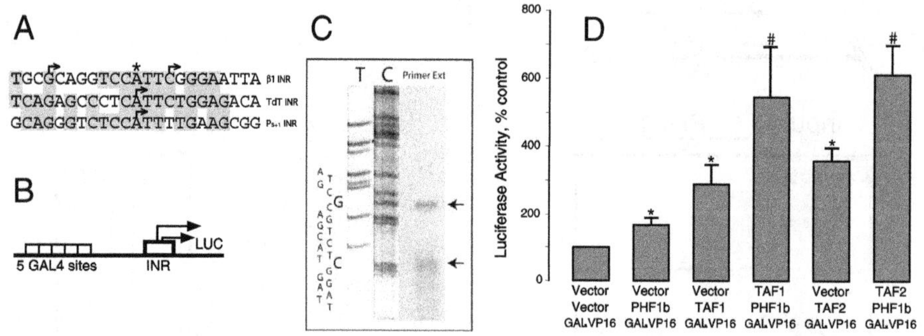

Figure 9 Study of the β_1-INR in COS cells. A) Sequence similarities between β_1-INR, TdT INR and the adeno-associated virus (AAV) P5+1 INR. Shadowed boxes highlight sequence identity. Arrows indicate transcription start sites. Star symbol indicates the major start site of β_1-INR in neocortical neurons (7). **B)** Depiction of a TATA-less synthetic promoter/reporter construct carrying a single β_1-INR with a GAL4 UAS (p5XG-β_1-INR-Luc). Promoter activity of the construct is regulated by co-expression of an upstream activator (GAL4-VP16). Arrows show the direction of transcription. **C)** Primer extension analysis of RNA from COS-7 cells transfected with the p5XG-β_1-INR-Luc construct. Primer extension products are separated on a sequencing gel. Sequencing reactions (dC and dT) were run alongside of primer extension products to determine the exact start sites for initiation. Top strand DNA sequence of β_1-INR is also shown next to sequencing lanes. Arrows indicate the major initiation sites in COS-7 cells. **D)** Co-activation of PHF1b transcriptional activity by TAF1 and 2. COS-7 cells were co-transfected with p5XG-β_1-INR-Luc, GAL4-VP16 and combinations of PHF1b, TAF1 and TAF2. 48 hours after transfection, cells were harvested and assayed for luciferase activity. Results shown are mean values ± SEM and normalized to protein content within each dish as well as to vector control (Vector+Vector+GAL-VP16 defined as 100%). "*" indicates significantly different from vector control ($p < 0.05$) as determined by 95% confidence interval. "#" indicates significantly different from PHF1b (Vector+PHF1b+GAL-VP16) ($p < 0.05$) as determined by 95% confidence interval.

into COS-7 cells. The GAL4-PHF1b fusions were recruited 200-bp upstream of the TK enhancer promoter at the GAL4 UAS (Figure 10) and luciferase reporter activity was measured. As seen in Figure 10, full length PHF1b fused to GAL4 functions as a strong repressor of

the TK enhancer promoter from a distance. To delineate the minimum domain required for repression, we tested both amino and carboxyl terminus deletions of PHF1b (Figure 3). A fusion protein containing both PHD fingers constitutes the most potent repressor of TK promoter

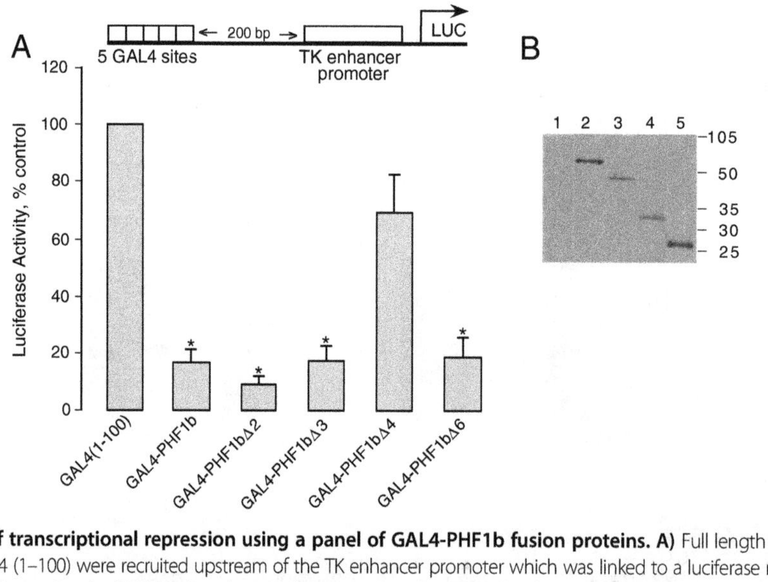

Figure 10 Investigation of transcriptional repression using a panel of GAL4-PHF1b fusion proteins. A) Full length PHF1b and truncated PHF1b versions fused to GAL4 (1–100) were recruited upstream of the TK enhancer promoter which was linked to a luciferase reporter gene (pG5-200tkLUC). GAL4 (1–100) contains the DNA binding domain that recognizes GAL4 regulatory sites. GAL4-PHF1b fusions were expressed from a CMV promoter. COS-7 cells were co-transfected with the reporter plasmid (pG5-200tkLUC) and the constructs as indicated. 48 hours after transfection, cells were harvested and assayed for luciferase activity. Results shown are mean values ± SEM and normalized to protein content within each dish as well as to vector control (pG5-200tkLUC+ GAL4 (1–100) defined as 100%). "*" indicates significantly different from vector control ($p < 0.05$) as determined by 95% confidence interval. **B)** GAL4-PHF1b fusion proteins are expressed in COS-7 cells as shown by Western analysis. Extracts of COS-7 cells mock transfected or expressing PHF1b constructs were analyzed by Western analysis using a GAL4 antisera. No proteins were detected in mock-transfected cells (1) and proteins were detected for cells transfected with PHF1b (2), PHF1bΔ4 (3), PHF1bΔ3 (4), PHF1bΔ6 (5). Molecular size markers are to the right.

activity (Figure 10, PHF1b Δ2). These results also show that each PHF1b PHD finger contains a potent repressor domain (Figure 10, PHF1b Δ3 and Δ6). Interestingly, deletion of the amino terminus with PHD finger I abolishes the repressive function of PHF1b (Figure 10, PHF1b Δ4). The expression levels of these transfected GAL4-PHF1b fusions are relatively similar in COS-7 cells and confirmed with immunoprecipitation analysis by using GAL4 antibodies (Figure 10B).

PHF1b co-immunoprecipitates with SUZ12, a PRC2 associated protein

In the PRC2 complex fraction, purified from HeLa and 293F cells, PHF1a is associated with PRC2 proteins [42,44]. We now asked whether neuronal PHF1b would also be part of PRC2 by determining whether it associates with any of the key proteins of the PRC2 complex. The SUZ12 antibody was chosen for co-immunoprecipitation analysis because this protein is an integral member of the PRC2 complex and because SUZ12 affinity columns have been successfully used to isolate EZH2-EED complexes found in the HeLa cell extract [44]. In the PHF1 immuno-precipitate, upon Western blot, the larger alternatively spliced isoform b of PHF1 is detected (see Figure 1, compare PHF1a and PHF1b) (Figure 11 A, lane 1 and 3). PHF1b is also the predominant isoform detected by standard Western analysis in rat neocortical neurons (Figure 12, panel 6). In the SUZ12 immunoprecipitate, PHF1b is detected (Figure 11A, lane 5) and likewise in the PHF1

immunoprecipitate, SUZ12 is detected confirming a potential association between the proteins in neurons (Figure 11B).

PHF1 proteins are highly expressed in the rat brain

Although PHF1a was present in the library, we did not identify PHF1a as a β_1-INR associating factor in yeast one-hybrid assays, even though it contains significant homology to the INR binding domain of PHF1b (Figure 2). Thus, it was hypothesized that the levels of PHF1a might differ from PHF1b in neurons. To understand whether there is a significant difference in the levels of alternatively spliced versions of PHF1, a PHF1 antibody was generated against a 20 amino acid peptide sequence that is common to both PHF1 isoforms (see Methods). Western blot analysis using the PHF1 antibody was then performed with nuclear extracts derived from primary cultured E18 rat neocortical neurons and adult rat brain. Two distinct protein bands of sizes 45 kD (PHF1a) and 60 kD (PHF1b) were observed (Figure 12, panel 6) with PHF1b being the predominate splice variant.

Given the fact that many GABA$_A$ receptors in the hippocampal formation are believed to contain β subunits [45], adult rat brain tissue was examined for the presence of PHF1 protein in regions where β1 subunit expression is expected to be high. Slices (Bregma −6.3mm) were stained with a PHF1 antibody as described above and in Methods. Hippocampal neurons show marked levels of PHF1 expression in the CA1 region, as well as the dentate gyrus (Figure 12, panels 2 and 3). PHF1 expression was also detected in the neocortex (data not shown).

Discussion

A human Polycomblike protein was discovered that associates with the initiator of the core *GABRB1* promoter. The PHF1b PHD zinc finger domain (C$_4$HC$_3$), HLH structure and the glycine-rich motif (SFPSGQGPGGG) of this protein are sufficient for specific DNA association at β_1-INR. Importantly, this discovery of a Polycomblike protein as a potential DNA recognition molecule for inhibitory receptor subunit expression sheds light on the important role of Polycomb group (PcG) proteins, whose mechanism for developmental regulation of transcription remains unknown [31,33,46]. In addition, our results may explain how the PcG/trxG complexes could be recruited to specific DNA sequences through protein-DNA interactions. PcG proteins were initially identified in *Drosophila* as proteins that are involved in maintaining the repression of homeotic genes necessary for anterior-posterior development [47]. PcG and trx-G are required for the maintenance of homeotic gene expression after the degradation of the gap and pair-rule proteins [47]. TrxG maintains expression of homeotic genes, whereas PcG factors maintain their repression [31].

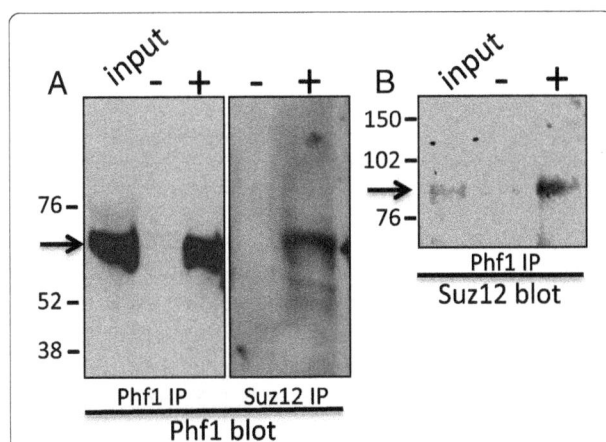

Figure 11 PHF1 and SUZ12 are co-immunoprecipitated from primary neocortical neurons, as shown by Western blot. Primary E18 cortical neurons, maintained seven days in culture, were lysed and immunoprecipitated (IP) with PHF1 (A lane 3, B lane 3), SUZ12 (A lane 5) and pre-immune (A lane 2, lane 4, B lane 2) antisera. Immune complexes were separated by sodium dodecyl sulfate polyacrylamide gel electrophoresis (SDS-PAGE) and transferred to nitrocellulose. PHF1 (**A**) or SUZ12 (**B**) proteins were identified by immunoblotting with either PHF1 (**A**) or SUZ12 (**B**) antisera. The molecular weight markers are shown to the left.

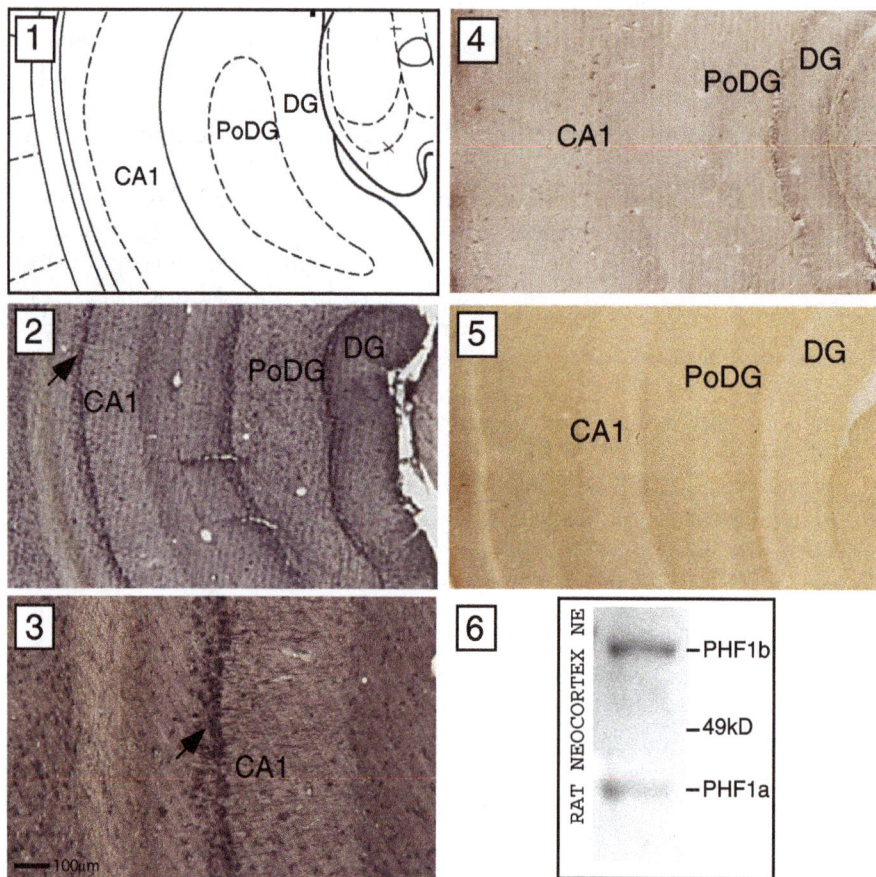

Figure 12 Immunodetection of PHF1 proteins in nuclear extracts of primary rat neocortical cultures and slices of adult rat hippocampus. Western analysis of PHF1a and PHF1b expression using nuclear extracts of rat neocortical neurons and a primary antibody raised against a PHF1 peptide present in both PHF1a and PHF1b **(panel 6)**. Relative size of PHF1 proteins is as indicated using relationship of migration pattern of putative PHF1a and b to position of marker proteins. Adult rat brains were sectioned coronally at Bregma −6.3mm **(as depicted in panel 1)** and treated with a primary antibody to PHF1 as described above. Positive immunostaining is indicated by brown-black precipitates **(panel 2 and 3)**. Regions of CA1 (field CA1 of hippocampus), DG (dentate gyrus) and PoDG (polymorph layer dentate gyrus) are indicated as references. Panel 2 displays high PHF1 immunoreactivity in the CA1 region. Arrow in panel 2 indicates area of CA1 region that was magnified (100×) in the display of panel 3. A dark scale bar at the bottom of panel 3 shows the virtual distance between two points. Hippocampal slices processed in parallel to the experimental were treated with the PHF1 antibody blocking peptide and secondary antibody **(shown in panel 4)**. A representative hippocampal slice processed in parallel treated only with the secondary antibody is displayed in **panel 5** as an additional control.

The function of PHD fingers is not well understood. Proteins containing PHD finger motifs are believed to drive chromatin remodeling [35] by affecting protein-DNA or protein-protein interactions. Recent reports contributed to our understanding of how this domain might function in the context of some well-characterized proteins. For example, acetyltransferase activity of CBP (CREB binding protein) is dependent upon an intact PHD finger [48]. Another report [49] has shown that ING2, a PHD protein and a putative tumor suppressor protein, binds to phosphoinositides (PtdinsPs) through its PHD finger domain. The PHD finger of ING2 is a PtdinsPs nuclear receptor and is involved in nuclear responses during DNA damage. Interestingly, we find that PHF1 (variants a and b) is a nuclear protein with nuclear localization determined by the PHD finger II (Figures 4, 5).

PHF1b may represent a different class of PtdinsPs nuclear receptor proteins that are also capable of specific DNA binding. Our DNA association studies show that the PHD finger II is not sufficient for DNA association on its own, but requires another adjacent 131 amino acid region, capable of forming a HLH [36]. Apart from containing the NLS, it is not clear how the PHD finger II contributes to the overall binding of DNA. Whether the PHD finger or the HLH motif of PHF1b makes contact with the β_1-INR-DNA remains to be determined. It is possible that the PHD finger itself may not be physically required for DNA binding but essential for modulating PHF1b's DNA binding recognition. Alternatively, we propose that PHD fingers may provide initial DNA sequence recognition by helping interaction with nucleosomes. A similar hypothesis has been proposed by

Ragvin et al. [50], who studied the function of the PHD finger in the context of a bromodomain. The authors show that both the bromodomain and PHD finger region of p300 are required for binding of acetylated nucleosomes *in vitro*. In this context, the PHD finger is thought to function as a co-recognizer of the nucleosomes or as a stabilizer of the bromodomain.

The functions of PcG and trxG proteins are mediated by overlapping Polycomb/Trithoraxgroup response elements (PRE/TRE) [31,51,52]. The mechanism behind target recognition of these sites still remains to be determined. Among the family of PcG and trxG, only three members have been shown to have specific DNA binding functions. PcG member PHO (a YY1 homolog) and two trxG proteins named GAGA and Zeste bind specific DNA sequences [53-57]. Our results suggest that PHF1b is another specific DNA binding protein of the PCL family that may function in a novel manner to recruit the PcG and trxG complexes to an INR sequence for effective control over pre-initiation complex formation at the core promoter region.

Results of PHF1b overexpression also show that activation of the human *GABRB1* promoter or a synthetic promoter containing a single β_1-INR can be positively regulated by PHF1b (Figures 6 and 9D). This is a surprising result given that PcG proteins are usually associated with transcriptional repression. It is intriguing that PHF1b can function as a positive and negative modulator of transcription in a manner similar to the function of the YY1 protein [23,58]. The positive or negative nature of YY1 regulation is also thought to be context dependent and achieved through the interactions with specific modulatory factors [58]. PHF1a/PHF1b and YY1 protein both share zinc finger domains required for DNA binding [26]. Interestingly, the β_1-INR is also similar to the core portion of the AAV P5+1 INR [26] promoter that is bound by YY1 (see Figure 9A). It remains to be determined whether these two initiator recognition proteins may recognize one another's binding sites to recruit different PcG complexes. The fact that YY1 has been implicated in gene regulation of neurons [59] and that *Gabrb1* is expressed early on in the germinal matrix of the embryonic rat nervous system [60] and in the adult rat brain [45], suggests that there may be a relationship between PHF1b and YY1 regulated transcription.

Both *Drosophila* PCL and PcG protein YY1 [61] interact with the mammalian members of RPD3 family of HDACs [62,63], suggesting an involvement in chromatin remodeling. Apart from being an INR binding protein, YY1 is also expressed in the *Xenopus* anterior neural tube during tailbud stage in embryos. Inhibition of *Xenopus* YY1 function resulted in embryos with anteroposterior axial patterning defects similar to over expression of *Xenopus*PcG genes *XPCL1/2*, *Xbmi1* and *XEZ*

[64-67]. Results of our GAL4-PHF1b fusion protein studies show that PHF1b is a strong repressor when recruited at a 200-bp distance from the TK enhancer promoter (Figure 10A). Repression by the PHF1b fusion protein is similar to that reported for the GAL4-YY1 fusion protein [23].

PHF1b-mediated repression is conferred by two PHD fingers that are also capable of repressing individually when they are fused to the GAL4 DNA binding domain (Figure 10; PHF1 Δ3 and Δ6). It has been shown that two PHD fingers of *Drosophila* Polycomblike protein are the target sites for RPD3 (histone deacetylase) interaction [62], which is consistent with our results where the repressive function of PHF1b is lost after deletion of the amino terminus of PHF1b containing the PHD finger I domain (Figure 10A; PHF1 Δ4).

The alternatively spliced version of PHF1, PHF1a, has been found to be associated with Enhancer of Zeste, EZH2 [42,44,68] to catalyze H3K27 trimethylation, which is essential for the maintenance of the repressive chromatin status of the HoxA gene [42]. The authors also found that the GAL4-PHF1b fusion protein is a strong repressor when it is recruited upstream of a TK promoter reporter gene. Unlike PHF1b, PHF1a has not been shown to bind any particular DNA sequence. Our results suggest, however, that neuronal PHF1b through its recognition of the β_1-INR may play an active role in stabilizing gene transcription rather than repression, consistent with a recent prediction for PHF1b interaction with the ATP-dependent chromodomain helicase DNA binding protein (CHD4) [69,70]. CHD4, when it is outside of the NuRD repressor complex, can function as an activator of transcription in association with p300 histone acetyltransferase [71].

Our results suggest that this may also be the case for PHF1b which immunoprecipitates with SUZ12, a key component of the repressive PRC2 complex (see Figure 11). In our studies, loss of PHF1b from *Gabrb1-p* (as measured by ChIP) is associated with a decrease in *Gabrb1* mRNA levels [34] and a decrease in monomethylated H3K27, without a subsequent increase in trimethylated H3K27 (Figure 8B). This finding suggests that either the monomethylated form may be uniquely associated with PHF1b binding to initiators or that there is an increase in di- and trimethylation that we have not yet detected with ChIP analysis. Recent studies of PHF1, and several other related genes, have revealed that PcG gene products can also be found associated with histone H3 trimethylated at lysine 36 (H3K36me3), a chromatin mark linked to transcriptionally active genes. These results suggest that the PCL family of proteins may facilitate recruitment of PcG proteins to previously active genes, leading to de novo gene silencing [72]. We are currently pursuing these studies in the laboratory to gain a better understanding of PHF1b gene regulation in the nervous system and its potential generalizability to the regulation of other gene products critical for brain development and disease.

From our studies, and taken together with the function of YY1 described above, we propose that binding of unique PcG factors such as PHF1b to the INR may be a key element to dynamically attract the chromatin remodeling machinery to the initiation site of a gene. It is here where stabilization of the pre-initiation complex is so critical for modulating rates of transcription. Unlike cells in many other regions of the body, in neurons small changes in the expression of membrane receptor proteins can have far-reaching effects on the activity of neural networks. Taken together with the finding that GABAergic excitation promotes differentiation of hippocampal progenitor cells [73], identification of a potential relationship between chromatin remodelers, receptor activation, and the transcription and/or repression of certain neurotransmitter receptor subunit genes opens a new area of investigation that may be extremely relevant to activity-dependent gene regulation in the nervous system.

Methods
Antibodies
PHF1(a and b) antibody (rabbit polyclonal) was raised against the peptide RPRLWEGQDVLARWTDGLLY by Research Genetics, Inc (Huntsville, AL, USA). Antibody against H3K27me1 (Cat No. 07–448, rabbit polyclonal) was purchased from Upstate (Millipore) (Billerica, MA, USA). H3K27me3 (Cat No. ab6002, mouse monoclonal)) and SUZ12 (Cat No. ab12073, rabbit polyclonal)) antibodies were obtained from Abcam Inc (Cambridge, MA, USA). A 1–200 to 1-500 dilution of antibodywas used for immunoprecipitation experiments. For Western analysis, a 1–1000 to 1-3000 dilution of antibody was used.

Chemicals
3-aminotriazole and GABA were purchased from Sigma-Aldrich (St. Louis, MO, USA). Yeast and tissue culture media were obtained from Invitrogen (Grand Island, NY, USA).

His3 Screening
The NLY2 strain of yeast carrying two integrated reporter genes (His3 and LacZ) was grown in YPDA media to make competent cells according to [74]. Forty µg of adult or neonatal human brain cDNA library (Clontech, constructed from 6X106 individual bacterial colonies) was transformed into competent yeast plated on minimal media (His-, Leu-) containing 10 mM 3-aminotriazole. Approximately 500 colonies were identified from the primary screen and tested for β-

galactosidase gene expression on X-gal containing plates. Blue colonies were isolated for further analysis in His3 growth screens. Plasmids that were recovered from both screens were transformed back into the original yeast strain to test plasmid linkage. A control experiment was also performed in yeast to verify that the DNA binding property of PHF1b (Genebank accession: BC008834) containing clones was specific to the β_1-INR. A chromosomally integrated reporter (lacZ) gene without the β_1-INR showed no activation from expression of isolated PHF1b (data not shown).

β-galactosidase activity
β-galactosidase activity and X-gal plate assays were performed as described in [75]. DNA sequencing was performed at the Boston University School of Medicine Genetic Core facility. Yeast strain NLY2 (gift of Dr. N. Lehming) (MATa Δgal4, gal80, ura3-52, his3-200, leu2-3, trp1, lys2) was used to integrate two reporter-carrying plasmids in yeast chromosomes. Reporter plasmids were constructed with two separate yeast-integrating vectors that carried Trp1 and Ura3 genes for chromosomal integration. A fragment containing three tandem initiator sites (TCGACTGCGCAGGTCCATTCGGGAAT TACT GCGCAGGTCCATTCGGGAATTA CTGCGCAGGTC CATTCGGGAATTAC) was inserted 40 nucleotides upstream of Gal1 and His3 TATA boxes. To determine the DNA binding function of PHF1b, the deletion constructs were made with pACT2 based candidate plasmids A4 and B37. PFU polymerase amplified PHF1b fragments were inserted into NcoI and XhoI restriction sites of the backbone vector. CMV-PHF1b was constructed by inserting full length human PHF1b cDNA in between Nhe1 and Xho1 sites of pCI-neo Vector (Promega). GABRB1-luciferase was previously described in [7]. 5XGAL4-INR-LUC is a derivative of the pGL2 vector (Promega). A fragment containing a single initiator with five upstream Gal4 sites was inserted in between the SmaI and BglII sites of pGL2. GAL4-VP16 expression was driven by a SV40 promoter and is described in [76]. CMV-DsRed-Nuclear and CMV-DsRed-Monomer were obtained from Clontech for nuclear localization studies. CMV-TAFII250 was a generous gift of Dr. R. Tjian. T7-TAFII150 [77] was a generous gift from Dr. R. G. Roeder and was converted to a CMV-TAFII150 with an insertion of the CMV promoter fragment (blunted BglII-SmaI). GFP fusion plasmids were constructed by inserting GFP (NheI-SalI) in between the CMV promoter and the PHF1b derivatives depicted in the figure. GAL4(1–100)/PHF1b fusions were constructed in a similar way by inserting the GAL4(1–100) fragment into the NheI and SalI sites between the CMV promoter and PHF1b fragments. All plasmids were confirmed by sequence analysis.

Primer extension analysis

Primer extension analysis of the p5XG-INR-LUC plasmid containing the β_1-INR was performed according to [40]. A luciferase specific primer (5'-CCATCCTCTAGA GGATAGAATGGC GCCGGG-3') was used for primer extension analysis. Total RNA was isolated from transfected COS cells containing the p5XG-INR-Luc plasmid and GAL4-VP16 activator plasmid for analysis.

Chromatin IP

ChIP assays were performed as previously described [78]. Five to 10 million cells were used for each assay and were split into three aliquots for immunoprecipitation in the presence and absence of PHF antibodies (200 × dilution). Genomic DNA (gDNA) was sheared to produce fragments of 300–500 bps. Average size was verified by agarose gel electrophoresis. Immunoprecipitatedg DNAs were isolated and dissolved in 100 μL TE to be used as templates for PCR amplification of a 213-bp fragment of the *GABRB1* promoter that contains the PHF1b binding site (β_1-INR). Primers 5'-AAGGGATTGAAATCTGTTGCCTG-3' (β_1-forward) and 5'-CCAAACTCTCTCGATTTTGTACT-3' (β_1-reverse) (rat β1: Genebankaccession: AC114826). 35S-labeled PCR products were separated on a 5% polyacrylamide gel and exposed to X-ray film (Kodak). PCR was also performed on gDNAs precipitated with rabbit IgG (Santa Cruz) as a negative control that was used for normalization. Figure 7C PCR detection was performed without radioactive isotope. Real-time PCR analysis (Figure 8) was performed using primers and probe designed with SciTools (IDT). *GABRB1-p* primers: sense (5'- TGTTTGCAAGGCACAAGGTGTC -3'), antisense (5'-TCTGCGAAGATTCAAGGAATGCAACT -3'); probe: 5'FAM- TCCATTCGGGAATTACTGCCCAGCCGCCGA -TAMRA3'. Thermocycling was done using the ABI7-900HT in a final volume of 20 μL. PCR parameters were 50°C for 2 min, 95°C for 15 min, 50 cycles of 95°C for 15 s, and 60°C for 1 min. Standard curves were generated from rat gDNA (Clonetech). Data were normalized as percentage of antibody/IgG signal after adjustment to input.

Culturing and transfection of primary rat neocortical neurons

Primary cortical and hippocampal neurons were derived from 18-day rat embryos and grown in media as described [7]. Cells were plated on 100 mm tissue culture dishes (1.33 brains per dish). The plating medium was replaced by a serum-free conditioned medium after one-hour incubation. Cultures were maintained for 7–9 days before being used for transfections or ChIP experiments.

Primary cell cultures were transfected using a modified calcium phosphate precipitation method [79]. Briefly, DNA and $CaCl_2$ was mixed with HeBs (137 mM NaCl, 5 mM KCI, 0.7 mM Na_2HPO_4, 7 H_2O, 7.5 mM dextrose, 21 mM HEPES, pH 7.14) and stored in the dark at room temperature for 25–30 min. Cultures were washed twice with DMEM (Invitrogen, Rockville, MD) and 250 μL of a DNA precipitate were added to each dish. CMV-PHF1b or CMV-vector DNA (10 μg) were transfected into each 100 mm dish (Nunc) with 5 μg of the *GABRB1*-luciferase promoter/reporter construct. Cultures were harvested and luciferase activity was measured [80].

Cell culture, transient transfection of COS-7 cells, fluorescent and confocal microscopy

COS-7 cells were grown in DMEM, penicillin/streptomycin, 10% fetal bovine serum (FBS), and 2 mM glutamine. COS-7 cells were grown to confluency in T flasks and treated with trypsin/EDTA. The cells were treated with 10 ml of media and seeded at 2X105/plate. After seeding (24 h), COS-7 cells were transfected using the FUGENE transfection reagent (Roche). 1.2 μl FUGENE/ 1 μg of DNA was used for each transfection. The expression of all plasmids used in our transfection studies was compared by Western analysis to control for nonspecific differences in functional assays that might be due to DNA quality or size of insert. Amount of DNA used in transfection assays was also based on moles rather than μg of vector DNA. After 48 hours, cells were assayed for luciferase activity (Promega kit and Victor 1420 detection system (Wallac)) or visualized with fluorescent microscopy. Luciferase counts were normalized independently to either total protein content or CMV-βgal activity. To prepare the cells for fluorescent microscopy, the plates were incubated 15 min in fixing solution: 4% paraformaldehyde, 25 mM HEPES, 150 mM NaCl, 1 mM $CaCl_2$, and 1 mM $MgCl_2$, washed 3× in PBS and then incubated in a quenching solution (PBS/50 mM NH_4) for 10 min. A PBS wash followed quenching. The cells were permeabilized with PBS/1% Triton X-100 for 5 min followed by a PBS wash. Transfected COS-7 cells were visualized using a fluorescent microscope (Zeiss Axioscope) and photographed using slide film (Kodak Elite II 400). Cells for confocal imaging were plated on glass coverslip dishes (MatTek Corp). Images of primary neurons were acquired using a Zeiss Axiovert 100M laser scanning confocal microscope with a C-Apochromat 40×/1.2 water immersion objective and an optical depth of 1 μm. An argon laser was used to detect GFP and a helium-neon laser was used to detect DsRed. The photomultiplier gain and pinhole aperture were kept constant.

Immunoprecipitation

Cortical cells were rinsed twice in ice-cold PBS and lysed in ice-cold lysate buffer (1% (v/v) Nonidet P-40, 0.1% (w/v) sodium dodecyl sulfate (SDS), 10% (v/v) glycerol, 50 mM, Tris HCl, pH 8, 150 mM NaCl with protease inhibitors (Roche)). Cell lysates were cleared by centrifugation

(20,000 g, 4°C, 10 min). The supernatants were incubated overnight with specific antibody or pre-immune serum. Then, protein A Sepharose beads were added for 2 hours. The beads were washed three times with lysate buffer and once with water. Proteins were eluted by boiling in sodium dodecyl sulfate polyacrylamide gel electrophoresis (SDS/PAGE) loading buffer and separated by SDS/PAGE before Western blotting.

Animal care

Adult male Sprague–Dawley rats (250-300 g) were purchased from Taconic Farms (Germantown, NY, USA) and housed individually with water and food available ad libitum. A 12-h light/dark cycle was maintained and all experiments were performed during the light cycle. All protocols were consistent with the guidelines of the National Institutes of Health and were approved by the Boston University School of Medicine Institutional Animal Care and Use Committee.

Tissue collection, sectioning and antibody staining

For immunohistochemistry, rats were euthanized with 100 mg/kg pentobarbital (i.p.). The animals were then perfused through the heart with 120 ml of 0.9% saline followed by 60 ml 2% paraformaldehyde in 0.1 M PBS, pH 7.3. The brains were removed and further fixed in 2% paraformaldehyde for 48 h at 4°C. Thirty-micron coronal serial sections were obtained using a vibratome (Energy Beam Sciences, Agawam, MA, USA) and placed in PBS until being processed by single-label immunohistochemistry. Brain sections were incubated in 4% normal rabbit serum (Jackson ImmunoResearch, West Grove, PA, USA) diluted in PBS for 45 min to prevent nonspecific binding. The sections were incubated overnight in primary rabbit antibody (PHF1) diluted 1:500 in PBS at 4°C. The incubation was followed by a 30 min wash in PBS. The sections were then incubated for 2 h in biotinylated goat anti-rabbit IgG (Vector Laboratories, Burlingame, CA, USA) diluted 1:500 in PBS. The sections were rinsed in PBS for 30 min, followed by incubation in avidin-biotin-peroxidase reagent (30 min) (ABC Elite; Vector). A final rinse in PBS preceded treatment with diaminobenzidine tetrachloride (DAB) containing H_2O_2 and nickel-enhancing solution for 10 min. Sections were mounted using slides and Slow Fade mounting media (Molecular Probes, Eugene OR, USA). Control sections were processed as described but without primary antibody or in combination with 5-fold excess of PHF blocking peptide for 2 hours before immunohistochemistry was performed.

Western blot analysis

Nuclear extract made from primary rat neocortical neurons [80] was electrophoresed on a 10% SDS-PAGE gel and transferred to a Biorad nylon filter (PVDF type) for Western blot analysis. The filter was probed with PHF1 antibody (1:3000 dilution) and the analysis was performed [81]. Immunoprecipitation of GAL4 fusion proteins was visualized using a polyclonal antibody raised against the GAL4 DNA binding domain (amino acids 1–147). GAL4 antibody was a kind gift Dr. Mark Ptashne.

Conclusions

We have demonstrated that the Polycomblike protein PHF1b binds to β1-INR to stimulate transcription, and that chronic exposure to GABA reduces PHF1 binding and H3K27 monomethylation associated with transcriptional activation. This strongly suggests that PHF1b, a protein involved in homeotic gene expression in Drosophila, may be a molecular transducer of GABAAR function and thus a component of GABA-mediated neurotransmission in the human central nervous system. We have also shown that PHF1b recognition of β1-INR is dependent on a plant homeodomain, an adjacent helix-loop-helix, and short glycine rich motif, and we propose that binding of PHF1b to β1-INR represents a critical step in chromatin remodeling that may be necessary for the modulation of certain forms of transcription. Given that the GABAAR contains recognition sites for a variety of agents used in the treatment of a range of brain disorders, we suggest that additional research into the role of PHF1b in the regulation of gene expression in neurons may potentially lead to the development of novel treatments for neurological and neuropsychiatric diseases such as epilepsy and anxiety.

Competing interest
The authors declare that they have no competing interests.

Authors' contributions
SS, YH, SCM, and SB carried out the molecular biological studies. SS drafted the manuscript. SJR edited the manuscript and wrote the response to reviewers. All authors read and approved the final manuscript.

Acknowledgements
We thank Dr. Marcia Ratner for assistance with Figure 12 during the preparation of the manuscript and Ms. Ramona Faris for her culturing expertise. We also thank Dr. Robert Saint for PHF1b cDNA and Drs. Daniel Roberts and Joseph Ozer for their valuable editorial input. YH was supported by the Program in Biomedical Neuroscience (PBN) at Boston University School of Medicine. SJR and DHF were funded by research grants from NIH {R01 NS050393-010A (SJR) and R01 AA11697-09 (DHF)}. DHF acknowledges NIAAA and NICHD for funding the study.

Author details
[1]Department of Pharmacology & Experimental Therapeutics, Laboratory of Molecular Neurobiology, Boston University School of Medicine, Boston, MA 02118, USA. [2]Department of Pharmacology & Experimental Therapeutics, Laboratory of Translational Epilepsy, Boston University School of Medicine, 72 East Concord Street, Boston, MA 02118, USA.

References
1. Rabow LE, Russek SJ, Farb DH: **From ion currents to genomic analysis: recent advances in GABA_A receptor research.** *Synapse* 1995, **21**:189–274.

2.   Brooks-Kayal AR, Shumate MD, Jin H, Rikhter TY, Coulter DA: **Selective changes in single cell GABAA receptor subunit expression and function in temporal lobe epilepsy.** *Nat Med* 1998, 4:1166–1172.

3.   Roberts DS, Raol YH, Bandyopadhyay S, Lund IV, Budreck EC, Passini MA, Wolfe JH, Brooks-Kayal AR, Russek SJ: **Egr3 stimulation of GABR$_A$4 promoter activity as a mechanism for seizure-induced up-regulation of GABA$_A$ receptor alpha4 subunit expression.** *Proc Natl Acad Sci USA* 2005, 102:11894–11899.

4.   Raol YH, Lund IV, Bandyopadhyay S, Zhang G, Roberts DS, Wolfe JH, Russek SJ, Brooks-Kayal AR: **Enhancing GABA$_A$ Receptor alpha 1 Subunit Levels in Hippocampal Dentate Gyrus Inhibits Epilepsy Development in an Animal Model of Temporal Lobe Epilepsy.** *J Neuroscience* 2006, 26:11342–11346.

5.   Hu Y, Lund IV, Gravielle MC, Farb DH, Brooks-Kayal AR, Russek SJ: **Surface expression of GABAA receptors is transcriptionally controlled by the interplay of cAMP-response element-binding protein and its binding partner inducible cAMP early repressor.** *J Biol Chem* 2008, 283:9328–9340.

6.   Lund IV, Hu Y, Raol YH, Benham RS, Faris R, Russek SJ, Brooks-Kayal AR: **BDNF selectively regulates GABAA receptor transcription by activation of the JAK/STAT pathway.** *Sci Signal* 2008, 1:ra9. http://www.ncbi.nlm.nih.gov/pubmed/18922788.

7.   Russek SJ, Bandyopadhyay S, Farb DH: **An initiator element mediates autologous downregulation of the human type A gamma -aminobutyric acid receptor beta 1 subunit gene.** *Proc Natl Acad Sci U S A* 2000, 97:8600–8605.

8.   Orphanides G, Lagrange T, Reinberg D: **The general transcription factors of RNA polymerase II.** *Genes Dev* 1996, 10:2657–2683.

9.   Roeder RG: **The role of general initiation factors in transcription by RNA polymerase II.** *Trends Biochem Sci* 1996, 21:327–335.

10. Hampsey M: **Molecular genetics of the RNA polymerase II general transcriptional machinery.** *Microbiol Mol Biol Rev* 1998, 62:465–503.

11. Sikorski TW, Buratowski S: **The Basal Initiation Machinery: Beyond the General Transcription Factors.** *Curr Opin Cell Biol* 2009, 21:344–351.

12. Smale ST, Kadonaga JT: **The RNA polymerase II core promoter.** *Annu Rev Biochem* 2003, 72:449–479.

13. Smale ST, Baltimore D: **The "initiator" as a transcription control element.** *Cell* 1989, 57:103–113.

14. Carcamo J, Buckbinder L, Reinberg D: **The initiator directs the assembly of a transcription factor IID-dependent transcription complex.** *Proc Natl Acad Sci U S A* 1991, 88:8052–8056.

15. Weis L, Reinberg D: **Accurate positioning of RNA polymerase II on a natural TATA-less promoter is independent of TATA-binding-protein-associated factors and initiator-binding proteins.** *Mol Cell Biol* 1997, 17:2973–2984.

16. Tora L: **A unified nomenclature for TATA box binding protein (TBP)-associated factors (TAFs) involved in RNA polymerase II transcription.** *Genes Dev* 2002, 16:673–675.

17. Verrijzer CP, Yokomori K, Chen JL, Tjian R: **Drosophila TAFII150: similarity to yeast gene TSM-1 and specific binding to core promoter DNA.** *Science* 1994, 264:933–941.

18. Verrijzer CP, Chen JL, Yokomori K, Tjian R: **Binding of TAFs to core elements directs promoter selectivity by RNA polymerase II.** *Cell* 1995, 81:1115–1125.

19. Shen WC, Green MR: **Yeast TAF(II)145 functions as a core promoter selectivity factor, not a general coactivator.** *Cell* 1997, 90:615–624.

20. Wang EH, Zou S, Tjian R: **TAFII250-dependent transcription of cyclin A is directed by ATF activator proteins.** *Genes Dev* 1997, 11:2658–2669.

21. Chalkley GE, Verrijzer CP: **DNA binding site selection by RNA polymerase II TAFs: a TAF(II)250-TAF(II)150 complex recognizes the initiator.** *Embo J* 1999, 18:4835–4845.

22. Baumann M, Pontiller J, Ernst W: **Structure and basal transcription complex of RNA polymerase II core promoter in the mammalian genome: an overview.** *Mol Biotechnol* 2010, 45:241–247.

23. Shi Y, Seto E, Chang LS, Shenk T: **Transcriptional repression by YY1, a human GLI-Kruppel-related protein, and relief of repression by adenovirus E1A protein.** *Cell* 1991, 67:377–388.

24. Cheriyath V, Roy AL: **Structure-function analysis of TFII-I. Roles of the N-terminal end, basic region, and I-repeats.** *J Biol Chem* 2001, 276:8377–8383.

25. He Y, Casaccia-Bonnefil P: **The Yin and Yang of YY1 in the nervous system.** *J Biochem* 2008, 106:1493–1502.

26. Galvin KM, Shi Y: **Multiple mechanisms of transcriptional repression by YY1.** *Mol Cell Biol* 1997, 17:3723–3732.

27. Strahl BD, Allis CD: **The language of covalent histone modifications.** *Nature* 2000, 403:41–45.

28. Orlando V: **Polycomb, epigenomes, and control of cell identity.** *Cell* 2003, 112:599–606.

29. Ehrenhofer-Murray AE: **Chromatin dynamics at DNA replication, transcription and repair.** *Eur J Biochem* 2004, 271:2335–2349.

30. Choi JK, Howe LJ: **Histone acetylation: truth of consequences?** *Biochem Cell Biol* 2009, 87:139–150.

31. Kennison JA: **The Polycomb and trithorax group proteins of Drosophila: trans-regulators of homeotic gene function.** *Annu Rev Genet* 1995, 29:289–303.

32. Margueron R, Reinberg D: **The Polycomb complex PRC2 and its mark in life.** *Nature* 2011, 469:343–349.

33. Simon J: **Locking in stable states of gene expression: transcriptional control during Drosophila development.** *Curr Opin Cell Biol* 1995, 7:376–385.

34. Pirrotta V: **PcG complexes and chromatin silencing.** *Curr Opin Genet Dev* 1997, 7:249–258.

35. Aasland R, Gibson TJ, Stewart AF: **The PHD finger: implications for chromatin-mediated transcriptional regulation.** *Trends Biochem Sci* 1995, 20:56–59.

36. Rost B, Liu J: **The PredictProtein server.** *Nucleic Acids Res* 2003, 31:3300–3304.

37. Coulson M, Robert S, Eyre HJ, Saint R: **The identification and localization of a human gene with sequence similarity to Polycomblike of Drosophila melanogaster.** *Genomics* 1998, 48:381–383.

38. Capili AD, Schultz DC, Rauscher IF, Borden KL: **Solution structure of the PHD domain from the KAP-1 corepressor: structural determinants for PHD, RING and LIM zinc-binding domains.** *Embo J* 2001, 20:165–177.

39. Pascual J, Martinez-Yamout M, Dyson HJ, Wright PE: **Structure of the PHD zinc finger from human Williams-Beuren syndrome transcription factor.** *J Mol Biol* 2000, 304:723–729.

40. Ma J, Ptashne M: **Deletion analysis of GAL4 defines two transcriptional activating segments.** *Cell* 1987, 48:847–853.

41. Lonie A, D'Andrea R, Paro R, Saint R: **Molecular characterisation of the Polycomblike gene of Drosophila melanogaster, a trans-acting negative regulator of homeotic gene expression.** *Development* 1994, 120:2629–2636.

42. Sarma K, Margueron R, Ivanov A, Pirrotta V, Reinberg D: **Ezh2 requires PHF1 to efficiently catalyze H3 lysine 27 trimethylation in vivo.** *Mol Cell Biol* 2008, 28:2718–2731.

43. Wu L, Rosser DS, Schmidt MC, Berk A: **A TATA box implicated in E1A transcriptional activation of a simple adenovirus 2 promoter.** *Nature* 1987, 326:512–515.

44. Cao R, Wang H, He J, Erdjument-Bromage H, Tempst P, Zhang Y: **Role of hPHF1 in H3K27 methylation and Hox gene silencing.** *Mol Cell Biol* 2008, 5:1862–1872.

45. Laurie DJ, Wisden W, Seeburg PH: **The distribution of thirteen GABAA receptor subunit mRNAs in the rat brain. III. Embryonic and postnatal development.** *J Neurosci* 1992, 12:4151–4172.

46. Brock HW, van Lohuizen M: **The Polycomb group–no longer an exclusive club?** *Curr Opin Genet Dev* 2001, 11:175–181.

47. Ingham PW: **The molecular genetics of embryonic pattern formation in Drosophila.** *Nature* 1988, 335:25–34.

48. Kalkhoven E, Teunissen H, Houweling A, Verrijzer CP, Zantema A: **The PHD type zinc finger is an integral part of the CBP acetyltransferase domain.** *Mol Cell Biol* 2002, 22:1961–1970.

49. Gozani O, Karuman P, Jones DR, Ivanov D, Cha J, Lugovskoy AA, Baird CL, Zhu H, Field SJ, Lessnick SL, Villasenor J, Mehrotra B, Chen J, Rao VR, Brugge JS, Ferguson CG, Payrastre B, Myszka DG, Cantley LC, Wagner G, Divecha N, Prestwich GD, Yuan J: **The PHD finger of the chromatin-associated protein ING2 functions as a nuclear phosphoinositide receptor.** *Cell* 2003, 114:99–111.

50. Ragvin A, Valvatne H, Erdal S, Arskog V, Tufteland KR, Breen K, AM OY, Eberharter A, Gibson TJ, Becker PB, Aasland R: **Nucleosome binding by the bromodomain and PHD finger of the transcriptional cofactor p300.** *J Mol Biol* 2004, 337:773–788.

51. Zuckerkandl E: **Sectorial gene repression in the control of development.** *Gene* 1999, 238:263–276.

52. Ringrose L, Rehmsmeier M, Dura JM, Paro R: **Genome-wide prediction of Polycomb/Trithorax response elements in Drosophila melanogaster.** *Dev Cell* 2003, 5:759–771.

53. Poux S, Horard B, Sigrist CJ, Pirrotta V: **The Drosophila trithorax protein is a coactivator required to prevent re-establishment of polycomb silencing.** *Development* 2002, **129**:2483–2493.

54. Brown JL, Mucci D, Whiteley M, Dirksen ML, Kassis JA: **The Drosophila Polycomb group gene pleiohomeotic encodes a DNA binding protein with homology to the transcription factor YY1.** *Mol Cell* 1998, **1**:1057–1064.

55. Mihaly J, Mishra RK, Karch F: **A conserved sequence motif in Polycomb response elements.** *Mol Cell* 1998, **1**:1065–1066.

56. Hur MW, Laney JD, Jeon SH, Ali J, Biggin MD: **Zeste maintains repression of Ubx transgenes: support for a new model of Polycomb repression.** *Development* 2002, **129**:1339–1343.

57. Rastelli L, Chan CS, Pirrotta V: **Related chromosome binding sites for zeste, suppressors of zeste and Polycomb group proteins in Drosophila and their dependence on Enhancer of zeste function.** *Embo J* 1993, **12**:1513–1522.

58. Thomas MJ, Seto E: **Unlocking the mechanisms of transcription factor YY1: are chromatin modifying enzymes the key?** *Gene* 1999, **236**:197–208.

59. Korhonen P, Huotari V, Soininen H, Salminen A: **Glutamate-induced changes in the DNA-binding complexes of transcription factor YY1 in cultured hippocampal and cerebellar granule cells.** *Brain Res Mol Brain Res* 1997, **52**:330–333.

60. Ma W, Barker JL: **Complementary expressions of transcripts encoding GAD67 and GABAA receptor alpha 4, beta 1, and gamma 1 subunits in the proliferative zone of the embryonic rat central nervous system.** *J Neurosci* 1995, **15**:2547–2560.

61. Atchison L, Ghias A, Wilkinson F, Bonini N, Atchison ML: **Transcription factor YY1 functions as a PcG protein in vivo.** *Embo J* 2003, **22**:1347–1358.

62. Tie F, Prasad-Sinha J, Birve A, Rasmuson-Lestander A, Harte PJ: **A 1 megadalton ESC/E(Z) complex from Drosophila that contains polycomblike and RPD3.** *Mol Cell Biol* 2003, **23**:3352–3362.

63. Yao YL, Yang WM, Seto E: **Regulation of transcription factor YY1 by acetylation and deacetylation.** *Mol Cell Biol* 2001, **21**:5979–5991.

64. Kwon HJ, Chung HM: **Yin Yang 1, a vertebrate polycomb group gene regulates antero-posterior neural patterning.** *Biochem Biophys Res Commun* 2003, **306**:1008–1013.

65. Yoshitake Y, Howard TL, Christian JL, Hollenberg SM: **Misexpression of Polycomb-group proteins in Xenopus alters anterior neural development and represses neural target genes.** *Dev Biol* 1999, **215**:375–387.

66. Barnett MW, Seville RA, Nijjar S, Old RW, Jones EA: **Xenopus Enhancer of Zeste (XEZ); an anteriorly restricted polycomb gene with a role in neural patterning.** *Mech Dev* 2001, **102**:157–167.

67. Kitaguchi T, Nakata K, Nagai T, Aruga J, Mikoshiba K: **Xenopus Polycomblike 2 (XPcl2) controls anterior to posterior patterning of the neural tissue.** *Dev Genes Evol* 2001, **211**:309–314.

68. O'Connell S, Wang L, Robert S, Jones CA, Saint R, Jones RS: **Polycomblike PHD fingers mediate conserved interaction with enhancer of zeste protein.** *J Biol Chem* 2001, **276**:43065–43073.

69. Scott MS, Barton GJ: **Probabilistic prediction and ranking of human protein-protein interactions.** *BMC Bioinformatics* 2007, **8**:239–260.

70. McDowall MD, Scott MS, Barton GJ: **PIPs: Human protein-protein interactions prediction database.** *Nucleic Acids Research* 2009, **37**. (Database issue):D651-6.

71. Williams CJ, Naito T, Arco PG, Seavitt JR, Cashman SM, De Souza B, Qi X, Keables P, Von Andrian UH, Georgopoulos K: **The chromatin remodeler Mi-2beta is required for CD4 expression and T cell development.** *Immunity* 2004, **20**:719–733.

72. Abed JA, Jones RS: **H3K36me3 key to Polycomb-mediated gene silencing in lineage specification.** *Nat Struct Mol Biol* 2012, **19**:1214–1215.

73. Tozuka Y, Fukuda S, Namba T, Seki T, Hisatsune T: **GABAergic excitation promotes neuronal differentiation in adult hippocampal progenitor cells.** *Neuron* 2005, **47**:803–815.

74. Sherman F, Fink GR, Hicks JB: *Laboratory course manual for methods in yeast genetics.* Cold Spring Harbor, New York: Cold Spring Harbor Laboratory; 1986.

75. Himmelfarb HJ, Pearlberg J, Last DH, Ptashne M: **GAL11P: a yeast mutation that potentiates the effect of weak GAL4-derived activators.** *Cell* 1990, **63**:1299–1309.

76. Sadowski I, Ma J, Triezenberg S, Ptashne M: **GAL4-VP16 is an unusually potent transcriptional activator.** *Nature* 1988, **335**:563–564.

77. Martinez E, Ge H, Tao Y, Yuan CX, Palhan V, Roeder RG: **Novel cofactors and TFIIA mediate functional core promoter selectivity by the human TAFII150-containing TFIID complex.** *Mol Cell Biol* 1998, **18**:6571–6583.

78. Kuo MH, Allis CD: **In vivo cross-linking and immunoprecipitation for studying dynamic Protein:DNA associations in a chromatin environment.** *Methods* 1999, **19**:425–433.

79. Xia Z, Dudek H, Miranti CK, Greenberg ME: **Calcium influx via the NMDA receptor induces immediate early gene transcription by a MAP kinase/ERK dependent mechanism.** *J Neurosci* 1996, **16**:5425–5436.

80. Lau GC, Saha S, Faris R, Russek SJ: **Up-regulation of NMDAR1 subunit gene expression in cortical neurons via a PKA-dependent pathway.** *J Neurochem* 2004, **88**:564–575.

81. Bailey D, O'Hare P: **Herpes simplex virus 1 ICP0 co-localizes with a SUMO-specific protease.** *J Gen Virol* 2002, **83**:2951–2964.

9

Reporting of drug induced depression and fatal and non-fatal suicidal behaviour in the UK from 1998 to 2011

Kyla H Thomas[1,4*], Richard M Martin[1], John Potokar[2], Munir Pirmohamed[3] and David Gunnell[1]

Abstract

Background: Psychiatric adverse drug reactions (ADRs) are distressing for patients and have important public health implications. We identified the drugs with the most frequent spontaneous reports of depression, and fatal and non-fatal suicidal behaviour to the UK's Yellow Card Scheme from 1998 to 2011.

Methods: We obtained Yellow Card data from the Medicines and Healthcare products Regulatory Agency for the drugs with the most frequent spontaneous reports of depression and suicidal behaviour from 1964 onwards. Prescribing data were obtained from the NHS Information Centre and the Department of Health. We examined the frequency of reports for drugs and estimated rates of reporting of psychiatric ADRs using prescribing data as proxy denominators from 1998 to 2011, as prescribing data were not available prior to 1998.

Results: There were 110 different drugs with ≥ 20 reports of depression, 58 with ≥10 reports of non-fatal suicidal behaviour and 33 with ≥5 reports of fatal suicidal behaviour in the time period. The top five drugs with the most frequent reports of depression were the smoking cessation medicines varenicline and bupropion, followed by paroxetine (a selective serotonin reuptake inhibitor), isotretinoin (used in acne treatment) and rimonabant (a weight loss drug). Selective serotonin reuptake inhibitors, varenicline and the antipsychotic medicine clozapine were included in the top five medicines with the most frequent reports of fatal and non-fatal suicidal behaviour. Medicines with the highest reliably measured reporting rates of psychiatric ADRs per million prescriptions dispensed in the community included rimonabant, isotretinoin, mefloquine (an antimalarial), varenicline and bupropion. Robust denominators for community prescribing were not available for two drugs with five or more suicide reports, efavirenz (an antiretroviral medicine) and clozapine.

Conclusions: Depression and suicide-related ADRs are reported for many nervous system and non-nervous system drugs. As spontaneous reports cannot be used to determine causality between the drug and the ADR, psychiatric ADRs which can cause significant public alarm should be specifically assessed and reported in all randomised controlled trials.

Keywords: Adverse drug reaction, Suicide, Non-fatal suicidal behaviour, Self injury, Depression, Yellow card, Adverse effects

Background

Adverse drug reactions (ADRs) cost the UK's NHS up to £2 billion each year [1]. In recent years there has been growing concern that certain prescribed medicines may be associated with psychiatric adverse drug reactions such as depression, non-fatal self-harm and suicide [2,3].

The occurrence of medication induced suicide is particularly distressing to the general public. In the UK, television programmes such as the British Broadcasting Company (BBC) programme "Secrets of Seroxat" which was first aired in October 2002 and "Dying for clear skin" shown in November 2012, have attracted record viewing figures and public response [4,5]. These documentaries focussed on the possible risk of suicide with the antidepressant paroxetine and isotretinoin (used to treat severe acne) and showed that drug- induced psychiatric ADRs have the potential to cause significant

* Correspondence: kyla.thomas@bristol.ac.uk
[1]School of Social and Community Medicine, University of Bristol, Canynge Hall 39 Whatley Road, Bristol BS8 2PS, UK
[4]Health and Wellbeing Division, Department for Children, Adults and Health, South Gloucestershire Council Badminton Road, Yate, Bristol, UK
Full list of author information is available at the end of the article

public alarm. This may lead to adverse health outcomes if unfounded safety concerns result in the reduced use of effective medicines. When a drug is first licensed for use in the general population, there is limited information about its possible adverse effects, as pre-marketing drug trials are underpowered to detect rare psychiatric ADRs such as suicide [6]. Therefore post marketing surveillance using spontaneous reporting systems is crucial, particularly for rare outcomes. However, only a small number of studies have systematically described the medicines which are associated with spontaneous reports of psychiatric ADRs [7-10]; to the best of our knowledge, this has never been done before in the UK.

The aim of this paper is to identify the drugs with the most frequent reporting of suspected psychiatric ADRs to the UK's Yellow Card Scheme from 1998 to 2011. We focus on depression and fatal and non-fatal suicidal behaviour. Although drug induced suicide is the psychiatric ADR that is most likely to cause significant public concern, we also include reports of depressive illness and non-fatal suicidal behaviour which are known to be important risk factors for completed suicide [11].

Methods

Yellow card data

The Yellow Card Scheme is used by the Medicines and Healthcare products Regulatory Agency (MHRA) to monitor the safety of currently licensed medicines and vaccines in the UK and is part of routine pharmacovigilance. Currently, health professionals (doctors, dentists, nurses, and pharmacists), coroners, patients, parents and carers are encouraged to report 'suspected' adverse drug reactions to the scheme using paper Yellow Cards or electronic reports (https://YellowCard.mhra.gov.uk accessed 27th February 2014).

We received preliminary data from the MHRA on all spontaneous reports to the Yellow Card Scheme from its creation in 1964 until the 25th January 2012 using the following Higher Level Terms (HLTs) from the Medical Dictionary for Regulatory Affairs (MedDRA): (a) Depressive disorders; and (b) Suicidal and self injurious behaviour. Details of the Preferred Terms (PTs) which are included in the HLTs are shown in Additional file 1. Due to the large number of drugs involved (Yellow Card reports of depressive disorders were received for 872 medicines, reports of non-fatal suicidal behaviour were received for 425 medicines and reports of fatal suicidal behaviour were received for 196 medicines) we requested detailed individual reports for drugs using the following pragmatically selected thresholds:

1. Twenty or more reports for depressive disorders with a non-fatal outcome.

2. Ten or more reports for suicidal and self injurious behaviour with a non-fatal outcome

3. Five or more reports for suicidal and self injurious behaviour with a fatal outcome

For reports of suicidal and self injurious behaviour associated with a fatal outcome (i.e. completed suicide), the MHRA also provided us with information regarding whether the medicine had also been taken in overdose; this is important as in some cases suicide may have been the result of the deliberate ingestion of excessive quantities of medicines (e.g. self poisoning with pain killers such as paracetamol and co-proxamol) and not actually an adverse effect of the drug. Additionally, new European Union (EU) legislation has amended the definition of the term adverse reaction to include unintended effects from unauthorised as well as authorised use of medication [12]. Age- and sex- specific data were provided in an aggregated format and were not available for individual reports. Data were anonymised, so the suspected ADR could not be linked to either the patient or the reporter. We obtained permission for use of Yellow Card data from the Independent Scientific Advisory Committee for MHRA database research. Ethics approval was not required for this study as Category 1b data are releaseable under the Freedom of Information Act (FOIA) 2000.

Prescribing data

Prescription cost analysis (PCA) data provide details of the number of items and the net ingredient cost of all prescriptions which have been dispensed in the community in England. Yearly prescription cost analysis data for England from 1998 to 2011 were obtained from the NHS Information Centre (http://www.hscic.gov.uk/prescribing accessed 13th September 2012) and used as crude proxy denominators for the yearly use of individual drugs. Individual drug data on the number of prescriptions dispensed were not available prior to 1998.

For drugs that were not commonly prescribed in the community (we defined this as <100 000 prescriptions in the 14 year study period) we also obtained data from 2008–2011 on hospital usage of medicines by acute trusts from the Commercial Medicines Unit of the Department of Health (cmu.dh.gov.uk). These data provided an estimation of yearly usage for those medicines that are more likely to be prescribed in hospitals than by general practitioners (GPs) in the community. Hospital usage data were not available prior to 2008.

Classification of medicines

We used the 2014 Anatomical Therapeutic Chemical (ATC) classification system to categorise the medicines [13]. Medicines are classified based on their main indication for use worldwide and there is only one ATC code for each route of administration.

We stratified the medicines into nervous system medications and non-nervous system medications according to their ATC classification to assess whether our psychiatric outcomes of interest were more likely to be reported for nervous system drugs than drugs which affect other systems. Although bupropion is only licensed for use as a smoking cessation medicine in the UK, its ATC code was changed in 2009 from ATC level 5 N07BA02 (under ATC level 4 N07BA- Drugs used in nicotine dependence) to N06AX12 (under ATC level 4 N06AX- Other antidepressants) to represent its main indication worldwide (personal communication WHO Collaborating Centre for Drug Statistics Methodology).

Statistical analyses
Stata version 12.0 (StataCorp, USA) and Excel 2007 (Microsoft, USA) were used for the analyses. We produced frequency tables for the drugs (all, nervous system and non nervous system drugs) with the most frequent reports of depression and non-fatal and fatal suicidal behaviour from 1998 to 2011. For drugs with reports of fatal suicidal behaviour we also examined the percentage of these reports that included ingestion of the specific medicine in an overdose (i.e. self-poisoning with the medicine).

We calculated overall rates of reporting of suspected ADRs per million prescriptions from 1998 to 2011 using the number of reports for each drug as the numerator and the number of prescriptions for each drug from the PCA data as the denominator [14]. Scatter plots of the reporting rates of depressive disorders versus non-fatal suicidal behaviour and versus suicide were created and Spearman's correlation coefficients were calculated to examine possible correlations between the rates of reporting of depression with non-fatal and fatal suicidal behaviour. We used Spearman's correlation coefficient as it is a non parametric method which does not assume that the data are normally distributed; this is particularly relevant in small samples.

Results
Psychiatric ADR reporting 1964–2012
Over the entire time period (1964 to 25th January 2012) there were 6800 Yellow Card reports (35.8% male) of depressive disorders, 3624 reports (42.5% male) of non-fatal suicidal behaviour and 664 reports (69.6% male) of suicide; these reports were 1.65% of all reports made to the database. The ratio of reports of non-fatal to fatal suicidal behaviour was 5.5: 1. Eighteen to 35 year olds accounted for 24.6% of reports of depressive disorders, 28.9% of reports of non-fatal suicidal behaviour and 29.7% of suicide reports. People aged 36 to 65 years

accounted for 47.7% of reports of depressive disorders, 43.8% of reports of non-fatal suicidal behaviour and 48.2% of suicide reports. Ten percent of reports of depressive disorders, 4.2% of non-fatal suicidal behaviour reports and 7.1% of suicide reports were from people aged ≥ 66 years.

Reports and prescribing 1998–2011
Using our thresholds, there were 110 different drugs with 20 or more Yellow Card reports of depressive disorders, 58 with 10 or more reports of non-fatal suicidal behaviour and 33 with five or more reports of suicide from January 1st 1998 to December 31st 2011.

For all drugs, the top five medicines for reports of depressive disorders were the smoking cessation medicines, varenicline (1st) and bupropion (2nd), paroxetine, a selective serotonin reuptake inhibitor (SSRI) antidepressant (3rd), isotretinoin, used in acne treatment (4th) and rimonabant, a weight loss drug (5th). The top five medicines for reports of non-fatal suicidal behaviour were paroxetine (1st), varenicline (2nd), the SSRI antidepressants citalopram (3rd) and fluoxetine (4th) and clozapine, an antipsychotic (5th). With the exception of varenicline and clozapine all of the drugs with the highest reporting of non-fatal suicidal behaviour are SSRIs. The drug with the most frequent reports of suicide was clozapine, an antipsychotic agent (1st), followed by three SSRIs, citalopram (2nd), fluoxetine (3rd) and paroxetine (4th) and a serotonin noradrenaline reuptake inhibitor (SNRI), venlafaxine (5th). Although bupropion and isotretinoin were in the top five for reports of depressive disorders, for reports of non-fatal suicidal behaviour, bupropion was ranked 7th and isotretinoin was ranked 11th. For suicide, bupropion was ranked 22nd and isotretinoin was ranked 7th. Although varenicline was ranked 1st for reports of depressive disorders and second for reports of non-fatal suicidal behaviour, for suicide it was ranked 6th. Unlike the other smoking cessation drugs, there were only 17 Yellow Card reports of depressive disorders, five reports of non-fatal suicidal behaviour and no reports of suicide for nicotine replacement therapy.

Figure 1 shows the distribution of the major drug classes of the top 20 medicines with the greatest number of Yellow Card reports of depressive disorders, non-fatal suicidal behaviour and suicide. Reports of psychiatric adverse reactions were most frequently observed for antidepressants (20% of drugs in the top 20 for reports of depressive disorders, 40% for reports of non-fatal suicidal behaviour and 45% for suicide reports). Antipsychotic agents were also commonly implicated (25% of suicide reports and 15% of reports of non-fatal suicidal behaviour) as well as anticonvulsants (10% of reports of depressive disorders and 15% of reports of non-fatal suicidal behaviour). Other drug classes such as smoking cessation drugs, weight loss medicines and antimalarials also had frequent

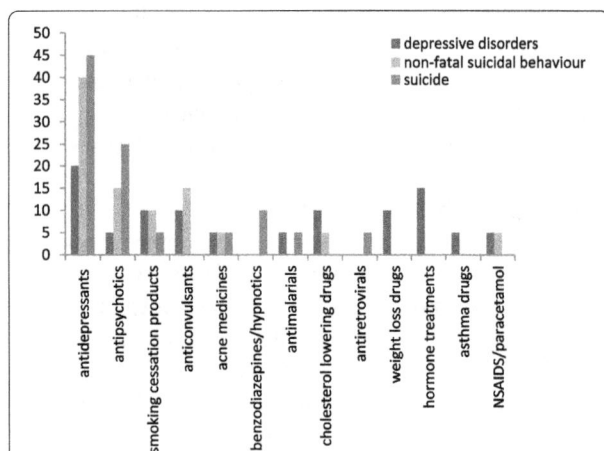

Figure 1 Distribution of major classes of the Top 20 medicines with the highest numbers of Yellow Card reports for depressive disorders and fatal and non-fatal suicidal behaviour.

Table 1 Percentage of Yellow Card reports for suicides where the implicated drug was taken in an episode of fatal self-poisoning from 1998 to 2011

Drug	Number of suicide reports	Percentage of overdose in suicide reports from 1998-2011
Aspirin	4	100.0
Tramadol	6	66.7
Zopiclone	13	61.5
Paracetamol	5	60.0
Diazepam	11	54.5
Amitryptiline	6	50.0
Temazepam	4	50.0
Co-proxamol	4	50.0
Quetiapine	13	46.2
Olanzapine	24	37.5
Venlafaxine	42	31.0
Sertraline	21	19.0
Citalopram	70	17.1
Bupropion*	6	16.7
Clozapine	78	12.8
Mirtazapine	17	11.8
Paroxetine	50	10.0
Varenicline	41	7.3
Escitalopram	15	6.7
Fluoxetine	58	5.2
Risperidone	24	4.2
Duloxetine	28	3.6
Isotretinoin	32	3.1
Aripiprazole	15	0.0
Mefloquine	8	0.0
Efavirenz	7	0.0
Infliximab	5	0.0
Flupenthixol	4	0.0

*Bupropion is licensed for use as an antidepressant in other countries but not the UK.

reports of psychiatric ADRs (smoking cessation medicines- 10% of reports of depressive disorders and non-fatal suicidal behaviour, 5% of suicide reports; weight loss medicines- 10% of reports of depressive disorders; and antimalarials- 5% of reports of depressive disorders and suicide).

With the exception of varenicline, bupropion and paroxetine, most of the top 10 drugs with reports of depressive disorders are treatments for non nervous system indications such as isotretinoin (an anti-acne preparation), rimonabant (an anti-obesity preparation), simvastatin (a lipid modifying agent), mefloquine (an antimalarial), levonorgestrel (a hormone), atorvastatin (a lipid modifying agent) and rofecoxib (an anti-inflammatory and antirheumatic product). However for reports of non-fatal and fatal suicidal behaviour, most of the top 10 drugs were nervous system drugs such as antidepressants, antipsychotics and the smoking cessation medicines.

The drugs (nervous system drugs versus non nervous system drugs) with reports of more than one psychiatric ADR stratified by ATC level 1 classification are listed in Additional file 2. Table 1 shows the percentage of Yellow Card reports of suicide which involved intentional overdose (i.e. deliberate ingestion of the medicines). Drugs that were commonly implicated in fatal overdose were aspirin, where 100% of suicide reports involved deliberate ingestion of the drug, followed by 66.7% for tramadol, a narcotic analgesic, 61.5% for zopiclone, a hypnotic medicine and 60% for paracetamol (an analgesic).

Rates of ADRs 1998–2011

In order to account for how often the drug is prescribed we describe reporting rates using community prescribing data next (Table 2). Although the SSRI antidepressants (paroxetine, fluoxetine and citalopram) had the most

frequent reports of depressive disorders and fatal and non-fatal suicidal behaviour, reporting rates were low as these drugs are widely prescribed. Additionally, simvastatin had a much lower reporting rate of depressive disorders than mefloquine (0.4 per million prescriptions versus 457 per million) although there was a similar number of reports (110 versus 105 respectively).

For medicines in the top 20 that were more commonly prescribed in secondary care such as efavirenz and clozapine, rates were re-calculated using hospital prescribing data for the most recent years. The rate of reporting for efavirenz was 27.4 per million hospital prescriptions

Table 2 Rates of Yellow Card adverse reports per million prescriptions dispensed for the top 20 drugs with the highest number of adverse reports for depressive disorders, non-fatal suicidal behaviour and suicide

	Drug	Number of reports	Overall rate per million prescriptions 1998-2011	95% confidence intervals
Depressive disorders				
Non-nervous system drugs	Rimonabant	190	773	667-891
	Isotretinoin	199	553	479-636
	Mefloquine	105	457	373-553
	Etonogestrel	51	82	61-108
	Sibutramine	55	25	19-33
	Levonorgestrel	86	14	12-18
	Desogestrel	64	9	7-12
	Rofecoxib	73	9	7-12
	Montelukast	45	5	3-6
	Atorvastatin	74	0.6	0.5-0.8
	Simvastatin	110	0.4	0.3-0.5
Nervous system drugs	Clozapine	50	630	468-831
	Bupropion*	483	330	301-361
	Varenicline	975	248	233-264
	Topiramate	61	18	14-23
	Levetiracetam	66	15	12-19
	Paroxetine	263	8	7-9
	Venlafaxine	57	2	2-3
	Fluoxetine	56	0.9	0.7-1.2
	Citalopram	56	0.7	0.5-0.9
Non-fatal suicidal behaviour				
Non-nervous system drugs	Rimonabant	74	30	236-378
	Isotretinoin	71	197	154-249
Nervous system drugs	Clozapine	132	1664	1393-1973
	Atomoxetine	126	230	192-274
	Varenicline	675	172	159-185
	Bupropion*	117	80	66-96
	Duloxetine	97	32	26-39
	Paroxetine	709	21	19-22
	Levetiracetam	69	16	12-20
	Topiramate	37	11	8-15
	Pregabalin	47	6	5-8
	Escitalopram	61	6	4-7
	Venlafaxine	113	4	3-5
	Risperidone	49	3	3-5
	Mirtazapine	67	3	3-4
	Olanzapine	48	3	2-4
	Citalopram	219	3	2-3
	Fluoxetine	161	3	2-3
	Sertraline	51	2	1-3
	Paracetamol	69	0.4	0.3-0.5

Table 2 Rates of Yellow Card adverse reports per million prescriptions dispensed for the top 20 drugs with the highest number of adverse reports for depressive disorders, non-fatal suicidal behaviour and suicide (Continued)

Suicide				
Non-nervous system drugs	Efavirenz	7	2312	930-4757
	Isotretinoin	32	89	61-126
	Mefloquine	8	35	15-69
Nervous system drugs	Clozapine	78	984	778-1227
	Varenicline	41	10	8-14
	Duloxetine	28	9	6-13
	Aripiprazole	15	9	5-14
	Risperidone	24	2	1-3
	Paroxetine	50	2	1-2
	Venlafaxine	42	1	1-2
	Olanzapine	24	1	0.9-2
	Escitalopram	15	1	0.8-2
	Quetiapine	13	1	0.6-2
	Fluoxetine	58	0.9	0.7-1
	Citalopram	70	0.8	0.7-1
	Mirtazapine	17	0.8	0.5-1
	Sertraline	21	0.8	0.5-1
	Zopiclone	13	0.2	0.1-0.4
	Diazepam	11	0.2	0.1-0.3
	Amitryptiline	6	0.1	0.03-0.2

*Bupropion is licensed for use as an antidepressant in other countries but not the UK.

for suicide (compared to 2312 per million community prescriptions) which would move efavirenz from 1st to 3rd place for non nervous system drugs associated with suicide (see Table 2). Clozapine had a reporting rate of 19.7 per million hospital prescriptions for depressive disorders (630 per million community prescriptions), 62.3 per million hospital prescriptions for non-fatal suicidal behaviour (1664 per million community prescriptions) and 36.3 per million hospital prescriptions for suicide (984 per million community prescriptions). Therefore clozapine remained at the top of the rankings for nervous system drugs with the highest reporting rate of suicide.

Figure 2 shows scatter plots of the reporting rates of non-fatal suicidal behaviour versus depressive disorders and suicide versus depressive disorders for nervous system versus non nervous system drugs (see Additional file 2). Clozapine and efavirenz were excluded as these drugs are not commonly prescribed in the community. For nervous system drugs there was positive correlation between reporting rates of non-fatal suicidal behaviour and depressive disorders (n = 14, Spearman's rho 0.88, p < 0.001) as well as for suicide and depressive disorders (n = 9 Spearman's rho 0.88, p < 0.01). For non- nervous

system drugs there was slightly weaker positive correlation between the rates for non-fatal suicidal behaviour and depression (n = 11, Spearman's rho 0.78, p < 0.01). Reports of depressive disorders and suicide were observed for only two non nervous system drugs so Spearman's rho was not calculated.

Discussion

Summary of findings

Reports of drug induced depression and fatal and non-fatal suicidal behaviour constitute a very small minority of total ADR reports. We found that the drugs with the highest frequency of Yellow Card reports of psychiatric ADRs included nervous system medicines such as the SSRI antidepressants, smoking cessation medicines varenicline and bupropion and the antipsychotic drug clozapine as well as non-nervous system drugs such as isotretinoin (used in acne treatment) and mefloquine (an antimalarial). Reports of depression were most frequently observed for non nervous system drugs; most reports of suicide and non-fatal suicidal behaviour involved nervous system medicines. Analgesics (such as paracetamol) and hypnotics/benzodiazepines were also likely to be implicated in reports of suicide but most of these deaths were reported to have

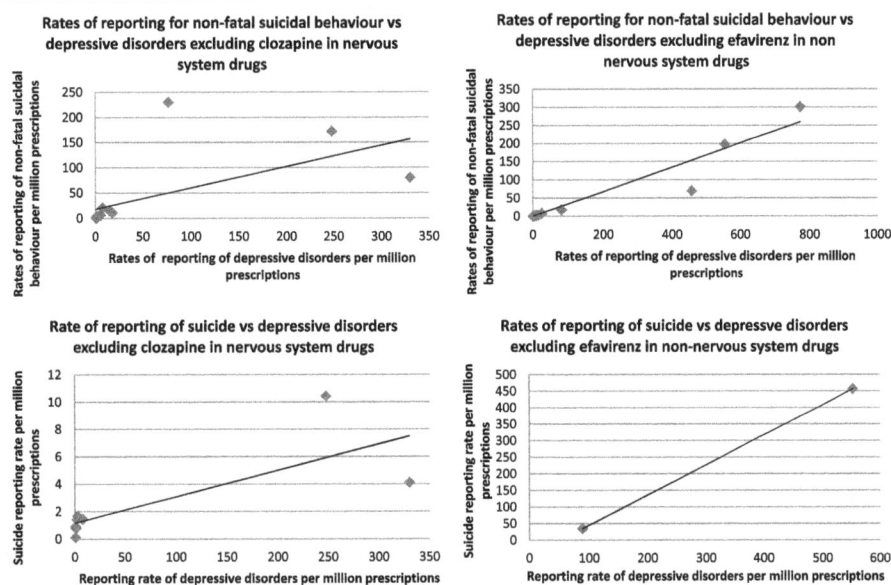

Figure 2 Scatter plots of reporting rates of suicide versus rates of depressive disorders and rates of non-fatal suicidal behaviour versus rates of depressive disorders for nervous system medicines (excluding clozapine) and non nervous system medicines (excluding efavirenz).

been caused by deliberate ingestion of excessive quantities of the drugs in overdose. Reporting rates for efavirenz and clozapine were much lower when data on hospital usage were used instead of community prescriptions as these drugs are not likely to be prescribed in a primary care setting. There was positive association between the reporting rates of self-harm and depression and suicide and depression for nervous system and non-nervous system drugs.

Strengths and limitations
This is the first study to systematically describe the reporting of depression and fatal and non-fatal suicidal behaviour to the UK's Yellow Card Scheme although it excludes other psychiatric adverse drug reactions, such as anxiety, psychosis and insomnia. Strengths include the 14 years of reporting and the inclusion of drug utilisation data (prescribing data) to calculate reporting rates. We examined the reports from all medicines that met pre-defined thresholds for inclusion and stratified the medicines by their ATC level 1 classification. The occurrence of Yellow Card reports of suspected ADRs with a specific drug does not indicate that the drug definitely caused the ADR as there are many factors that have to be taken into consideration when assessing causal relationships, such as the timing of when the drug was taken in relation to the outcome, the biological plausibility, the possible contribution of concomitant medication and the underlying disease [15].

Additionally, the reporting of ADRs using Yellow Cards is affected by the extent of use of a particular drug, whether the drug is newly licensed (i.e. length of time of

drug on the market) [16], stimulated reporting caused by safety warnings about a drug (notoriety bias) [17], adverse media publicity about a drug and the seriousness of the ADR [18]. In our study there were 5.5 times as many non-fatal suicidal behaviour as suicide reports, whereas the ratio of non-fatal self-harm to suicide in the general population is 30:1[19]. This is likely to have occurred because more serious (or fatal) adverse reactions are reported more often. Under-reporting is a serious issue; only 6% of ADRs in hospital and general practice are reported in the UK [20,21]. Also, drugs such as oral contraceptives and beta blockers which have long been recognised as associated with depression, were likely to have low numbers of reports in our study period, as Yellow Card reporting decreases the longer the drug has been available on the market [18]. Over the counter medicines, such as nicotine replacement therapy, may also be subject to under-reporting.

Due to the large numbers of drugs with reports of our psychiatric ADRs of interest, we used specific thresholds to request detailed individual reports. Although this approach is likely to have identified those medicines which would have potentially caused the most harm, it may have missed drugs which are rarely prescribed, but which have a high ratio of reports to prescriptions and drugs which have only recently been marketed with low consumption.

The number of Yellow Card reports received cannot be used to determine the actual incidence rate of an ADR as both the total number of reactions occurring and the number of patients who actually used the drug are unknown (although we used community prescribing data as a proxy). We used PCA data for the number of prescriptions dispensed in the community to estimate a rate of ADR reports per million prescriptions of the drug; this is a very crude estimation and did not include standardisation by age or sex or take account of the average duration of prescribing or the indication for which the drug was prescribed. Age and sex standardisation are important as most non-fatal suicidal behaviour occurs in women and at younger ages when general drug prescribing is rarer [22]. The importance of using proxy denominators to estimate reporting rates was shown by the stark contrast in the reporting rates of depression for mefloquine and simvastatin, although similar numbers of absolute reports were obtained for both medicines.

Certain drugs, such as efavirenz and clozapine are more often prescribed in hospitals, which resulted in underestimation of the denominator and over-estimation of reporting rates in our analyses using community prescriptions. Reporting rates were much lower when hospital prescribing data were used although these data were only available for a more limited time period. Additionally, clozapine is subject to extensive monitoring for adverse effects such as agranulocytosis; this would also increase the reporting of other unrelated adverse effects. Therefore the reporting pattern is likely to be very different for clozapine compared with other medicines for which reporting is truly spontaneous; limiting inference about possible causal associations.

Disproportionality analysis is another method that is often used to identify potential safety hazards or safety signals in spontaneous reporting data. Dal Pan et al. (2013) defined disproportionality as "the finding that a given adverse event/adverse drug reaction is reported for a particular drug more often than would be expected based on the number of reports of that adverse event/adverse drug reaction for all other drugs in the database" [23]. This method has several advantages over the use of proxy denominator data to calculate reporting rates because it is not affected by changes in the reporting of ADRs and does not require the use of external data sources [23]. Statistical methods for determining disproportionality include the use of the proportional reporting ratio (PRR), which can be interpreted in a similar manner to a risk ratio (i.e. a higher ratio indicates a stronger signal) [24]. However, the aim of this study was to provide a descriptive overview of the drugs associated with frequent Yellow card reports of depressive disorders and fatal and non-fatal self-harm as opposed to identifying new safety signals.

Evidence from other studies of worldwide spontaneous reporting systems

Few studies have examined the spontaneous reporting of psychiatric ADRs [7-10]. Robertson and Allison (2009)

used the Food and Drug Administration Adverse Event Reporting System (FDA AERS) to examine whether drugs associated with reports of suicidal ideation were also associated with reports of suicide attempts and found that many different classes of drugs were associated with both outcomes [10]. One recent study examined the reporting of psychiatric ADRs in the Swedish paediatric population using the Swedish Drug Information System (SWEDIS) database. In keeping with our analysis, this study found that isotretinoin, antiepileptics, SSRIs and montelukast (used in the treatment of asthma) were frequently associated with serious psychiatric ADRs [7]. Other frequently implicated drugs included vaccines, centrally working sympathomimetics and melatonin. An earlier study looked at reports to Canada's adverse drug reaction database from 1965 until the early 1990s. Adrenergic drugs (clonidine and methyldopa), beta blockers (propranolol), corticosteroids, benzodiazepines and oral contraceptives were associated with more than 10 reports of depression although none of these drugs featured prominently in our analysis, probably because we focussed on later years and reports of ADRs decrease the longer a particular drug has been on the market [8]. Vilhelmsson et al. (2011) looked at reports of psychiatric ADRs with antidepressant medication that were made to a consumer association in Sweden [9]. Depression was reported as an ADR for citalopram, escitalopram and paroxetine. Suicidal behaviour was reported as a psychiatric ADR for all included antidepressants, mainly SSRIs and serotonin noradrenaline reuptake inhibitors (SNRIs). These findings are also consistent with our analysis. Last, Aagaard and Hansen (2013) examined ADRs reported by consumers in Europe for nervous system medications including antiepileptics, antidepressants and smoking cessation medicines [25]. Most of the ADRs were reported for psychiatric disorders which also accounted for the majority of ADRs categorised as serious [25].

Other methods used to investigate psychiatric ADRs

There are three main explanations for the higher frequency of reports of depression and suicidal behaviour observed with certain drugs. First, the drug may have a causal role in triggering the adverse drug reaction. Second, the drug may have no causal role but is used in a condition which increases the risk of developing the adverse outcome, for example an association between antidepressants and suicide may be explained by the fact that depression itself is a risk factor for suicide [11]. Third, the drug may or may not have a causal role but there are reasons why patients, healthcare professionals and other individuals are more likely to send in a spontaneous report for the drug. For example, in the UK there was an increase in spontaneous reports of ADRs for paroxetine following adverse media publicity from the BBC Panorama programmes which suggested an association between paroxetine and suicidal behaviour [26]. In addition, the association between isotretinoin and inflammatory bowel disease observed in the FDA AERS has been explained by an excess of lawyer-initiated reports related to pending isotretinoin lawsuits [27]. Although spontaneous reporting systems are important for identifying previously unknown ADRs, RCTs and meta-analyses of RCTs are the preferred study designs for the evaluation of drug therapies, as if properly conducted, they provide the strongest evidence of causality between exposure to a particular drug and the outcome of interest [28]. The strongest evidence of adverse psychiatric ADRs comes from meta-analyses of placebo controlled randomised controlled trials (RCTs). These show increased risk of self-harm and suicidal thinking in children prescribed SSRIs such as paroxetine compared with placebo (3.7% vs 2.5%, RR 1.51:95% CI 0.62 to 3.69) [29]. Such evidence has resulted in regulatory action to restrict the use of SSRIs in young people in many countries. The authorisation for rimonabant was suspended by the European Medicines Agency in October 2008 because its adverse psychiatric effects, particularly depression, were felt to outweigh its benefits as a mildly effective weight loss drug [2]. These findings were also obtained from meta-analyses of randomised controlled trials and are in keeping with our findings of a high reporting rate of depression and non-fatal self-harm with rimonabant [30].

More recently, the MHRA in the UK and their equivalent in the US, the Food and Drug Administration (FDA), have issued warnings in relation to certain drugs such as varenicline, based on spontaneous reports of suspected ADRs in individual cases from the Yellow Card Scheme in the UK and its equivalent in the USA [31]. Prescription event monitoring studies have found conflicting results; a study carried out in New Zealand found that varenicline use was associated with more reports of suicide and suicidal ideation whereas a more recent study in England did not find any evidence for an increase in reports of depression and other neuropsychiatric adverse events with varenicline [32,33]. However, observational cohort studies have not found any definitive evidence that varenicline and bupropion are associated with increased suicidal behaviour [17,34].

In June 2009 the FDA requested the addition of information regarding neuropsychiatric adverse effects to the precautions section of montelukast prescribing information [35]. A review of Merck drug company trials failed to identify any completed suicides associated with its use [36], a finding supported by analysis of a large primary care database in the UK [37]. A meta-analysis of suicidal risk during treatment with clozapine also found a lower overall risk of suicidal behaviour associated with clozapine compared with other treatments for psychosis [38].

Although efavirenz has been associated with spontaneous reports of psychiatric ADRs, there was no clear evidence from a systematic review that patients taking efavirenz were at increased risk of suicide [39]. A recent review found little evidence for an increased risk of suicide and suicidal behaviour with antidepressants, antiepileptics, varenicline, montelukast and antipsychotics [40]. It is reassuring that, with the exception of SSRIs in young people, other study designs have not confirmed elevated risks of neuropsychiatric adverse effects for medicines with high numbers of spontaneous reports in our study.

Conclusions

Spontaneous Yellow Card reports of depression and suicide-related ADRs were obtained for many different classes of drugs including nervous system drugs such as antidepressants, antipsychotics and smoking cessation medicines, in addition to non- nervous system drugs such as weight loss medicines and drugs used in the treatment of acne. Although we could not examine emerging safety concerns for recently marketed drugs, it is reassuring that no new drugs were identified. As spontaneous reports of ADRs do not indicate causal associations between drugs and adverse reactions, we suggest that psychiatric adverse events which can cause significant public alarm such as suicide, suicidal behaviour and depression should be specifically monitored and reported in all randomised controlled trials.

Additional files

Additional file 1: List of Preferred Terms included in the Medical Dictionary for Regulatory Affairs Higher Level Terms (a) Depressive disorders and (b) Suicidal and self injurious behaviour.

Additional file 2: List of drugs with the most frequent reports of depressive disorders and fatal and non-fatal suicidal behaviour.

Competing interests
All authors have completed the Unified Competing Interest form at http://www.icmje.org/downloads/coi_disclosure.pdf (available on request from the corresponding author) and declare:
KHT has received support from the National Institute for Health Research for the submitted work, has no financial relationships with any organisations that might have an interest in the submitted work in the previous 3 years and has no other relationships or activities that could appear to have influenced the submitted work. RMM has no support for the submitted work, had specified relationship with the MHRA in the previous 3 years (is a member of the MHRA's Independent Scientific Advisory Committee for CPRD research and receives expenses and a small fee for meeting attendance and preparation for meetings) and has no other relationships or activities that could appear to have influenced the submitted work. DG had no support for the submitted work, had specified relationship with the MHRA in the previous 3 years (is a member of the MHRA's Pharmacovigilance Expert Advisory Group and receives travel expenses and a small fee for meeting attendance and preparation for meetings) and has no other relationships or activities that could appear to have influenced the submitted work. MP has no support for the submitted work, had specified relationship with the MHRA in the previous 3 years (is Chair of the Pharmacovigilance Expert Advisory Group of the Commission on Human Medicines and receives

travel expenses and a small fee for meeting attendance and preparation for meetings) and has no other relationships or activities that could appear to have influenced the submitted work. JP has no support for the submitted work, has no financial relationships with any organisations that might have an interest in the submitted work in the previous 3 years and has no other relationships or activities that could appear to have influenced the submitted work.

Authors' contributions

KT, DG and RMM conceived of the study. KT performed all of the statistical analyses. KT wrote the first draft of the manuscript. All authors contributed to the final draft of the manuscript and have read and approved of the final draft.

Acknowledgements

KHT was funded by a Doctoral fellowship award from the National Institute for Health Research (NIHR). The views expressed in this publication are those of the authors and not necessarily those of the NHS, the National Institute for Health Research or the Department of Health. MP and DG are NIHR Senior Investigators.

Author details

[1]School of Social and Community Medicine, University of Bristol, Canynge Hall 39 Whatley Road, Bristol BS8 2PS, UK. [2]The Academic Unit of Psychiatry, University of Bristol, Bristol, UK. [3]Centre for Drug Safety Science, University of Liverpool, Liverpool, UK. [4]Health and Wellbeing Division, Department for Children, Adults and Health, South Gloucestershire Council Badminton Road, Yate, Bristol, UK.

References

1. Pirmohamed M, James S, Meakin S, Green C, Scott AK, Walley TJ, Farrar K, Park BK, Breckenridge AM: Adverse drug reactions as cause of admission to hospital: prospective analysis of 18 820 patients. *BMJ* 2004, 329:15–19.
2. European Medicines Agency: The European Medicines Agency recommends suspension of the marketing authorisation of Acomplia. London, UK: European Medicines Agency; 2008.
3. Kuehn BM: Studies linking smoking-cessation drug with suicide risk spark concerns. *JAMA* 2009, 301:1007–1008.
4. BBC Panorama: The Secrets of Seroxat. 2002. http://news.bbc.co.uk/panorama/hi/front_page/newsid_8425000/8425414.stm.
5. BBC Three: Dying for clear skin. 2012. http://www.bbc.co.uk/programmes/p00xxy87.
6. Waller PC, Wood SM, Langman MJS, Breckenridge AM, Rawlins MD: Review Of Company Postmarketing Surveillance Studies. *BMJ* 1992, 304:1470–1472.
7. Bygdell M, Brunlöf G, Wallerstedt SM, Kindblom JM: Psychiatric adverse drug reactions reported during a 10-year period in the Swedish pediatric population. *Pharmacoepidemiol Drug Saf* 2012, 21:79–86.
8. Patten SB, Love EJ: Neuropsychiatric adverse drug reactions: passive reports to Health and Welfare Canada's Adverse Drug Reaction Database (1965-present). *Int J Psychiatry Med* 1994, 24:45–62.
9. Vilhelmsson A, Svensson T, Meeuwisse A, Carlsten A: What can we learn from consumer reports on psychiatric adverse drug reactions with antidepressant medication? Experiences from reports to a consumer association. *BMC Clin Pharmacol* 2011, 11:16.
10. Robertson HT, Allison DB: Drugs Associated with More Suicidal Ideations Are also Associated with More Suicide Attempts. *Plos One* 2009, 4:e7312.
11. Hawton K, van Heeringen K: Suicide. *The Lancet* 2009, 373:1372–1381.
12. European Parliament, Council of the European Union: Directive 2010/84/EU of the European Parliament and of the Council of 15 December 2010 amending, as regards pharmacovigilance, Directive 2001/83/EC on the Community code relating to medicinal products for human use. *Official J Eur Union* 2010, L348:74–79.
13. ATC/DDD Index 2014. http://www.whocc.no/atc_ddd_index/.
14. Speirs CJ: Prescription related adverse reaction profiles and their use in risk-benefit analysis. In *Iatrogenic diseases*. 3rd edition. Edited by D'Arcy PF, Griffin JP. Oxford: Oxford university press; 1986:93–101.
15. Bradford H: The environment and disease: association or causation? *ProcRSocMed* 1965, 58:295–300.

16. Pariente A, Daveluy A, Laribiere-Benard A, Miremont-Salame G, Begaud B, Moore N: Effect of date of drug marketing on disproportionality measures in pharmacovigilance: the example of suicide with SSRIs using data from the UK MHRA. *Drug Saf* 2009, 32:441–447.
17. Gunnell D, Irvine D, Wise L, Davies C, Martin RM: Varenicline and suicidal behaviour: a cohort study based on data from the General Practice Research Database. *BMJ* 2009, 339:b3805.
18. Davis S, King B, Raine JM: Spontaneous reporting- UK. In *Pharmacovigilance*. 2nd edition. Edited by Mann RD, Andrews EB. Chichester, West Sussex: John Wiley & Sons; 2007:199–215.
19. Martinez C, Rietbrock S, Wise L, Ashby D, Chick J, Moseley J, Evans S, Gunnell D: Antidepressant treatment and the risk of fatal and non-fatal self harm in first episode depression: nested case–control study. *BMJ* 2005, 330:389–393.
20. Hazell L, Shakir SAW: Under-Reporting of Adverse Drug Reactions: A Systematic Review. *Drug Safety* 2006, 29:385–396.
21. Martin RM, Kapoor KV, Wilton LV, Mann RD: Underreporting of suspected adverse drug reactions to newly marketed ("black triangle") drugs in general practice: observational study. *BMJ* 1998, 317:119–120.
22. Hawton K, Bergen H, Casey D, Simkin S, Palmer B, Cooper J, Kapur N, Horrocks J, House A, Lilley R, Noble R, Owens D: Self-harm in England: a tale of three cities - Multicentre study of self-harm. *Soc Psychiatr Psychiatr Epidemiol* 2007, 42:513–521.
23. Dal Pan GJ, Lindquist M, Gelperin K: Postmarketing Spontaneous Pharmacovigilance Reporting Systems. In *Textbook of Pharmacoepidemiology*. Chichester, UK: John Wiley & Sons Ltd; 2013:99–117.
24. Evans SJ, Waller PC, Davis S: Use of proportional reporting ratios (PRRs) for signal generation from spontaneous adverse drug reaction reports. *Pharmacoepidemiol Drug Saf* 2001, 10:483–486.
25. Aagaard L, Hansen EH: Adverse drug reactions reported by consumers for nervous system medications in Europe 2007 to 2011. *BMC Pharmacol Toxicol* 2013, 14:1–9.
26. Martin RM, May M, Gunnell D: Did intense adverse media publicity impact on prescribing of paroxetine and the notification of suspected adverse drug reactions? Analysis of routine databases, 2001–2004. *Br J Clin Pharmacol* 2006, 61:224–228.
27. Stobaugh DJ, Deepak P, Ehrenpreis ED: Alleged isotretinoin-associated inflammatory bowel disease: disproportionate reporting by attorneys to the Food and Drug Administration Adverse Event Reporting System. *J Am Acad Dermatol* 2013, 69:393–398.
28. Kim CJ, Berlin JA: The Use of Meta-analysis in Pharmacoepidemiology. In *Textbook of Pharmacoepidemiology*. Edited by Strom BL, Kimmel SE. West Sussex, England: John Wiley & Sons, Ltd; 2006:353–365.
29. Whittington CJ, Kendall T, Fonagy P, Cottrell D, Cotgrove A, Boddington E: Selective serotonin reuptake inhibitors in childhood depression: systematic review of published versus unpublished data. *The Lancet* 2004, 363:1341–1345.
30. Christensen R, Kristensen PK, Bartels EM, Bliddal H, Astrup A: Efficacy and safety of the weight-loss drug rimonabant: a meta-analysis of randomised trials. *The Lancet* 2007, 370:1706–1713.
31. Medicines and Healthcare products Regulatory Agency: Varenicline:adverse psychiatric reactions, including depression. *Drug Safety Update* 2008, 2:2–3.
32. Buggy Y, Cornelius V, Fogg C, Kasliwal R, Layton D, Shakir SA: Neuropsychiatric events with varenicline: a modified prescription-event monitoring study in general practice in England. *Drug Saf* 2013, 36:521–531.
33. Harrison-Woolrych M, Ashton J: Psychiatric Adverse Events Associated with Varenicline: An Intensive Postmarketing Prospective Cohort Study in New Zealand. *Drug Saf* 2011, 34:763–772.
34. Thomas KH, Martin RM, Davies N, Metcalfe C, Windmeijer F, Gunnell D: Smoking cessation treatment and the risk of depression, suicide and self-harm in the Clinical Practice Research Datalink: prospective cohort study. *BMJ* 2013, 347:f5704.
35. US Food and Drug Administration: Updated information on Leukotriene Inhibitors: Montelukast (marketed as Singulair), Zafirlukast (marketed as Accolate), and Zileuton (marketed as Zyflo and Zyflo CR). In *Book Updated information on Leukotriene Inhibitors: Montelukast (marketed as Singulair), Zafirlukast (marketed as Accolate), and Zileuton (marketed as Zyflo and Zyflo CR)*; 2009.
36. Philip G, Hustad C, Noonan G, Malice M-P, Ezekowitz A, Reiss TF, Knorr B: Reports of suicidality in clinical trials of montelukast. *J Allergy Clin Immunol* 2009, 124:691–696. e696.

37. Jick H, Hagberg KW, Egger P: **Rate of Suicide in Patients Taking Montelukast.** *Pharmacotherapy* 2009, **29**:165–166.

38. Hennen J, Baldessarini RJ: **Suicidal risk during treatment with clozapine: a meta-analysis.** *Schizophr Res* 2005, **73**:139–145.

39. Kenedi C, Goforth H: **A Systematic Review of the Psychiatric Side-Effects of Efavirenz.** *AIDS Behav* 2011, **15**:1803–1818.

40. Gibbons RD, Mann JJ: **Strategies for quantifying the relationship between medications and suicidal behaviour: what has been learned?** *Drug Saf* 2011, **34**:375–395.

10

Physiological and pharmacokinetic effects of oral 1,3-dimethylamylamine administration in men

Brian K Schilling[1*], Kelley G Hammond[1], Richard J Bloomer[1], Chaela S Presley[2] and Charles R Yates[2]

Abstract

Background: 1,3-dimethylamylamine (DMAA) has been a component of dietary supplements and is also used within "party pills," often in conjunction with alcohol and other drugs. Ingestion of higher than recommended doses results in untoward effects including cerebral hemorrhage. To our knowledge, no studies have been conducted to determine both the pharmacokinetic profile and physiologic responses of DMAA.

Methods: Eight men reported to the lab in the morning following an overnight fast and received a single 25 mg oral dose of DMAA. Blood samples were collected before and through 24 hours post-DMAA ingestion and analyzed for plasma DMAA concentration using high-performance liquid chromatography–mass spectrometry. Resting heart rate, blood pressure, and body temperature was also measured.

Results: One subject was excluded from the data analysis due to abnormal DMAA levels. Analysis of the remaining seven participants showed DMAA had an oral clearance of 20.02 ± 5 $L \cdot hr^{-1}$, an oral volume of distribution of 236 ± 38 L, and terminal half-life of 8.45 ± 1.9 hr. Lag time, the delay in appearance of DMAA in the circulation following extravascular administration, varied among participants but averaged approximately 8 minutes (0.14 ± 0.13 hr). The peak DMAA concentration for all subjects was observed within 3–5 hours following ingestion and was very similar across subjects, with a mean of ~ 70 $ng \cdot mL^{-1}$. Heart rate, blood pressure, and body temperature were largely unaffected by DMAA treatment.

Conclusions: These are the first data to characterize the oral pharmacokinetic profile of DMAA. These findings indicate a consistent pattern of increase across subjects with regards to peak DMAA concentration, with peak values approximately 15–30 times lower than those reported in case studies linking DMAA intake with adverse events. Finally, a single 25 mg dose of DMAA does not meaningfully impact resting heart rate, blood pressure, or body temperature.

Trial registration: NCT01765933

Keywords: 1,3-dimethylamylamine, Pharmacokinetics, Dietary supplements

Background

The stimulant 1,3-dimethylamylamine (DMAA; also known as methylhexaneamine) had been a component of many dietary supplements in the United States until the Food and Drug Administration warned retailers that DMAA did not have ample evidence of safety [1]. Little is known about the effects of oral administration of this compound in humans, but animal studies have indicated that the LD_{50} is 39 $mg \cdot kg^{-1}$ for intravenous [2] and 185 $mg \cdot kg^{-1}$ for intraperitoneal [3] administration. Dietary supplements containing DMAA were once widely available, with an estimated 440,000,000 servings of such supplements sold in recent years [4]. These doses are primarily as a component of "pre-workout" supplements marketed at those who exercise. The safety of this simple aliphatic amine has been called into question recently, partially based on case reports documented in New Zealand suggesting adverse outcomes following oral DMAA ingestion [5,6]. In these case studies, which cite cerebral hemorrhage following DMAA ingestion, individuals reported ingesting a single dose of DMAA (for its stimulant properties), often in conjunction with

* Correspondence: bschllng@memphis.edu
[1]Department of Health and Sport Sciences, The University of Memphis, 161 Roane Fieldhouse, 38152 Memphis, TN, USA
Full list of author information is available at the end of the article

caffeine and alcohol [5,6]. Contrary to these case studies, several prospective investigations to date using recommended doses have not shown any untoward side effects [7-12]. Despite this, DMAA has been banned in many countries, including the United States. The purpose of this study was to characterize the plasma concentration profile and associated physiological effects following a single 25 mg oral dose of DMAA.

Previously, Gee and coworkers [6] reported a patient that purportedly ingested two "tablets" containing DMAA (later confirmed by analysis to contain 278 mg of DMAA per "capsule": total dosage = 556 mg), along with 150 mg of caffeine and one can of beer. In a subsequent report [5], biochemical analysis of blood samples obtained from patients ingesting a 12.5 and 132 mg dose of DMAA indicated plasma DMAA concentrations of 760 ng·mL^{-1} (17 hours post-ingestion) and 1090 ng·mL^{-1} (1.66 hours post-ingestion). A third patient was noted to have a plasma DMAA concentration of 2310 ng·mL^{-1} (2 hours post-ingestion); however, no information was provided regarding the ingested dosage of DMAA. As indicated in these papers, it should be noted that other chemicals may have been taken along with the DMAA-containing products (e.g., alcohol, caffeine, phenethylamine, and cannabis).

As mentioned previously, DMAA is often ingested with caffeine for a proposed combined effect leading to greater arousal than either alone. Four studies are available that used this combination in a placebo-controlled design, and the health implications of DMAA in these studies has been unremarkable. In varying concentrations of caffeine and DMAA, there appears to be no effect on heart rate [8], while DMAA affected blood pressure and the rate-pressure product in a dose-dependent manner. These changes were not related to changes in norepinephrine or epinephrine, and caffeine/DMAA does not appear to be additive. Ergogenic effects of the combination of these substances on running performance have not yet been supported [7].

Whitehead et al. [12] assigned men to a placebo (n = 13) or a proprietary-blend supplement (Jack3d®;n = 12) condition, where subjects were directed to consume their assigned supplement on training days for the course of 10 weeks. No condition differences were noted for blood pressure, heart rate, or any variable of blood borne markers of health. Another sample of men (n = 7) consumed Jack3d®, while men (n = 4) and women (n = 2) consumed a different proprietary-blend supplement (OxyELITE Pro®) for two weeks [9]. In this open-label design, no significant chronic changes in heart rate, blood pressure, or rate pressure product noted for either product, although OxyELITE Pro® acutely increased systolic blood pressure. Since both of these products contain unique additional substances, it is difficult to ascribe responses to DMAA.

Finally, two studies examined OxyELITE Pro® in both acute [10] and chronic [11] conditions. Acutely, the supplement caused a significantly greater area under the curve for glycerol, free fatty acids, and kcal expenditure at rest. Heart rate, systolic blood pressure and rate pressure product were also higher with the supplement than the placebo [10]. Eight weeks of supplementation with the supplement or placebo did not demonstrate interactions for body weight, body composition, skinfold thickness, serum lipids or appetite [11].

To conclude on the safety profile of DMAA based solely on case reports would be problematic, in particular when accepting testimony from patients in uncontrolled environment, potentially under the influence of alcohol and other drugs. This is especially true in light of the fact that no prospective studies have shown these effects. Hence, the intent of the present study was to determine the pharmacokinetic profile of a single 25 mg oral dosage of DMAA alone through 24 hours post-ingestion. The results of this study, along with current available information, may provide a more comprehensive view of the effects of oral administration of this ingredient in humans.

Methods
Subjects and data collection
Eight healthy men (26 ± 4.1 y) were recruited to participate. Subjects met inclusion criteria by not currently smoking, and they did not have any self-reported cardiovascular or metabolic problems. Men were recruited so that there would be no possible gender effects, and since little is known about this ingredient, we thought it prudent to reduce potential confounding factors. Health history, drug and dietary supplement usage, and physical activity questionnaires were completed by all subjects and screened by an investigator to determine eligibility. Prior to participation, each subject gave written and verbal informed consent for procedures and publication of data in accordance with the procedures approved by the University of Memphis Institutional Review Board for Human Subjects Research (protocol approval number 2102). This trial is registered as NCT01765933. After giving informed consent, subjects had a dual x-ray absorptiometry (DXA) scan (Hologic QDR 4500, Bedford, MA) to measure fat mass and lean mass for descriptive purposes.

Subjects reported to the lab in the morning following an 8-hour overnight fast to minimize the possible effects of stomach contents. This is also similar to the instructions on some supplement labels. Subjects were asked to abstain from any dietary supplement containing DMAA for 72 hours prior to testing and also asked to refrain from strenuous physical activity for the 36 hours prior to testing. Following the measurement of resting heart rate (via 60 second palpation), blood pressure (standard manual procedures), and cutaneous temperature (forehead), in addition to collection of a fasting blood sample (as described below), subjects received 25 mg of DMAA in a cellulose capsule supplied by USPlabs (Dallas, TX). These are similar to capsules previously available commercially. The DMAA capsules used in this study were submitted for analysis to confirm the 25 mg dose. Mean concentration ($\pm$SD) of 10 capsules randomly selected from the same lot as the study capsules was 23.9 ± 1.9 mg. Subsequent measures of heart rate, blood pressure, and cutaneous temperature were obtained, and blood samples were taken at intervals over a 24 hour period (0.25, 0.5, 0.75, 1, 1.5, 2, 2.5, 3, 4, 5, 6, 8, 12, and 24 hr). Heart rate, blood pressure, and cutaneous temperature data were obtained to note the time effect on these variables [13]. Subjects remained in the lab for the first 8 hours of testing. They were given standardized meals for the 24- hour testing period (meals were consumed immediately after 3 and 6-hour draws, between 8 and 12-hour draws, and between 12 and 16 hours post-DMAA ingestion). They were instructed to have minimal physical activity, and return to the lab 8-hours fasted at the time of the 24-hour blood draw.

Blood collection and processing

Peripheral IV catheters (straight, 22 ga., length: 1" polyurethane) were inserted and secured prior to first blood draw and monitored throughout the first eight hours. The IV site was immediately covered with a transparent dressing to decrease the chance of infection and to allow for catheter monitoring. Venous blood samples (approximately 5 mL) were taken from subjects at intervals as described above. The first 0.5-1 mL of each sample was discarded to avoid contamination, the sample was collected, and the catheter was flushed with 2–3 ml of 0.9% saline solution. Blood samples at 12 and 24 hr were performed with standard needle venipuncture. Following collection, blood samples were processed accordingly with sodium heparin and plasma samples were stored at $-70°C$ until analyzed.

Plasma DMAA analysis

Plasma samples from the subjects were screened with high-performance liquid chromatography–mass spectrometry (an Agilent 1200 series HPLC [Agilent Technologies, Santa Clara, CA] with an ABSciex 3200 QTrap mass spectrometer [AB-Sciex, Foster City, CA]). Based on the properties of both DMAA and human plasma, we

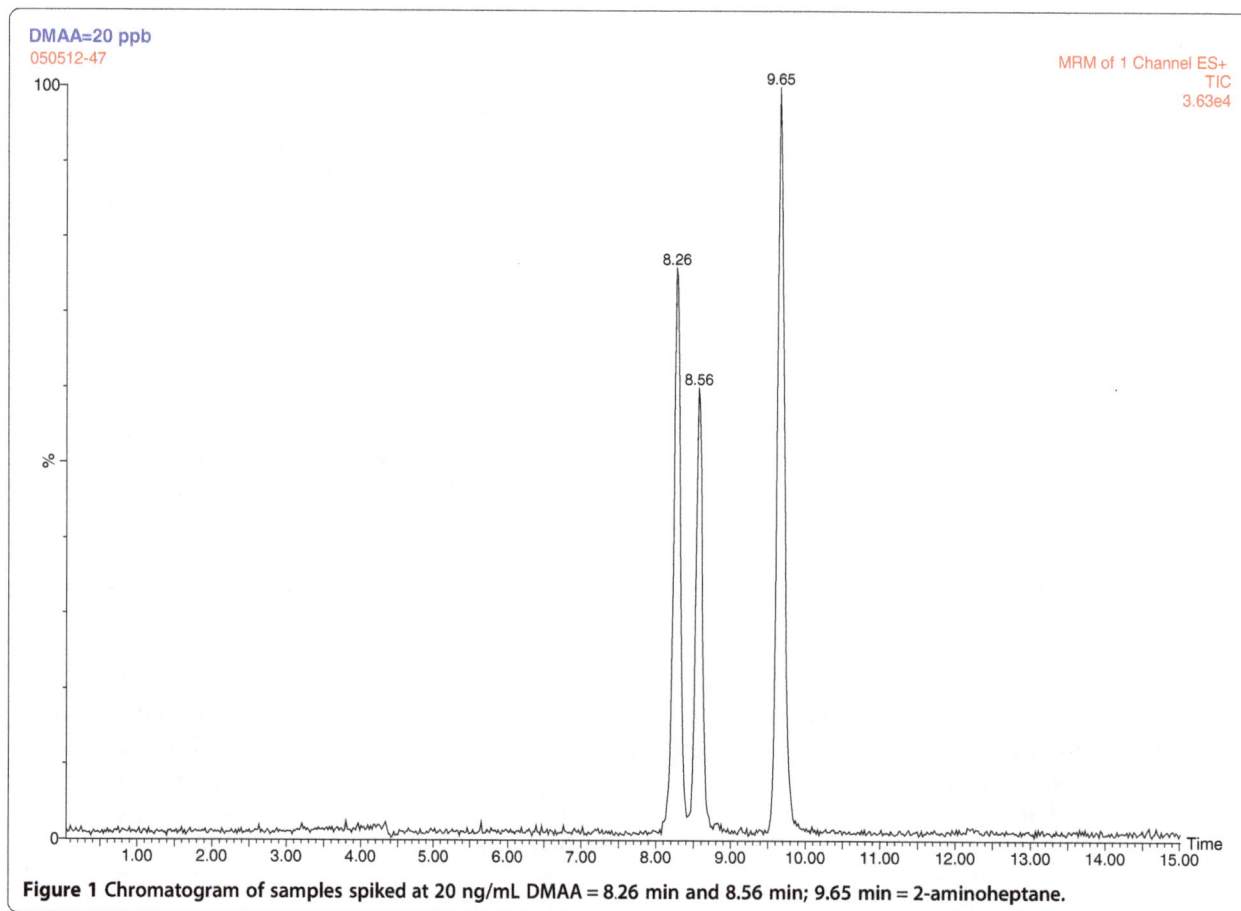

Figure 1 Chromatogram of samples spiked at 20 ng/mL DMAA = 8.26 min and 8.56 min; 9.65 min = 2-aminoheptane.

combined TCA precipitation with LC-MS-MS using analysis of DMAA in urine as reference [14,15], and 2-aminoheptane as an internal standard. In this method, the lower limit of quantitation (LLOQ) was estimated based on the lowest level in standard curve ($R^2 > 0.99$) (instrument sensitivity) and sample preparation. We forecasted that 5–50 ng/ml would cover the range of blood DMAA levels; therefore, we set up the accuracy experiment within 5–50 ng/ml-spiked levels. The LLOQ was 1–2 ng/ml (1 $ng·mL^{-1}$ average), and the average recovery was 92.4-97.4% when samples were spiked between 5–50 ng/ml; CV 0.9-6.8% between 5–50 ng/ml. Representative chromatograms are shown in Figures 1, 2 and 3. There is a double chromatographic peak of the racemic mixture that is made and sold commercially [14,15].

Pharmacokinetic analysis

DMAA plasma concentration-time data were evaluated using noncompartmental analysis in Phoenix WinNonlin software with adjustment for lag time after oral administration. The area under the plasma concentration-time curve from time 0 to infinity ($AUC_{0-\infty}$) was calculated using the trapezoidal rule extrapolated to time infinity. The terminal half-life ($t_{1/2}$) was calculated using $0.693/\lambda z$, with λz as the terminal rate elimination constant. Peak concentration (C_{max}), lag time (t_{lag}), time of maximum concentration (t_{max}), apparent volume of distribution during the terminal elimination phase (V_z/F), and oral clearance (CL/F) were also calculated.

Statistical analysis

Physiological response data (heart rate, blood pressure, temperature) were analyzed using a one-way repeated measures analysis of variance. The data are presented as mean ± SD. Statistical significance was set at $P \leq 0.05$, with Sidak post-hoc adjustments for multiple comparisons. Effect sizes were also calculated for selected pairwise comparisons, with corrections for correlations in repeated measures, and interpretation according to Hopkins [16].

Results

One participant had extremely high blood levels of DMAA, including a high baseline value of 131.1 $ng·mL^{-1}$ and a C_{max} of 266.2 $ng·mL^{-1}$ occurring at 24 hours. As

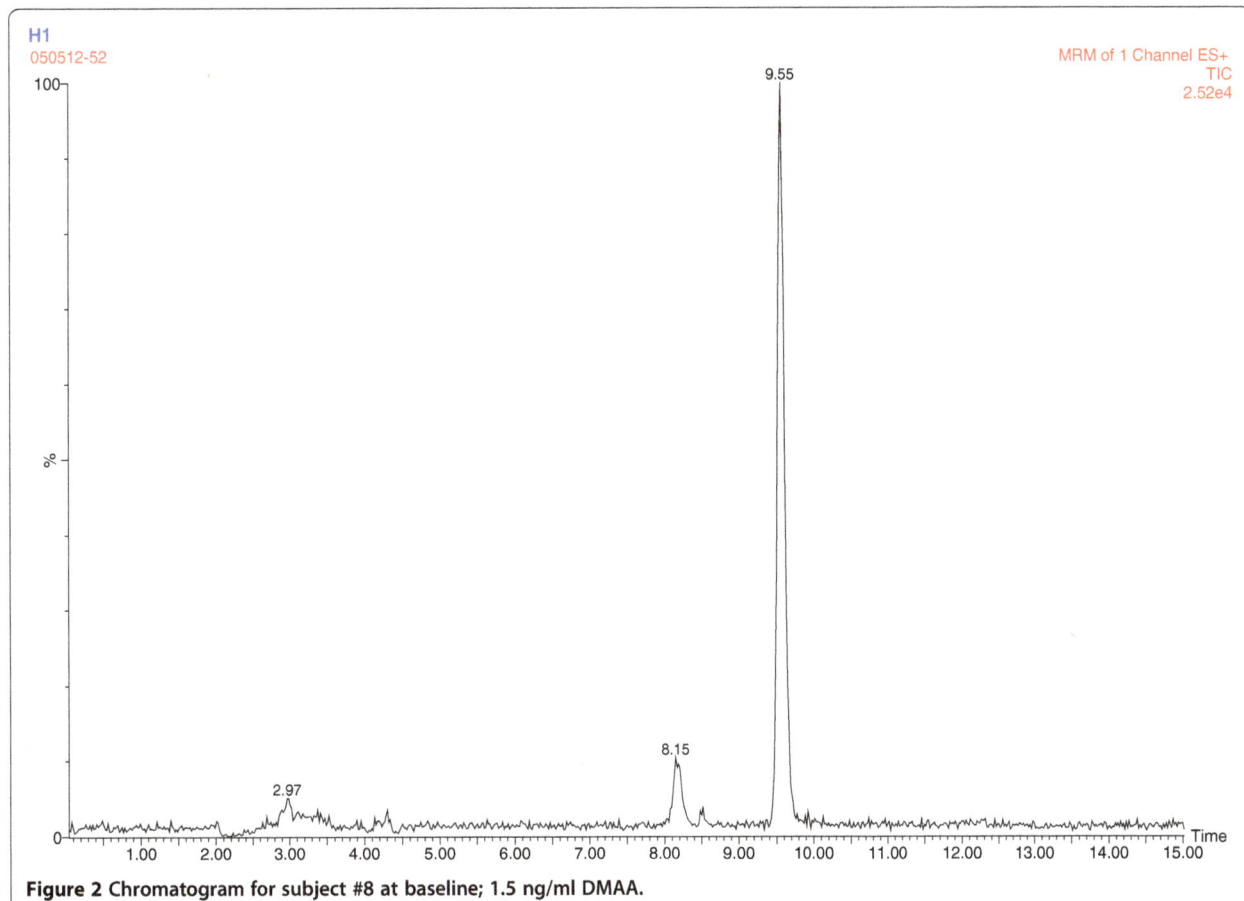

Figure 2 Chromatogram for subject #8 at baseline; 1.5 ng/ml DMAA.

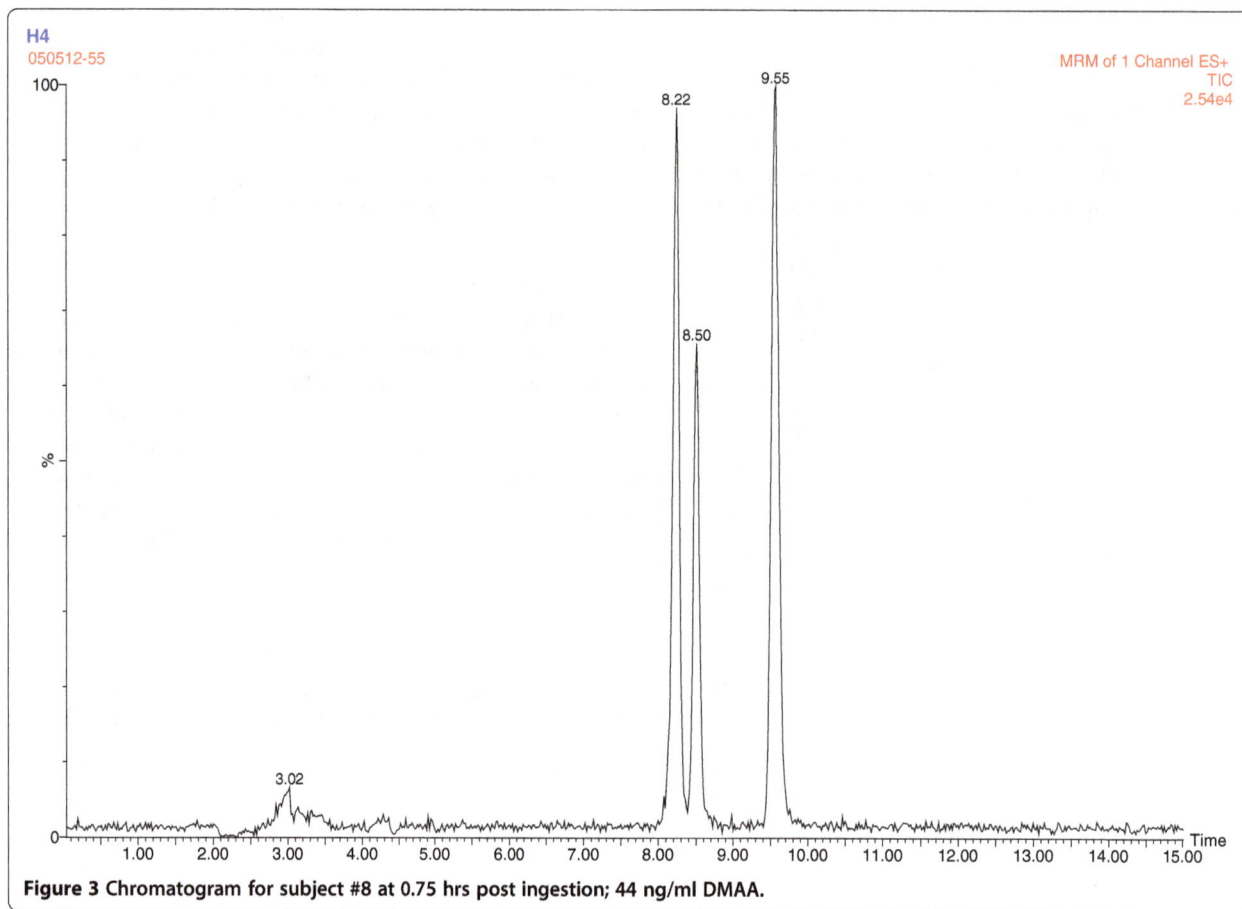

Figure 3 Chromatogram for subject #8 at 0.75 hrs post ingestion; 44 ng/ml DMAA.

the participant had rising blood levels throughout the experimental window, it was impossible to calculate a terminal half-life. Upon questioning, the subject denied taking a DMAA product within 72 hours of testing, so the reason for/source of the high levels is unknown and could not be attributed to a specific methodological issue. The physiological variables for this subject were comparable to the other participants, but the subject's DMAA t_{max} and C_{max} increased mean pharmacokinetic values by roughly 70% and 30%, respectively. Therefore, all data from the subject were excluded from the analysis. Subject characteristics for the seven subjects are presented in Table 1.

Physiological data
A significant time effect was observed for heart rate ($p < 0.000$; Figure 4), but no significant pairwise differences were noted. It should be noted that heart rate was slightly elevated at 12 hours post-ingestion (69.1 ± 2.9 BPM) compared to baseline (61.0 ± 3.2 BPM), with a large effect size of 1.9. A significant time effect ($p = 0.001$) was observed for temperature (Figure 5), with values significantly elevated 12-hours post-ingestion when

compared to two hours ($p = 0.025$, ES = 4.3) and three hours ($p = 0.009$, ES = 3.4). No changes were seen over time for blood pressure (Figure 6). Systolic blood pressure exhibited a moderate-to-large effect size (0.9) when comparing values at 24 hours post-ingestion (115 ± 3 mm Hg) vs. pre-ingestion (118 ± 3 mm Hg). There was a moderate effect size (0.5) when comparing diastolic blood pressure values at baseline (77 ± 4.4 mmHg) and at 0.25 hr post-ingestion (82 ± 3 mm Hg).

Pharmacokinetic data
Each subjects' pharmacokinetic parameters are shown in Table 2. Values for plasma DMAA of subjects peaked

Table 1 Participant descriptive information (n = 7)

	Age (y)	Lean body mass (kg)	Fat mass (kg)	Total body mass (kg)	% Fat
Mean	26.7	68.1	11.2	79.3	13.9
SD	4.3	6.0	4.9	8.3	4.8
Range	23-36	58.7-75.8	6.1-21.4	68.7-92.8	8.2-23.1

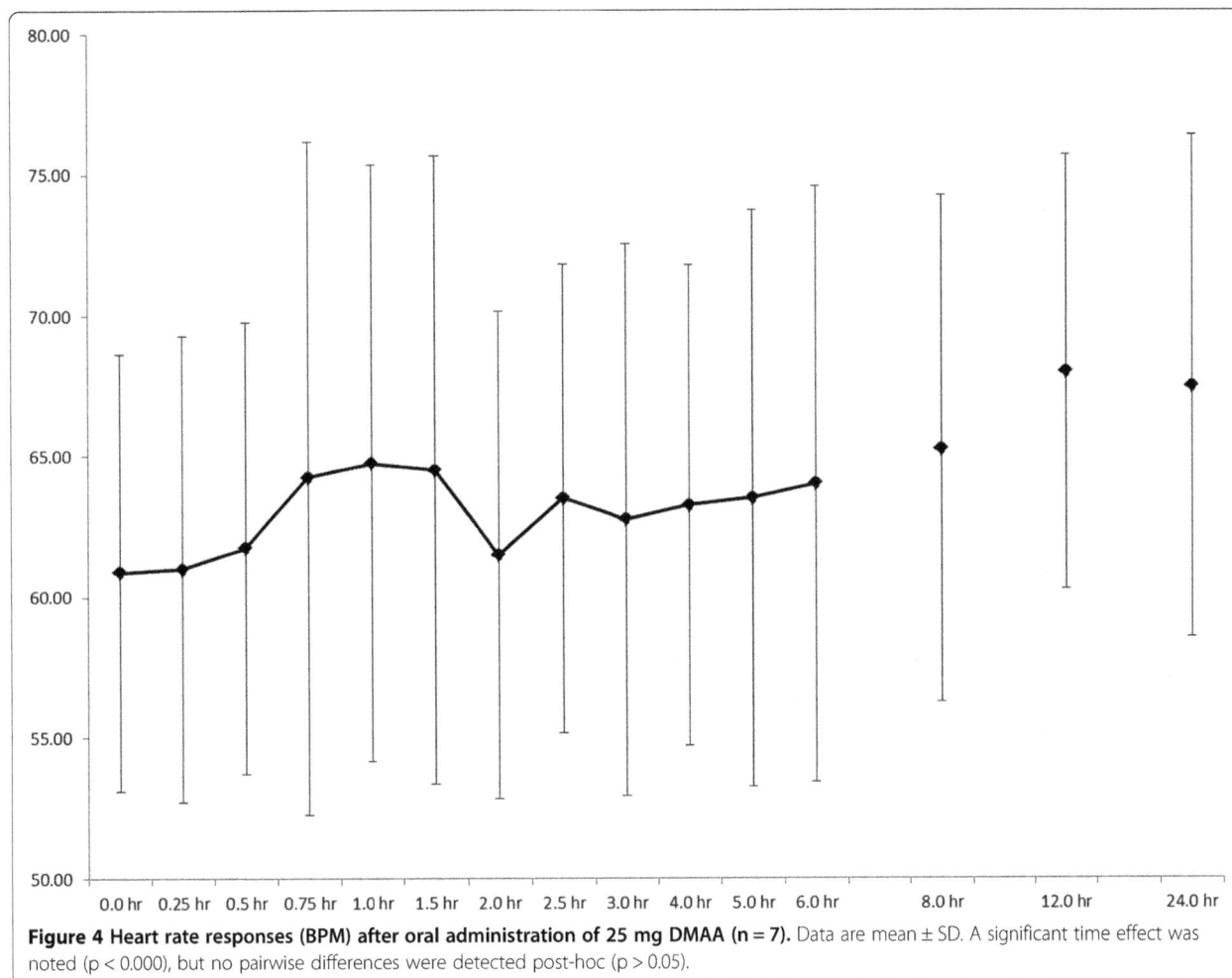

Figure 4 Heart rate responses (BPM) after oral administration of 25 mg DMAA (n = 7). Data are mean ± SD. A significant time effect was noted (p < 0.000), but no pairwise differences were detected post-hoc (p > 0.05).

at approximately 70 ng·mL^{-1}. The oral clearance was 20.02 ± 5 L·hr^{-1}, the oral volume of distribution was 236 ± 38 L, and terminal half-life was 8.45 ± 1.9 hr. Lag time varied among participants but averaged approximately 8 minutes (0.14 ± 0.13 hr). Individual and mean DMAA plasma-concentration time profiles are shown in Figure 7.

Discussion

The most important finding in this investigation is the relatively low plasma concentrations of DMAA corresponding to the 25 mg oral dose, and the lack of meaningful physiologic effects associated with the single dose. Since data from a standardized and verified dose of DMAA was not previously available, our findings shed light on the possible reason for the adverse outcomes noted in prior case reports citing DMAA use (*i.e.*, highly abusive dosages of this ingredient) [5,6]. Our data show a consistent pattern of increase across subjects with regards to peak plasma DMAA concentration, with peak

values approximately 15–30 times lower than those reported in the case studies—strongly questioning the accuracy of reporting by patients in the case reports [5,6]. It is hypothesized that patients in the case reports may have ingested dosages of DMAA that were approximately 15–30 times higher than what our subjects ingested (*i.e.*, 375 mg-750 mg). In fact, based on the time course of our peak response data (~5 hours post-ingestion), coupled with the times provided by Gee *et al.* [5,6] for blood sample collection from their patients (*i.e.*, before or after our noted peak concentration time), it is possible that our "15-30 times higher" estimation is quite low. The conclusions from our data are based on the assumption of linearity of DMAA PK, and that no previous DMAA was ingested by the participants. Also, no assumption of linearity can be made from our data since only one dose was used. The information regarding DMAA dosage as reported by patients in the work of Gee *et al.* [5,6] is not supported by our controlled laboratory analysis involving plasma sample analysis. If

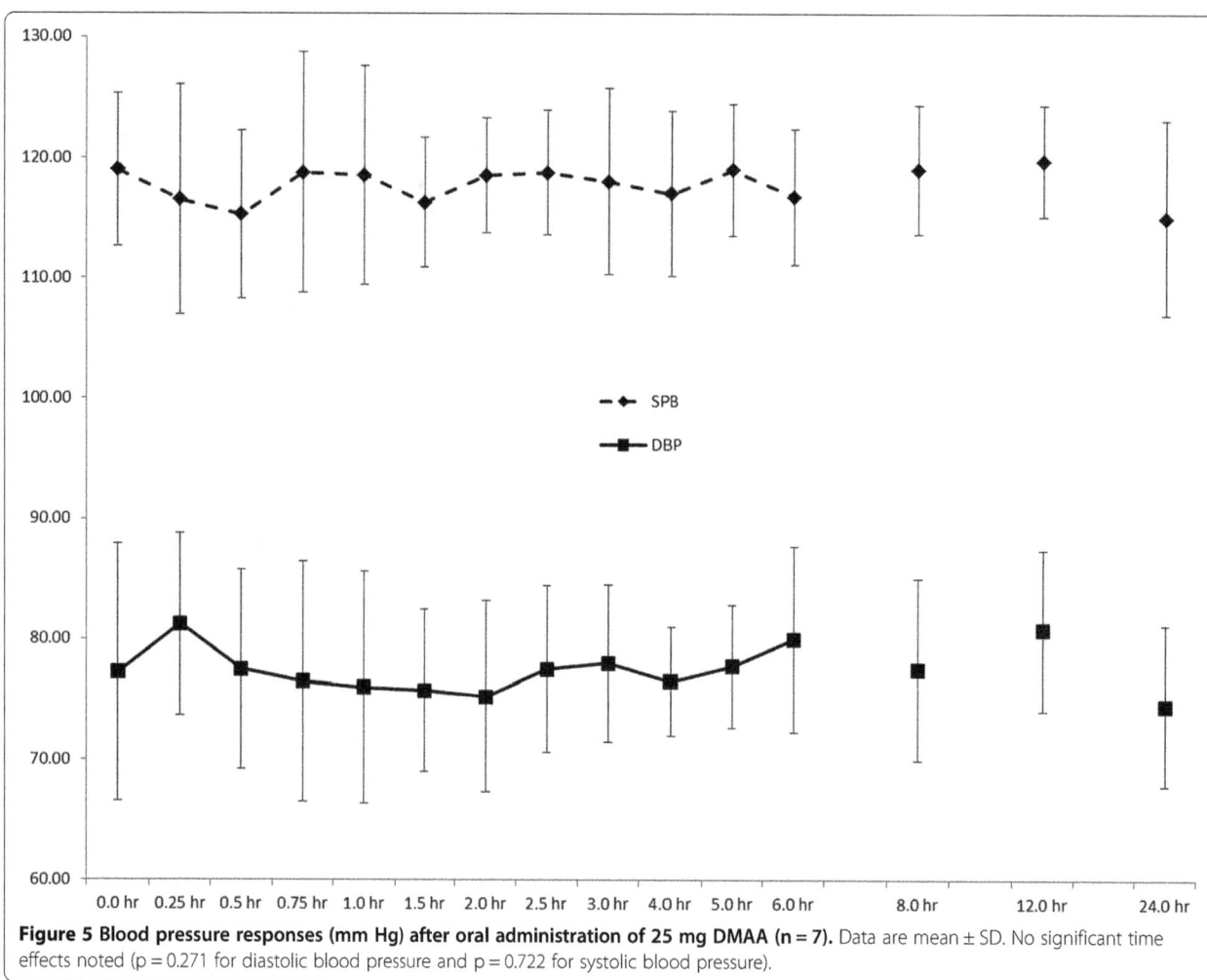

Figure 5 Blood pressure responses (mm Hg) after oral administration of 25 mg DMAA (n = 7). Data are mean ± SD. No significant time effects noted (p = 0.271 for diastolic blood pressure and p = 0.722 for systolic blood pressure).

these patients did in fact ingest such high dosages of DMAA (as directly indicated in the earlier report of Gee and coworkers, where the subject reportedly ingested 556 mg of DMAA) [6], it should not be surprising that such a blatant abuse resulted in untoward effects. This is particularly true when considering that these patients may have been using other chemicals along with the DMAA (*e.g.*, alcohol, caffeine, phenethylamine, cannabis). Indeed, the ingestion of other "stimulant-like" substances such as caffeine at a similarly high concentration taken as one dosage (*e.g.*, 2250 mg-4500 mg; assuming a typical intake of 150 mg) could be highly problematic.

The abnormal response of the one subject in our study cannot be readily explained. This subject did say that he was lightheaded immediately after the catheter placement, but this quickly subsided and was not present at the time of the DMAA administration. Since the subject denied taking DMAA within the 72-hour window preceding the experiment, it remains unclear why these values were so different from the other participants.

Compared to the commonly available stimulant caffeine, DMAA has a longer $t_{1/2}$, in this case 8.4 h vs. 5.4 hr for caffeine [17], as well as a shorter lag time of 0.14 h vs. 0.37 h for caffeine [17]. Previous reports have indicated that DMAA is absorbed over 4–12 hours [13]. It should be noted that caffeine also has interactive effects with oral contraceptives (increasing $t_{1/2}$) and other simultaneously ingested stimulants [17]. Examining the pharmacokinetics of combined DMAA/caffeine ingestion (as is commonly available in supplement formulations) could provide interesting data.

While a significant increase in temperature at 12-hours post-ingestion is noted in our data, the values are still within normal range of 36.1 to 37.8°C, suggesting little meaningful effect is present. The increase in temperature is likely attributable to the fact that subjects were out of the lab and reported back for testing, and that activity associated with leaving and returning to the lab slightly elevated temperature. These data are important to ensure that reports in the lay media of those

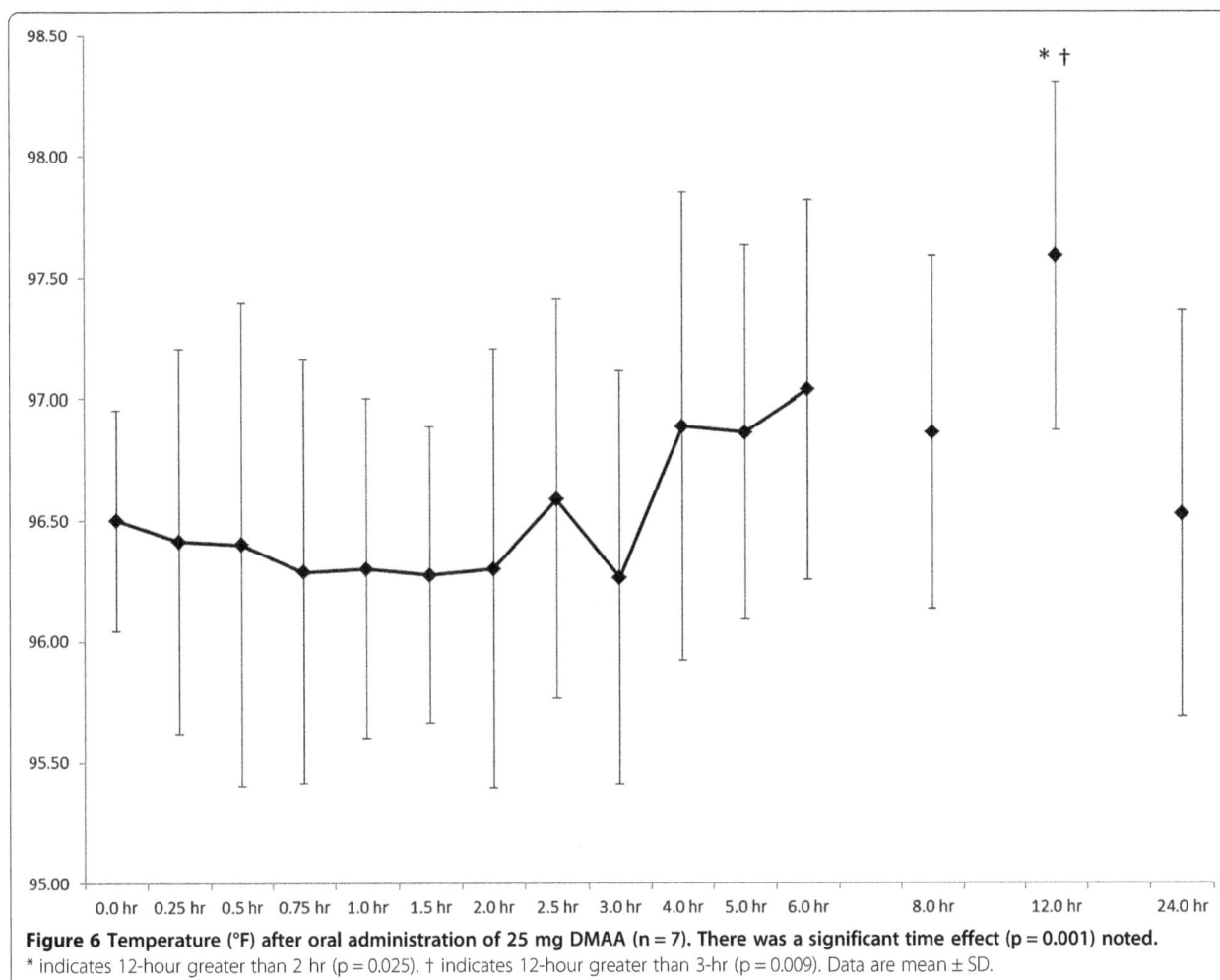

Figure 6 Temperature (°F) after oral administration of 25 mg DMAA (n = 7). There was a significant time effect (p = 0.001) noted. * indicates 12-hour greater than 2 hr (p = 0.025). † indicates 12-hour greater than 3-hr (p = 0.009). Data are mean ± SD.

reportedly taking DMAA suffering heat injury [18] can be contextualized. Further study of DMAA effects on temperature in the context of exercise and heat exposure is warranted.

Even with the significant time effect for heart rate, the grand mean was 64 bpm and the range was 50–88 bpm,

well within normal clinical values for healthy young men. Farney *et al.* [9] noted maximum increases of about 7 bpm 90 minutes after ingestion of OxyELITE Pro® (a supplement containing DMAA along with several other ingredients), which is more than the 3 bpm change we noted at the same time period after ingestion of

Table 2 Individual pharmacokinetic parameters after oral administration of 25 mg DMAA (n = 7)

Subject	$t_{1/2}$ (hr)	t_{lag} (hr)	t_{max} (hr)	C_{max} (ng·mL^{-1})	$AUC_{0-\infty}$ (hr ng·mL^{-1})	V_z/F (L)	Cl/F (L·hr^{-1})
2	7.84	0.0	2.5	82.85	1281.88	203.04	17.94
3	6.92	0.25	5.0	108.1	893.23	257.13	25.75
4	6.57	0.25	6.0	60.23	1136.17	191.87	20.24
5	7.13	0.25	2.0	63.14	818.91	289.05	28.09
6	9.29	0.0	4.0	76.68	1456.19	211.73	15.79
7	11.79	0.25	3.0	68.07	1420.82	275.29	16.19
8	9.660	0.0	2.5	76.69	1424.23	223.55	16.15
Mean	8.449	0.143	3.57	76.54	1204.550	235.95	20.02
SD	1.87788	0.134	1.48	16.09	262.89	37.82	5.00
%CV	22.22	93.71	41.46	21.02	21.83	16.03	24.96

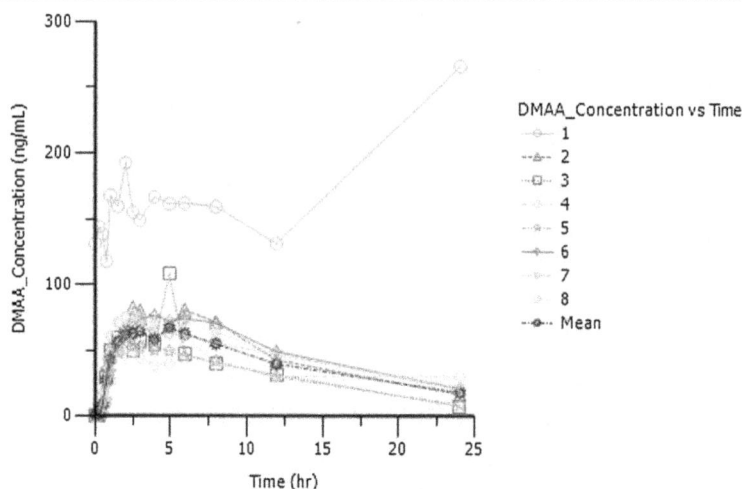

Figure 7 Individual and mean plasma concentration-time profiles after oral administration of 25 mg DMAA.

DMAA alone. Our heart rate data are more similar to McCarthy et al. [10], showing an increase of 4 bpm at 120 minutes post-ingestion of Jack3d® (another supplement containing DMAA along with other ingredients). It should be noted that McCarthy et al. [10] demonstrated an increase of about 4 bpm at 120 min post-ingestion of OxyELITE Pro®, similar to Farney et al. [9]. Our data are perhaps best compared with those of Bloomer et al. [8] who actually noted a decrease in heart rate of about 4 bpm and 3 bpm with ingestion of 50 mg and 75 mg of DMAA alone, respectively. Since all of these values are within normal ranges, it appears the effects of DMAA on heart rate are indeed minimal.

The lack of time effects for blood pressure is not surprising, and these values are within normal clinical ranges and well below values for hypertension. The systolic blood pressure grand mean was 118 mm Hg, with a range of 96–130 mm Hg. The diastolic blood pressure grand mean was 78 mm Hg, ranging from 60–88 mm Hg. Farney et al. [9] noted a significant increase in systolic blood pressure at 60, 90, and 120 post-ingestion of OxyELITE Pro®, but not Jack3d®. However, their maximum values were very similar for the two substances, and all of their values are similar to ours, aside from the greater baseline values for our study. McCarthy et al. [10] also had a significant time effect for OxyELITE Pro® on systolic blood pressure, and again their maximum values are similar to those herein. Study of nonproprietary concentrations of DMAA [8] demonstrated somewhat greater blood pressure effects for 50 and 75 mg (~8 and 12 mm Hg) than we noted for our 25 mg dose. Of the aforementioned studies, only Bloomer et al. [8] reported a significant increase in diastolic blood pressure, at both 50 and 75 mg doses, and at time points 30, 60, and 90 minutes post-ingestion.

Conclusions

We report for the first time the pharmacokinetic profile of oral DMAA. Based on our data, it appears that the concern over adverse health-related effects of DMAA is specific to the dosage ingested by the individual. When ingested at recommended doses (e.g., 25 mg), our data indicate minimal to no change in heart rate, blood pressure, or body temperature, and no adverse effects were noted. We also note a consistent pattern of increase across subjects concerning peak DMAA concentration, with mean peak values being <77 ng·mL^{-1}. This is approximately 15–30 times lower than plasma values reported by other investigators citing adverse outcomes following DMAA use. However, due to the case-study format of some of these adverse events, one cannot ignore possible drug interaction, errors in bioanalytical methods, differing bioavailability, or variability in exposure that might make this comparison difficult. Interpretation of our data would lead one to hypothesize that the adverse outcomes associated with DMAA use are simply due to the blatant abuse of this ingredient. Future research on DMAA may consider pharmacokinetic characterization of each individual diastereoisomer [14,15].

Competing interests

BKS, KGH and RJB have received research funding from USPlabs, including this study. These contracts paid for direct and indirect costs, as well as salary. USPlabs has also paid for the article-processing fee. This study was funded by USPlabs, who was consulted in the design of the study.

Authors' contributions

BKS and KGH were involved in the conception and design of the study, acquisition of data, analysis of data, and manuscript preparation. RJB was involved in the conception and design of the study, and manuscript preparation. CSP and CRY were involved in analysis of data and assistance with manuscript preparation. All authors read and approved the final manuscript.

Acknowledgements

The authors wish to acknowledge Mrs. Camille Myers and Mr. Tyler Farney for their assistance in data collection.

Author details

[1]Department of Health and Sport Sciences, The University of Memphis, 161 Roane Fieldhouse, 38152 Memphis, TN, USA. [2]University of Tennessee Health Sciences Center, Memphis, TN, USA.

References

1. U.S. Food and drug administration: http://www.fda.gov/NewsEvents/Newsroom/PressAnnouncements/ucm302133.htm.
2. Miya TS, Edwards LD: **A pharmacological study of certain alkoxyalkylamines.** *J Am Pharm Assoc* 1953, **42**:107–110.
3. Merck: **Monographs.** In *The Merck index.* 12th edition. Edited by Anonymous. New York: Merck; 1996:6166–6167.
4. Stars and stripes: http://www.stripes.com/news/military-probe-adding-to-skepticism-of-dmaa-1.167088.
5. Gee P, Tallon C, Long N, Moore G, Boet R, Jackson S: **Use of recreational drug 1,3-dimethylethylamine (DMAA) associated with cerebral hemorrhage.** *Ann Emerg Med* 2012, **60**(4):431–434.
6. Gee P, Jackson S, Easton J: **Another bitter pill: a case of toxicity from DMAA party pills.** *N Z Med J* 2010, **123**(1327):124–127.
7. Bloomer RJ, McCarthy CG, Farney TM, Harvey IC: **Effect of caffeine and 1,3-dimethylamylamine on exercise performance and blood markers of lipolysis and oxidative stress in trained men and women.** *J Caffeine Res* 2011, **1**(3):169–177.
8. Bloomer RJ, Harvey IC, Farney TM, Bell ZW, Canale RE: **Effects of 1,3-dimethylamylamine and caffeine alone or in combination on heart rate and blood pressure in healthy men and women.** *Phys Sportsmed* 2011, **39**(3):111–120.
9. Farney TM, McCarthy CG, Canale RE, Alleman RJ, Bloomer RJ: **Hemodynamic and hematologic profile of healthy adults ingesting dietary supplements containing 1,3-dimethylamylamine and caffeine.** *Nutr Metab Insights* 2012, **5**:1–12.
10. McCarthy CG, Farney TM, Canale RE, Alleman RJ, Bloomer RJ: **A finished dietary supplement stimulates lipolysis and metabolic rate in young men and women.** *Nutr Metab Insights* 2012, **5**:23–24.
11. McCarthy CG, Canale RE, Alleman RJ, Reed JP, Bloomer RJ: **Biochemical and anthropometric effects of a weight loss dietary supplement in healthy men and women.** *Nutr Metab Insights* 2012, **5**:1–14.
12. Whitehead PN, Schilling BK, Farney TM, Bloomer RJ: **Impact of a dietary supplement containing 1,3-dimethylamylamine on blood pressure and bloodborne markers of health: a 10-week intervention study.** *Nutr Metab Insights* 2012, **5**:33–34.
13. Venhuis BJ, de Kaste D: **Scientific opinion on the regulatory status of 1,3-dimethylamylamine (DMAA).** *Eur J Food Res Rev* 2012, **2**:93–100.
14. Perrenoud L, Saugy M, Soudan C: **Detection in urine of 4-methyl-2-hexaneamine, a doping agent.** *J Chromatogr B* 2009, **877**:3767–3770.
15. Vorce SP, Holler JM, Cawrse BM, Magluilo J: **Dimethylamylamine: a drug causing positive immunoassay results for amphetamines.** *J Anal Toxicol* 2011, **35**(3):183–187.
16. *A new view of statistics;a scale of magnitudes for effect statistics.* http://sportsci.org/resource/stats/index.html.
17. Csajka C, Haller CA, Benowitz NL, Verotta D: **Mechanistic pharmacokinetic modelling of ephedrine, norephedrine and caffeine in healthy subjects.** *Br J Clin Pharmacol* 2005, **59**(3):335–345.
18. **Stars and Stripes reports: Army study on DMAA will continue.** [http://www.stripes.com/news/army-study-of-dmaa-s-effect-on-soldiers-will-continue-1.176267]

11

Adverse drug reactions reported by consumers for nervous system medications in Europe 2007 to 2011

Lise Aagaard[1,3]* and Ebba Holme Hansen[2,3]

Abstract

Background: Reporting of adverse drug reactions (ADRs) has traditionally been the sole province of healthcare professionals. In the European Union, more countries have allowed consumers to report ADRs directly to the regulatory agencies. The aim of this study was to characterize ADRs reported by European consumer for nervous system medications.

Methods: ADRs reported by consumers for nervous system medications (ATC group N) from 2007 to 2011 and located in the European ADR database, EudraVigilance, were analysed. Data were categorized with respect to age and sex, category and seriousness of reported ADRs and medications. The unit of analysis was one ADR.

Results: We located 4766 ADRs reported for nervous system medications, and one half of these were serious including 19 deaths. Less than 5% of ADRs were reported in children. Totally, 58% of ADRs were reported for women, 42% for men. The majority of reported ADRs were of the types "nervous system disorders" (18% of total ADRs) followed by "psychiatric disorders" (18% of total ADRs) and "general disorders" (15% of total ADRs) which also were the system organ classes in which the majority of serious ADRs were found. ADR reports encompassed medicines from the therapeutic groups: antiepileptics (ATC group N03) (36% of total ADRs), parasympathomimetics (ATC group N07) (22% of total ADRs) and antidepressants ATC group N06A (9% of total ADRs). Antiepileptics were the therapeutic group with the highest share of serious ADRs (60%) followed by antidepressants (15%). Many serious ADRs were reported for pregabalin and varenicline.

Conclusions: The majority of ADRs from nervous system mediations reported by consumers that were identified from the EudraVigilance database were serious. The value of consumer reports in pharmacovigilance still remains unclarified.

Keywords: Adverse drug reactions, Nervous system medications, Pharmacovigilance, Consumers, EudraVigilance

Background

Reporting of adverse drug reactions (ADRs) to national databases has traditionally been the sole province of health care professionals [1]. In order to strengthen the systems in some countries, consumers have also been allowed to report ADRs directly to the regulatory agencies [2]. Consumers can provide first-hand information about their experience with medicines and may therefore constitute a valuable information source [1,2]. The weakness of consumer ADR reports is the lack of medical confirmation, which might impede the interpretation of ADR causation [2]. Only few studies have analysed consumer reports submitted to ADR databases, but over the last years studies analysing ADRs reported to national pharmacovigilance databases have been published [3,4]. Medawar and Herxheimer investigated ADR reports on the risk of dependence and suicidal behaviour from paroxetine from UK consumers and healthcare professionals, respectively [5]. In 2011, McLernon et al. published a study investigating the characteristics of consumer ADRs reported in UK

* Correspondence: laagaard@health.sdu.dk
[1]Clinical Pharmacology, Institute of Public Health, Faculty of Health Sciences, University of Southern Denmark, J.B. Winsløws Vej 19, DK - 5000 Odense C, Denmark
[3]Danish Pharmacovigilance Research Project (DANPREP), Copenhagen, Denmark
Full list of author information is available at the end of the article

from 2008 to 2009 [6]. In Sweden, it has been possible for consumers to ADR report directly to the non-profit organization KILEN since 1978 [2], and research conducted on these data has been published in several papers and reports [7-10]. Experience with consumer reporting (2004 to 2007) in the Netherlands was recently published showing differences in the categories of seriousness and outcome of the reported ADRs between patients and healthcare professionals [11]. A study from Denmark analysing differences in ADR reporting patterns between consumers and healthcare professionals (2004 to 2006) showed that patients were more likely to report ADRs from nervous and psychiatric medications, that patients' share of reports on serious ADRs was comparable to that of physicians, and that patients provided new and unknown information about ADRs [12]. Analysis of consumer reports of suspected ADRs submitted voluntarily to the website of a Danish consumer magazine showed that consumers reported ADRs for nervous systems medications and that patients report rather unspecific symptoms, as they use lay terms to describe reactions [13]. Patients also reported several ADRs, which prescribers may not consider serious but may be troublesome to patients and therefore patients find worthy of reporting [13]. The published consumer studies which all were conducted on national datasets showed that consumers are willing to report many ADRs for nervous system medications, but we do not know to which extent the above findings are generaliserable to populations in other countries. Since 2012, researchers were allowed access to ADR data in the EU ADR database, EudraVigilance (EV) and this has opened for cross-national analysis based on a standardised reporting format [14]. The objective of this study was to investigate ADR reports submitted by consumers for nervous system medications in Europe during the first 5 years of electronic reporting to the EV ADR database.

Methods

Setting

EudraVigilance (EV) is the central database of reports of suspected spontaneous ADR reports and ADRs reported in clinical trials for all medicinal products authorized in the European Economic Area (EEA) [15]. In compliance with the EU pharmacovigilance legislation, ADRs are reported to EV by regulatory agencies in member states where the ADR occurred. EV was set up in December 2001 to facilitate the electronic reporting of ADRs in the EEA. Data should be transmitted in accordance with the ICH E2B (R2) standard [15]. The minimum information required for an ADR report to enter the EV database is the following parameters: type of reporter, patient, at least one suspected active substance/medicinal product, and at least one suspected ADR (Volume 9A) [15]. The EV database is not publically accessible, and authorisation for data access

was given by the European Medicines Agency. By 2012, consumer reporting was officially accepted in 5 European countries: Denmark, the Netherlands, Norway, Sweden and the United Kingdom [1]. Before July 2012, countries were only requested to forward serious consumer ADR reports to the EV database [16].

Study design

The study comprised all ADR reports occurring from 2007 to 2011, located in the EV database and reported by consumers for nervous system medications (ATC group N). The content of the reports was analysed with respect to seriousness, categories of ADRs classified by system organ class (SOC) and medications. The unit of analysis was one ADR. Patients' age was dichotomized into two groups: children (0-17-year-olds) and adults (18 +).

Material

ADR information was provided for this study in anonymous form with encrypted identification [8]. Data extraction and data analyses of the raw material were comprehensive and time-consuming. Information was extracted from the ADR database on the date reports were received; category of persons submitting the reports; and criteria of seriousness and medications for which the ADRs were reported. The reported ADRs were coded according to type and seriousness using CIOMS (Council for International Organizations of Medical Sciences) criteria by academic staff in the national regulatory agencies [16]. ADR data was placed at the disposal of this study in anonymous form with encrypted identification of the medicine user. Data were extracted from the EV database in Microsoft Excel files using the following criteria: patient's sex and age, medicines (active substance), adverse drug reaction and severity. EMA has to ensure that, in complying with regulation (EC) 1049/2001, the protection of privacy and integrity of individuals is guaranteed, and therefore individual country specific ADR information was not disclosed [17]. The material comprised all ADRs reports from consumers reported to the EV database from 2007 to 2011. Data were extracted from the EV database and delivered to us as several large Excel files. Data comprised all ADR reports form consumers located in the EV database by 14 March 2012. In STATA® (statistical software package) the Excel files were merged into one major file and the ADR reports were searched for duplicates. Data analysis including coding of ADR reports was conducted in an Access database. Each ADR report may refer to one or more suspected ADR (s) as well as to one or more medicinal products. In this study we included ADRs reported for medications, which were listed as suspect drug by the reporter, meaning that the reporter suspected this drug and not the concomitant medicine to have caused the ADR.

Table 1 Fatal consumer cases reported for nervous systems medications in Europe, 2007 to 2011

Case no.	Medicine (s)	ATC group	Adverse drug reaction (s)	Sex (M/F)	Age
1	Diamorphine	N02AA09	Sudden death	F	18+
2	Metamizole	N02BB02	Agranulocytosis	F	18+
			Leukopenia		
			Multi-organ failure		
			Sepsis/septic shock		
3	Morphine	N02AA01	Cerebrovascular accident	F	18+
4	Oxycodone	N02AA05	Intentional overdose/suicidal ideation	M	18+
5	Apomorphine	N04BC07	Pneumonia	M	NA
6	Apomorphine	N04BC07	Intestinal haemorrhage	M	NA
			Pneumonia aspiration		
7	Apomorphine	N04BC07	Anaemia	F	18+
			Haematocrit decreased		
			Red blood cell sedimentation rate increased		
8	Apomorphine	N04BC07	Death	F	NA
9	Apomorphine	N04BC07	Death	F	18+
10	Apomorphine	N04BC07	Death	F	NA
11	Apomorphine	N04BC07	Death	F	18+
12	Carbidopa/levodopa Entacapone, Rotigotine	N04BA02	Death	M	18+
13	Clomethiazole	N05CM02	Leucocytosis	F	NA
			Pyrexia		
			Musculoskeletal stiffness		
			Neuroleptic malignant syndrome		
14	Clozapine	N05AH02	Cardiac failure	F	18+
			Somnolence		
15	Citalopram	N06AB04	Fatigue/malaise	F	NA
16	Duloxetine	N06AX21	Deafness	F	18+
			Abasia		
			Urinary tract infection		
			Septic shock		
			Urosepsis		
			Hyponatraemia		
			Neoplasm malignant		
			Aphasia		
			Urinary incontinence		
			Renal failure		
17	Trimipramine	N06AA06	Asthenia	M	18+
			Depressed level of consciousness/sedation		
			Tachyphrenia		
			Completed suicide		
			Dependence		
			Indifference		

Table 1 Fatal consumer cases reported for nervous systems medications in Europe, 2007 to 2011 *(Continued)*

18	Amitriptyline	N06AA09	Toxicity to various agents	M	NA
19	Rivastigmine	N06DA03	Lung infection	F	18+
			Mood altered/aggression		

M: male, F: female, NA:no information available.

Classification of ADRs by type

The different types of reported ADRs were classified according to the *Medical Dictionary for Regulatory Activities* (MedDRA) System Organ Class (SOC) [18]. Serious ADRs were defined as: fatal, life-threatening, requiring hospitalisation or prolongation of existing hospitalisation, resulting in persistent or significant disability/incapacity in the reporter's assessment, in a congenital anomaly/birth defect and other medically important conditions. All other ADRs are classified as non-serious [18].

Classification of medications by anatomical therapeutic chemical (ATC) group

The ATC system is a system for classifying medicinal products according to their primary constituent, the organ or system on which they act and their chemical, pharmacological and therapeutic properties [19]. Medicinal products are classified at five different levels. The medicines are divided into 14 main groups (first level), with one pharmacological/therapeutic subgroup (second level), and the fifth level is the chemical substance [18]. As the ADR data provided by EMA did not contain any information about ATC codes, these were added manually to the data file. The medicinal products reported are referenced based on their active substance and in this article we present ADR data at ATC level 1 and 5 [19].

Results

From 2007 to 2011, a total of 7434 consumer ADR reports containing information about 35349 ADRs was located in EV. Of these, 4766 ADRs were submitted for nervous system medications. In total, 51% of ADRs were classified as serious and of these 19 fatal cases were reported. The characteristics of the fatal cases are displayed in Table 1. The largest number of fatal cases (n = 8) was reported for apomorphine (ATC group N04) followed by five fatal cases reported for antidepressants (ATC group N06). Totally, 58% of ADRs were reported for women and 42% for men. Less than 5% of ADRs were reported in children.

ADRs by type and seriousness

Table 2 shows the distribution of reported ADRs by SOC. In total, consumers reported 26 ADR categories. The largest shares of ADRs were reported for the SOCs: nervous system disorders (18% of total ADRs), psychiatric disorders (18% of total ADRs); and general disorders and administration site conditions (15% of total ADRs).

The largest share of serious ADRs was of the type psychiatric disorders (23% of serious) followed by nervous system disorders (17% of serious) and ADRs of the general type (12% of ADRs).

ADRs by therapeutic groups

Table 3 displays the number of ADRs reported by consumers distributed on therapeutic groups and seriousness. Reports encompassed medicines from the therapeutic groups: antiepileptics (ATC group N03) (36%),

Table 2 Number of consumer adverse drug reactions for nervous system medications in Europe by type and seriousness, 2007 to 2011

System organ class (descending order)	Number (serious)
Psychiatric disorders	868(547)
Nervous system disorders	847(424)
General disorders and administration site conditions	736(303)
Gastrointestinal disorders	651(199)
Investigations	251(151)
Skin and subcutaneous tissue disorders	236(118)
Musculoskeletal and connective tissue disorders	219(96)
Injury, poisoning and procedural complications	145(93)
Eye disorders	142(65)
Respiratory, thoracic and mediastinal disorders	123(69)
Cardiac disorders	79(57)
Vascular disorders	74(58)
Metabolism and nutrition disorders	69(44)
Renal and urinary disorders	60(38)
Ear and labyrinth disorder	56(29)
Infections and infestations	50(29)
Reproductive system and breast disorders	44(15)
Blood and lymphatic system disorders	21(21)
Social circumstances	19(14)
Surgical and medical procedures	18(17)
Hepatobiliary disorders	17(15)
Immune system disorders	16(10)
Neoplasm benign, malignant and unspecified	10(10)
Endocrine disorders	9(9)
Congenital, familial and genetic disorders	2(2)
Pregnancy, puerperium and perinatal conditions	2(2)
Total	4766 (2433)

Table 3 Consumer adverse drug reactions (N) for nervous system medications in Europe by therapeutic group and seriousness (in parentheses), 2007 to 2011

Therapeutic group (ATC level 2)	Substance	Total (serious)
Anaesthetics (N01)	Articaine	1(1)
	Bupivacaine	4(4)
	Fentanyl	24(24)
	Propofol	2(2)
	Sevoflurane	2(2)
	Sufentanil	4(4)
Total N01		37(37)
Analgesics (N02)	Buprenorphine	24(24)
	Codeine	14(14)
	Diamorphine	3(3)
	Dihydroergotamine	27(27)
	Ergotamine	2(2)
	Flupirtine	6(6)
	Frovatriptan	2(2)
	Hydromorphone	22(22)
	Metamizole	20(20)
	Methylergometrine	2(2)
	Methysergide	25(25)
	Morphine	6(6)
	Oxycodone	56(56)
	Paracetamol	42(42)
	Phenazone	8(8)
	Pizotifen	2(2)
	Propyphenazone	7(7)
	Sumatriptan	3(3)
	Tilidine	11(10)
	Tramadol	62(57)
Total N02		344(338)
Antiepileptic drugs (N03)	Carbamazepine	142(142)
	Clonazepam	13(13)
	Gabapentin	53(53)
	Lamotrigine	78(78)
	Levetiracetam	2(2)
	Oxcarbazepine	36(36)
	Phenytoin	6(6)
	Phenobarbital	4(4)
	Pregabalin	1510(1510)
	Topiramate	6(6)
	Valproate	17(17)
	Zonisamide	3(3)
Total N03		1870(1870)
Antiparkinson drugs (N04)	Amantadine	9(9)

Table 3 Consumer adverse drug reactions (N) for nervous system medications in Europe by therapeutic group and seriousness (in parentheses), 2007 to 2011 *(Continued)*

Therapeutic group (ATC level 2)	Substance	Total (serious)
	Apomorphine	45(45)
	Benserazide	1(1)
	Bromocriptine	26(26)
	Cabergoline	1(1)
	Carbidopa	43(43)
	Entacapone	39(39)
	Levodopa	44(44)
	Piribedil	1(1)
	Pramipexole	17(17)
	Procyclidine	7(7)
	Rasagiline	15(15)
	Rotigotine	1(1)
	Ropinirole	15(15)
Total N04		264(264)
Antipsychotics (N05A)	Amisulpride	1(1)
	Aripiprazole	19(19)
	Bromperidol	8(8)
	Chlorpromazine	7(7)
	Chlorprothixene	23(23)
	Clozapine	71(71)
	Flupentixol	1(1)
	Fluspirilene	2(2)
	Haloperidol	12(12)
	Levomepromazine	9(9)
	Lithium	18(18)
	Melperone	7(7)
	Olanzapine	23(23)
	Perphenazine	12(12)
	Pipamperone	3(3)
	Quetiapine	46(46)
	Risperidone	37(37)
	Sulpiride	7(7)
	Thioridazine	6(6)
	Tiapride	6(6)
	Zuclopenthixol	21(21)
Total N05A		339(339)
Anxiolytics (N05B)	Alprazolam	17(17)
	Bromazepam	14(14)
	Chlordiazepoxide	2(2)
	Clorazepate	9(9)
	Diazepam	19(19)
	Lorazepam	74(74)
	Oxazepam	8(8)

Table 3 Consumer adverse drug reactions (N) for nervous system medications in Europe by therapeutic group and seriousness (in parentheses), 2007 to 2011 *(Continued)*

Total N05B		143(143)
Hypnotics and sedatives (N05C)	Butalbital	5(5)
	Clomethiazole	5(5)
	Flunitrazepam	1(1)
	Melatonin	4(4)
	Zaleplon	3(3)
	Zolpidem	14(14)
	Zopiclone	12(12)
Total N05C		44(44)
Antidepressants (N06A)	Agomelatine	29(29)
	Amitriptyline	11(11)
	Bupropion	7(7)
	Citalopram	38(38)
	Clomipramine	5(5)
	Duloxetine	27(27)
	Doxepin	1(1)
	Escitalopram	25(25)
	Fluoxetine	14(14)
	Imipramine	1(1)
	Mirtazapine	18(18)
	Nortriptyline	6(6)
	Opipramol	28(28)
	Paroxetine	21(21)
	Sertraline	22(22)
	Trimipramine	7(7)
	Venlafaxine	217(177)
Total N06A		477(437)
Psychostimulants (N06B)	Caffeine	16(16)
	Methylphenidate	61(61)
Total N06B		77(77)
Anti-dementia drugs (N06D)	Memantine	2(2)
	Rivastigmine	50(50)
Total N06D		52(52)
Parasympathomimetics (N07)	Disulfiram	11(11)
	Methylnaltrexone	2(2)
	Nicotine	91(91)
	Varenicline	1017(135)
Total N07		1121(239)
Total ATC group N		4766(2433)

parasympathomimetics (ATC group N07) (22%) and antidepressants ATC group N06A (9%). Except from parasympathomimetics, the majority of ADRs were serious. In particular, a large number of ADRs were reported for prebagalin (n = 1510) and varenicline (n = 1017). The most commonly reported ADRs for venlafaxine were anxiety, restlessness, paraesthesia and sleep disorder. Table 4 displays characteristics of serious ADRs reported for pregabaline. In total, 50 ADR categories were reported; the most frequently reported ADRs were drug ineffective/drug effect decreased (n = 83), dizziness (n = 78), pain (n = 61), somnolence (n = 56) and fatigue (n = 54). Table 5 displays the characteristics of serious ADRs reported for varenicline. The largest number of reported ADRs was musculoskeletal pain (n = 9), sleep disorder (n = 7), chest disorder/pain (n = 7), depression (n = 6) and suicidal behavior/ideation (n = 6).

Discussion

This is the first study to systematically analyse ADRs for nervous system medications reported by consumers to the EV database. Almost all ADRs, except for those reported for parasympathomimetics, were serious and several fatal cases were reported. Reported ADRs were predominantly of the type nervous and psychiatric disorders and general disorders. The majority of ADRs were reported for pregabalin, varenicline and venlafaxine.

ADRs by type and seriousness

The most frequently reported ADRs for nervous system medications were of the type nervous and psychiatric disorders and this finding was expected due to the mechanism of action of the reported nervous system medications. Additionally, a large number of ADRs of the type general disorders and administration site conditions and gastrointestinal disorders were reported, and this finding was also in line with results in previous consumer studies [5-13]. More than one half of reported ADRs were serious, however this reporting pattern was not surprising, since countries were not requested to report non-serious ADRs to the EV database during the study period [16].

ADRs by therapeutic groups

The largest number of ADRs was reported for antiepileptics and antidepressants, which can be explained by the frequent use of these medications in adults [20]. A high number of ADRs were reported for varenicline but only few were serious. In 2007, based on consumer reports in the USA, there was a high media attention on the increased risk of serious ADRs such as suicidal ideation and occasional suicidal behaviour, erratic behaviour and drowsiness reported for varenicline leading to black box warnings in the USA (July 2009) [21]. The ADR signal was later confirmed in a meta-analysis [22]. The high number of ADRs reported for varenicline by European consumers could have been stimulated by this media attention; however, the majority of reported ADRs were

Table 4 Serious adverse drug reactions reported for pregabalin by European consumers, 2007 to 2011

Adverse drug reaction(s)	N
Drug ineffective/drug effect decreased	83
Dizziness	78
Pain	61
Somnolence	56
Fatigue	54
Weight changes	47
Abdominal pain	39
Nausea	36
Headache	35
Vision blurred	28
Insomnia	24
Muscle spasms	24
Oedema	24
Gait disturbance	23
Myalgia	21
Hyperhidrosis	20
Appetite changes	18
Dry mouth	18
Malaise	17
Pruritus	17
Constipation	16
Disturbance in attention	16
Depression	15
Rash	15
Balance disorder	14
Memory impairment	14
Paraesthesia	14
Vertigo	14
Withdrawal syndrome	14
Accidental exposure	13
Diarrhoea	13
Feeling abnormal	13
Speech disorder	13
Anxiety	12
Arthralgia	12
Feeling drunk	12
Tremor	12
Eye swelling	11
Nasal congestion	11
Burning sensation	10
Erectile dysfunction	10
Urinary tract disorder	10

Table 4 Serious adverse drug reactions reported for pregabalin by European consumers, 2007 to 2011 *(Continued)*

Vomiting	10
Others (n < 10)	492
Total	1510

non-serious. For pregabalin a large number of the ADRs "drug ineffective/drug effect decreased" were reported, probably because this side effect can easily be assessed, and is very obvious compared to many other types of ADRs. To evaluate whether ADRs reported for pregabalin and varenicline can act as early warning for new ADR signals more in-depth analysis of the ADR reports should be conducted.

Strengths and limitations of this study

The strength of this study is that data comprised all ADRs reported by consumers in Europe, which were

Table 5 Serious adverse drug reactions reported for varenicline by European consumers, 2007 to 2011

Adverse drug reaction(s)	N
Musculoskeletal pain	9
Sleep disorder	7
Chest discomfort/pain	7
Depression	6
Suicidal behaviour/ideation	6
Nausea	5
Rash	4
Aggression	3
Mood altered/mood swings	3
Feeling abnormal	3
Headache	3
Oropharyngeal blistering/pain	3
Anxiety	2
Hallucination	2
Tearfulness	2
Fatigue	2
Pyrexia	2
Epilepsy	2
Movement disorder	2
Muscle spasms/weakness	2
Abdominal discomfort/pain	2
Erythema	2
Hypersensitivity	2
Others (n < 2)	53
Total	135

forwarded to the EV database during a five-year period and present in the database by March 2012. A major limitation to this study is that we do not know to which extent the causality of these ADRs can be confirmed, and this has implications for the interpretation of the findings [2]. The value of consumer reports in detection of new ADR signals remains unclarified due to the lack of information about causality. In this study, we did not evaluate the validity of the consumer reports since we only had access to the data entered into the EV database and not the original reports. Spontaneous reporting systems suffer from various barriers, such as incomplete recognition of ADRs, administrative barriers to reporting and low data quality, all of which may result in underreporting of important serious and rare events [2]. ADRs that are non-serious or already known may be overreported; however, this study provides information on reported ADRs, and this information contributes to broadening the knowledge on medicine safety. Before July 2012 countries were only obliged to report serious consumer reports to EV, which may explain the large number of serious ADRs found, and the low number of non-serious consumer reports. Therefore there may be additional non-serious consumer ADR reports present in the regulatory agencies. With the new pharmacovigilance regulation that came into force in July 2012 the share of serious consumer reports in EV will probably decline although the total number of consumer reports is expected to increase.

Hence, it is not possible to generalize from data reported to the EV database to the other EU member states. Spontaneous reports are an important source of information about new and previously unrecognized ADRs, and the value of spontaneous reporting schemes lies in their ability to act as hypothesis-generating procedures [2]. Therefore, EMA should continue to systematically survey and analyse ADRs reported by consumers in order to signal previously unknown ADRs. Another important issue to be investigated in future studies is to which extent individuals suffering from ADRs later recover from the reported reactions.

Conclusion

The majority of ADRs from nervous system mediations reported by consumers that were identified from the EudraVigilance database were serious. The value of consumer reports in pharmacovigilance still remains unclarified.

Competing interests

The authors have not received reimbursements, fees, funding, or salary from an organization that may in any way gain or lose financially from the publication of this manuscript, either now or in the future. The authors do not hold stocks or shares in an organization that may in any way gain or lose financially from the publication of this manuscript. The authors do not hold or plan to apply for any patents relating to the content of the manuscript. The authors have not received reimbursements, fees, funding, or salary from an organization that holds or has applied for patents relating to the content of the manuscript. The authors declare no other non-financial competing interests.

Authors' contribution

LA and EHH designed the study, analysed data and wrote the first version of the manuscript. LA carried out the sampling. Both authors saw and approved the final version of the manuscript. No sources of funding were used to assist in the preparation of this study.

Acknowledgements

The authors would like to thank the European Medicines Agency for providing data and MSc Jesper Frederiksen for assistance with data handling.

Author details

[1]Clinical Pharmacology, Institute of Public Health, Faculty of Health Sciences, University of Southern Denmark, J.B. Winsløws Vej 19, DK - 5000 Odense C, Denmark. [2]Section for Social and Clinical Pharmacy, Department of Pharmacy, Faculty of Health and Medical Sciences, University of Copenhagen, Copenhagen, Denmark. [3]Danish Pharmacovigilance Research Project (DANPREP), Copenhagen, Denmark.

References

1. van Hunsel F, Härmark L, Pal S, Olsson S, van Grootheest K: **Experiences with adverse drug reaction reporting by patients: an 11-country survey.** van Hunsel F, Härmark L, Pal S, Olsson S, van Grootheest K. *Drug Saf* 2012, **35**:45–60.
2. Blenkinsopp A, Wilkie P, Wang M, Routledge PA: **Patient reporting of suspected adverse drug reactions: a review of published literature and international experience.** *Br J Clin Pharmacol* 2006, **63**:148–156.
3. Hawcutt DB, Mainie P, Riordan A, Smyth RL, Pirmohamed M: **Reported paediatric adverse drug reactions in the UK 2000–2009.** *Br J Clin Pharmacol* 2012, **73**:437–446.
4. Durrieu G, Palmaro A, Pourcel L, Caillet C, Faucher A, Jacquet A, Ouaret S, Perault-Pochat MC, Kreft-Jais C, Castot A, Lapeyre-Mestre M, Montastruc J: **First French experience of ADR reporting by patients after a mass immunization campaign with Influenza A (H1N1) pandemic vaccines: a comparison of reports submitted by patients and healthcare professionals.** *Drug Saf* 2012, **35**:845–854.
5. Medawar C, Herxheimer A: **A comparison of adverse drug reactions from professionals and users, relating to risk of dependence and suicidal behaviour with paroxetine.** *Int J Risk Saf Med* 2004, **16**:5–19.
6. McLernon DJ, Bond CM, Hannaford PC, Watson MC, Lee AJ, Hazell L, Avery A: **Adverse drug reaction reporting in the UK: a retrospective observational comparison of yellow card reports submitted by patients and healthcare professionals.** *Drug Saf* 2010, **33**:775–788.
7. KILEN: *Consumer reports on medicines (CRM) – consensus document.* ; 2000. Available at http://www.kilen.org/indexe.htm (last accessed 21 March 2013).
8. Health Action International Europe: *Patient reporting of adverse drug reactions – seminar report*; 2005. Available at http://www.haiweb.org/docs2005/final_report.doc (last accessed 21 March 2013).
9. Vilhelmsson A, Svensson T, Meeuwisse A, Carlsten A: **What can we learn from consumer reports on psychiatric adverse drug reactions with antidepressant medication? Experiences from reports to a consumer association.** *BMC Clin Pharmacol* 2011, **25**:11.
10. Vilhelmsson A, Svensson T, Meeuwisse A, Carlsten A: **Experiences from consumer reports on psychiatric adverse drug reactions with antidepressant medication: a qualitative study of reports to a consumer association.** *BMC Pharmacol Toxicol.* 2012, **13**:19.
11. De Langen J, Van Hunsel F, Passier A, de Jong-van den Berg L, van Groothest K: **Adverse drug reaction reporting by patients in the Netherlands. Three years of experience.** *Drug Saf* 2008, **31**:515–554.
12. Aagaard L, Nielsen LH, Hansen EH: **Consumer reporting of adverse drug reactions. A retrospective analysis of Danish adverse drug reaction database from 2004 to 2006.** *Drug Saf* 2009, **32**:1067–1074.

13. Aagaard L, Hansen EH: **Consumers' reports of suspected adverse drug reactions volunteered to a consumer magazine.** *Br J Clin Pharmacol* 2010, **69:**317–318.

14. *EU directive of the European Parliament and of the council amending Directive 2001/83/EC as regards information to the general public on medicinal products subject to medical prescription. COM (2012) 48 final.* Brussels. 10.2.2012. Available at: http://eur-lex.europa.eu/index.htm (last accessed 21 March 2013).

15. European Medicines Agency: *Note for guidance – EudraVigilance Human – Processing of safety messages and individual case safety reports (ICSRs). EMA/H/20665/04/Final Rev. 2.* Available at: http://eudravigilance.ema.europa.eu/human/euPoliciesAndDocs03.asp (last accessed 21 March 2013).

16. **Volume 9. Pharmacovigilance: medicinal products for human use and veterinary products.** Available at http://ec.europa.eu/enterprise/pharmaceuticals/eudralex/homev9.htm (last accessed 3 April 2012).

17. Office Journal of the European Commission: *Regulation (EC) No 1049/2001 of the European Parliament and of the Council of 30 May 2001 regarding public access to European Parliament, Council and Commission. L 145/43.* Available at: *www.europarl.europa.eu/register/pdf/r1049_en.pdf* (last accessed 21 March 2013).

18. **MedDRA.** Available at http://www.meddramsso.com (last accessed 5 May 2012).

19. **WHO collaboration centre for drug statistics methodology.** 2007. Available at http://www.whocc.no/atc_ddd_index/ (last accessed 3 April 2012).

20. **Danish national registry of medicinal products statistics.** http://www.medstat.dk/ (last accessed 3 April 2012).

21. FDA: **FDA requires new box warnings for the smoking cessation drugs Chantix and Zyban.** Available at: http://www.fda.gov/Drugs/DrugSafety/DrugSafetyPodcasts/ucm170906.htm (last accessed 21 March 2013).

22. Singh S, Loke YK, Spangler JG, Furberg CD: **Risk of serious adverse cardiovascular events associated with varenicline: a systematic review and meta-analysis.** *CMAJ* 2011, **83:**1359–1366.

12

Effects of cytarabine on activation of human T cells – cytarabine has concentration-dependent effects that are modulated both by valproic acid and all-trans retinoic acid

Elisabeth Ersvaer[1,2]*, Annette K Brenner[1], Kristin Vetås[1], Håkon Reikvam[1] and Øystein Bruserud[1,3]

Abstract

Background: Cytarabine is used in the treatment of acute myeloid leukemia (AML). Low-dose cytarabine can be combined with valproic acid and all-trans retinoic acid (ATRA) as AML-stabilizing treatment. We have investigated the possible risk of immunotoxicity by this combination. We examined the effects of cytarabine combined with valproic acid and ATRA on *in vitro* activated human T cells, and we tested cytarabine at concentrations reached during *in vivo* treatment with high doses, conventional doses and low doses.

Methods: T cells derived from blood donors were activated *in vitro* in cell culture medium alone or supplemented with ATRA (1 μM), valproic acid (500 or 1000 μM) or cytarabine (0.01-44 μM). Cell characteristics were assessed by flow cytometry. Supernatants were analyzed for cytokines by ELISA or Luminex. Effects on primary human AML cell viability and proliferation of low-dose cytarabine (0.01-0.5 μM) were also assessed. Statistical tests include ANOVA and Cluster analyses.

Results: Only cytarabine 44 μM had both antiproliferative and proapoptotic effects. Additionally, this concentration increased the CD4:CD8 T cell ratio, prolonged the expression of the CD69 activation marker, inhibited CD95L and heat shock protein (HSP) 90 release, and decreased the release of several cytokines. In contrast, the lowest concentrations (0.35 and 0.01 μM) did not have or showed minor antiproliferative or cytotoxic effects, did not alter activation marker expression (CD38, CD69) or the release of CD95L and HSP90, but inhibited the release of certain T cell cytokines. Even when these lower cytarabine concentrations were combined with ATRA and/or valproic acid there was still no or minor effects on T cell viability. However, these combinations had strong antiproliferative effects, the expression of both CD38 and CD69 was altered and there was a stronger inhibition of the release of FasL, HSP90 as well as several cytokines. Cytarabine (0.01-0.05 μM) showed a dose-dependent antiproliferative effect on AML cells, and in contrast to the T cells this effect reached statistical significance even at 0.01 μM.

Conclusions: Even low levels of cytarabine, and especially when combined with ATRA and valproic acid, can decrease T cell viability, alter activation-induced membrane-molecule expression and decrease the cytokine release.

Keywords: T cells, Cytarabine, All-trans retinoic acid, Valproic acid, Acute myeloid leukemia

* Correspondence: elisabeth.ersver@hib.no
[1]Institute of Clinical Science, University of Bergen, Bergen, Norway
[2]Institute of Biomedical Laboratory Sciences, Bergen University College, Nygårdsgaten 112, P.O. Box 7030, N-5020 Bergen, Norway
Full list of author information is available at the end of the article

Background

Intensive anticancer therapy causes an acute and severe panleukopenia, including T lymphopenia, that may last for 2-4 weeks [1], and after hematopoietic reconstitution these patients usually develop a $CD4^+$ T cell defect that may persist for several months especially in adults [2]. This persisting T cell defect has been described both after conventional chemotherapy as well as after autologous and allogeneic stem cell transplantation. All these three therapeutic strategies are used in the treatment of acute myeloid leukemia (AML), and early lymphocyte recovery after such intensive treatment then predicts superior relapse-free survival. This observation suggests that early immunological events [3-6] and possibly also cancer- or AML-related inflammation [7] are important for AML cell survival and proliferation after chemotherapy.

Even though AML is an aggressive malignancy and intensive chemotherapy eventually in combination with stem cell transplantation is the most effective antileukemic therapy [8], many elderly or unfit patients cannot receive this treatment due to an unacceptable risk of severe toxicity and early treatment-related mortality. These patients will either receive supportive care alone or in combination with low-toxicity AML-stabilizing chemotherapy [8]. One such low-toxicity AML stabilizing chemotherapy is single-drug, low-dose subcutaneous cytarabine injections usually administered as daily treatment for 10 days with 4-6 weeks intervals; this treatment can eventually be combined with oral all-trans retinoic acid (ATRA) and valproic acid, i.e. a histone deacetylase inhibitor [9-14]. Previous *in vivo* clinical studies have shown that the triple combination of low-dose cytarabine, ATRA and valproic acid has immunomodulatory effects through a normalization of the increased pretherapy levels of circulating Treg cells, whereas the levels of Th17 cells are not affected by the treatment [15]. However, very little is known both about the acute and long-term effects of such treatment on the T cell system and whether T cell toxicity affects its antileukemic efficiency. In the present study we therefore investigated the *in vitro* effects of various cytarabine concentrations, valproic acid and ATRA on activated T cells.

Methods

Cell donors and preparation of peripheral blood mononuclear cells

The studies were approved by the local Ethics Committee (Regional Ethics Committee III, University of Bergen, Bergen, Norway) and buffy coats were derived from healthy blood donors after informed consent. Peripheral blood mononuclear cells (PBMC) were isolated by density gradient separation (Ficoll-Hypaque; NyCoMed, Oslo, Norway; specific density 1.077) from buffy coats from seven healthy blood donors (median age 29 years; 3 male

and 4 female). Viability, proliferation and cytokine release was examined for all individuals, CD4:CD8 ratio and expression of activation markers were investigated only for 3 randomly selected individuals.

Drugs

Cytarabine (Cytosine β-D-arabinofuranoside; Sigma-Aldrich, USA) was dissolved in ddH_2O to obtain a concentration of 400 μM before aliquoted, ATRA (Sigma-Aldrich; Oslo, Norway) was dissolved in 96% ethanol to 1 mM and valproic acid (Desitin Arzneimittel GmbH, Hamburg, Germany) was diluted in saline to 60 mM. All drugs were stored at -80°C. Drugs were thawed on the same day they were used in experiments and based on previous studies of *in vivo* levels the drugs were tested at the following concentrations that are relevant to low-toxicity AML treatment: valproic acid 1000 μM and 500 μM [16], cytarabine 0.35 μM and 0.01 μM [17-19], and ATRA 1 μM [20-22]. Cytarabine was also tested at 44 μM and 1 μM corresponding to high-dose therapy [23,24]. The relevance of these 4 cytarabine concentrations with regard to the levels reached *in vivo* is discussed in detail below in the Discussion section.

Cell culture

PBMC were suspended in pre-warmed X-Vivo 10® medium (BioWhittaker, Cambridge, MA, USA) with 10% FBS (Lonza Braine, Belgium) and cultured in 24-well culture plates at a final concentration of 0.5×10^6 cells/mL (viability and proliferation analyses) or 1×10^6 cells/mL (analysis of activation markers). T lymphocytes were activated by 0.6 μg/mL of mouse anti-human CD3 (Pelicluster, Amsterdam, The Netherlands) and 0.4 μg/mL of mouse anti-human CD28 (Pelicluster). Drugs were prepared from frozen stock solutions the same day as the experiments. Cultures were incubated at 37°C in a humidified atmosphere of 5% CO_2 before cells/supernatants were harvested.

Flow cytometric analysis of viability, proliferation and membrane molecule expression

Flow cytometry was performed by FACS Canto II. For each sample at least 20 000 $CD5^+$ lymphocytes were counted. All results were analyzed by FlowJo software (Tree Star, Inc., OR, USA).

Proliferation and viability assay

PBMC dissolved in PBS were stained strictly according to the manufacturer's instructions in the CellTrace Violet Cell Proliferation Kit (Invitrogen); thereafter cells were washed and cultures prepared as described above. The cells were harvested after 4 days and washed in ice-cold PBS before being resuspended in Annexin V Bindings buffer (BD Biosciences, Trondheim, Norway) and stained for 15 minutes with LIVE/DEAD Far Red Fixable Dead

Cell Stain (Invitrogen, Oregon, USA). Annexin V conjugated with Alexa488 (Invitrogen, Oregon, USA) and anti-human CD5 conjugated with PE-CY7 (clone L17F12; BD) was added, cells were further incubated for 15 minutes and thereafter washed in ice-cold 1% BSA/PBS before four-color flow cytometric analysis.

Analysis of CD4/CD8 ratio and activation marker expression

Cells were harvested after 20, 44 and 68 hours of culture, thereafter washed in ice-cold 1% BSA/PBS followed by 10 minutes of incubation in 200 µg/ml of Fc-receptor blocking agent (Octagam, Octapharma Ltd, Coventry, UK) before the following anti-human antibodies were added; FITC-conjugated anti-CD5 (L17F12; BD Biosciences), V500-conjugated anti-CD8 (RPA-T8; BD Biosciences), PerCPCy5.5-conjugated anti-CD4 (RPA-T4; BD Pharmingen), PE-conjugated anti-CD25 (M-A251; BD Biosciences), PE-CY7-conjugated anti-CD69 and APC-conjugated anti-CD38. Cells were incubated with antibodies on ice for 20 minutes, washed once in 1% BSA/PBS and finally analyzed by flow cytometry.

Analysis of soluble mediator concentrations
Luminex analyses

Culture supernatants were harvested after 4 days and stored at -80°C until analyzed. Cytokine levels were determined by Human Cytokine Panel A Fluorokine® Multianalyte Profiling (MAP) Kit (LUH000; R&D Systems, Abingdon, UK). All analyses were performed strictly according to the manufacturer's instructions. Standard curves were constructed by using the mean of duplicate determinations, and differences between duplicates were generally <10% of the mean. The minimal detectable levels were IFNγ 1.27 pg/mL, TNF-α 1.5 pg/mL, G-CSF 1.48 pg/mL, GM-CSF 1.98 pg/mL, VEGF 1.84 pg/mL, bFGF 4.91 pg/mL, IL1RA 10.91 pg/mL, IL1α 0.36 pg/mL, IL1β 0.57 pg/mL, IL2 2.23 pg/mL, IL4 4.46 pg/mL, IL5 0.71 pg/mL, IL6 1.11 pg/mL, IL8 1.97 pg/mL (CXCL8), IL10 0.30 pg/mL, IL17 1.1 pg/mL, CCL2 (MCP-1) 0.47 pg/mL, CCL3 (MIP-1α) 1.45 pg/mL, CCL4 (MIP-1β) 0.74 pg/mL, CCL5 (RANTES) 1.91 pg/mL, CXCL5 (ENA-78) 4.14 pg/mL.

Enzyme-linked immuno-sorbent analyses (ELISA)

Supernatants were harvested and stored as described above. Mediator levels were determined by HSP90α human EIA kit (ADI-EKS-895; Enzo Life Sciences, Exeter, UK), HSP70 high sensitivity ELISA kit (ADI-EKS-715; Enzo Life Science) TRAIL/TNFSF10 immunoassay (Quantikine, R&D Systems), human CD95/Fas Ligand/TNFSF6 immunoassay (Quantikine, R&D Systems). All analyses were performed strictly according to the manufacturer's instructions. Standard curves were constructed based on the mean of duplicate determinations, and differences between

duplicates were generally <10% of the mean. The minimal detectable levels were HSP90 0.05 ng/mL, HSP70 0.09 ng/mL, FasL 2.26 pg/mL, TRAIL 2.86 pg/mL.

AML patient samples and analyses

The effect of low-doses cytarabine were also tested on primary human AML cells from 48 consecutive patients (median age 67 years; range 24-83 years; 23 female and 25 male). Our strategy for recruitment of consecutive patients has been described in detail previously [25]. All patients were tested at the time of diagnosis before they eventually received antileukemic treatment. The AML cells were isolated from peripheral blood using density gradient separation (Lymphoprep; Axis Shield, Oslo, Norway) and contained at least 90% blasts. For cell viability measurement, AML cells (2×10^5 cells/well) were incubated in flat-bottomed microtiter plates (200 µl/well; Costar 3596 culture plates; Costar, Cambridge, MA, USA) in Stem Span SFEM™ medium (Stem Cell Technologies; Vancouver, BC, Canada) at 37°C in a humidified 5% CO_2 incubator for 40 hours before the percentage of viable cells was determined by flow cytometry after staining with propidium iodide (PI) and Annexin V. Furthermore, for the proliferation assay 5×10^4 AML cells/well were cultured in flat-bottomed microtiter plates (200 µl/well) in Stem Span for six days prior to addition of 37 kBq of ^{3}H-thymidine (Perkin Elmer) to each well and incubated for 18 hours before cells were harvested and radioactive activity determined. The medium used in the proliferation assay was supplemented with the growth factors (20 ng/ml) G-CSF, SCF and Flt3l.

Statistical analyses

Statistical comparisons were made by using GraphPad PRISM (version 5.0, GraphPad Software, Inc., USA) with repeated measures ANOVA (within-subjects ANOVA or ANOVA for correlated samples) with Dunnett's Multiple Comparison Test (post-test). Differences were regarded as significant when $p < 0.05$. Cluster analyses were performed by the use of J-Express 2011 analysis suite (MolMine AS, Bergen, Norway). The AML cell data were analysed with the IBM Statistical Package for the Social Sciences (SPSS) version 21 using pair sampled t-test and the Wilcoxon signed rank test to compare drug-containing and drugfree cultures.

Results
ATRA and low doses of valproic acid do not affect viability and proliferative capacity of activated normal T cells, whereas cytarabine has a dose-dependent antiproliferative and proapoptotic effect

PBMC derived from healthy blood donors (n = 7) were activated *in vitro* with anti-CD3 plus anti-CD28 during 4 days of culture in medium alone or medium supplemented with ATRA 1 µM, valproic acid 500 and 1000 µM or cytarabine 0.01-44 µM. The viability (Figure 1; Annexin-PI assay) and proliferation (Figure 2; the CellTrace Violet Cell proliferation assay) of CD5$^+$ T cells were then analyzed by flow cytometry. ATRA and valproic acid (500 µM) did not cause any statistically significant alteration of T cell viability or proliferation. A small, but statistically significant, decrease in proli

feration was detected after exposure to valproic acid (1000 µM). In contrast, cytarabine caused a dose-dependent reduction both in viability and proliferation. An increased fraction of apoptotic cells was then detected together with the decreased viability in the cytarabine-containing cultures; an observation suggesting that the decreased viability is caused by drug-induced apoptosis.

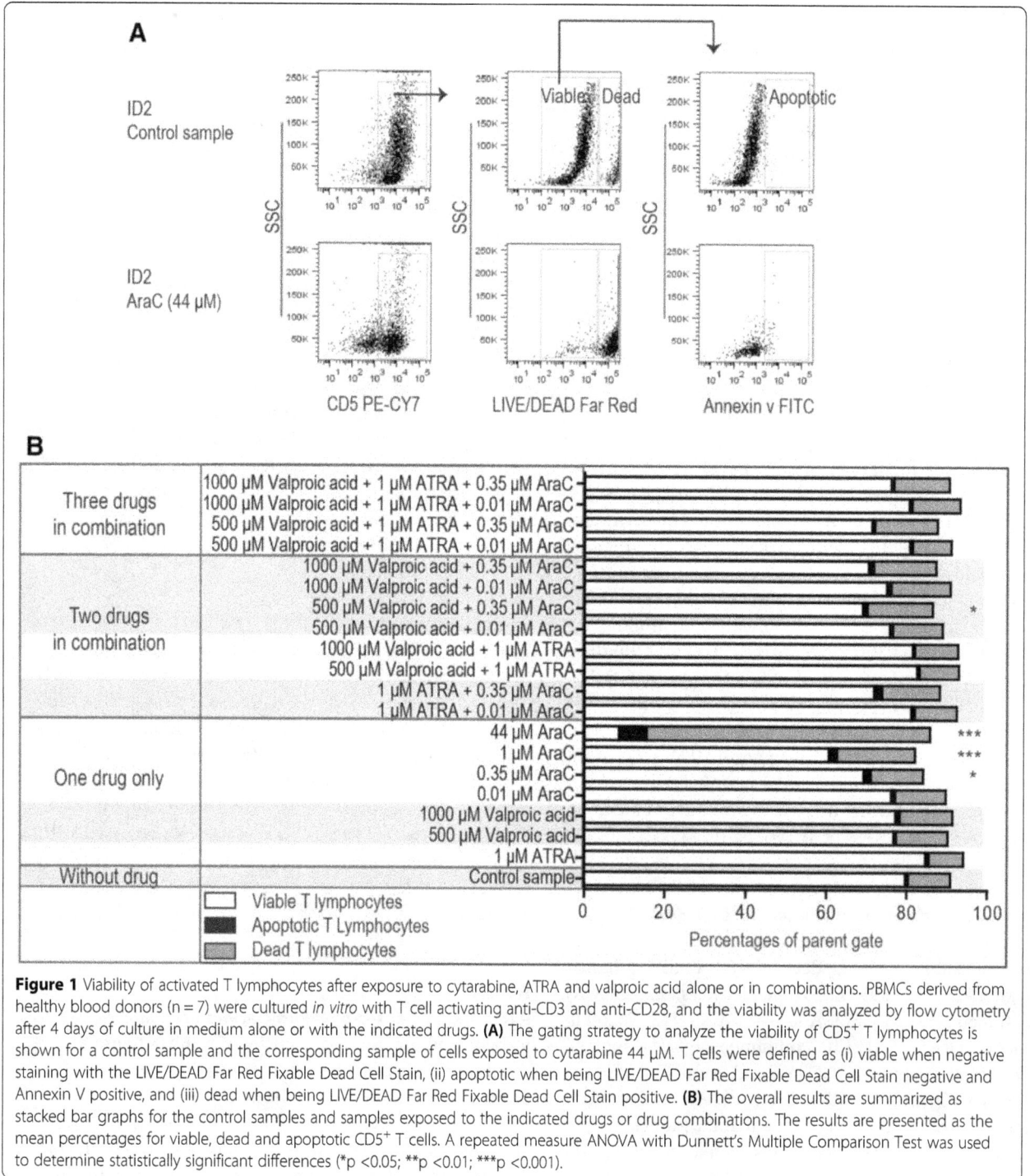

Figure 1 Viability of activated T lymphocytes after exposure to cytarabine, ATRA and valproic acid alone or in combinations. PBMCs derived from healthy blood donors (n = 7) were cultured in vitro with T cell activating anti-CD3 and anti-CD28, and the viability was analyzed by flow cytometry after 4 days of culture in medium alone or with the indicated drugs. **(A)** The gating strategy to analyze the viability of CD5$^+$ T lymphocytes is shown for a control sample and the corresponding sample of cells exposed to cytarabine 44 µM. T cells were defined as (i) viable when negative staining with the LIVE/DEAD Far Red Fixable Dead Cell Stain, (ii) apoptotic when being LIVE/DEAD Far Red Fixable Dead Cell Stain negative and Annexin V positive, and (iii) dead when being LIVE/DEAD Far Red Fixable Dead Cell Stain positive. **(B)** The overall results are summarized as stacked bar graphs for the control samples and samples exposed to the indicated drugs or drug combinations. The results are presented as the mean percentages for viable, dead and apoptotic CD5$^+$ T cells. A repeated measure ANOVA with Dunnett's Multiple Comparison Test was used to determine statistically significant differences (*p <0.05; **p <0.01; ***p <0.001).

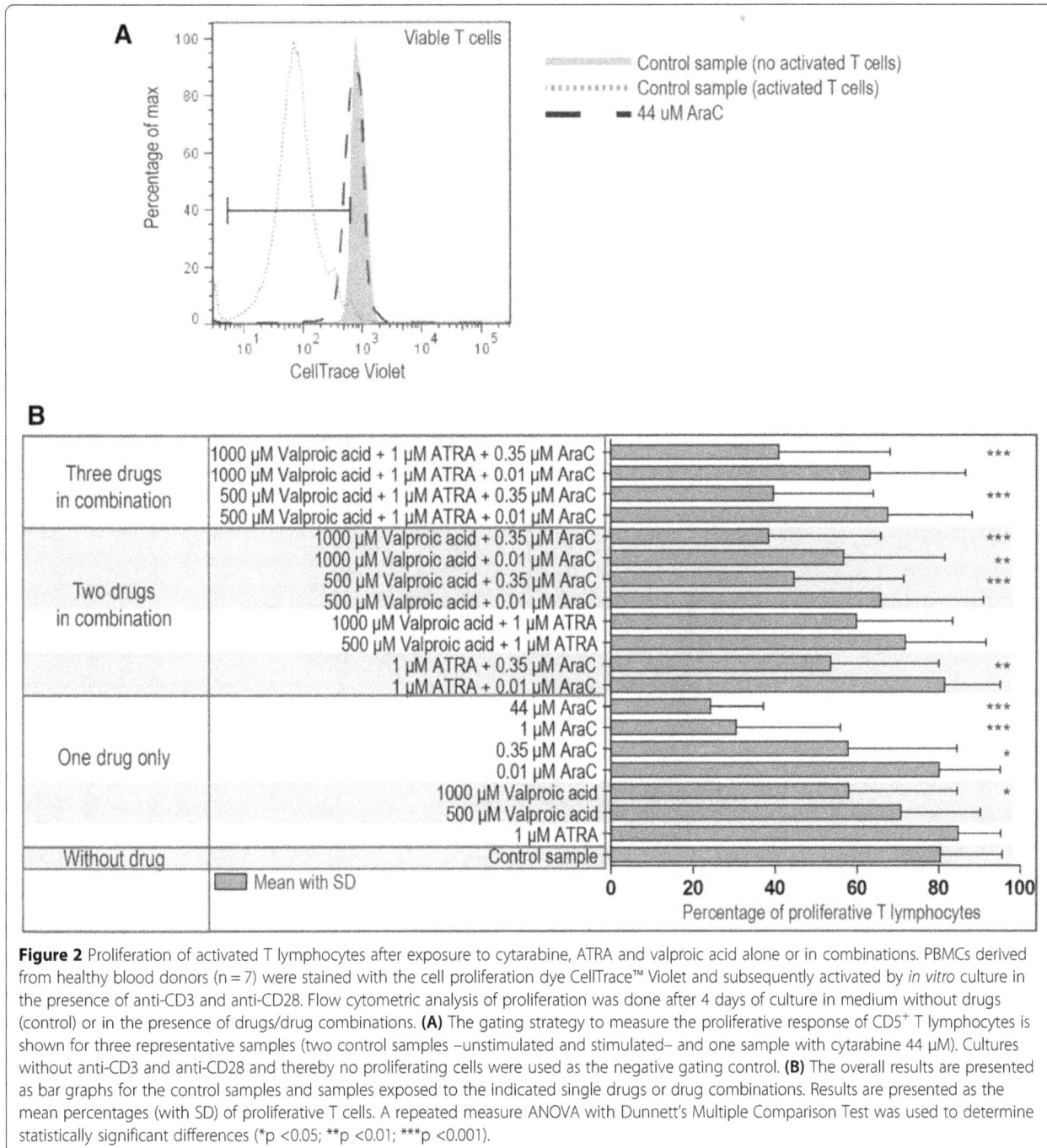

Figure 2 Proliferation of activated T lymphocytes after exposure to cytarabine, ATRA and valproic acid alone or in combinations. PBMCs derived from healthy blood donors (n = 7) were stained with the cell proliferation dye CellTrace™ Violet and subsequently activated by *in vitro* culture in the presence of anti-CD3 and anti-CD28. Flow cytometric analysis of proliferation was done after 4 days of culture in medium without drugs (control) or in the presence of drugs/drug combinations. **(A)** The gating strategy to measure the proliferative response of CD5$^+$ T lymphocytes is shown for three representative samples (two control samples –unstimulated and stimulated– and one sample with cytarabine 44 μM). Cultures without anti-CD3 and anti-CD28 and thereby no proliferating cells were used as the negative gating control. **(B)** The overall results are presented as bar graphs for the control samples and samples exposed to the indicated single drugs or drug combinations. Results are presented as the mean percentages (with SD) of proliferative T cells. A repeated measure ANOVA with Dunnett's Multiple Comparison Test was used to determine statistically significant differences (*p <0.05; **p <0.01; ***p <0.001).

Valproic acid increases the antiproliferative effect of cytarabine on normal human T cells

As described above, normal PBMC were activated in the presence of various drug combinations (Figures 1 and 2). Proliferation and viability was not altered for cultures containing various combinations of ATRA and valproic acid, and ATRA alone did not alter the antiproliferative or proapoptotic effects of cytarabine.

Valproic acid 500 and 1000 μM was also combined with cytarabine 0.01 and 0.35 μM; these cytarabine concentrations correspond to the *in vivo* levels reached during low-dose cytarabine treatment when the drug can be combined with ATRA and valproic acid [15,26,27]. Cytarabine 0.01 μM alone did not have any antiproliferative effect but a statistically significant antiproliferative effect was observed when cytarabine at this concentration was combined with valproic acid 1000 μM (Figure 2). Similarly, when cytarabine at a higher concentration of 0.35 μM was present together with valproic acid an increased antiproliferative effect was observed with valproic acid at both 1000 μM and 500 μM. Finally, dual or triple drug combinations did not have significant effects on T cell viability, the only exception being cytarabine 0.35 μM in combination with valproic acid 500 μM (Figure 1).

The CD4:CD8 ratio is altered only by high-dose cytarabine but not by ATRA, valproic acid or low-dose cytarabine
Normal PBMCs derived from 3 healthy individuals were activated as described above in the presence of various

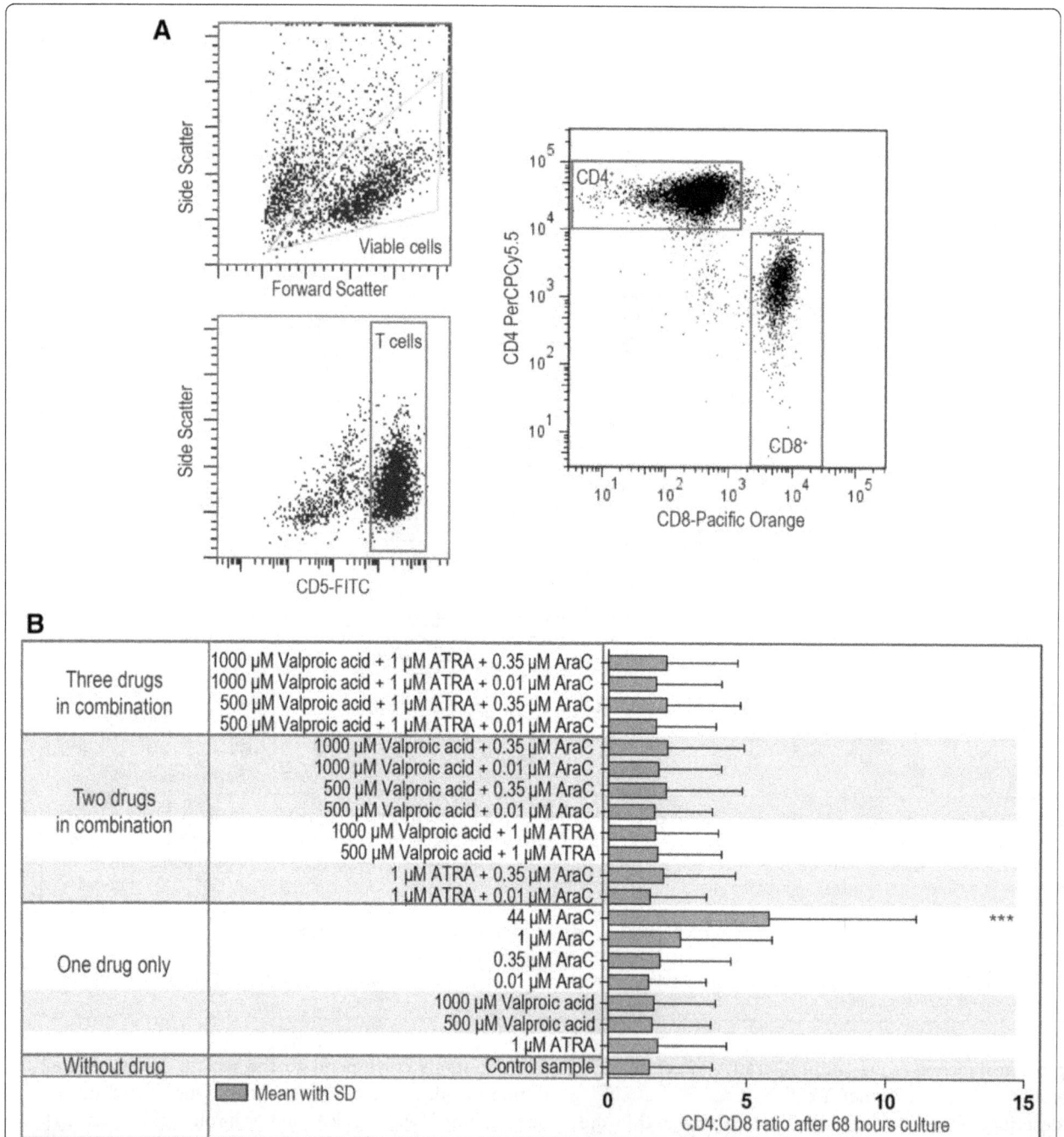

Figure 3 The CD4:CD8 ratio of activated T lymphocytes after exposure to cytarabine, ATRA and valproic acid alone or in combination. PBMCs derived from three healthy blood donors were activated by anti-CD3 plus anti-CD28 during 3 days of *in vitro* culture before flow cytometric analysis of the CD4:CD8 ratio. Cultures were prepared without drugs, with single drugs or with drug combinations. **(A)** The figure shows the gating strategy for estimation of CD4+CD5+ and CD8+CD5+ T cells lymphocytes in a representative experiment. **(B)** The overall results are presented as bar graph (mean ratio with SD) for the drugfree control cultures and cultures prepared with the indicated single drugs or drug combinations. A repeated measure ANOVA with Dunnett's Multiple Comparison Test was used to determine statistically significant differences (*p <0.05; **p <0.01; ***p <0.001).

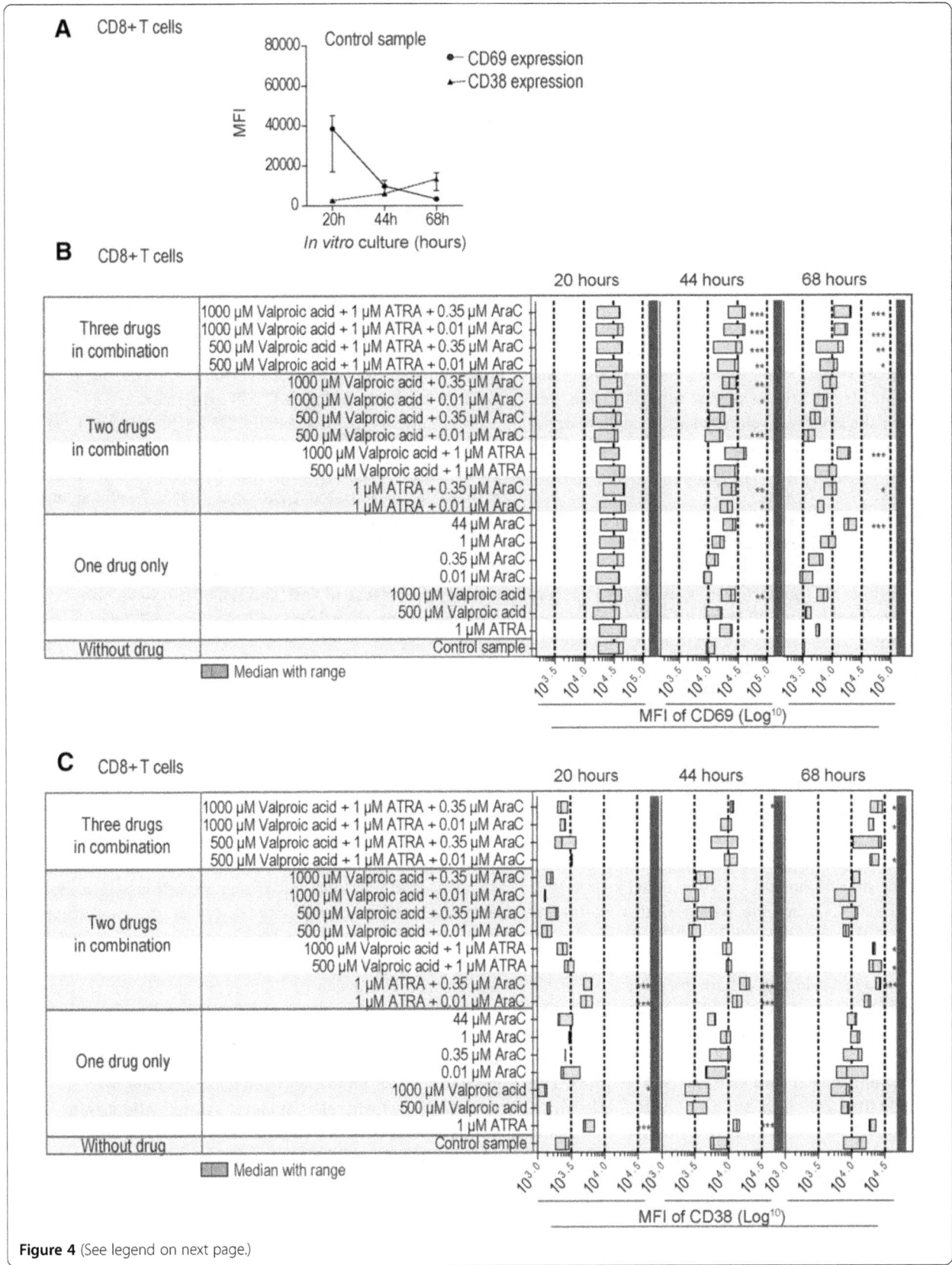

Figure 4 (See legend on next page.)

(See figure on previous page.)
Figure 4 Expression of the CD69 and CD38 activation markers by anti-CD3 plus anti-CD28 activated CD8$^+$ T lymphocytes – effects of cytarabine, ATRA and valproic acid tested alone or in combination. PBMCs derived from three healthy donors were activated during *in vitro* culture with anti-CD3 and anti-CD28, and flow-cytometric analysis of surface CD69 and CD38 expression was performed after 20, 44, and 68 hours of culture. **(A)** The figure shows the mean fluorescence intensity (MFI) of surface CD69 and CD38 expression by CD8$^+$CD5$^+$ T lymphocytes in drugfree control cultures after 20, 44, and 68 hours (median and range, three experiments). **(B)** The overall results for CD69 expression are presented as bar graph (median MFI and range) for CD8$^+$CD5$^+$ T lymphocytes cultured *in vitro* for 20, 44, and 68 hours in the presence of the indicated single drugs or drug combinations. **(C)** The overall results for CD38 expression are presented as bar graph (median MFI and range) for CD8$^+$CD5$^+$ T lymphocytes cultured *in vitro* for 20, 44, and 68 hours in the presence of the indicated single drugs or drug combinations. Repeated measures ANOVA with Dunnett's Multiple Comparison Test was for the statistical analyses (*p <0.05; **p <0.01; ***p <0.001).

drug combinations. Only cytarabine (0.35, 1.0 and 44 µM) caused a dose-dependent reduction both in viability and proliferation. Proliferation, but not viability, was altered for cultures containing several of the dual or triple drug combinations. However, the CD4:CD8 ratio was significantly increased only by the highest cytarabine concentration of 44 µM whereas the ratio was not altered when the cells were cultured with single drugs at the other concentrations or any dual or triple drug combination (Figure 3).

ATRA and valproic acid alters the expression of the CD69 and CD38 activation markers by CD4$^+$ and CD8$^+$ normal T cells whereas cytarabine has only minor effects

In our experimental model CD69 showed an expected high early expression after 20 hours of culture with anti-CD3 plus anti-CD28 both for CD4$^+$ and CD8$^+$ T cells, and thereafter it decreased gradually when tested after 44 and 68 hours. In contrast, CD38 showed a gradual increase for both T cell subsets during the same period after activation (3 healthy individuals tested).

Even though ATRA 1 µM and valproic acid 500 and 1000 µM had no or only minor effects on T cell proliferation and viability as well as the CD4:CD8 ratio, both drugs prolonged the expression of CD69 both for CD4$^+$ and CD8$^+$ T cells, and significantly increased expression was detected after 44 hours (3 healthy individuals tested, Figures 4 and 5). Cytarabine had a similar increasing effect on CD69 expression for both T cell subsets but only when testing the highest concentration (44 µM). The drugs showed additive enhancing effects on CD69 expression both for CD4$^+$ and CD8$^+$ T cells when testing double or triple combinations, and highly significant differences could then be detected (i) for CD4$^+$ T cells when combining ATRA and valproic acid 500 µM; and (ii) especially for CD4$^+$ cells but also CD8$^+$ T cells when ATRA/valproic acid were combined with low cytarabine concentrations (0.01 and 0.35 µM, p <0.001).

ATRA and valproic acid had opposite effects on CD38 expression by activated T cells; ATRA increased the expression whereas valproic acid decreased the early expression of this marker both for CD4$^+$ and CD8$^+$ T cells. None of these effects were detected after 68 hours. In contrast, cytarabine did not alter CD38 expression for

any concentration tested (0.01, 0.35, 1 and 44 µM). The ATRA-induced enhancement was only maintained in the presence of cytarabine (both for CD4$^+$ and CD8$^+$ T cells) but not in the presence of ATRA alone. Finally, the valproic acid-induced reduction of CD38 levels was maintained in the presence of cytarabine and the triple combinations did not alter CD38 expression.

Cytarabine 44 µM decreased CD25 expression of CD4$^+$ T cells but only after 68 hours of culture (p <0.05). No other single drug or drug combinations altered CD25 expression by activated CD8$^+$ and CD4$^+$ T cells at any time point tested (data not shown).

The combination of cytarabine, valproic acid and ATRA reduces the release of FasL and HSP90 but have only weak effects on the release of TRAIL and HSP70 by activated T cells

Normal PBMC derived from 7 healthy individuals were activated with anti-CD3 and anti-CD28 and cultured for 4 days *in vitro* with or without valproic acid, ATRA or/ and cytarabine alone or in combination before supernatant levels of FasL, TRAIL HSP70 and HSP90 were determined (Figure 6). Both valproic acid and cytarabine caused a dose-dependent reduction of HSP90 and FasL. However, the reduction in single-drug cultures was relatively small and the most significant decreases were seen for drug combinations and strong reductions were then seen even when combining drugs at concentrations (cytarabine 0.01 and 0.35 µM, valproic acid 500 µM) that did not cause significant reductions when tested alone. In contrast, the drugs had either no significant or only weak effects on the release of TRAIL and HSP70.

Only high cytarabine concentrations show a broad inhibitory effect on the cytokine release profile by activated T cell whereas high-level valproic acid as well as combinations of low valproic acid-cytarabine levels inhibits the release of a minor cytokine subset

PBMC derived from 7 healthy individuals were cultured with anti-CD3 plus anti-CD28 for 4 days before supernatant cytokine levels were determined for cultures prepared in medium alone and medium with ATRA 1 µM, valproic acid 500 and 100 µM, and cytarabine 0.01, 0.35, 1 and 44 µM. Each drug was tested alone and in the dual

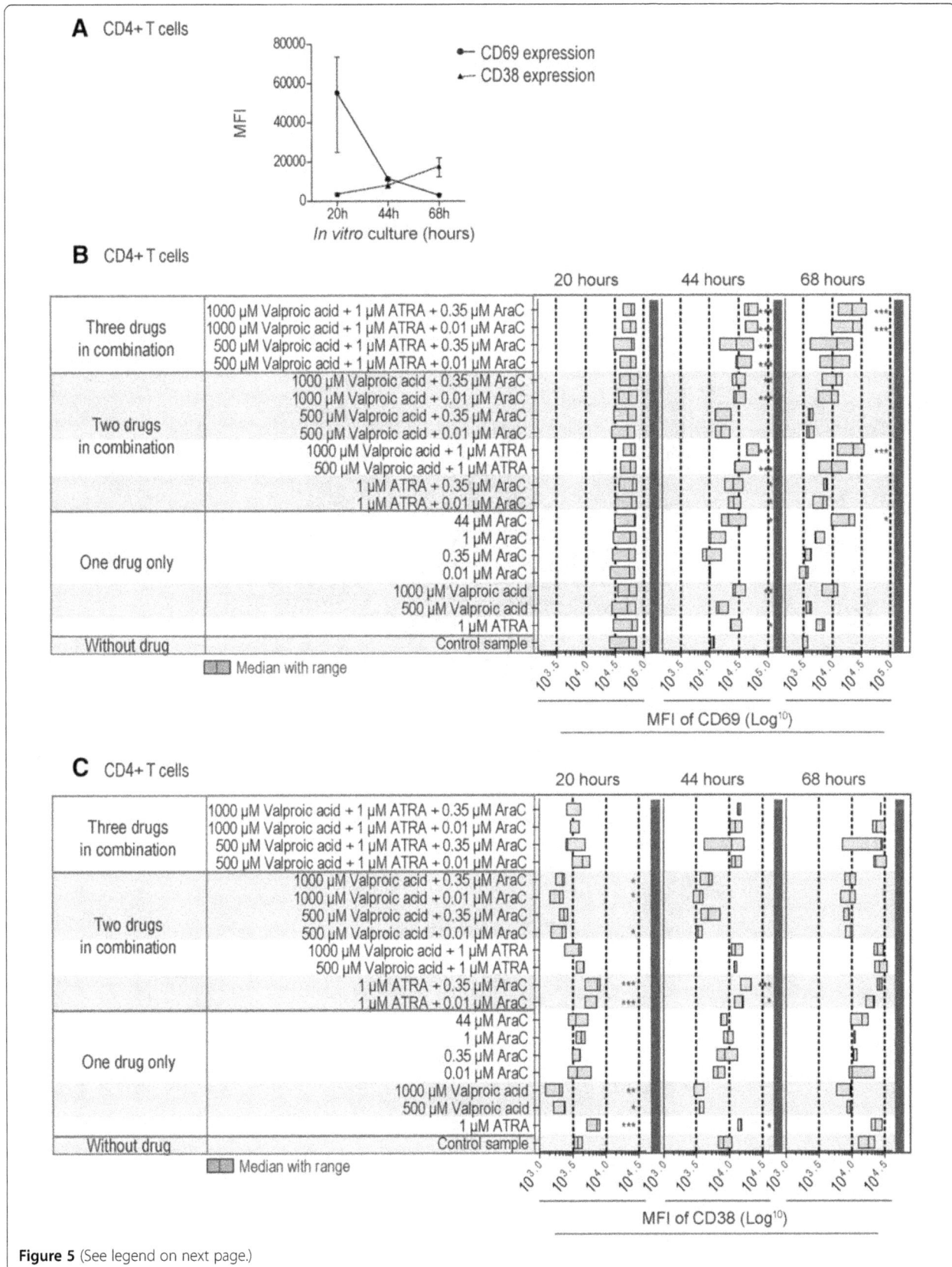

Figure 5 (See legend on next page.)

(See figure on previous page.)

Figure 5 Expression of the CD69 and CD38 activation markers by anti-CD3 plus anti-CD28 activated CD4$^+$ T lymphocytes – effects of cytarabine, ATRA and valproic acid tested alone or in combination. PBMCs derived from three healthy donors were activated during *in vitro* culture with anti-CD3 and anti-CD28, and flow-cytometric analysis of surface CD69 and CD38 expression was performed after 20, 44, and 68 hours of culture. **(A)** The figure shows the mean fluorescence intensity (MFI) of surface CD69 and CD38 expression by CD4$^+$CD5$^+$ T lymphocytes in drug-free control cultures after 20, 44, and 68 hours (median and range, three experiments). **(B)** The overall results for CD69 expression are presented as bar graph (median MFI and range) for CD4$^+$CD5$^+$ T lymphocytes cultured *in vitro* for 20, 44, and 68 hours in the presence of the indicated single drugs or drug combinations. **(C)** The overall results for CD38 expression are presented as bar graph (median MFI and range) for CD4$^+$CD5$^+$ T lymphocytes cultured *in vitro* for 20, 44, and 68 hours in the presence of the indicated single drugs or drug combinations. Repeated measures ANOVA with Dunnett's Multiple Comparison Test was for the statistical analyses (*p <0.05; **p <0.01; ***p <0.001).

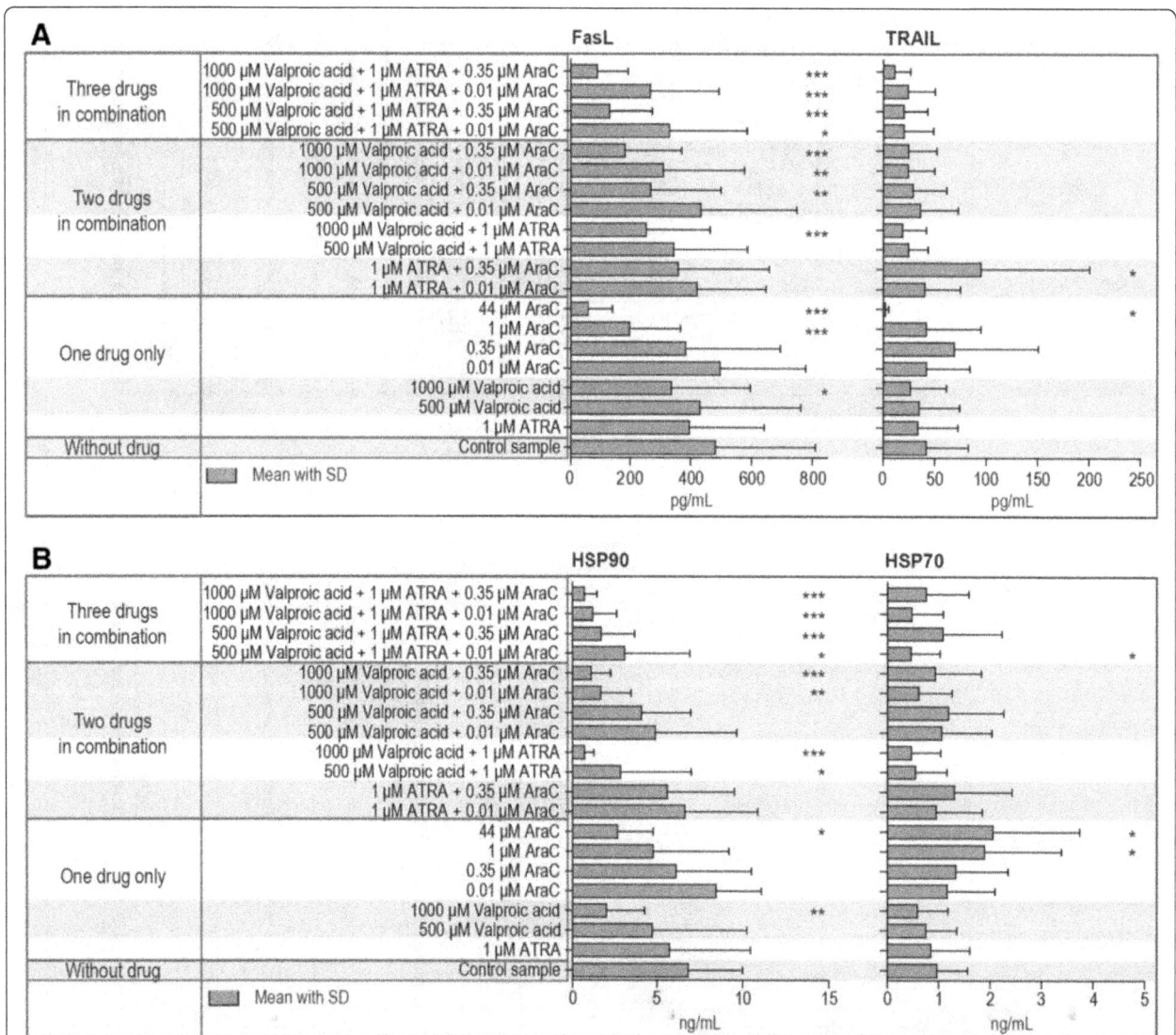

Figure 6 The release of FasL, TRAIL, HSP70 and HSP90 by anti-CD3 plus anti-CD28 activated normal T cells – effects of cytarabine, ATRA and valproic acid tested alone or in combination. The supernatant concentrations of FasL, TRAIL, HSP90 and HSP70 were determined after 4 days of PBMC culture with anti-CD3 plus anti-CD28. Cultures were prepared in medium alone or together with the single drugs or drug combinations indicated in the figures. **(A)** The upper figure presents the FasL (left panel) and TRAIL (right panel) levels, the lower figure **(B)** presents the levels of HSP90 (left panel) and HSP70 (right panel). All results are presented as the mean with SD. Repeated measures ANOVA with Dunnett's Multiple Comparison Test against control samples were used for statistical analyses (*p <0.05; **p <0.01; ***p <0.001).

or triple combinations used throughout the study. The overall cytokine results are presented in Additional file 1: Tables S1-S4, and the results are summarized in a two-ways hierarchical cluster analysis including 20 cytokines and in addition FasL, TRAIL, HSP70 and HSP90 (Figure 7). We investigated the levels of (i) the immunoregulatory cytokines IFNγ and TNFα; (ii) the growth factors G-CSF, GM,-CSF, VEGF and bFGF; (iii) the chemokines CCL2-5 and CXCL5; and (iv) the interleukins IL1α, IL1β, IL2, IL4-6, IL8, IL10 and IL17. For this two-way hierarchical cluster analysis the cytokine levels in drug-containing

cultures were made relative to the level in the corresponding drugfree control, and the mean relative level of each drug-cytokine combination was used for the analysis that included the 24 soluble mediators and the 19 single drug/drug combinations. The drugs/drug combinations formed three main clusters:

- Only cytarabine 44 µM reduced the levels of a majority of the soluble mediators (Figure 7 right margin, lower and upper middle mediator clusters), including HSP90 as well as several chemokines

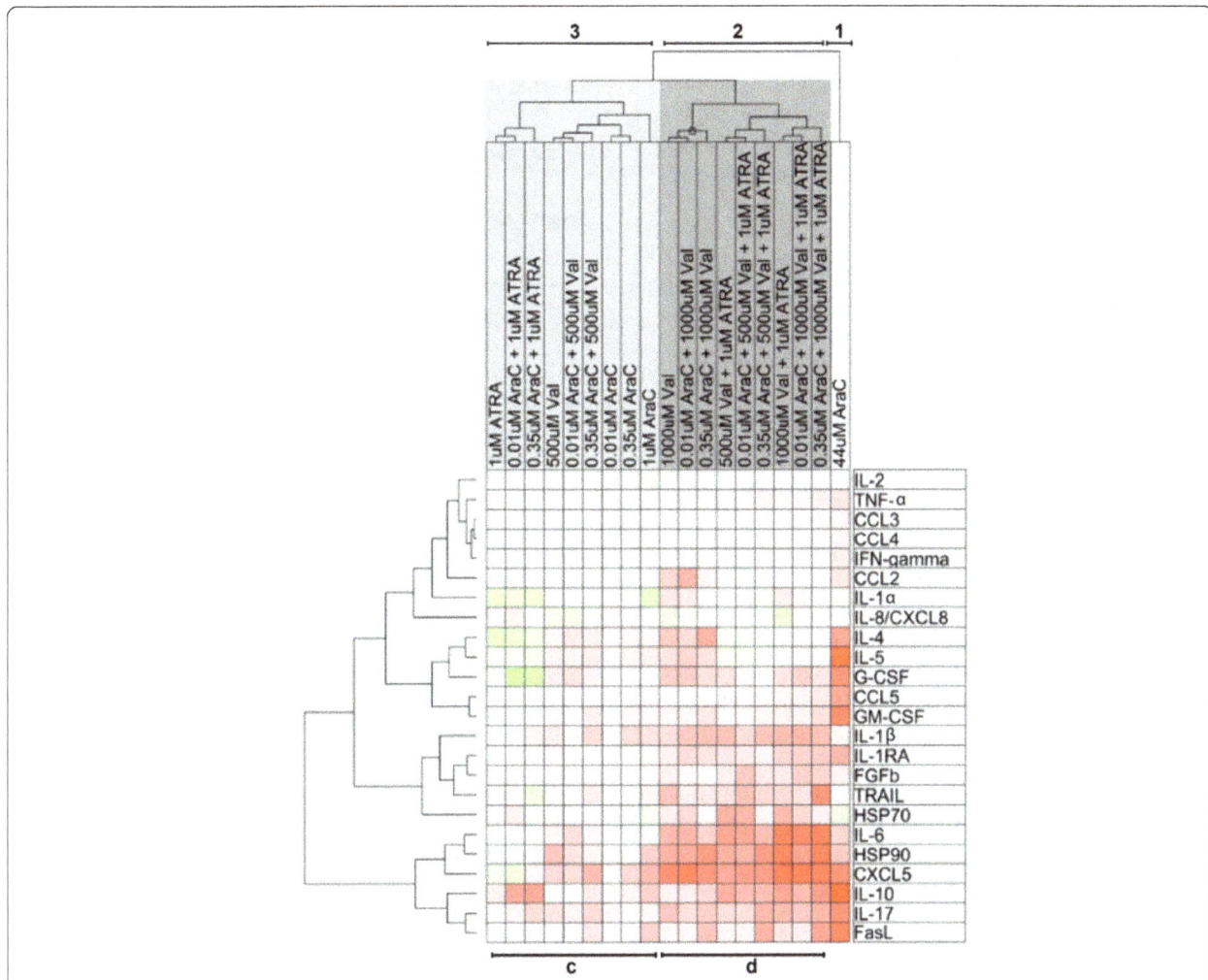

Figure 7 The soluble release profile by activated T cells is altered by valproic acid, ATRA and cytarabine – a two-ways hierarchical cluster analysis. PBMCs derived from 7 healthy individuals were cultured with the T cell activating signal anti-CD3 plus anti-CD28 for 4 days before supernatants were harvested and cytokine levels determined. The cells were then cultured in drugfree control cultures and together with ATRA 1 µM, valproic acid 500 and 100 µM, and cytarabine 0.01, 0.35, 1 and 44 µM, and each drug was also tested in dual or triple combinations as indicated at the top of the figure. The overall results are presented in detail in Additional file 1: Table S1-S4. The results from a two-ways hierarchical cluster analysis including FasL, TRAIL, HSP70 and HSP90 together with 20 cytokines are presented in the figure. We investigated the levels of (i) the immunoregulatory cytokines IFNγ and TNFα; (ii) the growth factors G-CSF, GM,-CSF, VEGF and bFGF; (iii) the chemokines CCL2-5 and CXCL5; and (iv) the interleukins IL1α, IL1β, IL1RA, IL2, IL4-6, IL8, IL10 and IL17. The cytokines formed 4 main clusters as indicated on the left margin of the figure. The analysis included the 19 single drug/drug combinations used throughout the study and the various drugs/drug combinations formed three main clusters.

(CCL5, CXCL5) and immunoregulatory cytokines (IL4-6, IL10, IL17).

- A second cluster was mainly formed by (i) all triple combinations, (ii) the two valproic acid + ATRA combinations and (iii) valproic acid 1000 µM tested alone or in combination with low-level cytarabine. This cluster was characterized by decreased release of the lower mediator cluster similar to cytarabine 44 µM and in addition a relatively weak effect for the lower middle cluster.
- For the other drugs/combinations we only observed weak and divergent effects.

Thus, only high cytarabine levels show a broad and strong inhibition of the T cell cytokine response, whereas high valproic acid levels 1000 µM as well as all triple combinations of low-level cytarabine, low-level valproic acid and ATRA inhibit the release of a defined subset of T cell derived mediators.

Low cytarabine concentrations show little effect on patient cell viability but significantly reduce their proliferation capability

We investigated the effect of low-dose cytarabine on cell viability and proliferation for AML cells derived from 48 consecutive patients. As described previously the AML cell viability varies widely between patients after in vitro incubation due to spontaneous in vitro apoptosis [28], and the median viability in our drug-free control cultures was 34% (range 2-64%) in the control samples. We investigated cytarabine 0.5, 0.05 and 0.01 µM (Figure 8A), and the viability was significantly reduced only for the two highest drug concentrations (0.5 µM, median viability 26%, p <0.001; 0.05 µM, median viability 32%, p =0.030). In contrast, all three cytarabine concentrations reduced AML cell proliferation significantly. The median radioactivity corresponded to 5900 counts per minute (cpm) for the drugfree controls (range <1000 – 179200), the activity was only 600 cpm for cytarabine 0.5 µM (p <0.001), 900 cpm for cytarabine 0.05 µM (p <0.001) and 1800 cpm for cytarabine 0.01 µM (p <0.001) (Figure 8B).

Discussion

Low-toxicity AML-stabilizing treatment is now tried for patients who are unfit for intensive and potentially curative therapy. The HDAC inhibitor valproic acid has been investigated as an antileukemic agent in several clinical studies, usually in combination with ATRA [15] and/or low-dose cytotoxic agents [29]. Three phase II clinical studies have shown that the combination of valproic acid, ATRA and low-dose cytarabine [15,26,27] has low clinical toxicity and can induce complete remission for a minority and disease stabilization for a larger subset of elderly and unfit patients. Despite low clinical toxicity,

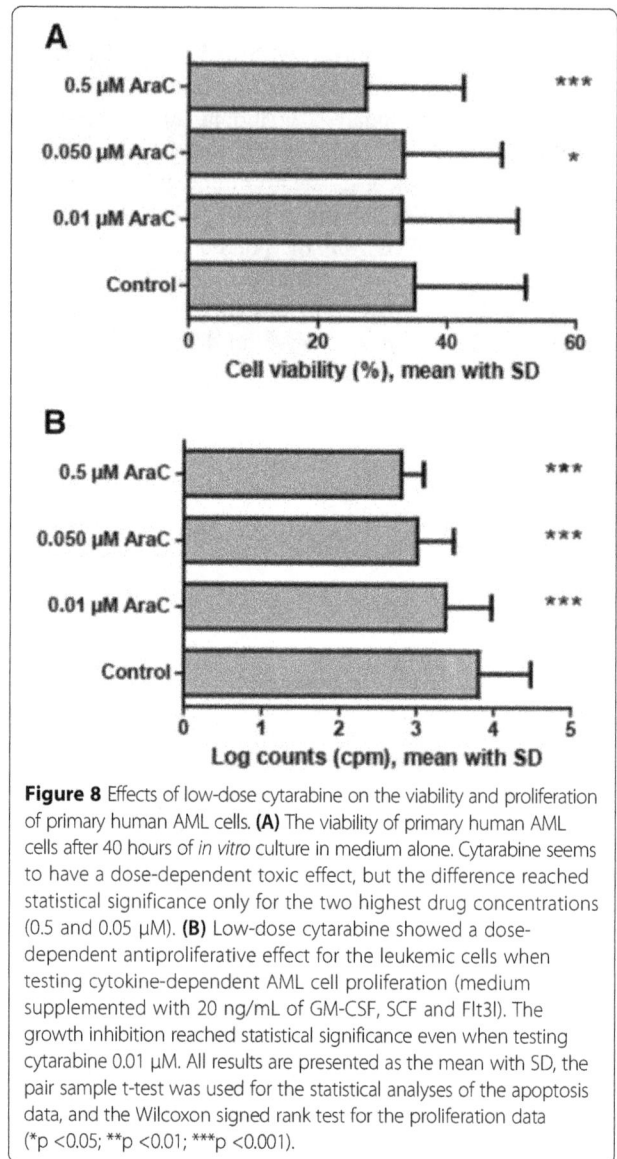

Figure 8 Effects of low-dose cytarabine on the viability and proliferation of primary human AML cells. **(A)** The viability of primary human AML cells after 40 hours of in vitro culture in medium alone. Cytarabine seems to have a dose-dependent toxic effect, but the difference reached statistical significance only for the two highest drug concentrations (0.5 and 0.05 µM). **(B)** Low-dose cytarabine showed a dose-dependent antiproliferative effect for the leukemic cells when testing cytokine-dependent AML cell proliferation (medium supplemented with 20 ng/mL of GM-CSF, SCF and Flt3l). The growth inhibition reached statistical significance even when testing cytarabine 0.01 µM. All results are presented as the mean with SD, the pair sample t-test was used for the statistical analyses of the apoptosis data, and the Wilcoxon signed rank test for the proliferation data (*p <0.05; **p <0.01; ***p <0.001).

our in vitro results suggest that the treatment may have immunosuppressive effects as we observed decreased T cell viability, reduced T cell proliferation, altered activation-induced expression of membrane molecules and reduced cytokine release (see Table 1 for summary).

Cytarabine is commonly used in AML therapy and is then used at single doses ranging from 10 mg/m^2 up to 3000 mg/m^2 [30]. The systemic serum levels therefore show a wide variation depending both on the single dose, the administration form and the gender with faster clearance in males [30]. Firstly, the daily doses commonly used in induction treatment of human AML are 100-200 mg/m^2; the drug can then be given as intermittent injections or as continuous infusions and the clearance is also influenced by the pretreatment leukemia blast count in the blood. The average steady state levels

Table 1 A summary of pharmacological effects on T cell activation; studies of high cytarabine concentrations alone, low cytarabine levels and low cytarabine levels in combination with ATRA and/or valproic acid

Parameter	High cytarabine levels (44 and 1.0 µM)	Low cytarabine levels (0.35 and 0.01 µM)	Low cytarabine levels (0.35 and 0.01 µM) combined with ATRA 1 µM and/or valproic acid (500 and 1000 µM)
T cell viability	Decreased, apoptosis induction	Decreased only for 0.35 µM	No significant effect for most combinations
T cell proliferation	Decreased	Decreased only for 0.35 µM	A highly significant decrease for combinations with cytarabine 0.35 µM
CD4:CD8 ratio	Decreased	No effect	No effect
CD69 expression	Prolonged expression, especially for CD8+ but also CD4+ cells	No effect both for CD4+ and CD8+ cells	CD4+ cells: Increased by ATRA and decreased by valproic acid, no effect when combining these two drugs. The ATRA effect maintaining when combined with cytarabine. CD8+ cells: Increased by ATRA and valproic acid, the increase was also seen in combinations with cytarabine.
CD38 expression	No effect	No effect both for CD4+ and CD8+ cells	CD4+ cells: Increased by ATRA and decreased by valproic acid, the ATRA effect maintained in the presence of cytarabine. CD8+ cells: Increased by ATRA and decreased by valproic acid, the ATRA effect maintained in combinations.
FasL release	Decreased	No effect	Strong decrease in all combinations also with cytarabine 0.01 µM
TRAIL release	Minor decrease only at 44 µM	No effect	Minor effects
HSP90 release	Decreased	No effect	Strong decrease both for cytarabine 0.35 and 0.01 µM
HSP70	Increased	No effect	No effect for all except one combination
Cytokine release; hierarchical cluster analysis including 24 soluble mediators	Decreased levels for two out of 4 main clusters including 9 cytokines, including the cluster showing decreased levels for the drug combinations.	Only minor effects	Decreased levels only for one out of the four main clusters, including 4 cytokines

during continuous infusions in one study were 0.4 and 0.8 µM for 100 and 200 mg/m^2/day, respectively [31]. Levels will be higher when giving these daily doses as injections. Secondly, the drug may also be used at single doses up to 3 g/m^2 twice daily administered as short-time infusions and resulting in peak concentrations during a 3-hours infusion averaging 50-100 µM [30,31]. Finally, cytarabine is used as low-toxicity subcutaneous injections (10-20 mg/m^2) once or twice daily usually for a 10 days period with 4-6 weeks intervals [15]; the steady state levels are then below 0.1 µM [30,32-35] and the peak levels after a subcutaneous injection of 10 mg/m^2/12 hours can be up to 0.2-0.5 µM [18]. In our present study we therefore investigated the concentrations (i) 44 µM that corresponds to peak levels during high-dose treatment; (ii) 1 µM that is reached when using the conventional doses of 100-200 mg/m^2; and (iii) and 0.35 and 0.01 µM that correspond to levels reached early after and during steady state of low-dose treatment.

Cytarabine effects on T cell activation were concentration-dependent; decreased viability was only seen for the higher concentrations and this is in accordance with previous studies suggesting that cytarabine has cytotoxic effects only at concentrations above 100 nM [30]. However, cytarabine had immunoregulatory effects even at lower level. Several of our present observations suggest that the cytarabine effects on activated T cells at least partly differ between T cell subsets. This is supported both by (i) the altered CD4:CD8 ratio after exposure to high cytarabine levels, (ii) the differences between CD4+ and CD8+ T cells with regard to cytarabine effects on CD38 and CD69 expression during T cell activation; and (iii) previous studies describing that *in vivo* treatment with our triple combination causes normalization of the increased pre-therapy levels of circulating Treg cells, whereas the levels of circulating Th17 cells are not affected by the treatment [15].

Cytarabine decreased AML cell viability only when tested at 0.5 and 0.05 µM but not at the lowest concentration, whereas the drug inhibited AML cell proliferation even at 0.01 µM. In contrast, T cell proliferation was inhibited only at cytarabine concentrations ≥0.35 µM. Thus, based on the proliferation studies we conclude that primary AML cells are more susceptible to cytarabine than normal T cells; suggesting that there is a therapeutic window for cytarabine treatment that makes it possible to achieve antileukemic effects *in vivo* before severe T cell toxicity occurs.

Our *in vitro* studies showed that valproic acid alone affected T cell activation but only for a minority of our experimental models and usually when testing the highest concentration of 1000 μM that corresponds to a level slightly above the recommended therapeutic serum level [15]. ATRA did not affect T cell activation in most of our studies. However, both drugs contributed to the effects of the triple combination of T cell activation, and in several of our models highly significant immunomodulatory effects were seen only when testing the triple combination.

Early lymphoid reconstitution after intensive and potentially curative antileukemic therapy is associated with decreased risk of later AML relapse, suggesting that post-treatment immunological events are clinically important to maintain disease control and complete hematological remission after end of treatment [36,37]. This association between early lymphoid reconstitution and survival has also been observed after conventional intensive chemotherapy [3], autotransplantation [4] and allotransplantation [5,6]. The mechanisms behind this association are not known [38], but taken together these observations suggest that not only allogeneic but also autologous antileukemic T cell reactivity after intensive treatment or autotransplantation is clinically important.

To the best of our knowledge no previous studies have investigated whether such autologous antileukemic T cell reactivity is important also in patients receiving AML-stabilizing treatment, e.g. the combination of ATRA, valproic acid and cytarabine. There are two major differences between AML patients receiving intensive treatment and patients receiving our low-toxicity triple combination: (i) most patients receiving stabilizing treatment do not achieve complete hematological remission, and (ii) these patients will often receive continued therapy until disease progression. Furthermore, many AML patients have severe leucopenia, including T lymphopenia [16]. During the continued AML-stabilizing treatment most of these patients thus have a combined AML-induced quantitative and treatment-induced qualitative T cell effect. Most of the patients who respond to the treatment do not show increased leukocyte counts [16,39]. If antileukemic immune reactivity is important for the efficiency of AML-stabilizing treatment similar to its effect in patients receiving intensive therapy, the immunosuppressive effects described in our present study may influence the efficiency of this treatment. The question should be addressed in future clinical studies, and one should then especially investigate whether the effect differs between various T cell subsets.

Three clinical studies have previously investigated the antileukemic effect of low-dose cytarabine, ATRA and valproic acid [13,39,40], but the question of immunosuppression was only addressed in one of them [39]. This study showed that even though the drug-induced immunosuppression may be important for the antileukemic efficiency of AML-stabilizing (see above), the triple combination does not seem to have a major impact on the risk of complicating infections in responders to the treatment as these patients usually stayed outside hospital without severe infections as long as the disease was stable without signs of AML progression [39]. However, it should be emphasized that these patients were treated with even a lower cytarabine dose than commonly used for low-dose cytarabine treatment [39], and in contrast to the other two studies ATRA was administered as an intermittent therapy with 2 weeks of treatment at 12 weeks intervals. Our studies suggest that clinically relevant immunosuppression may occur if standard low-dose cytarabine or continuous ATRA therapy is used.

The valproic acid-ATRA-cytarabine combination altered T cell release of several soluble mediators. Firstly, FasL (CD95L) and TNF-related apoptosis-inducing ligand (TRAIL or APO2) may mediate autocrine activation-induced cell death (AICD) to maintain self-tolerance and suppress immune responses [41,42], but soluble CD95L may also induce non-apoptotic signals that promote cell migration [43]. The effects of single drugs and especially our triple combination on FasL release suggest that the treatment may alter cell trafficking. Secondly, the intracellular chaperones HSP90 and HSP70 can be released extracellularly and will then have immunomodulatory effects [44-47]; these effects may be affected by the altered HSP90 levels during T cell activation in the presence of our triple combination. Finally, both cytarabine, valproic acid and ATRA affected the release of several interleukins and chemokines by activated T cells. Taken together these observations suggest that the antileukemic triple combination not only has direct effects on T cells, but probably also indirect effects on other immunocompetent cells mediated by the altered release of soluble mediators during T cell activation.

Conclusions

Both previous *in vivo* studies and the present *in vitro* studies suggest that the triple combination of low-dose cytarabine, ATRA and valproic acid has immunomodulatory effects, and as discussed above these effects may differ between various T cell subsets. The triple combination has direct effects on the T cells, but it may also affect other immunocompetent cells through the altered release of soluble mediators during T cell activation. This possible risk of immunosuppression should be further investigated in future clinical studies.

Additional file

Additional file 1: Table S1. Supernatant levels of immunomodulatory cytokines and growth factors. Table S2. Supernatant levels of chemokines. Table S3. Supernatant levels of Interleukins (IL-1 – IL-5). Table S4. Supernatant levels of Interleukins (IL-6 – IL-17).

Abbreviations
AML: Acute myeloid leukemia; ATRA: All-trans retinoic acid; ELISA: Enzyme-linked immuno-sorbent analyses (ELISA); HSP: Heat shock protein; PBMC: Peripheral blood mononuclear cells.

Competing interests
The authors declare that they have no competing interests.

Authors' contributions
EE, AKB and KV designed and performed experiments, analyzed data and wrote the manuscript. HR performed cluster analyses, interpreted the data and revised the manuscript. ØB conceived and guided the study, and wrote the manuscript. All authors read and approved the final manuscript.

Acknowledgements
This work was supported by Helse-Vest and Norwegian Cancer Society. The technical assistance of Kristin Paulsen is highly appreciated. Parts of the ELISA and Luminex results are based upon the work done by the following bachelor-students: Hilde V. Edvardsen, Trude B. Grannes, Marthe D. Johnsen, Janicke Danielsen and Trude Nordal.

Author details
[1]Institute of Clinical Science, University of Bergen, Bergen, Norway. [2]Institute of Biomedical Laboratory Sciences, Bergen University College, Nygårdsgaten 112, P.O. Box 7030, N-5020 Bergen, Norway. [3]Department of Medicine, Haukeland University Hospital, Bergen, Norway.

References
1. Liseth K, Sjo M, Paulsen K, Bruserud O, Ersvaer E. Early pre-engraftment, functional, in vitro responsiveness of T lymphocytes in allotransplanted, acute leukemia patients: proliferation and release of a broad profile of cytokines, possibly predictive of graft-versus-host disease. Eur Cytokine Netw. 2010;21(1):40–9.
2. Mackall C, Fry T, Gress R, Peggs K, Storek J, Toubert A, et al. Background to hematopoietic cell transplantation, including post transplant immune recovery. Bone Marrow Transplant. 2009;44(8):457–62.
3. Behl D, Porrata LF, Markovic SN, Letendre L, Pruthi RK, Hook CC, et al. Absolute lymphocyte count recovery after induction chemotherapy predicts superior survival in acute myelogenous leukemia. Leukemia. 2006;20(1):29–34.
4. Porrata LF, Litzow MR, Tefferi A, Letendre L, Kumar S, Geyer SM, et al. Early lymphocyte recovery is a predictive factor for prolonged survival after autologous hematopoietic stem cell transplantation for acute myelogenous leukemia. Leukemia. 2002;16(7):1311–8.
5. Parkman R, Cohen G, Carter SL, Weinberg KI, Masinsin B, Guinan E, et al. Successful immune reconstitution decreases leukemic relapse and improves survival in recipients of unrelated cord blood transplantation. Biol Blood Marrow Transplant. 2006;12(9):919–27.
6. Kim DH, Sohn SK, Won DI, Lee NY, Suh JS, Lee KB. Rapid helper T-cell recovery above 200 x 10 6/l at 3 months correlates to successful transplant outcomes after allogeneic stem cell transplantation. Bone Marrow Transplant. 2006;37(12):1119–28.
7. Colotta F, Allavena P, Sica A, Garlanda C, Mantovani A. Cancer-related inflammation, the seventh hallmark of cancer: links to genetic instability. Carcinogenesis. 2009;30(7):1073–81.
8. Smith M, Barnett M, Bassan R, Gatta G, Tondini C, Kern W. Adult acute myeloid leukemia. Crit Rev Oncol Hematol. 2004;50(3):197–222.
9. Fredly H, Reikvam H, Gjertsen BT, Bruserud O. Disease-stabilizing treatment with all-trans retinoic acid and valproic acid in acute myeloid leukemia: serum hsp70 and hsp90 levels and serum cytokine profiles are determined by the disease, patient age, and anti-leukemic treatment. Am J Hematol. 2012;87(4):368–76.
10. Schlenk RF, Frohling S, Hartmann F, Fischer JT, Glasmacher A, del Valle F, et al. Phase III study of all-trans retinoic acid in previously untreated patients 61 years or older with acute myeloid leukemia. Leukemia. 2004;18(11):1798–803.
11. Kuendgen A, Knipp S, Fox F, Strupp C, Hildebrandt B, Steidl C, et al. Results of a phase 2 study of valproic acid alone or in combination with all-trans retinoic acid in 75 patients with myelodysplastic syndrome and relapsed or refractory acute myeloid leukemia. Ann Hematol. 2005;84 Suppl 1:61–6.
12. Raffoux E, Chaibi P, Dombret H, Degos L. Valproic acid and all-trans retinoic acid for the treatment of elderly patients with acute myeloid leukemia. Haematologica. 2005;90(7):986–8.
13. Bug G, Ritter M, Wassmann B, Schoch C, Heinzel T, Schwarz K, et al. Clinical trial of valproic acid and all-trans retinoic acid in patients with poor-risk acute myeloid leukemia. Cancer. 2005;104(12):2717–25.
14. Venditti A, Stasi R, Del Poeta G, Buccisano F, Aronica G, Bruno A, et al. All-trans retinoic acid and low-dose cytosine arabinoside for the treatment of 'poor prognosis' acute myeloid leukemia. Leukemia. 1995;9(7):1121–5.
15. Fredly H, Gjertsen BT, Bruserud O. Histone deacetylase inhibition in the treatment of acute myeloid leukemia: the effects of valproic acid on leukemic cells, and the clinical and experimental evidence for combining valproic acid with other antileukemic agents. Clinical epigenetics. 2013;5(1):12.
16. Ryningen A, Stapnes C, Lassalle P, Corbascio M, Gjertsen BT, Bruserud O. A subset of patients with high-risk acute myelogenous leukemia shows improved peripheral blood cell counts when treated with the combination of valproic acid, theophylline and all-trans retinoic acid. Leuk Res. 2009;33(6):779–87.
17. Yamauchi T, Kawai Y, Kishi S, Goto N, Urasaki Y, Imamura S, et al. Monitoring of intracellular 1-beta-D-arabinofuranosylcytosine 5'-triphosphate in 1-beta-D-arabinofuranosylcytosine therapy at low and conventional doses. Jpn J Cancer Res. 2001;92(5):546–53.
18. Ishikura H, Sawada H, Okazaki T, Mochizuki T, Izumi Y, Yamagishi M, et al. The effect of low dose Ara-C in acute nonlymphoblastic leukaemias and atypical leukaemia. Br J Haematol. 1984;58(1):9–18.
19. Ueda T, Matsuyama S, Yamauchi T, Kishi S, Fukushima T, Tsutani H, et al. Clinical pharmacology of intermediate and low-dose cytosine arabinoside (ara-C) therapy in patients with hematologic malignancies. Adv Exp Med Biol. 1998;431:647–51.
20. Trus MR, Yang L, Suarez Saiz F, Bordeleau L, Jurisica I, Minden MD. The histone deacetylase inhibitor valproic acid alters sensitivity towards all trans retinoic acid in acute myeloblastic leukemia cells. Leukemia. 2005;19(7):1161–8.
21. Ertesvag A, Engedal N, Naderi S, Blomhoff HK. Retinoic acid stimulates the cell cycle machinery in normal T cells: involvement of retinoic acid receptor-mediated IL-2 secretion. J Immunol. 2002;169(10):5555–63.
22. Breitman TR, Selonick SE, Collins SJ. Induction of differentiation of the human promyelocytic leukemia cell line (HL-60) by retinoic acid. Proc Natl Acad Sci U S A. 1980;77(5):2936–40.
23. DeAngelis LM, Kreis W, Chan K, Dantis E, Akerman S. Pharmacokinetics of ara-C and ara-U in plasma and CSF after high-dose administration of cytosine arabinoside. Cancer Chemother Pharmacol. 1992;29(3):173–7.
24. Hiddemann W. Cytosine arabinoside in the treatment of acute myeloid leukemia: the role and place of high-dose regimens. Ann Hematol. 1991;62(4):119–28.
25. Bruserud O, Hovland R, Wergeland L, Huang TS, Gjertsen BT. Flt3-mediated signaling in human acute myelogenous leukemia (AML) blasts: a functional characterization of Flt3-ligand effects in AML cell populations with and without genetic Flt3 abnormalities. Haematologica. 2003;88(4):416–28.
26. Corsetti MT, Salvi F, Perticone S, Baraldi A, De Paoli L, Gatto S, et al. Hematologic improvement and response in elderly AML/RAEB patients treated with valproic acid and low-dose Ara-C. Leuk Res. 2011;35(8):991–7.
27. Lane S, Gill D, McMillan NA, Saunders N, Murphy R, Spurr T, et al. Valproic acid combined with cytosine arabinoside in elderly patients with acute myeloid leukemia has in vitro but limited clinical activity. Leuk Lymphoma. 2012;53(6):1077–83.
28. Ryningen A, Ersvaer E, Oyan AM, Kalland KH, Vintermyr OK, Gjertsen BT, et al. Stress-induced in vitro apoptosis of native human acute myelogenous leukemia (AML) cells shows a wide variation between patients and is associated with low BCL-2:Bax ratio and low levels of heat shock protein 70 and 90. Leuk Res. 2006;30(12):1531–40.

29. Fredly H, Stapnes Bjornsen C, Gjertsen BT, Bruserud O. Combination of the histone deacetylase inhibitor valproic acid with oral hydroxyurea or 6-mercaptopurin can be safe and effective in patients with advanced acute myeloid leukaemia—a report of five cases. Hematology. 2010;15(5):338–43.

30. Hubeek I, Kaspers G-JL, Ossenkoppele GJ, Peters GJ. Deoxynucleoside analogs in cancer therapy. In: Peter GJ, editor. Cancer Drug Discovery and Development. 2006. p. 119–52. View at Google Scholar.

31. Cole N, Gibson BE. High-dose cytosine arabinoside in the treatment of acute myeloid leukaemia. Blood Rev. 1997;11(1):39–45.

32. Papayannopoulou T, de Ron Torrealba A, Veith R, Knitter G, Stamatoyannopoulos G. Arabinosylcytosine induces fetal hemoglobin in baboons by perturbing erythroid cell differentiation kinetics. Science. 1984;224(4649):617–9.

33. Fleming RA, Capizzi RL, Rosner GL, Oliver LK, Smith SJ, Schiffer CA, et al. Clinical pharmacology of cytarabine in patients with acute myeloid leukemia: a cancer and leukemia group B study. Cancer Chemother Pharmacol. 1995;36(5):425–30.

34. Kreis W, Chaudhri F, Chan K, Allen S, Budman DR, Schulman P, et al. Pharmacokinetics of low-dose 1-beta-D-arabinofuranosylcytosine given by continuous intravenous infusion over twenty-one days. Cancer Res. 1985;45(12 Pt 1):6498–501.

35. Spriggs D, Griffin J, Wisch J, Kufe D. Clinical pharmacology of low-dose cytosine arabinoside. Blood. 1985;65(5):1087–9.

36. Williams KM, Hakim FT, Gress RE. T cell immune reconstitution following lymphodepletion. Semin Immunol. 2007;19(5):318–30.

37. Auletta JJ, Lazarus HM. Immune restoration following hematopoietic stem cell transplantation: an evolving target. Bone Marrow Transplant. 2005;35(9):835–57.

38. Obeid M, Tesniere A, Panaretakis T, Tufi R, Joza N, van Endert P, et al. Ecto-calreticulin in immunogenic chemotherapy. Immunol Rev. 2007;220:22–34.

39. Fredly H, Ersvaer E, Kittang AO, Tsykunova G, Gjertsen BT, Bruserud O. The combination of valproic acid, all-trans retinoic acid and low-dose cytarabine as disease-stabilizing treatment in acute myeloid leukemia. Clinical epigenetics. 2013;5(1):13.

40. Cimino G, Lo-Coco F, Fenu S, Travaglini L, Finolezzi E, Mancini M, et al. Sequential valproic acid/all-trans retinoic acid treatment reprograms differentiation in refractory and high-risk acute myeloid leukemia. Cancer Res. 2006;66(17):8903–11.

41. Monleon I, Martinez-Lorenzo MJ, Monteagudo L, Lasierra P, Taules M, Iturralde M, et al. Differential secretion of Fas ligand- or APO2 ligand/TNF-related apoptosis-inducing ligand-carrying microvesicles during activation-induced death of human T cells. J Immunol. 2001;167(12):6736–44.

42. Martinez-Lorenzo MJ, Anel A, Gamen S, Monle nl, Lasierra P, Larrad L, et al. Activated human T cells release bioactive Fas ligand and APO2 ligand in microvesicles. J Immunol. 1999;163(3):1274–81.

43. Tauzin S, Chaigne-Delalande B, Selva E, Khadra N, Daburon S, Contin-Bordes C, et al. The naturally processed CD95L elicits a c-yes/calcium/PI3K-driven cell migration pathway. PLoS Biol. 2011;9(6), e1001090.

44. Calderwood SK, Theriault JR, Gong J. Message in a bottle: role of the 70-kDa heat shock protein family in anti-tumor immunity. Eur J Immunol. 2005;35(9):2518–27.

45. Chen T, Cao X. Stress for maintaining memory: HSP70 as a mobile messenger for innate and adaptive immunity. Eur J Immunol. 2010;40(6):1541–4.

46. Barreto A, Gonzalez JM, Kabingu E, Asea A, Fiorentino S. Stress-induced release of HSC70 from human tumors. Cell Immunol. 2003;222(2):97–104.

47. Broquet AH, Thomas G, Masliah J, Trugnan G, Bachelet M. Expression of the molecular chaperone Hsp70 in detergent-resistant microdomains correlates with its membrane delivery and release. J Biol Chem. 2003;278(24):21601–6.

Clinical coding of prospectively identified paediatric adverse drug reactions – a retrospective review of patient records

Jennifer R Bellis[1*], Jamie J Kirkham[2], Anthony J Nunn[3] and Munir Pirmohamed[4]

Abstract

Background: National Health Service (NHS) hospitals in the UK use a system of coding for patient episodes. The coding system used is the International Classification of Disease (ICD-10). There are ICD-10 codes which may be associated with adverse drug reactions (ADRs) and there is a possibility of using these codes for ADR surveillance. This study aimed to determine whether ADRs prospectively identified in children admitted to a paediatric hospital were coded appropriately using ICD-10.

Methods: The electronic admission abstract for each patient with at least one ADR was reviewed. A record was made of whether the ADR(s) had been coded using ICD-10.

Results: Of 241 ADRs, 76 (31.5%) were coded using at least one ICD-10 ADR code. Of the oncology ADRs, 70/115 (61%) were coded using an ICD-10 ADR code compared with 6/126 (4.8%) non-oncology ADRs (difference in proportions 56%, 95% CI 46.2% to 65.8%; p < 0.001).

Conclusions: The majority of ADRs detected in a prospective study at a paediatric centre would not have been identified if the study had relied on ICD-10 codes as a single means of detection. Data derived from administrative healthcare databases are not reliable for identifying ADRs by themselves, but may complement other methods of detection.

Keywords: Adverse drug reaction, Paediatrics, Medical coding

Background

National Health Service (NHS) hospitals in the UK use a system of coding alongside the length of hospital stay to determine the chargeable cost of care for each patient. The coding system used is the International Classification of Disease (ICD-10). The process of coding is by case note review, undertaken by trained coders. It relies on diagnoses, procedures and other events being written down by the clinical team caring for the patient. The data are submitted to become part of the national hospital episode statistics (HES) for the NHS in England and are used for research and planning.

There are ICD-10 codes which may be associated with adverse drug reactions (ADRs). Although these codes can also be associated with overdose and medication

errors, there is a possibility of using ICD-10 codes for ADR surveillance. Previous studies in the adult population have identified ADRs or ADEs either by retrospective case note review or by prospective monitoring, and then reviewed the ICD-10 codes for these cases; these studies showed that, in the majority of cases, ADRs and ADEs had not been coded properly [1-3]. Other studies have used ICD-10 codes to determine ADR or ADE incidence followed by a review of the case note record to confirm the accuracy of the code. This method can identify false positives but does not allow the investigator to estimate how many ADRs have been missed by using ICD codes for their identification [4-7]. A previous paediatric study identified ADR cases by searching for the relevant ICD codes and compared these with spontaneously reported cases. They found that not all ADRs were identified by both methods and concluded that neither method in isolation was reliable for ADR surveillance [8].

* Correspondence: jennifer.bellis@alderhey.nhs.uk
[1]Research & Development, Alder Hey Children's NHS Foundation Trust, Liverpool, UK
Full list of author information is available at the end of the article

In this study, we aimed to determine whether prospectively identified ADRs in a paediatric population could have been detected via review of ICD-10 codes.

Methods

The electronic records of children in whom a total of 241 ADRs had been prospectively identified in an earlier study, were reviewed. The aim was to determine whether an ICD-10 code related to the ADR had subsequently been added to their electronic admission abstract.

The methodology of the prospective study in which the 241 ADRs were initially detected has been described previously [9], here a brief summary is provided. The study duration was 12 months (2008–2009) and the participants were children admitted to a paediatric tertiary referral centre (Alder Hey Children's NHS Foundation Trust). A prospective review of each unplanned admission was undertaken by a member of a multi-disciplinary research team which comprised a paediatrician, a paediatric nurse and a pharmacist. The total number of reviews undertaken by each team member and the types of patients in each caseload were similar. The research team reviewed medication taken in the two weeks prior to admission alongside the reason for admission to determine whether the admission was partly or entirely related to an ADR. The severity, causality and avoidability of each suspected ADR were subsequently evaluated by the research team. The records of the patients identified in this study as having experienced an ADR were examined in order to undertake the retrospective study described below.

For each ADR, the following information was obtained from the prospective study dataset to meet the specific objectives of this retrospective study: patient identification, suspected drug(s), ADR description (usually a symptom), ADR type, severity and causality. ADR type was defined as either Type A (augmented) resulting from an exaggeration of a drug's normal pharmacological actions or Type B (bizarre) which are novel responses that are not expected from the known pharmacological actions of the drug [10]. ADR severity was classified according to an adaptation of the Hartwig scale [11]; 1 - No change in treatment with suspected drug, 2 - Drug dosing or frequency changed, without antidote or treatment, 3 - Required treatment, or drug administration discontinued, 4 - Resulted in patient transfer to higher level of care, 5 - Caused permanent harm or significant haemodynamic instability, 6 - Directly or indirectly resulted in patient death. ADR causality was assessed using the Liverpool Causality Assessment Tool (LCAT) and the outcome could be unlikely, possible, probable or definite [12].

The electronic admission abstract for each patient identified through the earlier prospective study as having experienced at least one ADR was examined and a record was made of whether the ADR(s) and/or their signs

and symptoms had been coded using ICD-10 and if so, which code(s) had been used.

At Alder Hey, clinical coding is undertaken by a non-clinical team of trained individuals. There were two types of code relevant to ADRs: external cause codes Y40-Y59 (adverse effects in therapeutic use) for example, *'Y42 Hormones (including synthetic, antagonists)'* (Table 1) and codes including the word 'drug induced' for example: *'T88.6 Drug-induced anaphylaxis', 'E16.0 Drug induced hypoglycaemia without coma'*. Codes for drug-induced complications were listed in the relevant chapters of the ICD-10 handbook according to the system affected – for example *'E16.0 Drug induced hypoglycaemia without coma'* was listed in Chapter IV: Endocrine, nutritional and metabolic diseases [13]. We refer to all of these here as 'ICD-10 ADR codes'. A record was made of whether the ADR signs and symptoms had been coded using ICD-10 with no acknowledgment of their drug cause, for example a drug-induced rash recorded as *'D69.0 Allergic purpura'*. We refer to these as 'ICD-10 sign and symptom codes'.

A Chi-square test for difference in proportions was used to determine whether there were any differences in the characteristics of coded and uncoded ADRs.

This study used routinely collected clinical data in an anonymized format. The Chair of the Liverpool Paediatric

Table 1 ICD-10 codes which may apply to adverse drug events or adverse drug reactions

Code	Description
Y40	Systemic antibiotics
Y41	Other systemic anti-infectives/antiparasitics
Y42	Hormones (including synthetic, antagonists)
Y43	Primarily systemic agents
Y44	Agents primarily affecting blood constituents
Y45	Analgesics/antipyretics/anti-inflammatories
Y46	Antiepileptics/antiParkinsonism drugs
Y47	Sedatives, hypnotics, antianxiety drugs
Y48	Anaesthetics, therapeutic gases
Y49	Psychotropic drugs
Y50	CNS stimulants
Y51	Drugs affecting autonomic nervous system
Y52	Agents primarily affecting cardiovascular system
Y53	Agents primarily affecting gastrointestinal system
Y54	Agents affecting water/mineral balance/uric acid
Y55	Agents affecting muscle/respiratory system
Y56	Topical agents affecting skin, ENT, dental
Y57	Other and unspecified medicaments
Y58	Bacterial vaccines
Y59	Other vaccines/biologicals

Y40-Y59 external cause codes (adverse effects in in therapeutic use).

Clinical coding of prospectively identified paediatric adverse drug reactions – a retrospective review...

131

LREC informed us that this study did not require individual patient consent or review by an Ethics Committee.

Results

Of the 241 ADRs evaluated in this retrospective study, 76 (31.5%) were coded using at least one ICD-10 ADR code, two reactions had two codes (Table 2). One reaction was incorrectly coded; a skin reaction to topical dimeticone, was coded as 'Y53.1 Other antacids and anti-gastric-secretion drugs'.

A large proportion of ADRs in the prospective study [2] occurred in patients under the care of the oncologists; we refer to these as oncology ADRs and to the remaining ADRs as non-oncology. There were 126 non-oncology ADRs and 115 oncology ADRs. Of the 126 non-oncology ADRs, 6 (4.8%) were coded using an ICD-10 ADR code. Of the 115 oncology reactions, 70 (61%) were coded using an ICD-10 ADR code (difference in proportions 56%, 95% CI (46.2% to 65.8%); p < 0.001). Without exception, the code 'Y43.3 other antineoplastic drugs' was used to indicate adverse effects which had occurred secondary to the therapeutic use of oncology drugs.

The signs and symptoms of 212/241 (88%) ADRs were acknowledged by ICD-10 sign and symptom code(s). These 212 ADRs cases were made up of 107 oncology cases of which 70 also had an ADR code and 104 non-oncology cases of which 4 also had an ADR code. There were a variety of ICD-10 codes used for the same reaction type (Additional file 1: Table S1). There were 20/126 (15.9%) non-oncology ADRs and 8/115 (7.0%) oncology ADRs not acknowledged by either an ICD-10 ADR code or an ICD-10 sign and symptom code.

Considering oncology and non-oncology reactions together, coded ADRs were not more likely to be type A than type B reactions (difference in proportions 3%, 95% CI: –3.0% to 8.9%, p = 0.26). Coded ADRs were not more likely to be of severity 1, 2 and 3 than those of severity 4 and 5 (difference in proportions 6%, 95% CI –0.1% to 11.9%, p = 0.07). Finally, coded ADRs were more likely to be definite and probable ADRs than possible ADRs

(difference in proportions 47%, 95% CI 32.3% to 59.7%; p < 0.001).

Discussion

This retrospective study of electronic patient records demonstrates that the majority of ADRs detected in a prospective cohort study at a paediatric tertiary care centre would not have been identified if the study had relied on ICD-10 codes as a single means of detection. The use of ICD10 ADR codes was infrequent. The use of ICD-10 sign and symptom codes was more frequent but a wide variety of codes were used for the same ADR type. When undertaking research which uses data derived from administrative healthcare databases it is essential to first consider the reliability of those data.

The limitations of this study relate to those of the prospective cohort study in which the ADR cases were identified. The recording of a medication history for each participant relied on parents and/or patients recalling and communicating accurately all medicines administered prior to admission. Clearly there was scope for errors and omissions in this process. The detection of suspected ADRs by the study team relied on two things: a) signs and symptoms associated with the ADR being recorded by the clinical team looking after the patient; and b) the study team suspecting a link between signs and symptoms recorded and the medicines administered before admission. Where signs and symptoms were not recorded or the study team missed the link, the ADR was not highlighted and an evaluation of how it had been coded could not be undertaken.

In previous studies of ICD-10 coding for ADRs and ADEs in the adult population, the reported rate of coding was 2.0-6.8% [1,2]. Here, a higher rate of ICD-10 codes being used to record ADRs (31.5%) was found. This can be explained by the high proportion of oncology ADRs that were coded using an ICD-10 ADR code. The two main reasons for this were: a) the oncology unit was using a structured admission proforma for unplanned admissions presenting with febrile neutropenia

Table 2 ADRs coded using ICD-10 ordered by reaction frequency (n = 76, two reactions had two codes)

Description of reaction (s)	ICD –10 code	Number of reactions
ADRs secondary to chemotherapy: neutropenia, anaemia, thrombocytopenia, immunosuppression, deranged liver function tests, mouth ulcers, nausea, vomiting, diarrhoea, back pain, fever, deranged renal function	Y43.3 Other antineoplastic drugs	70
Rash secondary to penicillinVomiting secondary to penicillin	Y40.0 Penicillins	2
Hyperglycaemia secondary to dexamethasone	Y42.7 Androgens and anabolic congeners	2
Anaemia, immunosuppression, thrombocytopenia, neutropenia	Z51.2 Other chemotherapy	1
Hypoglycaemia secondary to insulin	E16.0 Drug induced hypoglycaemia without coma	1
Irritability following pneumococcal and DTP vaccines	T88.1 Other complications following immunization	1
Irritability following pneumococcal and DTP vaccines	Y59.9 Vaccine or biological substance, unspecified	1

(one of the most common ADRs in this study); this proforma was also used to record details of other drug-related problems and b) there were specifically trained, non-clinical, coding staff assigned to the oncology unit. If we consider the non-oncology ADRs only, the rate of ADR coding (4.8%) is more comparable to that in adult studies.

As a result of the system by which coding is undertaken, there are reasons why ADRs may not be coded using an ICD-10 ADR code. An ADR cannot be coded if it is not identified and subsequently recorded by the clinical team; this relies on many factors including the ability of the clinical team to identify an ADR and record it as such. It is interesting to note that ADRs which were classified as probable or definite in this study were more likely to have been coded using an appropriate ICD-10 ADR code. This suggests that a more confident causality assessment by the clinician is more likely to lead to a case-note entry which is picked up by coders.

Many ADRs which were not coded using an ICD-10 ADR code had their signs and symptoms coded (Additional file 1: Table S1). The ICD-10 sign and symptom codes for each reaction were recorded to explore whether any of these codes were commonly being used for ADR cases and if so, whether they could provide an additional means of ADR detection. However, there was inconsistency in coding. For example, amongst the non-oncology ADRs, 15 different ICD-10 codes were associated with 18 cases of immunosuppression. The diversity of sign and symptom codes used would have limited their usefulness for the detection of ADRs in our cohort of patients.

Conclusions

In summary, the use of ICD-10 codes to identify ADRs leading to admission at a paediatric tertiary care centre is not currently a reliable method of pharmacovigilance but may complement other approaches. A standardised approach to the use of administrative healthcare data for the identification of adverse drug events has the potential to improve the reliability of this method [14].

Additional file

Additional file 1: Table S1. ADRs only acknowledged by ICD 10 signs and symptom codes.

Competing interests

None of the authors have any competing interests to declare. MP chairs the Pharmacovigilance Expert Advisory Group for the MHRA and is a Commissioner on Human Medicines. AJN is a member of MHRA Paediatric Medicines Expert Advisory Group, a member of the European Medicines Agency Paediatric Committee (PDCO) and a temporary advisor to WHO.

Authors' contributions

JRB, JJK, AJN and MP conceived and designed the study, JRB collected the data, JRB and JJK analysed the data, JRB, JJK, AJN and MP wrote the paper. All authors read and approved the final manuscript.

Acknowledgements

This report presents independent research funded by the National Institute for Health Research (NIHR) under its Programme Grants for Applied Research scheme (RP-PG-0606-1170). The views expressed in this publication are those of the authors and not necessarily those of the NHS, the NIHR or the DH.

Author details

[1]Research & Development, Alder Hey Children's NHS Foundation Trust, Liverpool, UK. [2]Department of Biostatistics, University of Liverpool, Liverpool, UK. [3]Department of Women's & Child Health, University of Liverpool, Liverpool, UK. [4]Department of Molecular and Clinical Pharmacology, University of Liverpool, Liverpool, UK.

References

1. Juntti-Patinen L, Kuitunen T, Pere P, Neuvonen PJ: **Drug-related visits to a district hospital emergency room.** *Basic Clin Pharmacol Toxicol* 2006, **98**:212–217.
2. Brvar M, Fokter N, Bunc M, Mozina M: **The frequency of adverse drug reaction related admissions according to method of detection, admission urgency and medical department specialty.** *BMC ClinPharmacol* 2009, **9**(8).
3. Hohl C, Kuramoto L, Yu E, Rogula B, Stausberg J, Sobolev B: **Evaluating adverse drug event reporting in administrative data from emergency departments: a validation study.** *BMC Health Serv Res* 2013, **13**:473.
4. Schlienger RG, Oh PI, Knowles SR, Shear NH: **Quantifying the costs of serious adverse drug reactions to antiepileptic drugs.** *Epilepsia* 1998, **39**(Suppl 7):S27–S32.
5. Backstrom M, Mjorndal T, Dahlqvist R: **Under-reporting of serious adverse drug reactions in Sweden.** *Pharmacoepidemiol Drug Saf* 2004, **13**:483–487.
6. Hougland P, Xu W, Pickard S, Masheter C, Williams SD: **Performance of international classification of diseases, 9th revision, clinical modification codes as an adverse drug event surveillance system.** *Med Care* 2006, **44**:629–636.
7. Hodgkinson MR, Dirnbauer NJ, Larmour I: **Identification of adverse drug reactions using the ICD-10 Australian modification clinical coding surveillance.** *J Pharm Prac Res* 2009, **39**:19–23.
8. Batz A, Bondon-Guitton E, Durrieu G, Lapeyre-Mestre M, Petiot D, Montastruc J: **Using PMSI database to identify adverse drug reactions in a pediatric university hospital.** *Fundamental Clin Pharmacol* 2011, **25**:65.
9. Gallagher RM, Mason JR, Bird KA, Kirkham JJ, Peak M, Williamson PR, Nunn AJ, Turner MA, Pirmohamed M, Smyth RL: **Adverse drug reactions causing admission to a paediatric hospital.** *PLoS One* 2012, **7**:e50127.
10. Rawlins MD, Thompson JW: **Pathogenesis of adverse drug reactions.** In *Textbook of adverse drug reactions.* Edited by Davies DM. Oxford: Oxford University Press; 1977.
11. Hartwig SC, Siegel J, Schneider PJ: **Preventability and severity assessment in reporting adverse drug reactions.** *Am J Hosp Pharm* 1992, **49**:2229–2232.
12. Gallagher RM, Kirkham JJ, Mason JR, Bird KA, Williamson PR, Nunn AJ, Turner MA, Smyth RL, Pirmohamed M: **Development and inter-rater reliability of the Liverpool adverse drug reaction causality assessment tool.** *PLoS One* 2011, **6**:e28096.
13. International statistical classification of diseases and related health problems 10th revision. http://apps.who.int/classifications/icd10/browse/2008/en.
14. Hohl CM, Karpov A, Reddekopp L, Stausberg J: **ICD-10 codes used to identify adverse drug events in administrative data: a systematic review.** *J Am Med Inform Assoc* 2014, **21**:547–557.

14

Arylamine *N*-acetyltransferase polymorphisms in Han Chinese patients with ankylosing spondylitis and their correlation to the adverse drug reactions to sulfasalazine

Zhi-duo Hou[1], Zheng-yu Xiao[1], Yao Gong[1], Yu-ping Zhang[1] and Qing Yu Zeng[2*]

Abstract

Background: Polymorphisms of Arylamine *N*-acetyltransferase (*NAT*) that contribute to diverse susceptibilities of some autoimmune diseases are also linked to the metabolism of several drugs including sulfasalazine (SSZ). The aim of this study was to investigate the distribution of *NAT* polymorphisms in Han Chinese patients with ankylosing spondylitis (AS) and their correlation to sulfasalazine-induced adverse drug reactions (ADRs).

Methods: Arylamine *N*-acetyltransferase 1 (*NAT1*) and arylamine *N*-acetyltransferase 2 (*NAT2*) genotypes were determined in 266 AS patients who received SSZ treatment and 280 healthy controls. The correlation between *NAT* polymorphisms and SSZ-induced ADRs was analyzed.

Results: The co-occurrence frequency of *NAT2* fast acetylator genotype and *NAT1*10/NAT1*10* genotype was lower in AS patients than in controls. No positive correlations were detected between *NAT* polymorphisms and AS clinical features. The prevalence of SSZ-induced ADRs and drug withdrawal was 9.4% and 7.1%, respectively. The frequencies of overall ADRs, dose-related ADRs, and termination of drug treatment because of intolerance were higher in the *NAT2* slow acetylator genotype carriers than in the fast-type carriers and in those with co-existence of *NAT1* and *NAT2* slow acetylator genotypes. Furthermore, the ADRs emerged earlier in the AS cases carrying both *NAT1* and *NAT2* slow acetylator genotypes.

Conclusions: The prevalence of co-occurring *NAT2* fast acetylator genotype and *NAT1*10/NAT1*10* genotype was lower in AS patients than in controls. The *NAT2* slow acetylator genotype and co-existing *NAT1* and *NAT2* slow acetylator genotypes appear to be associated with higher risks of SSZ-induced ADRs.

Keywords: Arylamine *N*-acetyltransferases, Genetic polymorphism, Sulfasalazine, Ankylosing spondylitis, Adverse drug reactions

Background

Sulfasalazine (SSZ) is one of the disease-modifying anti-rheumatic drugs (DMARDs) and has been widely used for the treatment of ankylosing spondylitis (AS) in China for years [1]. Though the efficacy of SSZ in treating AS is still under debate, Chinese rheumatologists prefer to prescribe SSZ for the treatment of AS because of its good cost-effectiveness ratio. Nevertheless, the therapy is often terminated in about 14–38% of AS patients receiving SSZ treatment because of adverse drug reactions (ADRs) [2-4]. There is currently no effective method of identifying a patient's susceptibility to SSZ-induced ADRs. Thus, predicting the therapeutic response of AS patients to SSZ is of great importance for individualized therapies of AS.

SSZ is constituted by 5-aminosalicylic acid (5-ASA) and sulfapyridine (SP). SP is considered to be an active component for the therapy of AS [5], and is related to ADRs such as nausea, vomiting, and headache [6], while 5-ASA is effective for the treatment of inflammatory

* Correspondence: qyzeng@stu.edu.cn
[2]Research Unit of Rheumatology, Shantou University Medical College, No.22 Xin Ling Road, Shantou 515041, Guangdong Province, China
Full list of author information is available at the end of the article

bowel disease and is related to ADRs such as diarrhea [7]. When orally administered, SSZ is metabolized into SP and 5-ASA in the presence of the gut microbiota [8,9]. SP is almost completely absorbed and metabolized to N-acetyl-SP predominantly by hepatic arylamine N-acetyltransferase 2 (NAT2), while only about 20–30% of 5-ASA is absorbed and metabolized to N-acetyl-5-ASA by arylamine N-acetyltransferase 1 (NAT1), the rest being eliminated in the feces [9,10]. Therefore, arylamine N-acetyltransferases (NATs) play an important role in the metabolism of SP and 5-ASA.

Humans have two functional NAT genes (NAT1 and NAT2) and a pseudogene (NATP), all found on chromosome 8p22 [11]. Genetic mutations of NAT1 and NAT2 result in amino acid substitutions of their protein products, and may lead to altered gene expression and activity of the NAT enzyme [11-14]. These changes were shown to contribute to increased susceptibility to a range of disorders including autoimmune diseases [15-20] and carcinomas [21-24], but were also linked to the differences in the ability to N-acetylate certain drugs including SSZ [6,10,25-29]. In this study, we investigated the genotypes of the two human NATs in Han Chinese patients with AS versus healthy controls and also the potential correlation between NAT polymorphisms and SSZ-induced ADRs.

Methods
Subjects
Two hundred and sixty-six consecutive cases of AS from the First Affiliated Hospital of Shantou University Medical College were studied during the period of 2004–2010. All patients were diagnosed based on the Modified New York Criteria of AS [30]. All patients were treated with SSZ at a dose of 1.5–3.0 g/day (Shanghai Zhongxi Sunve Pharmaceutical Co., Ltd, China). Non-steroidal anti-inflammatory drugs were prescribed as needed. Two hundred and eighty healthy volunteers served as the healthy controls. All subjects were Han Chinese residing in Shantou, China. This study was approved by the Institutional Ethics Committee of Shantou University Medical College, and written informed consent was obtained from all participants.

Determination of NAT genetic polymorphisms
Genomic DNA was extracted from peripheral blood samples with the QIAamp Blood Kit (QIAGEN, Hilden, Germany) and stored at −80°C. Genetic polymorphisms of NAT1 (NAT1*4, NAT1*3, NAT1*10, NAT1*11) and NAT2 (NAT2*4, NAT2*5, NAT2*6, NAT2*7) were determined using the polymerase chain reaction-restriction fragment length polymorphism (PCR-RFLP) method [24,31]. The NAT genotypes of a number of samples were confirmed through direct DNA sequencing for quality control purposes. Subjects were classified as NAT1 fast acetylator

genotype carriers (those with at least one NAT1*10 allele) or NAT1 slow acetylator genotype carriers (those without NAT1*10 allele) [24]. Individuals carrying at least one wild-type allele (NAT2*4 allele) were classified as NAT2 fast acetylator genotype carrier, and those carrying the mutant allele (NAT2*5, *6, *7) were classified as NAT2 slow acetylator genotype carriers [32].

Observation of clinical features
Clinical features observed included age of onset, duration of disease, joint involvement (classified into two types: axial joint involvement only, and both axial and peripheral joint involvements), incidence of radiological hip involvement, and HLA-B27 status.

Assessment of ADRs
All patients were followed up for more than 2 years and SSZ-induced ADRs were monitored. ADRs and severe ADRs were defined according to the criteria proposed by Edwards et al. [33]. ADRs were classified into six types: dose-related (Augmented), non-dose-related (Bizarre), dose-related and time-related (Chronic), time-related (Delayed), withdrawal (End of use), and failure of therapy (Failure). The causality assessment of suspected ADRs was determined as described previously [33]. ADRs were classified as being "certain", "probable", "possible", "unlikely", "conditional", and "unassessable". All ADRs noted in this study were "certain", "probable", or "possible".

Statistical analysis
Data were analyzed using SPSS 19.0 statistical software. Departure from the Hardy–Weinberg equilibrium was tested by the chi-squared test. Frequencies of the alleles, genotypes, acetylator genotypes, and co-occurrence of NAT1 with NAT2 acetylator genotypes in each group were compared using chi-squared test or the Fisher's exact test as appropriate. Age of onset and duration of disease in each group were compared using t-test, one-way ANOVA test or Kruskal Wallis test as appropriate. Odds ratio (OR) and a 95% confidence interval (95% CI) were estimated from logistic regression models to test for associations between the risk of SSZ-induced ADRs and the NAT acetylator genotypes. Binary logistic regression analysis was used to identify the variables (NAT acetylator genotype, dose, age, sex, and NSAIDs combination) that provided an important contribution towards the variability of SSZ-induced ADRs and to adjust for confounding variables by analysis of covariates. The prevalence of drug treatment termination because of SSZ-induced ADRs in each group was compared using the chi-squared test or the Fisher's exact test as appropriate. Differences in the duration of ADRs occurring in each group were compared using the Mann–Whitney U test. $P < 0.05$ was considered statistically significant.

Results

Subject characteristics

Of the AS patients, 219 were male and 47 were female. The positive rate of HLA-B27 in patients was 90.2%. The mean age was 27.8 ± 9.1 years and the mean disease duration was 6.8 ± 5.7 years. The control group included 221 male and 59 female healthy volunteers with a mean age of 35.1 ± 10.0 years.

NAT polymorphisms in AS patients and healthy controls

The distribution of NAT1 and NAT2 gene polymorphisms in AS patients and healthy controls is shown in Table 1. The allele frequencies of both AS patients and healthy controls were consistent with the Hardy–Weinberg equilibrium ($P > 0.05$). No significant differences between the AS and control group were found for the distribution of alleles, genotypes, and acetylator genotypes when NAT1 and NAT2 polymorphisms were analyzed independently. However, the co-occurrence frequency of the NAT2 fast acetylator genotype and NAT1*10/NAT1*10 genotype was lower in AS patients than in controls (6.4% vs 11.4%, $P = 0.04$, OR = 0.53, 95% CI 0.29–0.98).

Correlations between NAT polymorphisms and clinical features of AS

The age of onset, duration of disease, joint involvement types, incidence of radiological hip involvement, and the positive rate of HLA-B27 were not significantly different in each NAT genotype or NAT acetylator genotype group among the AS patients ($P > 0.05$).

SSZ-induced ADRs

SSZ-induced ADRs occurred in 25 cases (9.4%) of AS (Table 2). Among these, 16 patients (64.0%) experienced dose-related ADRs; eight patients (32.0%) experienced non-dose-related ADRs, and one patient (4.0%) experienced time-related ADR. The dose-related ADRs observed in this study included nausea, anorexia, abdominal pain, diarrhea, epigastric discomfort, dizziness, elevation of serum liver enzyme levels, and chest congestion. Non-dose-related ADRs included rash, oral ulcer, and leukopenia. One patient with cacospermia was classified as having time-related ADR. No serious ADRs were found in the AS group of patients. SSZ therapy was terminated because of SSZ-induced ADRs in 19 AS patients (7.1%). Of these, 10 patients (52.6%) withdrew from SSZ therapy because of dose-related ADRs; eight patients (42.1%) because of non-dose-related ADRs, and one patient (5.3%) because of time-related ADR. The mean duration of SSZ therapy from the time when the first ADR occurred was 19 days (range 3–450 days). Most ADRs occurred within 12 weeks after the start of SSZ treatment (23 cases, 92.0%).

Correlations of NAT polymorphisms and SSZ-induced ADRs

Correlations between NAT acetylator genotypes and SSZ-induced ADRs are shown in Table 3. The incidence of overall ADRs in patients carrying the NAT2 slow acetylator genotype was 18.5% (10/54) and was significantly higher than patients carrying the NAT2 fast acetylator genotype (7.1%, 15/212, $P = 0.013$, OR = 2.99, 95% CI 1.26–7.09). The incidence of dose-related ADRs in patients carrying the NAT2 slow acetylator genotype was also higher than in patients carrying the fast acetylator genotype (16.7% vs 3.3%, $P = 0.002$, OR = 5.17, 95% CI 1.79–14.92). No significant difference in the incidence of non-dose-related ADRs was found between the NAT2 fast and NAT2 slow acetylator genotype groups (3.3% vs 1.9%, $P > 0.05$). The prevalence of drug treatment termination owing to ADRs or dose-related ADRs was higher in the NAT2 slow acetylator genotype carriers than in the fast-type carriers (14.8% vs 5.2%, $P = 0.032$ and 13.0% vs 1.4%, $P = 0.001$, respectively).

The incidences of overall ADRs, dose-related ADRs, and non-dose-related ADRs in patients carrying the NAT1 fast acetylator genotype were 8.1% (11/136), 4.4% (6/136), and 3.7% (5/136) respectively, similar to 10.8% (14/130), 7.7% (10/130), and 2.3% (3/130) in patients carrying the NAT1 slow acetylator genotype ($P > 0.05$). The prevalence of drug treatment termination owing to overall ADRs or dose-related ADRs was slightly higher in the NAT1 slow acetylator genotype carriers than in the fast-type carriers (8.5% vs 5.9%, and 5.4% vs 2.2%, respectively). However, the difference was not significant ($P > 0.05$).

The incidences of both overall ADRs and dose-related ADRs were higher in patients carrying both the NAT1 slow acetylator genotype and the NAT2 slow acetylator genotype than in the other carriers (26.3% vs 6.6%, $P < 0.001$, OR = 5.07, 95% CI 2.08–12.37 and 23.7% vs 3.1%, $P < 0.001$, OR = 9.52, 95% CI 3.20–28.30). The prevalence of drug treatment termination owing to overall ADRs or dose-related ADRs was also higher in the carriers of both NAT1 slow acetylator genotype and NAT2 slow acetylator genotype than in the other carriers (21.1% vs 4.8%, $P = 0.002$ and 18.4% vs 1.3%, $P < 0.001$, respectively). The mean duration of SSZ treatment when the first ADR occurred in patients carrying both the NAT1 slow acetylator genotype and the NAT2 slow acetylator genotypes was 8 days (range 3–128 days), shorter than that of 33 days (range 10–450 days) in the carriers of other acetylator genotypes ($P = 0.003$). No significant differences in the frequencies of non-dose-related ADRs were found among carriers of any NAT1 and NAT2 acetylator genotype combinations ($P > 0.05$).

Only one patient was identified that experienced time-related ADR and carried NAT1 slow acetylator (NAT1*3/NAT1*3) and NAT2 fast acetylator (NAT2*4/NAT2*6) genotypes.

Table 1 Distribution of *NAT* polymorphisms in AS patients and healthy controls

Alleles/Genotypes/Acetylator genotypes		AS		HC		χ^2	P
		N	%	N	%		
NAT1 Alleles	*NAT1*4*	268	50.4	261	46.6	1.55	0.21
	*NAT1*3*	101	19.0	108	19.3	0.02	0.90
	*NAT1*10*	159	29.9	188	33.6	1.71	0.19
	*NAT1*11*	4	0.7	3	0.5	-	0.72*
	Total	532		560			
NAT1 Genotypes	*NAT1*4/NAT1*4*	75	28.2	65	23.2	1.78	0.18
	*NAT1*4/NAT1*3*	39	14.7	48	17.1	0.63	0.43
	*NAT1*4/NAT1*10*	77	28.9	80	28.6	0.01	0.92
	*NAT1*4/NAT1*11*	2	0.8	3	1.1	-	1.00*
	*NAT1*3/NAT1*3*	14	5.2	14	5.0	0.02	0.89
	*NAT1*3/NAT1*10*	34	12.8	32	11.4	0.24	0.63
	*NAT1*3/ NAT1*11*	0	0	0	0	-	-
	*NAT1*10/NAT1*10*	23	8.6	38	13.6	3.33	0.07
	*NAT1*10/NAT1*11*	2	0.8	0	0	-	-
	*NAT1*11/NAT1*11*	0	0	0	0	-	-
	Total	266		280			
NAT1 Acetylator Genotypes	Fast	136	51.1	150	53.6	0.33	0.57
	Slow	130	48.9	130	46.4		
	Total	266		280			
NAT2 Alleles	*NAT2*4*	310	58.3	340	60.7	0.68	0.41
	*NAT2*5*	18	3.4	18	3.2	0.02	0.88
	*NAT2*6*	134	25.2	129	23.0	0.69	0.41
	*NAT2*7*	70	13.1	73	13.1	0.00	0.95
	Total	532		560			
NAT2 Genotypes	*NAT2*4/NAT2*4*	98	36.8	110	39.3	0.35	0.56
	*NAT2*4/NAT2*5*	9	3.4	10	3.6	0.01	0.91
	*NAT2*4/NAT2*6*	70	26.3	71	25.4	0.07	0.80
	*NAT2*4/NAT2*7*	35	13.2	39	13.9	0.07	0.79
	*NAT2*5/NAT2*5*	0	0	1	0.4	-	-
	*NAT2*5/NAT2*6*	6	2.3	2	0.7	-	0.17*
	*NAT2*5/NAT2*7*	3	1.1	4	1.4	-	1.00*
	*NAT2*6/NAT2*6*	18	6.8	18	6.4	0.03	0.87
	*NAT2*6/NAT2*7*	22	8.2	20	7.1	0.24	0.62
	*NAT2*7/NAT2*7*	5	1.9	5	1.8	-	1.00*
	Total	266		280			
NAT2 Acetylator Genotypes	Fast	212	79.7	230	82.1	0.53	0.47
	Slow	54	20.3	50	17.9		
	Total	266		280			
NAT2 fast acetylator genotype plus *NAT1*10/NAT1*10*		17	6.4	32	11.4	4.24	0.04

*Results of Fisher's exact test; AS = Ankylosing Spondylitis; HC = healthy control; *NAT1* = Arylamine *N*-acetyltransferases 1; *NAT2* = Arylamine *N*-acetyltransferases 2; N = Number; χ^2 = Chi-squared test.

Table 2 Clinical features and *NAT* polymorphisms in 25 AS patients who experienced SSZ-induced ADRs

ADR types*	Cases	SSZ Dose (g/day)	ADR	Termination of Drug therapy	NAT2		NAT1	
					Genotypes	Acetylatorgenotypes	Genotypes	Acetylatorgenotypes
Dose-related	Case 1	3.0	Nausea	No	NAT2*4/NAT2*7	Fast	NAT1*10/NAT1*10	Fast
	Case 2	3.0	Nausea, anorexia	No	NAT2*4/NAT2*5	Fast	NAT1*3/NAT1*10	Fast
	Case 3	1.5	Abdominal pain	Yes	NAT2*4/NAT2*6	Fast	NAT1*4/NAT1*10	Fast
	Case 4	3.0	Diarrhea	Yes	NAT2*7/NAT2*7	Slow	NAT1*4/NAT1*4	Slow
	Case 5	3.0	Diarrhea	No	NAT2*5/NAT2*7	Slow	NAT1*4/NAT1*4	Slow
	Case 6	3.0	Epigastric discomfort	No	NAT2*4/NAT2*4	Fast	NAT1*4/NAT1*10	Fast
	Case 7	1.5	Epigastric discomfort	Yes	NAT2*4/NAT2*7	Fast	NAT1*4/NAT1*10	Fast
	Case 8	1.5	Increase in transaminases	Yes	NAT2*6/NAT2*7	Slow	NAT1*4/NAT1*4	Slow
	Case 9#	2.25	Increase in transaminases	Yes	NAT2*6/NAT2*7	Slow	NAT1*4/NAT1*3	Slow
	Case 10	2.25	Dizziness	No	NAT2*6/NAT2*7	Slow	NAT1*3/NAT1*3	Slow
	Case 11	1.5	Dizziness	Yes	NAT2*6/NAT2*6	Slow	NAT1*4/NAT1*4	Slow
	Case 12	1.5	Dizziness	Yes	NAT2*5/NAT2*6	Slow	NAT1*4/NAT1*4	Slow
	Case 13	1.5	Dizziness	Yes	NAT2*4/NAT2*7	Fast	NAT1*10/NAT1*10	Fast
	Case 14	1.5	Dizziness	Yes	NAT2*6/NAT2*6	Slow	NAT1*4/NAT1*4	Slow
	Case 15	3.0	Dizziness	No	NAT2*4/NAT2*4	Fast	NAT1*4/NAT1*4	Slow
	Case 16	1.5	Chest congestion	Yes	NAT2*5/NAT2*6	Slow	NAT1*4/NAT1*3	Slow
Non-dose-related	Case 17	2.25	Leukopenia	Yes	NAT2*4/NAT2*6	Fast	NAT1*4/NAT1*4	Slow
	Case 18	1.5	Rash	Yes	NAT2*6/NAT2*6	Slow	NAT1*4/NAT1*4	Slow
	Case 19	1.5	Rash	Yes	NAT2*4/NAT2*6	Fast	NAT1*3/NAT1*10	Fast
	Case 20	1.5	Rash	Yes	NAT2*4/NAT2*6	Fast	NAT1*4/NAT1*11	Slow
	Case 21	3.0	Rash	Yes	NAT2*4/NAT2*4	Fast	NAT1*4/NAT1*10	Fast
	Case 22	3.0	Rash	Yes	NAT2*4/NAT2*4	Fast	NAT1*3/NAT1*10	Fast
	Case 23	2.25	Oral ulcer	Yes	NAT2*4/NAT2*4	Fast	NAT1*10/NAT1*10	Fast
	Case 24	2.25	Oral ulcer	Yes	NAT2*4/NAT2*4	Fast	NAT1*4/NAT1*10	Fast
Time-related	Case 25#	2.25	Cacospermia	Yes	NAT2*4/NAT2*6	Fast	NAT1*3/NAT1*3	Slow

*ADRs were classified into six types: dose-related, non-dose-related, dose-related and time-related, time-related, withdrawal (End of use), and failure of therapy; #Case 9 was observed to have elevated serum liver enzyme levels at day 138 and case 25 had cacospermia at day 450 after the start of SSZ treatment; ADRs = Adverse Drug Reactions; NAT1 = Arylamine N-acetyltransferases 1; NAT2 = Arylamine N-acetyltransferases 2; SSZ = Sulfasalazine.

Discussion

This study showed that the *NAT* genotype appeared not to correlate with the development of AS or the clinical features of AS such as age of onset, duration of disease, joint involvements, incidence of radiological hip involvement, or positive status of HLA-B27. However, the frequency of co-occurrence of the *NAT2* fast acetylator genotype and the *NAT1*10/NAT1*10* genotype was significantly lower in AS patients than in healthy controls ($P = 0.04$, OR = 0.53, 95% CI 0.29–0.98). This suggests that the co-occurrence of the *NAT2* fast acetylator genotype and the *NAT1*10/NAT1*10* genotype is likely to reduce

one-half the risk of AS in the Chinese Han population. It was reported that partial linkage disequilibrium exists between the *NAT1*10* allele and the *NAT2* fast acetylation genotype, and a reduced risk for bladder cancer was identified in carriers of these co-existing genotypes [34]. Because the sample size of our study was relatively small, further investigation should be conducted to reveal the biological significance of the partial linkage disequilibrium between the *NAT1*10* allele and the *NAT2* fast acetylation genotype in the development of AS.

In the current study, the most common SSZ-induced ADR were gastrointestinal reactions (nausea and diarrhea),

Table 3 Associations between *NAT* acetylator genotypes and SSZ-induced ADRs

	NAT2 acetylator genotype		NAT1 acetylator genotype		Co-existence of NAT1 and NAT2 acetylator genotypes	
	Fast	Slow	Fast	Slow	NAT1 slow plus NAT2 slow	Non NAT1 slow plus NAT2 slow
Total ADRs	7.1%(15/212)	18.5%(10/54)	8.1%(11/136)	10.8%(14/130)	26.3%(10/38)	6.6%(15/228)
P*	0.013		0.45		<0.001	
OR*	2.99				5.07	
95% CI*	1.26-7.09				2.08-12.37	
Drug therapy termination rate due to ADRs	5.2%(11/212)	14.8%(8/54)	5.9%(8/136)	8.5%(11/130)	21.1%(8/38)	4.8%(11/228)
P	0.032#		0.41		0.002#	
Dose-related ADR	3.3%(7/212)	16.7%(9/54)	4.4%(6/136)	7.7%(10/130)	23.7%(9/38)	3.1%(7/228)
P*	0.002		0.27		<0.001	
OR*	5.17				9.52	
95% CI*	1.79-14.92				3.20-28.30	
Drug therapy termination rate due to dose-related ADRs	1.4%(3/212)	13.0%(7/54)	2.2%(3/136)	5.4%(7/130)	18.4%(7/38)	1.3%(3/228)
P	0.001#		0.21#		<0.001#	
Non-dose-related ADR	3.3%(7/212)	1.8%(1/54)	3.7%(5/136)	2.3%(3/130)	2.6%(1/38)	3.1%(7/228)
P*	0.58		0.51		0.88	

*Results of binary logistic regression analysis after adjusting for dose, age, sex, and NSAIDs combination; #Results of Fisher's exact test; OR = odds ratio; CI = confidence interval; ADRs = Adverse Drug Reactions; *NAT1* = Arylamine *N*-acetyltransferases 1; *NAT2* = Arylamine *N*-acetyltransferases 2; SSZ = Sulfasalazine.

followed by rash, dizziness, and elevated levels of serum liver transaminases. Hematological disturbances (leukopenia) and cacospermia were rarely seen. These characteristics were similar to those reported in previous studies [9,35]. It was also reported that most SSZ-induced ADRs occurred within the first 12 weeks of SSZ treatment [36]. In our study, most ADRs (92%) also occurred within the first 12 weeks. However, one patient (case 9) was observed to have elevated serum liver enzyme levels at day 138 and another patient (case 25) had cacospermia at day 450 after the start of SSZ treatment. This indicates it is important to monitor the ADRs during the first 12 weeks of SSZ treatment. However, liver function tests need to be carried out beyond 12 weeks. Morphological examination and motility tests for sperm are also important for male patients.

The association between single nucleotide polymorphisms (SNPs) and *NAT* expression has been described in previous reports [11-14]. For example, 341 T > C (I114T) and 590G > A (R197Q) reduce NAT2 catalytic activities, whereas 481C > T (L161L) do not. *NAT* polymorphisms linked to the differences in the ability to *N*-acetylate SSZ have been identified [6,10,25-29]. However, it is still not clear whether the genetic variants of *NAT1* and *NAT2* underlie the patients' response to SSZ. Previous studies identified a strong association between *NAT2* polymorphisms and SSZ-induced ADRs [20,31,37-39] and this association was thought to have an effect on the efficacy of SSZ [26,39]. However, others suggested that *NAT1* and

NAT2 polymorphisms played no roles in predicting responses to SSZ or related toxicities [40,41]. In our study, the frequencies of overall ADRs and dose-related ADRs of SSZ were higher in the *NAT2* slow acetylation genotype group than in the *NAT2* fast-type group. The ORs were 2.99 (95% CI 1.26–7.09) and 5.17 (95% CI 1.79–14.92), respectively, indicating that the *NAT2* slow acetylator genotype may be a risk factor for ADRs, especially the dose-related ADRs of SSZ. In addition, the prevalence of SSZ treatment terminations owing to overall ADRs or dose-related ADRs was also higher in the *NAT2* slow acetylator genotype carriers as compared with that in the *NAT2* fast-type carriers (14.8% vs 5.2%, P = 0.032 and 13.0% vs 1.4%, P = 0.001). In our study, non-dose-related ADRs only occurred in one patient carrying the *NAT2* slow acetylator genotype. Therefore, it is difficult to evaluate the contribution of the *NAT2* acetylation genotype to non-dose-related ADRs of SSZ.

The NAT1 function is also widely variable in human populations, although the effects of its genetic polymorphisms are not generally as marked as those of NAT2 [12,13,42]. The current study provided little evidence of correlation between *NAT1* acetylator genotypes and the risk of SSZ-induced ADRs by *NAT1* single-gene analysis. However, the co-existence of the *NAT1* slow acetylator genotype and the *NAT2* slow acetylator genotype conferred a 5-fold greater risk for overall ADRs, and a 9-fold greater risk for dose-related ADRs as compared with other acetylator genotype carriers. The termination of SSZ treatment owing to overall ADRs or dose-related ADRs was more commonly seen in AS patients carrying the NAT1 slow and NAT2 slow acetylator genotypes. Additionally, the onset of ADRs was earlier in patients with co-existing the NAT1 slow and NAT2 slow acetylator genotypes than that for other acetylator genotype carriers (8 vs 33 days, P = 0.003). These findings allow the identification of patients at a possible risk of SSZ-induced ADRs or subsequent terminations of SSZ treatment. It is also important to note that a multi-gene analysis approach is still worthwhile in pharmacogenetic studies even if no positive correlations are found via a single gene analysis.

Similar to the findings of other studies involving Asians such as Chinese and Japanese populations [19,43], our results showed the prevalence of the NAT2 slow acetylator genotype was 20.3% in Han Chinese patients with AS, which is significantly lower than that reported for Western populations (40–70%) [13]. This might explain why SSZ-induced ADRs are much less prevalent among the Chinese (9.4% in our study population) and the Japanese (11.1%) [37] as compared with Western populations (22.7-53.5%) [2,9,35,40]. However, the statistical power is relatively low because of the low frequency of the NAT2 slow acetylator genotype in our study population. It is a challenge to evaluate correlations between NAT polymorphisms and SSZ-induced ADRs without bias. Thus, studies of multiethnicity and larger populations are required.

Conclusions

The co-occurrence of the NAT2 fast acetylator genotype and the NAT1*10/NAT1*10 genotype is less frequent in AS patients compared with healthy controls in the Han Chinese population. The NAT2 slow acetylator genotype and co-existing NAT1 and NAT2 slow acetylator genotypes appear to be associated with higher risks of SSZ-induced ADRs.

Abbreviations
NAT: Arylamine N-acetyltransferases; NAT1: Arylamine N-acetyltransferases 1; NAT2: Arylamine N-acetyltransferases 2; AS: Ankylosing Spondylitis; ADRs: Adverse Drug Reactions; SSZ: Sulfasalazine; DMARDs: Disease-Modifying Antirheumatic Drugs; OR: Odds Ratio; CI: Confidence Interval.

Competing interests
The authors declare that they have no competing interests.

Authors' contributions
QYZ conceived the study. QYZ, ZDH, and ZYX designed the study. QYZ, ZDH, ZYX, YG, and YPZ collected data and performed data analysis. ZDH drafted the manuscript. All authors read and approved the final manuscript.

Acknowledgments
This study was supported primarily by a grant from the Department of Science and Technology of Guangdong Province (No. 2004B33701014) and Shantou University Medical College (No. LC0401). The funders had no role in study design, data collection and analysis, decision to publish, or preparation of the manuscript.

Author details
[1]Department of Rheumatology, the First Affiliated Hospital of Shantou University Medical College, No.57 Chang Ping Road, Shantou 515041, Guangdong Province, China. [2]Research Unit of Rheumatology, Shantou University Medical College, No.22 Xin Ling Road, Shantou 515041, Guangdong Province, China.

References
1.   Zeng QY: Ankylosing spondylitis in Shantou, China: 15 years' clinical experience. J Rheumatol 2003, 30(8):1816–1821.
2.   Dougados M, Maetzel A, Mijiyawa M, Amor B: Evaluation of sulphasalazine in the treatment of spondyloarthropathies. Ann Rheum Dis 1992, 51(8):955–958.
3.   Clegg DO, Reda DJ, Abdellatif M: Comparison of sulfasalazine and placebo for the treatment of axial and peripheral articular manifestations of the seronegative spondylarthropathies: a Department of Veterans Affairs cooperative study. Arthritis Rheum 1999, 42(11):2325–2329.
4.   Schmidt WA, Wierth S, Milleck D, Droste U, Gromnica-Ihle E: Sulfasalazine in ankylosing spondylitis: a prospective, randomized, double-blind placebo-controlled study and comparison with other controlled studies. Z Rheumatol 2002, 61(2):159–167.
5.   Taggart AGP, McEvoy FHR, Bird H: Which is the active moiety of sulfasalazine in ankylosing spondylitis? A randomized, controlled study. Arthritis Rheum 1996, 39(8):1400–1405.
6.   Tanigawara Y, Kita T, Aoyama N, Gobara M, Komada F, Sakai T, Kasuga M, Hatanaka H, Sakaeda T, Okumura K: N-acetyltransferase 2 genotype-related sulfapyridine acetylation and its adverse events. Biol Pharm Bull 2002, 25(8):1058–1062.
7.   Moum B: Which are the 5-ASA compound side effects and how is it possible to avoid them. Inflamm Bowel Dis 2008, 14(Suppl 2):S212–S213.
8.   Klotz U: Clinical pharmacokinetics of sulphasalazine, its metabolites and other prodrugsof 5-aminosalicylic acid. Clin Pharmacokinet 1985, 10(4):285–302.
9.   Plosker GL, Croom KF: Sulfasalazine: a review of its use in the management of rheumatoid arthritis. Drugs 2005, 65(13):1825–1849.
10. Kuhn UD, Anschutz M, Schmucker K, Schug BS, Hippius M, Blume HH: Phenotyping with sulfasalazine - time dependence and relation to NAT2 pharmacogenetics. Int J Clin Pharmacol Ther 2010, 48(1):1–10.
11. Vatsis KP, Weber WW, Bell DA, Dupret JM, Evans DA, Grant DM, Hein DW, Lin HJ, Meyer UA, Relling MV, Sim E, Suzuki T, Yamazoe Y: Nomenclature for N-acetyltransferases. Pharmacogenetics 1995, 5(1):1–17.
12. Walker K, Ginsberg G, Hattis D, Johns DO, Guyton KZ, Sonawane B: Genetic polymorphism in N-Acetyltransferase (NAT): Population distribution of NAT1 and NAT2 activity. J Toxicol Environ Health B Crit Rev 2009, 12(5–6):440–472.
13. Meyer UA, Zanger UM: Molecular mechanisms of genetic polymorphisms of drug metabolism. Annu Rev Pharmacol Toxicol 1997, 37:269–296.
14. Hein DW: N-acetyltransferase SNPs: emerging concepts serve as a paradigm for understandingcomplexities of personalized medicine. Expert Opin Drug Metab Toxicol 2009, 5(4):353–366.
15. Pawlik A, Ostanek L, Brzosko I, Gawroska-Szklarz B, Brzosko M, Dabrowska-Zamojcin E: Increased genotype frequency of N-acetyltransferase 2 slow acetylation inpatients with rheumatoid arthritis. Clin Pharmacol Ther 2002, 72(3):319–325.
16. Baranska M, Trzcinski R, Dziki A, Rychlik-Sych M, Dudarewicz M, Skretkowicz J: The role of N-acetyltransferase 2 polymorphism in the etiopathogenesis of inflammatory bowel disease. Dig Dis Sci 2011, 56(7):2073–2080.
17. Mikuls TR, Levan T, Gould KA, Yu F, Thiele GM, Bynote KK, Conn D, Jonas BL, Callahan LF, Smith E, Brasington R, Moreland LW, Reynolds R, Gaffo A, Bridges SL Jr: Interactions of cigarette smoking with NAT2 polymorphisms on rheumatoid arthritis risk in African Americans. Arthritis Rheum 2012, 64(3):655–664.
18. Tamer L, Tursen U, Eskandari G, Ates NA, Ercan B, Yildirim H, Atik U: N-acetyltransferase 2 polymorphisms in patients with Behcet's disease. Clin Exp Dermatol 2005, 30(1):56–60.
19. Kiyohara C, Washio M, Horiuchi T, Tada Y, Asami T, Ide S, Takahashi H, Kobashi G, Kyushu Sapporo SLE (KYSS) Study Group: Cigarette smoking, N-acetyltransferase 2 polymorphisms and systemic lupuserythematosus in a Japanese population. Lupus 2009, 18(7):630–638.

20. Gunnarsson I, Kanerud L, Pettersson E, Lundberg I, Lindblad S, Ringertz B: Predisposing factors in sulphasalazine-induced systemic lupus erythematosus. *Br J Rheumatol* 1997, **36**(10):1089–1094.

21. García-Closas M, Malats N, Silverman D, Dosemeci M, Kogevinas M, Hein DW, Tardón A, Serra C, Carrato A, García-Closas R, Lloreta J, Castaño-Vinyals G, Yeager M, Welch R, Chanock S, Chatterjee N, Wacholder S, Samanic C, Torà M, Fernández F, Real FX, Rothman N: NAT2 slow acetylation, GSTM1 null genotype, and risk of bladder cancer: results from the Spanish Bladder Cancer Study and meta-analyses. *Lancet* 2005, **366**(9486):649–659.

22. Zhang J, Qiu LX, Wang ZH, Wang JL, He SS, Hu XC: NAT2 polymorphisms combining with smoking associated with breast cancer susceptibility: a meta-analysis. *Breast Cancer Res Treat* 2010, **123**(3):877–883.

23. Butcher NJ, Minchin RF: Arylamine N-acetyltransferase 1: a novel drug target in cancer development. *Pharmacol Rev* 2012, **64**(1):147–165.

24. Bell DA, Stephens EA, Castranio T, Umbach DM, Watson M, Deakin M, Elder J, Hendrickse C, Duncan H, Strange RC: Polyadenylation polymorphism in the acetyltransferase 1 gene (NAT1) increases risk of colorectal cancer. *Cancer Res* 1995, **55**(16):3537–3542.

25. Kita T, Sakaeda T, Adachi S, Sakai T, Aoyama N, Hatanaka H, Kasuga M, Okumura K: N-Acetyltransferase 2 genotype correlates with sulfasalazine pharmacokinetics after multiple dosing in healthy Japanese subjects. *Biol Pharm Bull* 2001, **24**(10):1176–1180.

26. Kumagai S, Komada F, Kita T, Morinobu A, Ozaki S, Ishida H, Sano H, Matsubara T, Okumura K: N-Acetyltransferase 2 Genotype-Related Efficacy of Sulfasalazine in patients with Rheumatoid Arthritis. *Pharm Res* 2004, **21**(2):324–329.

27. Chen B, Zhang WX, Cai WM: The influence of various genotypes on the metabolic activity of NAT2 in a Chinese population. *Eur J Clin Pharmacol* 2006, **62**(5):355–359.

28. Ma JJ, Liu CG, Li JH, Cao XM, Sun SL, Yao X: Effects of NAT2 polymorphism on SASP pharmacokinetics in Chinese population. *Clin Chim Acta* 2009, **407**(1–2):30–35.

29. Daly AK: Pharmacogenomics of adverse drug reactions. *Genome Med* 2013, **5**(1):5.

30. van der Linden S, Valkenburg HA, Cats A: Evaluation of diagnostic criteria for ankylosing spondylitis. A proposal for modification of the New York criteria. *Arthritis Rheum* 1984, **27**(4):361–368.

31. Chen M, Xia B, Chen B, Guo Q, Li J, Ye M, Hu Z: N-acetyltransferase 2 slow acetylator genotype associated with adverse effects of sulphasalazine in the treatment of inflammatory bowel disease. *Can J Gastroenterol* 2007, **21**(3):155–158.

32. Tanaka E, Taniguchi A, Urano W, Yamanaka H, Kamatani N: Pharmacogenetics of disease-modifying anti-rheumatic drugs. *Best Pract Res Clin Rheumatol* 2004, **18**(2):233–247.

33. Edwards IR, Aronson JK: Adverse drug reactions: definitions, diagnosis, and management. *Lancet* 2000, **356**(9237):1255–1259.

34. Cascorbi I, Roots I, Brockmoller J: Association of NAT1 and NAT2 polymorphisms to urinary bladder cancer: significantly reduced risk in subjects with NAT1*10. *Cancer Res* 2001, **61**(13):5051–5056.

35. Braun J, van der Horst-Bruinsma IE, Huang F, Burgos-Vargas R, Vlahos B, Koenig AS, Freundlich B: Clinical efficacy and safety of etanercept versus sulfasalazine in patients with ankylosing spondylitis: a randomized, double-blind trial. *Arthritis Rheum* 2011, **63**(6):1543–1551.

36. Amos RS, Pullar T, Bax DE, Situnayake D, Capell HA, McConkey B: Sulphasalazine for rheumatoid arthritis: toxicity in 774 patients monitored for one to 11 years. *Br Med J (Clin Res Ed)* 1986, **293**(6544):420–423.

37. Tanaka E, Taniguchi A, Urano W, Nakajima H, Matsuda Y, Kitamura Y, Saito M, Yamanaka H, Saito T, Kamatani N: Adverse effects of sulfasalazine in patients with rheumatoid arthritis are associated with diplotype configuration at the N-acetyltransferase 2 gene. *J Rheumatol* 2002, **29**(12):2492–2499.

38. Soejima M, Kawaguchi Y, Hara M, Kamatani N: Prospective study of the association between NAT2 gene haplotypes and severe adverse events with sulfasalazine therapy in patients with rheumatoid arthritis. *J Rheumatol* 2008, **35**(4):724.

39. Sabbagh N, Delaporte E, Marez D, Lo-Guidice JM, Piette F, Broly F: NAT2 genotyping and efficacy of sulfasalazine in patients with chronic discoidlupus erythematosus. *Pharmacogenetics* 1997, **7**(2):131–135.

40. Ricart E, Taylor WR, Loftus EV, O'Kane D, Weinshilboum RM, Tremaine WJ, Harmsen WS, Zinsmeister AR, Sandborn WJ: N-acetyltransferase 1 and 2 genotypes do not predict response or toxicity to treatment with mesalamine and sulfasalazine in patients with ulcerative colitis. *Am J Gastroenterol* 2002, **97**(7):1763–1768.

41. Kitas GD, Farr M, Waterhouse L, Bacon PA: Influence of acetylator status on sulphasalazine efficacy and toxicity inpatients with rheumatoid arthritis. *Scand J Rheumatol* 1992, **21**(5):220–225.

42. Wang D, Para MF, Koletar SL, Sadee W: Human N-acetyltransferase 1 *10 and *11 alleles increase protein expression through distinct mechanisms and associate with sulfamethoxazole-induced hypersensitivity. *Pharmacogenet Genomics* 2011, **21**(10):652–664.

43. Xie HG, Xu ZH, Ou-Yang DS, Shu Y, Yang DL, Wang JS, Yan XD, Huang SL, Wang W, Zhou HH: Meta-analysis of phenotype and genotype of NAT2 deficiency in Chinese populations. *Pharmacogenetics* 1997, **7**(6):503–514.

15

Effect of airway acidosis and alkalosis on airway vascular smooth muscle responsiveness to albuterol

Jose E Cancado[1†], Eliana S Mendes[1*†], Johana Arana[1], Gabor Horvath[2], Maria E Monzon[1], Matthias Salathe[1†] and Adam Wanner[1†]

Abstract

Background: *In vitro* and animal experiments have shown that the transport and signaling of β_2-adrenergic agonists are pH-sensitive. Inhaled albuterol, a hydrophilic β_2-adrenergic agonist, is widely used for the treatment of obstructive airway diseases. Acute exacerbations of obstructive airway diseases can be associated with changes in ventilation leading to either respiratory acidosis or alkalosis thereby affecting albuterol responsiveness in the airway. The purpose of this study was to determine if airway pH has an effect on albuterol-induced vasodilation in the airway.

Methods: Ten healthy volunteers performed the following respiratory maneuvers: quiet breathing, hypocapnic hyperventilation, hypercapnic hyperventilation, and eucapnic hyperventilation (to dissociate the effect of pH from the effect of ventilation). During these breathing maneuvers, exhaled breath condensate (EBC) pH and airway blood flow response to inhaled albuterol ($\Delta\dot{Q}_{aw}$) were assessed.

Results: Mean ± SE EBC pH (units) and $\Delta\dot{Q}_{aw}$ ($\mu l.min^{-1}.mL^{-1}$) were 6.4 ± 0.1 and 16.8 ± 1.9 during quiet breathing, 6.3 ± 0.1 and 14.5 ± 2.4 during eucapnic hyperventilation, 6.6 ± 0.2 and -0.2 ± 1.8 during hypocapnic hyperventilation ($p = 0.02$ and <0.01 vs. quiet breathing), and 5.9 ± 0.1 and 2.0 ± 1.5 during hypercapnic hyperventilation ($p = 0.02$ and <0.02 vs quiet breathing).

Conclusions: Albuterol responsiveness in the airway as assessed by $\Delta\dot{Q}_{aw}$ is pH sensitive. The breathing maneuver associated with decreased and increased EBC pH both resulted in a decreased responsiveness independent of the level of ventilation. These findings suggest an attenuated response to hydrophilic β_2-adrenergic agonists during airway disease exacerbations associated with changes in pH.

Trial registration: Registered at clinicaltrials.gov: NCT01216748.

Keywords: Airway surface liquid pH, Airway blood flow, Respiratory alkalosis, Respiratory acidosis, Albuterol

Background

In vitro and animal experiments have shown that transport of and signaling by β_2-adrenergic agonist are pH-sensitive. At acidic pH, the transport of β_2-adrenergic agonists across the airway epithelium is decreased [1], β_2-adrenergic receptor function is impaired [2,3], endothelial function is diminished [4-6], and systemic vascular smooth muscle tone is increased [7]. Conversely, epithelial β_2-adrenergic agonist transport is increased at alkaline pH [1]. The effects of alkalosis on β_2-adrenergic receptor function, endothelial function and systemic vascular smooth muscle tone are less clear, with studies showing minimal or no changes in β_2-adrenergic signaling [5], but an increase in vascular smooth muscle tone [7].

Inhaled albuterol, a hydrophilic β_2-adrenergic agonist, is widely used for the treatment of obstructive airway disease. Acute exacerbations of obstructive airway diseases can be associated with changes in ventilation leading to either respiratory acidosis or alkalosis. The

---

* Correspondence: emendes@med.miami.edu

†Equal contributors

[1]Division of Pulmonary, Allergy, Critical Care and Sleep Medicine, University of Miami School of Medicine, Miami, FL 33136, USA

Full list of author information is available at the end of the article

resulting changes in airway pH could have an effect on albuterol responsiveness. We therefore sought to test the hypothesis that the magnitude of vasodilation in the airway caused by inhaled albuterol could be altered by changes in airway pH. To investigate this possibility, we determined the effect of airway surface pH on airway blood flow ($\dot{Q}_{aw}$) responsiveness to inhaled albuterol in healthy subjects by manipulating airway pH through ventilatory maneuvers. Healthy subjects were chosen because the required respiratory maneuvers would be difficult to impose on patients with airflow obstruction. $\dot{Q}aw$ was chosen as a "biomarker" of albuterol responsiveness because airflow responses would only be marginally sensitive to albuterol in healthy subjects.

Methods

Subjects

Ten healthy lifetime non-smokers participated in the study. The exclusion criteria were as follows: *1)* a physician diagnosis of cardiovascular or pulmonary disease; *2)* the use of cardiovascular or airway medication; *3)* a body mass index >30; and *4)* a forced expiratory volume in 1 second (FEV_1) < 80% of predicted and FEV_1-to-forced vital capacity ratio < 0.7. All subjects had been free of an acute respiratory infection for at least 4 weeks before beginning the study, and no subject had an acute respiratory infection during the study. The study was approved by the Western Institutional Review Board and by the Human Subjects Research Office at the University of Miami. A signed informed consent was obtained from the subjects. The study is registered at clinicaltrials.gov: NCT01216748.

Measurements

Airway blood flow ($\dot{Q}aw$)

A previously validated soluble inert gas uptake method was used to measure $\dot{Q}_{aw}$ [8,9]. The subjects first inhaled room air to total lung capacity. After exhaling 500 mL, they rapidly re-inhaled the same volume of a pre-mixed gas consisting of 10% dimethylether (DME), balance nitrogen. After a predetermined breathhold time, the subjects then exhaled through a critical flow orifice to standardize the expiratory flow. During the entire maneuver, the instantaneous concentrations of DME and nitrogen were measured at the airway opening with a mass spectrometer (Perkin-Elmer; Pomona, CA). The maneuver was performed with two breathhold times each of 5 and 15 sec in random order. The DME concentration (F_{DME}) at the end of phase 1 of the nitrogen wash-in curve (defining a virtual anatomical dead space, V_D) was obtained. The difference in F_{DME} between the two breathhold times (ΔF_{DME}) multiplied by V_D was used to calculate DME uptake ($\dot{V}_{DME}$) over the intervening 10 sec. From $\dot{V}_{DME}$, the mean DME concentration between the two breathholds (F_{mDME}) and the solubility

coefficient for DME in blood and tissue (α), was calculated using the Fick principle ($\dot{Q}_{aw} = \dot{V}_{DME}/(\alpha \cdot F_{mDME})$. $\dot{Q}_{aw}$ was normalized for V_D; therefore, V_D cancels out and wasn't measured. $\dot{Q}_{aw}$ was expressed as $\mu l.min^{-1}.mL^{-1}$, where $\mu l.min^{-1}$ reflects blood flow and mL reflects the virtual anatomical deadspace. At each $\dot{Q}_{aw}$ determination, data from two 5 sec and two 15 sec breathholds were analyzed. A $\dot{Q}_{aw}$ determination took less than 5 min.

Blood pressure and arterial oxygen saturation (SaO_2) by pulse-oximetry were monitored at each measurement point. Mean systemic arterial pressure (perfusion pressure for airway blood flow) was calculated as diastolic pressure plus 1/3 pulse pressure.

Spirometry

For spirometry (Forced Expired Volume in one second/FEV1, Forced Vital Capacity/FVC, FEV_1/FVC), a Koko spirometer was used (Ferraris Respiratory, Louisville, CO). The tracing with the highest FVC of three forced vital capacity maneuvers was analyzed. Predicted normal values were taken from Crapo et al [10]. The values were expressed in absolute values and percent of predicted.

Exhaled Breath Condensate (EBC) pH was obtained as recommended by an American Thoracic Society/European Respiratory Society task force [11]. The EBC samples were collected with the condenser temperatures close to 0°C. We determined EBC pH immediately following sample collection without argon purging [12], using a Thermo Orion 3 Star pH Meter and Micro pH Electrode (Thermo Scientific Orion Inc., Carlsbad, CA). During the different breathing maneuvers, EBC samples were collected by directing the subject's exhaled breath into a pre-cooled (-10°C) tube for 5 min, using the disposable R-tubes® from Respiratory Research System (Charlottesville, VA). Over this period of time, approximately 0.5-1 mL of condensate was collected. For further standardization, the subjects were not allowed to drink or eat for at least one hour before the EBC samples were collected [13,14].

Ventilation

Compressed air was lead through a calibrated airflow regulator (Dakota Instruments, Orangeburg, NY) and an anesthesia bag to a one-way valve at the mouthpiece. During the ventilatory maneuvers, the airflow was adjusted to keep the anesthesia bag from collapsing or overinflating until a steady state was reached [15]. The airflow was read at that point and expressed as $l.min^{-1}$. The system had a deadspace of 100 mL between the mouthpiece and the valve separating inspiration from expiration. Subjects wore a nose clip for all measurements.

Respiratory maneuvers

Different respiratory maneuvers were used to change airway pH as reflected by EBC pH.

The same measurements were made in all subjects during quiet breathing, hypercapnic hyperventilation, hypocapnic hyperventilation and eucapnic hyperventilation. To induce hypercapnic hyperventilation, we employed a modification of a previously described procedure [15]. While monitoring S_aO_2 using pulse oximetry and end-tidal CO_2 by mass-spectrometry (Perkin-Elmer, Pomona, CA) on a breath by breath basis, CO_2 was bled into the inspired air to achieve an end-tidal pCO_2 of at least 55 mmHg, expected to result in a decrease in systemic pH of about 0.1 pH units. For hypocapnic hyperventilation, the subjects were instructed to breathe fast and deep until their end-tidal pCO_2 fell to 30 mmHg, corresponding to a systemic pH increase of about 0.1 pH units. For eucapnic hyperventilation, the subjects were instructed to increase their ventilation to the highest level of ventilation recorded in the previous two hyperventilation maneuvers, while CO_2 was bled into the inspired air to maintain end-tidal pCO_2 at 40 mmHg. This maneuver was used to separate the effect of ventilation from the effect of pH on albuterol responsiveness. The same mouthpiece set-up was used for the measurement of $\dot{Q}_{aw}$, EBC pH, and ventilation.

Protocol

The subjects were instructed to abstain from ingesting alcoholic beverages the night before each study day and not to ingest caffeinated drinks for at least 12 hours before the study. The subjects were also instructed not to use phosphodiesterase type 5 inhibitors for 12 hours before coming to the laboratory.

There were 6 visit days. On day 1, informed consent was obtained and the subjects underwent a physical examination to ensure good general health. In females, a urine pregnancy test was performed to rule out current pregnancy. Then, spirometry was performed to ensure normal lung function. For technical reasons, EBC pH, $\dot{Q}_{aw}$ responses to albuterol and the level of ventilation could not be assessed simultaneously during the breathing maneuvers. Therefore, these parameters were measured during different breathing maneuvers on different days in random order (quiet breathing, hypercapnic hyperventilation, hypocapnic hyperventilation and eucapnic hyperventilation.

Exhaled breath condensate collection

For each respiratory maneuver, the subjects breathed at the respective ventilatory level for 2 minutes followed by a 5 minutes EBC collection while maintaining the same breathing pattern.

Determination of ventilation

This was done during the different respiratory maneuvers as described for the EBC collection. Ventilation was measured during the 5 min steady state period.

$\dot{Q}_{aw}$ response to albuterol

This was done during the four breathing protocols as described above. During the 5 min steady state breathing period, $\dot{Q}_{aw}$ was first measured with a short break in the breathing maneuver. After resuming the designated breathing maneuver, the subjects inhaled albuterol (180 µg) delivered by a metered dose inhaler using a holding chamber during a brief interruption of the breathing maneuver. The subjects then continued to perform the prescribed respiratory maneuver for another 5 min. $\dot{Q}_{aw}$ was again measured 15 min after drug administration during quiet breathing. Albuterol responsiveness was expressed as the difference between pre- and post albuterol $\dot{Q}_{aw}$ ($\Delta\dot{Q}_{aw}$).

Statistical analysis

Values are presented as mean ± standard error (SE). Differences between the groups were analyzed by a nonparametric Kruskal-Wallis ANOVA test followed, when significant, by the Mann-Whitney U test for comparisons between groups. Values were expressed as mean ± SE and a p value less than 0.05 was accepted as a statistically significant difference. All statistics were analyzed with SPSS software (Statistical Product and Services Solutions, version 18.0; SPSS Inc., Chicago, IL).

Results

The demographics and baseline characteristics of study participants are shown in Table 1, consistent with good cardiovascular and respiratory health. All subjects completed the protocol.

Table 1 Demographics and baseline characteristics of study participants (visit 1)

	Subjects
N	10
Mean age (range), yr	37 ± 8 (24-53)
Sex (M/F)	3 / 7
Heart rate, beats/min	65 ± 12
Systolic BP, mmHg	106 ± 5
Diastolic BP, mmHg	68 ± 4
SAT O_2	99 ± 1
FEV_1, liters	3.26 ± 0.61
FEV_1, %predicted	104 ± 1

Values are mean ± SE.
N = number of subjects; M, male; F, female; BP, blood pressure; SAT O_2, arterial oxygen saturation measured by pulse oximetry; FEV_1, forced expiratory volume in 1 second.

Ventilation and EBC pH

The levels of ventilation at the time of albuterol administration during the four respiratory maneuvers are shown in Table 2. Hypercapnia and hypocapnia changed EBC pH, while eucapnic hyperventilation had no effect on EBC pH. Thus, it was possible to unlink the level of ventilation from the changes in EBC pH, which presumably is a reflection of airway surface liquid pH.

Airway blood flow response to albuterol

Mean systemic blood pressure and oxygen saturation were not different at the $\dot{Q}_{aw}$ measurement points (baseline, pre-albuterol and post albuterol). The lack of changes in mean systemic blood pressure obviated the need to express the airway blood flow responses as airway blood flow conductance. Vasodilator responses therefore were reported as $\Delta\dot{Q}_{aw}$.

Baseline mean $\dot{Q}_{aw}$ values were similar before the four breathing maneuvers and remained unchanged during the subsequent breathing maneuvers as reflected by the pre-albuterol values (Table 3). All subjects had similar albuterol response to the different breathing maneuvers. Albuterol increased mean $\dot{Q}_{aw}$ significantly, by 46.2 and 33.8% 15 min post drug inhalation during quiet breathing and eucapnic hyperventilation, respectively (Table 3, Figure 1). In contrast, albuterol had no effect on mean $\dot{Q}_{aw}$ during hypercapnic hyperventilation (4.9%) or hypocapnic hyperventilation (-1.3%) maneuvers, which were associated with a decrease or increase in EBC pH.

Discussion

The purpose of this study was to determine if respiratory acidosis and alkalosis have an effect on the physiological response to inhaled albuterol in airway tissue and if the effect is related to the ventilation-associated changes in airway pH as reflected by exhaled breath condensate (EBC) pH. In order to demonstrate the role of pH in the observed changes in albuterol responsiveness associated with respiratory acidosis and alkalosis, it was necessary to unlink the changes in EBC pH from the changes in ventilation. This was done by comparing quiet breathing with eucapnic hyperventilation, where ventilation changes while pH is

Table 2 Ventilation and exhaled breath condensate pH during respiratory maneuvers

Challenges	$\dot{V}$ (L · min^{-1})	EBC pH (units)
Quiet breathing	14.4 ± 4.2	6.39 ± 0.14
Eucapnic hyperventilation	35.5 ± 3.4*	6.31 ± 0.08
Hypocapnic hyperventilation	35.2 ± 3.3*	6.59 ± 0.15**
Hypercapnic hyperventilation	24.4 ± 2.9*	5.88 ± 0.14**

$\dot{V}$, ventilation.
EBC, exhaled breath condensate.
*p < 0.05 vs. quiet breathing.
**p < 0.02 vs. quiet breathing.

kept constant. Albuterol responsiveness was the same during the two maneuvers, suggesting that hyperventilation per se did not alter albuterol responsiveness. Likewise, the preserved albuterol responsiveness during eucapnic hyperventilation ruled out the possibility that cooling and drying of the airway could have been the cause of the blunted albuterol responsiveness during respiratory alkalosis and acidosis. Eucapnic hyperventilation was investigated last in order to be able to reproduce the highest level of ventilation achieved in any of the other maneuvers. We therefore are confident that ventilation per se had no effect on albuterol responsiveness. The level of ventilation during quiet breathing was higher than one would have expected in healthy subjects at rest (mean 14.4 L·min^{-1}). It has previously been reported that wearing a nose clip and breathing through a mouthpiece increases tidal volume and minute ventilation [16]. In addition, the breathing setup we used for our study included a 100 mL deadspace, another stimulus for increasing tidal volume and respiratory rate.

In our study, the intended target of albuterol was airway vascular smooth muscle contained in the airway wall. Since the different respiratory maneuvers by themselves had no effect on $\dot{Q}_{aw}$ we were able to assess the effect of respiratory acidosis and alkalosis on albuterol responsiveness. In some systemic vascular beds, hypercapnic acidosis causes relaxation and hypocapnic alkalosis causes constriction, resulting in corresponding blood flow changes [5]. The airway circulation appears not to be subject to this regulation at least in the range of pCO_2 changes seen in the present study in which changes in pH had no effect on $\dot{Q}_{aw}$; however, they affected albuterol responsiveness. We allowed 5 min for albuterol absorption during the four breathing maneuvers, and measured $\dot{Q}_{aw}$ 15 min after drug inhalation. This was done because in previous studies we found that the maximum response typically occurs after 15 min while a vasodilator response to inhaled albuterol is already seen after 5 min [17].

We found that both airway alkalosis and acidosis attenuated albuterol responsiveness. The pH-sensitivity of albuterol responsiveness could have been related to a combination of several factors, including absorption and transport of albuterol from the airway surface to the airway vascular smooth muscle, β_2-adrenergic receptor function, vascular endothelial function or vascular smooth muscle responsiveness. In vitro and animal experiments suggest that all of these functions can be pH-dependent.

Acidosis

The majority of the currently used β_2-adrenergic bronchodilators, including albuterol, cannot freely diffuse across the epithelial cell membrane because they are hydrophilic and carry a transient or permanent positive

Table 3 Effects of respiratory maneuvers on airway blood flow ($\dot{Q}_{aw}$)

		Pre-maneuver $\dot{Q}_{aw}$	$\dot{Q}_{aw}$ during steady state	$\dot{Q}_{aw}$ 15 min post albuterol
Quiet breathing	Mean ± SE	38.1 ± 1.4	37.2 ± 1.5	53.7 ± 2.1*
	Median	37.7	35.7	54.3
	25% quartile	33.8	34.1	46.9
	75%quartile	42.1	41.9	58.7
Eucapnic hyperventilation	Mean ± SE	41.8 ± 4.3	42.6 ± 4.3	56.4 ± 4.0*
	Median	40.7	42.7	49.7
	25% quartile	34.8	34.8	46.7
	75% quartile	48.8	48.8	61.7
Hypocapnic hyperventilation	Mean ± SE	42.9 ± 2.8	45.2 ± 3.4	45.1 ± 2.9
	Median	40.1	42.2	43.7
	25% quartile	37.2	35.0	38.8
	75% quartile	49.1	49.7	54.1
Hypercapnic hyperventilation	Mean ± SE	42.1 ± 2.4	44.8 ± 3.8	46.7 ± 4.0
	Median	37.5	44.7	43.7
	25% quartile	35.5	34.1	38.4
	75% quartile	46.2	57.1	52.2

$\dot{Q}_{aw}$ is expressed in $\mu l.min^{-1}.mL^{-1}$. * $p < 0.05$ vs. steady state.

charge at physiological pH. Thus, the epithelium of the airway becomes a barrier to these agents, requiring cellular or paracellular transport across the epithelial lining of the airway to reach their intended target tissues including airway vascular smooth muscle. We have previously demonstrated the existence of an organic cation transport machinery in the human airway epithelium and showed that this process is largely mediated by the organic cation/carnitine transporter OCTN2, which is likely involved in the delivery of inhaled hydrophilic cationic bronchodilators to the airway tissue [1]. We showed that cationic drug uptake is pH dependent, with about 3-fold lower rates at an acidic pH (5.7) than alkaline pH (8.2). This mechanism could have been fully or

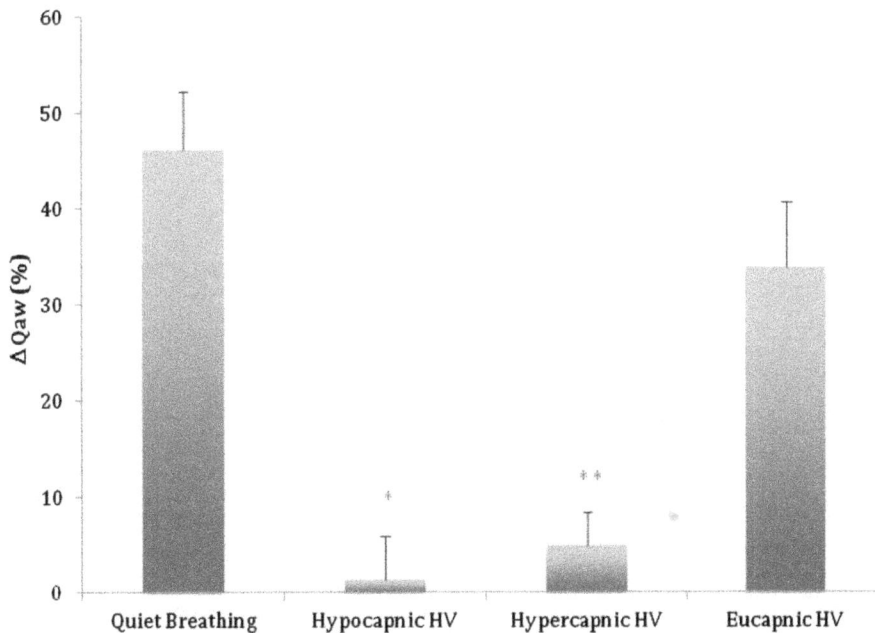

Figure 1 Relative albuterol-induced changes in airway blood flow ($\Delta\dot{Q}_{aw}$) during four breathing maneuvers. Values are mean ± SE. *p < 0.01 and ** p < 0.02 vs quiet breathing and eucapnic hyperventilation.

partially responsible for the blunted albuterol responsiveness during respiratory acidosis associated with a decreased airway surface liquid pH. We have also shown that albuterol crosses the airway epithelium via the paracellular route [18]. The paracellular pathway can also mediate pH-dependent permeability to pH-dependent changes in negative charges.

It has also been reported that acidosis can cause rapid desensitization and uncoupling of β_2-adrenergic receptors [2], possibly leading to albuterol unresponsiveness as seen in the present investigation.

Albuterol-induced vasodilation is endothelium-dependent, involving endothelial relaxant factors including nitric oxide [19]. Although the observations on the effects of intracellular and extracellular acidosis and pCO_2 on endothelial function have not been consistent, the majority of studies have shown that acidosis can impair endothelial function [4-6]. It is likely that airway surface liquid pH is a reflection of extracellular pH, but changes in both extracellular and intracellular pH have been implicated in the effect of acidosis on endothelial function. Thus, endothelial dysfunction could have had a role in the blunted albuterol responsiveness in our study. Finally, airway vascular smooth muscle function could be directly affected by acidosis. In particular, acidosis can lead to smooth muscle cell hyperpolarization, which in turn could attenuate albuterol-induced vasodilation [5].

Alkalosis

Respiratory alkalosis also attenuated albuterol-induced vasodilation in our study. *In vitro*, alkalosis increases the transport of organic cations such as albuterol across the airway epithelium via the transcellular and paracellular routes [18]. Alkalosis may also increase β_2-adrenergic receptor ligand binding [3]. Finally, alkalosis has been shown to cause endothelium-dependent vasodilation without altering endothelial nitric oxide synthase function [5]. All of these actions would be expected to potentiate inhaled albuterol-induced vasodilation. The mechanistic explanation for our observation that respiratory alkalosis has the same attenuating effect on albuterol responsiveness as acidosis remains unclear at this time.

Conclusions

Patients with airway disease are likely to have highly variable airway surface liquid pH and adrenergic airway smooth muscle responsiveness [20-23]. Therefore, we decided to investigate the pH dependence of β_2-adrenergic responsiveness as a marker of albuterol responsiveness in healthy subjects with normal β_2-adrenergic smooth muscle responsiveness in whom the airway surface liquid pH can be artificially manipulated. From a clinical perspective, airway smooth muscle would have been a more meaningful airway wall target to assess responsiveness to inhaled albuterol. However, healthy subjects do not have an increased

airway smooth muscle tone and responses to albuterol would have been too small to study the effects of respiratory acidosis and alkalosis. We chose not to include patients with asthma or COPD in the investigation because they have a blunted airway blood flow response to albuterol due to endothelial dysfunction [18], and because measuring airflow responses by pulmonary function testing would have been technically difficult under the experimental conditions of the study.

Our *in vivo* observation showed that both respiratory acidosis and alkalosis blunt albuterol responsiveness in the airway wall, although it is not known whether the effect is driven by intracellular or extracellular pH or pCO_2 and which of the above-mentioned mechanisms may be involved. In this study we found that albuterol responsiveness as assessed by $\dot{Q}_{aw}$ in the airway is blunted by acidosis and alkalosis, using $\dot{Q}_{aw}$ as a bioassay. It remains to be shown whether the clinical benefits of inhaled albuterol, i.e., bronchodilation may be less than expected during acute respiratory acidosis and alkalosis, which can be associated with exacerbations of asthma and COPD.

Competing interests
The authors declare that they have no competing interests.

Authors' contributions
AW: Conception and design, analysis and interpretation of data, drafting of the manuscript, critical revision of the manuscript for important intellectual content, supervision and final approval of the version to be published. MS: Conception and design and manuscript editing. ESM: Acquisition of data, statistical analysis, and interpretation of data. JEC: Acquisition and analysis of data, GH: Conception and design of the study. MEM: Sample analysis and interpretation. JA: Acquisition of data. All authors read and approved the final manuscript.

Authors' information
Matthias Salathe and Adam Wanner are senior authors contributed equally to this paper.

Funding
The study was supported by NIH 1R01HL060644.

Author details
[1]Division of Pulmonary, Allergy, Critical Care and Sleep Medicine, University of Miami School of Medicine, Miami, FL 33136, USA. [2]Department of Pulmonology, Semmelweis University School of Medicine, Budapest, Hungary.

References
1. Horvath G, Schmid N, Fragoso MA, Schmid A, Conner GE, Salathe M, et al. Epithelial organic cation transporters ensure pH dependent drug absorption in the airway. Am J Respir Cell Mol Biol. 2007;36:53–60.
2. Davies AO. Rapid desensitization and uncoupling of human beta-adrenergic receptors in an *in vitro* model of lactic acidosis. J Clin Endocrinol Metab. 1984;59:398–405.
3. Modest VE, Butterworth JF. Effect of pH and lidocaine on beta-adrenergic receptor binding: interaction during rescucitation. Chest. 1995;108:1373–9.
4. Crimi E, Taccone FS, Infante T, Scoletta S, Crudele V, Napoli C. Effects if intracelular acidosis on endotelial function: an overview. J Crit Care. 2012;27:108–18.

5. Celotto AC, Capellini CF, Baldo CF, Dalio MB, Rodriguez AJ, Evora PRB. Effects of acid-base imbalance on vascular reactivity. Braz J Med Biol Res. 2008;41:439–45.

6. Nagy S, Harris MB, Ju H, Bhatia J, Venema RC. pH and nitric synthase activity and expression in bovine endothelial cells. Acta Pediatr. 2006;95:814–7.

7. Kontos HA, Wei EP, Raper AJ, Patterson JL. Local mechanism of CO_2 action of cat pial arterioles. Stroke. 1977;8:226–9.

8. Wanner A, Mendes ES, Atkins ND. A simplified noninvasive method to measure airway blood flow in humans. J Appl Physiol. 2006;100:1674–8.

9. Scuri M, McCascill V, Chediak AD, Abraham WM, Wanner A. Measurement of airway blood flow with dimethylether: validation with microspheres. J Appl Physiol. 1995;79:1386–90.

10. Crapo RO, Morris AH, Gardner RM. Reference spirometric values using techniques and equipment that meet ATS recommendations. Am Rev Respir Dis. 1981;123:659–64.

11. Horvath G, Hunt J, Barnes PJ. On behalf of the ATS/ERS Task Force on Exhaled Breath Condensate. Eur Respir J. 2005;26:523–48.

12. Paget-Brown AO, Ngamtrakulpanit L, Smith A, Bunyan D, Hom S, Nguyen A, et al. Normative data for pH of exhaled breath condensate. Chest. 2006;129:426–30.

13. Wells K, Vaughan J, Pajewski TN, Hom S, Ngamtrakulpanit L, Smith A, et al. Exhaled breath condensate pH assays are not influenced by oral ammonia. Thorax. 2005;60:27–31.

14. Effros RM, Casaburi R, Su J, Dunning M, Torday J, Biller J, et al. The effects of volatile salivary acids and bases on exhaled breath condensate pH. Am J Respir Crit Care Med. 2006;173:386–92.

15. Gilbert IA, McFadden ER. Airway cooling and rewarming. J Clin Invest. 1992;90:699–704.

16. Bloch KE, Barandun J, Sackner MA. Effect of mouthpiece breathing on cardiorespiratory response to intense exercise. Am J Respir Crit Care Med. 1995;151:1087–92.

17. Onorato DJ, Demirozu MC, Breitenbucher A, Atkins ND, Chediak AD, Wanner A. Airway mucosal blood flow in man: response to adrenergic agonists. Am J Respir Crit Care Med. 1994;149:1132–7.

18. Unwalla HJ, Horvath G, Roth FD, Conner GE, Salathe M. Albuterol modulates its own transepithelial flux via changes in paracellular permeability. Am J Respir Cell Mol Biol. 2012;46:551–8.

19. Wanner A, Mendes ES. Airway endothelial dysfunction in asthma and COPD: a challenge for future research. Am J Respir Crit Care Med. 2010;182:1344–51.

20. Hunt JF, Fang K, Malik R, Snyder A, Malhotra N, Platts-Mills TA, et al. Endogenous airway acidification. Implications for asthma pathophysiology. Am J Respir Crit Care Med. 2000;161:694–9.

21. Kodric M, Shah A, Fabbri L, Confalonieri M. An investigation of airway acidification in asthma using induced sputum. Am J Respir Crit Care Med. 2007;175:905–10.

22. McShane D, Davies JC, Davies MG, Bush A, Geddes DM, Alton EW. Airway surface pH in subjects with cystic fibrosis. Eur Respir J. 2003;21:37–42.

23. Brieva J, Wanner A. Adrenergic airway vascular smooth muscle responsiveness in healthy and asthmatic subjects. J Appl Physiol. 2001;90:665–9.

16

Effects of early life exposure to ultraviolet C radiation on mitochondrial DNA content, transcription, ATP production, and oxygen consumption in developing *Caenorhabditis elegans*

Maxwell CK Leung[1,2], John P Rooney[1,2], Ian T Ryde[1], Autumn J Bernal[2], Amanda S Bess[1,2], Tracey L Crocker[1], Alex Q Ji[1] and Joel N Meyer[1,2*]

Abstract

Background: Mitochondrial DNA (mtDNA) is present in multiple copies per cell and undergoes dramatic amplification during development. The impacts of mtDNA damage incurred early in development are not well understood, especially in the case of types of mtDNA damage that are irreparable, such as ultraviolet C radiation (UVC)-induced photodimers.

Methods: We exposed first larval stage nematodes to UVC using a protocol that results in accumulated mtDNA damage but permits nuclear DNA (nDNA) repair. We then measured the transcriptional response, as well as oxygen consumption, ATP levels, and mtDNA copy number through adulthood.

Results: Although the mtDNA damage persisted to the fourth larval stage, we observed only a relatively minor ~40% decrease in mtDNA copy number. Transcriptomic analysis suggested an inhibition of aerobic metabolism and developmental processes; mRNA levels for mtDNA-encoded genes were reduced ~50% at 3 hours post-treatment, but recovered and, in some cases, were upregulated at 24 and 48 hours post-exposure. The mtDNA polymerase γ was also induced ~8-fold at 48 hours post-exposure. Moreover, ATP levels and oxygen consumption were reduced in response to UVC exposure, with marked reductions of ~50% at the later larval stages.

Conclusions: These results support the hypothesis that early life exposure to mitochondrial genotoxicants could result in mitochondrial dysfunction at later stages of life, thereby highlighting the potential health hazards of time-delayed effects of these genotoxicants in the environment.

Keywords: *Caenorhabditis elegans*, Mitochondrial DNA damage, Mitochondrial dysfunction, Ultraviolet C radiation, Early life exposure, Genotoxicity

* Correspondence: joel.meyer@duke.edu
[1]Nicholas School of the Environment, Duke University, Durham, NC, USA
[2]Integrated Toxicology and Environmental Health Program, Duke University, Durham, NC, USA

Background

In recent years, potential environmental effects on mitochondrial biology have attracted increasing research interest [1,2]. Mitochondrial DNA (mtDNA) is more sensitive than nuclear DNA (nDNA) to exposure to some chemicals, perhaps due to the absence of chromatin packing and many DNA repair pathways in mitochondria [3]. The high lipid content of the mitochondrial membranes and the slightly negative charge of the mitochondrial matrix also attract lipophilic or positively charged compounds to mitochondria [4]. Furthermore, non-genotoxic mitochondrial toxicants might disrupt mitochondrial function and indirectly cause mtDNA damage via generation of reactive oxygen species [5].

Theoretical considerations and some empirical data suggest that mtDNA damage that occurs at different stages of human life may lead to very different physiological effects. Since the quality of mitochondria in differentiated tissues depends on the quality of mitochondria in their precursors, mitochondrial damage in the early stages of human development may potentially affect mature tissue function. For example, mitochondrial toxicities exerted by developmental exposure to anti-HIV drugs in humans and laboratory models [6] demonstrate the importance of normal mtDNA biology during development.

The mitochondrial biology of Caenorhabditis elegans is generally similar to that of humans [7]. The genome is 13,794 base pairs in length (Additional file 1: Figure S1), compared to 16,649 in humans. The genes encoded appear to be identical; while an *atp-8* gene has not been definitively identified in C. elegans, it is probably present with an unusual sequence, as is the case in other nematodes [8]. There are also indications that the developmental biology of mitochondria is similar in C. elegans and humans: C. elegans [7,9,10], like humans [11,12], shows a large increase in mtDNA copy number with age as well as a switch from anaerobic to aerobic metabolism during development. Thus, C. elegans offers a useful model for the *in vivo* study of mitochondrial biology, as well as the response to toxicants [13].

Recent work by Furda et al. [14] demonstrated that persistent mtDNA damage can lead to mitochondrial dysfunction, but the response was dependent on the type of DNA damage incurred. We recently described a serial ultraviolet C radiation (UVC) exposure protocol that resulted in a large amount of irreparable mtDNA damage in C. elegans, but permitted the repair of the nDNA damage [15]. UVC creates photodimers almost exclusively, and previous *in vitro* evidence [16,17] suggests that such damage might inhibit mtDNA replication and transcription *in vivo*. In this work, we investigated the hypothesis that early life exposure to serial UVC results in later life mitochondrial dysfunction.

Methods

C. elegans culture and exposures

C. elegans were cultured and exposed to UVC during the L1 stage, largely as previously described [15]. Briefly, synchronized L1 larvae were produced by overnight hatch in M9 medium following bleach-sodium hydroxide isolation of eggs as previously described [18]. The L1 larvae were placed on peptone-free (to prevent inadvertent microbial growth) K agar plates with or without 5 μg/mL ethidium bromide (EtBr) for 48 h without food at 20°C. Half of the plates were also exposed to 7.5 J/m^2 UVC radiation at 0, 24, and 48 h as described [15], and then transferred to OP50-seeded plates. The UVC exposure protocol is based on the fact that UVC-induced DNA damage is quickly repaired in the nuclear but not mitochondrial genome [15,19], thus allowing for accumulation of mitochondrial DNA damage while permitting repair of nuclear DNA. This protocol results in no larval growth delay prior to the L4 stage [15]. The transgenic strain PE255 expressing firefly luciferase as an *in vivo* reporter for ATP level [20] was generously provided by Dr. Cristina Lagido (University of Aberdeen, UK). The wildtype strain N2 was obtained from *Caenorhabditis* Genetics Center (University of Minnesota), which is funded by the NIH National Center for Research Resources (NCRR).

Microarray experiments

N2 nematodes were sampled for RNA isolation at 3 h after the first UVC exposure, 1 h prior to the second exposure, 1 h prior to the third exposure, and 3 h after the third exposure, and transferred to OP50 plates (schematic presented in Figure 1). Transfer to OP50 plates and isolation for freezing were accomplished by washing nematodes off of plates into a 15 mL tube with K-medium, pelleting by centrifugation, followed by two additional cycles of resuspension and centrifugation as described [19]. Nematodes were frozen by dripping 3,000-5,000 pelleted nematodes suspended in about 500 μl K-medium into liquid nitrogen, and stored at –80°C. The pellets were ground into fine powder with a liquid nitrogen-cooled mortar and pestle and RNA was extracted using an RNeasy kit (Qiagen, Valencia, CA, USA). RNA was quantified with a NanoDrop 8000 spectrophotometer (Thermo Scientific/NanoDrop, Wilmington, DE, USA) and analyzed for integrity with an Agilent 2100 BioAnalyzer G2939A (Agilent Technologies, Santa Clara, CA, USA). These exposures were carried out seven times. The seven replicates generated a total "n" of between 4 and 6 for each treatment and timepoint, after excluding samples lost due to insufficient mRNA quality or principle components analysis-based identification of outliers.

Gene expression analysis was conducted using Affymetrix /C. elegans/ GeneChip® arrays (Affymetrix, Santa Clara, CA). Hybridization targets were prepared with

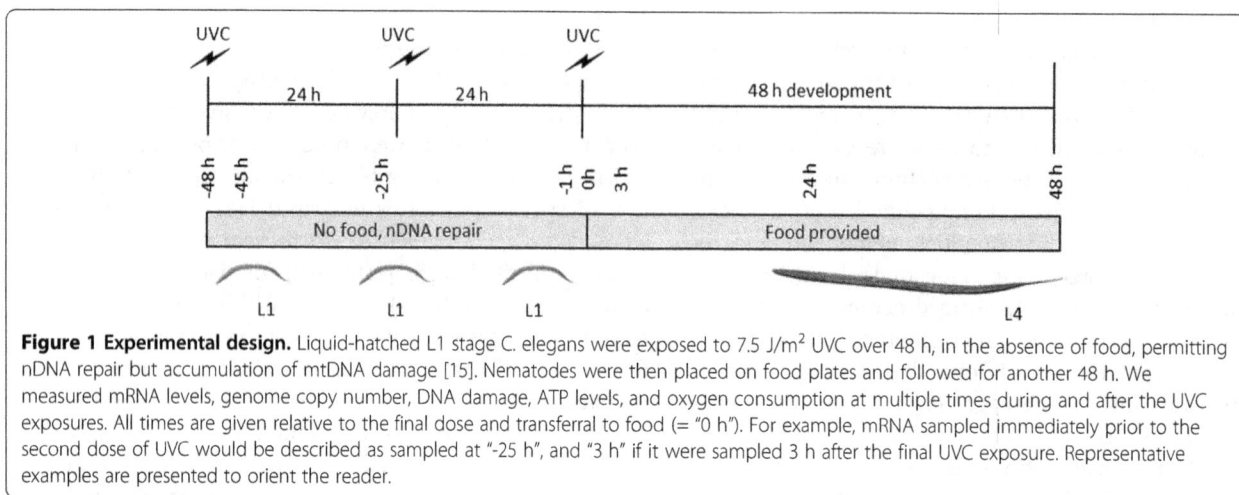

Figure 1 Experimental design. Liquid-hatched L1 stage C. elegans were exposed to 7.5 J/m² UVC over 48 h, in the absence of food, permitting nDNA repair but accumulation of mtDNA damage [15]. Nematodes were then placed on food plates and followed for another 48 h. We measured mRNA levels, genome copy number, DNA damage, ATP levels, and oxygen consumption at multiple times during and after the UVC exposures. All times are given relative to the final dose and transferral to food (= "0 h"). For example, mRNA sampled immediately prior to the second dose of UVC would be described as sampled at "-25 h", and "3 h" if it were sampled 3 h after the final UVC exposure. Representative examples are presented to orient the reader.

MessageAmp™ Premier RNA Amplification Kit (Applied Biosystems/Ambion, Austin, TX) from total RNA, hybridized to GeneChip® C. elegans Genome Arrays in Affymetrix GeneChip® hybridization oven 645, washed in Affymetrix GeneChip® Fluidics Station 450 and scanned with Affymetrix GeneChip® Scanner 7 G according to standard Affymetrix GeneChip® Hybridization, Wash, and Stain protocols (Affymetrix, Santa Clara,CA). Microarray data have been deposited in the National Center for Biotechnology Information's GEO and are accessible through GEO series accession number GSE38997.

Microarray data preprocessing, normalization, error modeling, and initial visualization
We used Principal Components Analysis (PCA) followed by pairwise correlation analysis on unfiltered data to identify outlier samples. Data preprocessing, normalization, and error modeling were performed with Rosetta Resolver® after grouping biological replicates. The resulting fold-changes and p-values were used for Cytoscape analyses (described below).

GeneSpring-based analysis of microarray data
We used GeneSpring version GX11 (Agilent) to carry out ANOVA, PCA analysis, gene ontology (GO) enrichment analysis, and some visualization.

Interactome-based analysis of microarray data
Cytoscape (version 2.8.2) was used to overlay microarray data onto two interactomes: the high-confidence WI8 interactome compiled by the Vidal lab [21], and an interactome built by joining four previously-described interactomes: the integrated_function_network from the Vidal lab [21]; an interactome that we assembled previously [19] based on the BIND database [22] and Zhong and Sternberg [23] interactome; the "core" interactome described by Lee et al. [24]; and the higher-probability interactome generated

by Alexeyenko and Sonnhammer [25] using a probability of functional coupling cut-off of 0.75. These networks are referred to herein as "WI8" and "Union4" and are composed of 2500 nodes and 3706 edges, and 14334 nodes and 346484 edges, respectively. The Union4 interactome is presented as Additional file 2 in .sif format. jActiveModules (version 2.23, [26]) was used to find, via greedy searching, the top 10 modules with a maximum overlap of 0.3, as identified at a search depth of 1 and maximum depth from start nodes of 2 (with the WI8 interactome) or 1 (with the Union4 interactome). The resulting subnetworks were analyzed for Gene Ontology enrichment with the BiNGO (version 2.44) plugin [27]. We assessed overrepresentation using the hypergeometric test with the Benjamini and Hochberg False Discovery Rate multiple testing correction and significance level of 0.05, testing each cluster versus the entire annotation and identifying altered GO Biological Processes.

mtDNA and nDNA copy number measurements
mtDNA copy number was measured in N2 and PE255 nematodes using a modification of the real-time PCR assay described by Bratic et al. [28]; this assay is based on a plasmid DNA-based standard curve and so generates actual rather than relative copy numbers. The only change to the assay was the use of 2-fold rather than 10-fold dilutions in the standard curve. nDNA copy number was measured using primers designed with Primer 3 [29]: forward - 5'-GCC GAC TGG AAG AAC TTG TC-3'; reverse - 5'-GCG GAG ATC ACC TTC CAG TA-3'. These primers amplify a 164 bp region of the gene W09C5.8 (cox-4). Nuclear copy number was determined by creating a standard curve for the nuclear DNA based on young adult (24 h post-L4) glp-1 mutant nematodes raised at 25°C. At this temperature, this strain has a fixed number of cells since it has no germline proliferation [30] and C. elegans somatic cells do not divide in

adulthood [31]. We based the standard curve on the calculation that adults lacking germ cell proliferation would contain 3134 genomic copies [32,33]. Real-time PCR was carried out in a 7300 Real Time PCR System (Applied Biosystems), under the following conditions: 2 min at 50°C, 10 min at 95°C, 40 cycles of 15 sec at 95°C and 60 sec at 60°C. A dissociation curve was calculated for each sample at the end of each profile. The 25 μl PCR reactions contained 12.5 μl of SYBR Green PCR Master Mix (Applied Biosystems), 8.5 μl H_2O, 2 μl of target-specific primers at 400 nM final concentration, and 2 μl of nematode lysate obtained as described [34]. The ABI PRISM 7300 Sequence Detection System Software, Version 1.1 (Applied Biosystems) was used to carry out data analysis. All samples were run in triplicate and triplicates were averaged prior to analysis.

DNA damage measurements

nDNA and mtDNA damage were evaluated using a QPCR-based method as previously described [35] except that mtDNA damage was normalized to mtDNA copy number based on measurements obtained using the real-time method described above.

mRNA levels

mRNA levels of five mitochondrial electron transport chain (ETC) complex subunits, including two mitochondria-encoded genes (*ctb-1* and *nd-5*) and three nucleus-encoded genes (*C34B2.8*, *D2030.4* and *K09A9.5*), were measured using real-time PCR. mRNA levels of the nuclear-encoded *polg-1* gene, which encodes the *C. elegans* mitochondrial DNA polymerase γ, were also measured. 250 ng of mRNA isolated from *C. elegans* as described above was converted to cDNA using the Qiagen Omniscript Reverse Transcription kit. Real time PCR was carried out with a 7300 Real Time PCR System as described above except that the extension temperatures were 62°C for *ctb-1* and *nd-5*, and 60°C for C34B2.8, D2030.4 and K09A9.5. The average mRNA fold change of each target gene was calculated by comparing the CT (cycle threshold) of the target gene to that of the housekeeping genes *cdc-42* and *pmp-3* [36]. Primers were based on the literature (*ctb-1*, *polg-1*, and *nd-5* from [28]) except that we used an annealing temperature of 62° rather than 60°C, were designed using Primer 3, or were recommended by Dr. Marni Falk (University of Pennsylvania: C34B2.8, D2030.4 and K09A9.5). The experiment was carried out twice for a total "n" of 3–5 except when the microarray samples were used in which case the "n" was 5–7 from 5–7 experiments. Unpublished primers were as follows: *cdc-42*, forward - 5'- GAG AAA AAT GGG TGC CTG AA-3', reverse - 5'-CTC GAG CAT TCC TGG ATC AT-3' (101 bp); pmp-3, forward - 5'- GTT CCC GTG TTC ATC ACT CAT-3', reverse - 5'- ACA CCG TCG AGA AGC TGT AGA-3' (115 bp); D2030.4, forward - 5'- GCG

AGA TGA AGG CTA CTT GG-3', reverse - 5'-GGT GCA TTT TGG GTT TGG-3' (115 bp); K09A9.5, forward - 5'-AGT CAT CAT CAA GGC CAT CC-3', reverse - 5'-TTG TTG GGA TGT CAA TAC CG-3' (185 bp); C34B2.8, forward - 5'- CTT TTC CGA AGC TTG TCT GG-3', reverse - 5'-CTT GGC CAA CAA TTT GAG C-3' (197 bp). All samples were run in duplicate or triplicate and replicates were averaged prior to analysis.

ATP assay

Steady-state ATP levels were determined by the luminescence level of the PE255 strain [20,37]. Luminescence was measured in a 96-well microplate reader (FLUOstar OPTIMA, BMG Labtech, Ortenberg, Germany) with approximately 300 nematodes per well (in 100 μl) in the visible spectral range between 300 and 600 nm (firefly luciferase typically emits at 550–570 nm). An automated dispenser delivered 50 μl of luminescence buffer to each well, consisting of citrate phosphate buffer pH 6.5, 0.1 mM D-luciferin, 1% DMSO and 0.05% triton-X (all final concentrations). Three separate experiments with 3–5 replicates total at each timepoint were conducted.

Oxygen consumption measurement

Oxygen consumption over 2 minutes was measured in PE255 nematodes in an oxygen chamber (782 Oxygen Meter, Strathkelvin Instruments, North Lanarkshire, Scotland) as described [38]. *C. elegans* were washed with K medium and counted using a nematode sorter (COPAS, Union Biometrica, Holliston, MA). Three separate experiments with 2 replicate plates per timepoint per dose each were conducted (1–4 samples per plate were measured and averaged), resulting in a total n = 4–6. Each replicate contained 1000 nematodes for the 0, 3, and 24 h time points and 500 nematodes for the 48 h time point.

Statistical analysis

All data except the microarray data were analyzed using Statview© for Windows (Version 5.0.1, SAS Institute Inc., Cary, NC). "Treatment," "time," and "experiment" were treated as independent variables in two- or three-way ANOVA analyses. When warranted based on initial ANOVA analyses, posthoc comparisons were carried out using Fisher's Protected Least Significant Differences (FPLSD) test. Since oxygen consumption and ATP levels increased dramatically during larval development, and we wished to test for proportional differences based on treatment, we log-transformed those data prior to analysis. However, non-log-transformed data were plotted to avoid obscuring the large developmental changes that occurred. A p-value of less than 0.05 was considered statistically significant. Throughout the manuscript, error bars indicate the standard error of the mean.

Results

Transcriptomic response during and 3 h after UVC exposures

We examined the transcriptomic response to a UVC exposure protocol that results in high levels of mtDNA damage but allows for repair of the nDNA damage that is also induced [15]. Since EtBr, a specific inhibitor of mtDNA replication [39], exacerbates the response of *C. elegans* to such mtDNA damage [15], we also exposed half of the nematodes to EtBr. We considered the possibility that co-exposure to EtBr and UVC would lead to increased DNA damage compared to UVC alone due to photosensitization [40,41]; however, we did not detect any difference in DNA damage with EtBr co-exposure (Additional file 1: Figure S2). In a parallel experiment, we also measured mtDNA copy number throughout the exposure. The mtDNA copy number did not change in control nematodes, nor was there a marked change in mtDNA copy

number due to UVC during the exposure (Additional file 1: Figure S2).

We sampled mRNA at 4 timepoints (3 h after the first UVC exposure or "-45 h"; 1 h prior to the second exposure or –25 h; 1 h prior to the final exposure, and 3 h after the final exposure and being placed on food: Figure 1). At each timepoint, nematodes were sampled that had been exposed to UVC, EtBr, both, or neither (controls). The "n" was 4–6 samples per timepoint per treatment, each generated from different experiments (separated in time).

Most differentially expressed transcripts (DETs) were associated with time. Three-factor ANOVA (time, UVC, EtBr with Benjamini-Hochberg correction) identified 10095 genes that showed differential expression over time, using a cut-off of $p < 0.001$ (which results in 10 differentially expressed genes expected by chance). Only 1447 DETs resulted from EtBr treatment, and 36 DETs resulted from

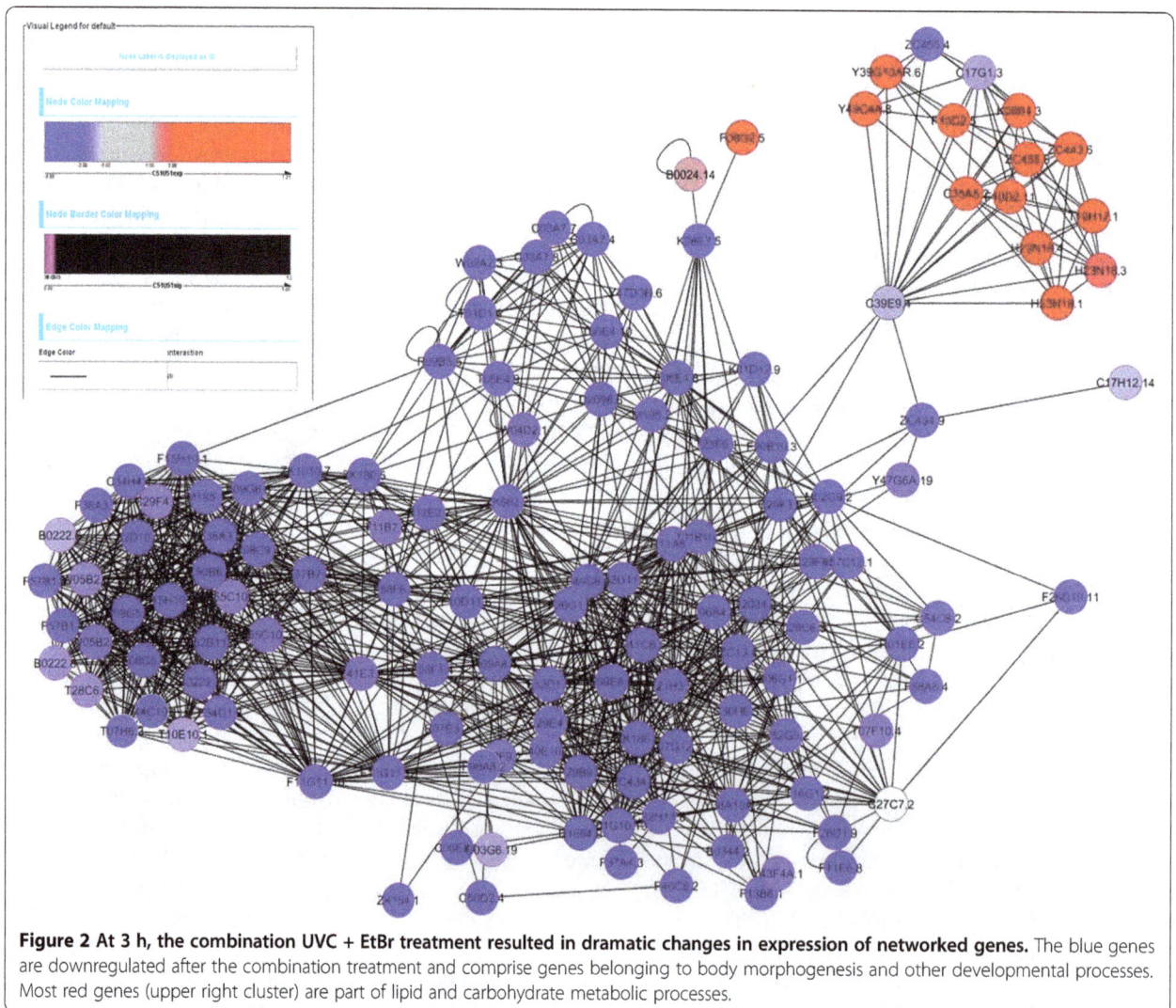

Figure 2 At 3 h, the combination UVC + EtBr treatment resulted in dramatic changes in expression of networked genes. The blue genes are downregulated after the combination treatment and comprise genes belonging to body morphogenesis and other developmental processes. Most red genes (upper right cluster) are part of lipid and carbohydrate metabolic processes.

UVC. At this cut-off only three genes demonstrated altered responses to EtBr based on time (i.e., a time x EtBr interaction), six genes demonstrated a time-dependent response to UVC, and no genes were identified for which the response to UVC was dependent on the presence of EtBr or EtBr and time. PCA results also indicated a very strong effect of time. PCA and detailed ANOVA results for the global dataset are presented in Additional file 1: Figure S3. Since we were most interested in the combined effect of prolonged inhibition of mtDNA replication and mtDNA damage, and since the presence of food is likely to alter mitochondrial function and response to stressors, we also carried out ANOVA on the 3 h timepoint samples only. However, we found no significant (p < 0.05) UVC x EtBr interactions for any genes at 3 h.

At 3 h, all three treatments resulted in many DETs associated with many developmental processes. Shown in Figure 2 is one of the most altered gene networks ("neighborhoods") identified by jActiveModules at 3 h when comparing the combination treatment to control nematodes; BiNGO-based GO enrichment analysis identified developmental processes as a top altered process. Similar GO results were obtained using GeneSpring to characterize DETs detected by ANOVA. Furthermore, the combination treatment led to greater alterations in expression of developmental genes compared to either treatment alone (e.g., Additional file 1: Figure S4). This is consistent with our previous observation of developmental delay after both treatments, which was strongest in the combination [15].

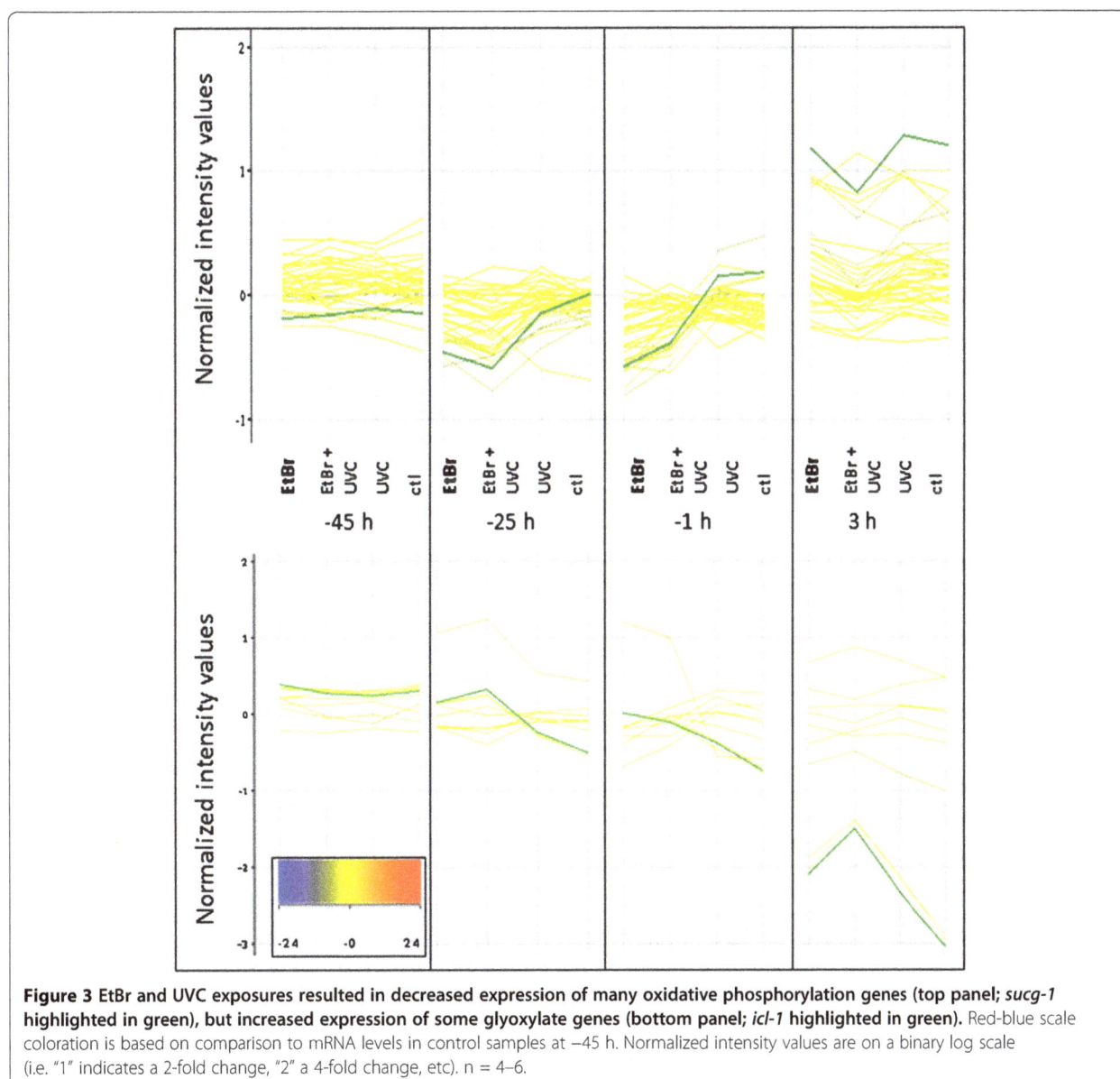

Figure 3 EtBr and UVC exposures resulted in decreased expression of many oxidative phosphorylation genes (top panel; *sucg-1* highlighted in green), but increased expression of some glyoxylate genes (bottom panel; *icl-1* highlighted in green). Red-blue scale coloration is based on comparison to mRNA levels in control samples at −45 h. Normalized intensity values are on a binary log scale (i.e. "1" indicates a 2-fold change, "2" a 4-fold change, etc). n = 4–6.

We hypothesized that persistent mtDNA damage would lead to reduced (via damage-mediated inhibition of the mitochondrial RNA polymerase) or upregulated (compensatory) expression of genes coding for mitochondrial proteins, both from the mitochondrial and nuclear genomes. Using published lists of mitochondrial genes [42], we found that at timepoints later than 3 h, some transcripts for oxidative phosphorylation decreased in the presence of EtBr, and this effect was often exacerbated by UVC (Figure 3). Furthermore, several genes in the glyoxylate pathway were induced by EtBr and EtBr + UVC at several timepoints; many of these same transcripts were also decreased in abundance across treatments at 3 h (after food addition) (Figure 3). We observed no statistically significant differences in mitochondrial-encoded transcripts (not shown), but since these are poorly represented on the platform that we used, we also carried out additional real time PCR-based analyses (see below).

Based on the role of mitochondrial fusion, fission, and autophagy in responding to UVC-induced mtDNA damage [15], we examined expression specifically of genes in these pathways. We observed a small increase in expression of some autophagy genes at −25 and −1 h, along with an inhibition of the decrease observed in many autophagy genes at 3 h, after food was available (Additional file 1: Figure S5). There was either no change or a small increase in fusion and fission genes after EtBr and EtBr +UVC, only at 3 h (Additional file 1: Figure S5).

While of less relevance for this manuscript, the transcriptomic responses to EtBr and UVC alone are interesting in their own right. The DETs (defined liberally as $p < 0.05$ and fold-change >1.2, based on Rosetta Resolver values) for each pairwise treatment comparison at each timepoint are provided in Additional file 3. The short-term (−45 h) response was stronger in terms of number of regulated genes for UVC than EtBr, but the reverse was true thereafter. This suggests that UVC led to a more robust signaling response, but EtBr altered more biological processes over time or that the response was slower due to the kinetics of uptake of EtBr. The most altered gene

ontologies observed for UVC exposure were stress response and aging. EtBr treatment alone altered expression of many development-related genes (as described earlier) but also led to a dramatic induction of many xenobiotic metabolism genes, in particular cytochrome P450s (some of which were induced 50 to 100-fold: Additional file 1: Figure S6), but also including p-glycoprotein and glutathione S-transferase genes (Additional file 3). Some xenobiotic metabolism genes, however, were down-regulated by EtBr (e.g., cyp-35A3, ugt-37, and gst-25; Additional file 3). Finally, of all DNA repair genes that we identified previously [34], only one was strongly upregulated by any treatment at any time: pme-4 (Additional file 1: Figure S7).

We next carried out additional experiments to test whether mitochondrial function was in fact altered, as suggested by the transcriptomic data, and whether the mild alterations in levels of mtDNA- and nuclear genome-encoded genes would persist to later timepoints.

mtDNA damage was persistent to the L4 stage (48 h timepoint)

Immediately (0 h) after the third UVC exposure, 2.7 ± 0.1 mitochondrial and 1.1 ± 0.1 nuclear DNA lesions per 10 kilobases were detected in larval C. elegans (Figure 4). nDNA damage dropped to 0.4 ± 0.1 at 3 h post-exposure, and to 0.0 ± 0.1 in 48 h. The mtDNA lesions, in contrast, persisted at 1.8 ± 0.2 and 0.7 ± 0.2 at 3 and 48 h, respectively. These results suggest a dilution of the UVC-induced DNA damage due to replication of the nuclear and mitochondrial genomes throughout C. elegans development, since the kinetics of photodimer removal in nuclear and mitochondrial DNA in C. elegans would not explain this rate of reduction [15,19,34].

Measurement of mtDNA and nDNA copy number throughout development

We used RT-PCR to establish a baseline of mtDNA and nDNA copy number in N2 nematodes (Table 1). As previously observed [9,28], mtDNA copy number increased

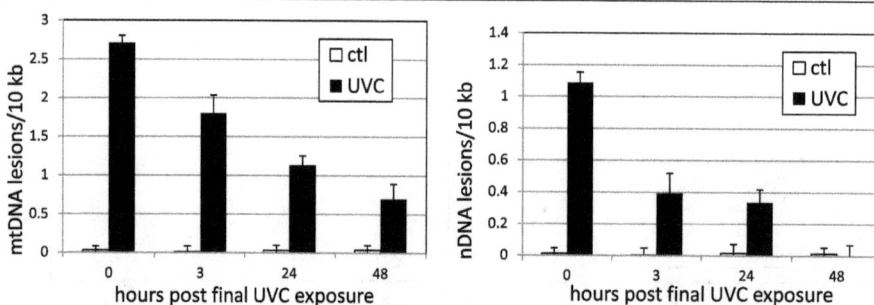

Figure 4 Exposure to UVC resulted in persistent mtDNA damage in larval C. elegans. Main effects of treatment, time, genome, and all interactions were significant ($p \le 0.0002$). At 0, 3, and 24 h after the last exposure, DNA damage was statistically significant in both genomes. At 48 h, DNA damage was detected in mtDNA ($p = 0.0009$) but not nDNA ($p = 0.82$). Note different y-axis scales. n = 4–11 in two experiments.

Table 1 Nuclear and mitochondrial DNA copy number in wildtype (N2) *C. elegans* raised ay 20 C, starting from eggs laid on k agar plates, ± standard error of the mean

Developmental stage	nDNA copy number	mtDNA copy number (x10^4)	mtDNA:nDNA ratio
Egg, 0 h (n=6)	92±36	4.12±1.30	948±498
Hatch, 13 h (n=15)	890±23	6.26±0.16	71±3
Mid-L1, 21 h (n=7)	1155±57	9.96±0.58	87±4
Mid-L2, 33.5 h (n=7)	1492±119	14.00±1.45	94±7
L2/L3, 38 h (n=8)	2000±140	20.17±1.77	101±4
Early L3, 41 h (n=8)	2856±235	29.23±2.72	103±5
Late L3, 44 h (n=8)	3242±245	38.63±3.18	119±6
L3/L4, 47 h (n=7)	3967±273	48.39±3.55	123±6
Early L4, 50.7 h (n=8)	4805±205	56.12±4.02	116±5
Late L4, 54.3 (n=12)	5552±325	73.99±7.43	131±7
L4/young adult, 58 h (n=10)	6496±228	102.77±4.81	159±8
Early young adult, 66 h (n=12)	7430±550	126.49±12.18	174±13
Late young adult, 66 h (n=11)	7737±310	123.57±12.15	157±12
Adult, 70 h (n=12)	9456±315	140.72±6.10	152±10

"0 h" refers to eggs laid within a 1 h period and immediately collected frozen. "n" indicates the number of individual eggs or nematodes lysed and separately analyzed.

significantly late in development. In contrast to those previous reports, we saw only a slight increase in mtDNA copy number in early larval stages that did not keep pace with nDNA replication, resulting in a >10-fold decrease in mtDNA:nDNA ratio from freshly laid eggs to hatched L1s. This ratio then roughly doubled by adulthood. These studies were performed on eggs laid on plates during 1 h, so that "0 h" refers to eggs frozen within 1 h of being laid. Since our subsequent experiments were carried out on nematodes that were raised from eggs that were age-synchronized via bleach-sodium hydroxide isolation of eggs and liquid hatch, we also compared mtDNA copy number after one or two days without food in M9 medium (comparable to the conditions used for the serial UVC exposure). The egg prep resulted in a decrease of ~50% in mtDNA copy number in the growth-arrested L1s, but copy number returned to normal by the L3 stage (data not shown; also compare Table 1 with Additional file 1: Figure S2).

UVC exposure affected mtDNA copy number but not nDNA copy number

Because somatic cell division and development are invariant in *C. elegans* [31], nDNA copy number serves as a proxy for developmental stage. Despite the development-related transcriptomic responses we observed and the mild developmental delay that we previously documented at this dose of serial UVC [15], we did not detect a reduction in nDNA copy number during this experiment ($p = 0.82$ for main effect of treatment, $p < 0.0001$ for main effect of time; $p = 0.37$ for interaction; Figure 5).

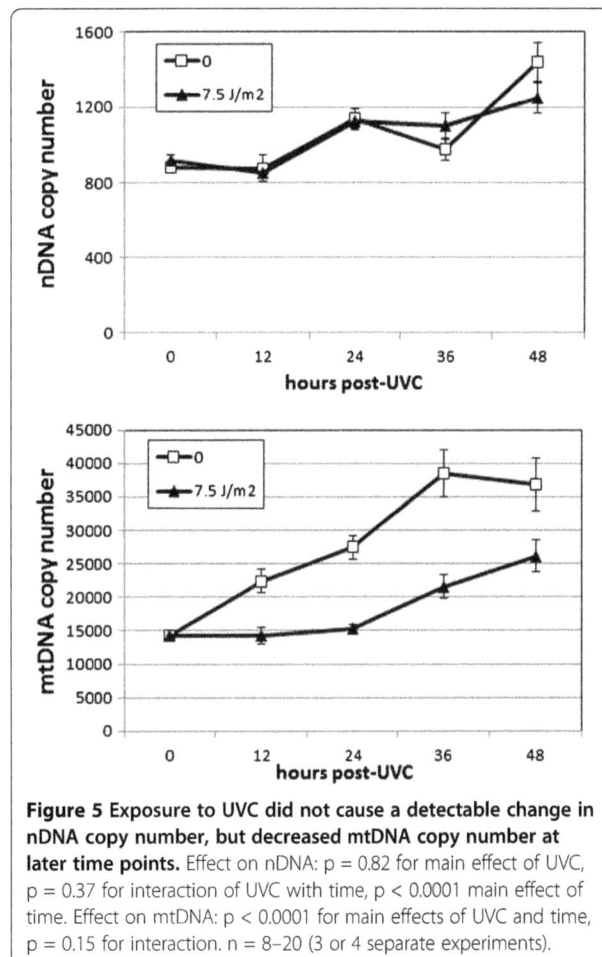

Figure 5 Exposure to UVC did not cause a detectable change in nDNA copy number, but decreased mtDNA copy number at later time points. Effect on nDNA: $p = 0.82$ for main effect of UVC, $p = 0.37$ for interaction of UVC with time, $p < 0.0001$ main effect of time. Effect on mtDNA: $p < 0.0001$ for main effects of UVC and time, $p = 0.15$ for interaction. n = 8–20 (3 or 4 separate experiments).

Nonetheless, preliminary experiments suggested that adult egg reproduction (i.e., at later timepoints) was affected by the UVC treatment.

In contrast, and as hypothesized based on the *in vitro* ability of UVC-induced photodimers to inhibit DNA polymerase γ [16], mtDNA copy number was decreased at all later timepoints (p < 0.0001 for main effects of time and treatment; p = 0.048 for interaction; timepoints past 0 h p < 0.05 UVC vs control by FPLSD; Figure 5).

These experiments were carried out in the PE255 strain, in order to permit comparison to the ATP data derived from that strain (see below). However, we observed similar results (no effect on nDNA copy number, decreased mtDNA copy number) in preliminary experiments with N2 and *glp-1* strains as well (data not shown).

UVC exposure altered expression of mtDNA- and nDNA-encoded mRNAs

We also hypothesized that UVC-induced mtDNA damage would inhibit the mitochondrial RNA polymerase [17], resulting in a decrease in mtRNAs. Because our microarray platform has few probes for mtDNA-encoded genes, we examined those samples using RT-PCR analysis. At 3 h, but not earlier, mRNA levels for the mtDNA-encoded genes *ctb-1* and *nd-5* were decreased ~50% after exposure to UVC or UV + EtBr, without a change in mRNA levels for 4 nDNA-encoded mRNAs (*C34B2.8*, *D2030.4* and *K09A9.5*, coding for ETC (Complex I) components, and *polg-1*, coding for the mitochondrial DNA polymerase γ) (Additional file 1: Figure S8). However, formal statistical comparisons of each gene at each timepoint could not be

carried out due to the lack of a significant time x treatment x gene interaction.

Next, to determine whether this change was persistent through development, we repeated the experiments and measured mRNA levels for the same genes at 0, 3, 12, 24, and 48 h post-exposure. We observed lower amounts of the mtDNA-encoded mRNAs at 0–12 h (Figure 6). However, we also detected a significant increase in mRNA levels for all of the examined transcripts at 24 and 48 h, including an 8-fold induction of *polg-1* at 48 h post-exposure (Figure 6). Finally, we replicated this experiment in the PE255 strain, with somewhat different results. In the PE255 nematodes, the mtDNA and most nDNA-encoded ETC component mRNAs were generally lower at nearly all timepoints after UVC; only *polg-1* was induced, but to a lesser extent than in the N2 nematodes (Additional file 1: Figure S9).

UVC exposure resulted in a delayed decrease in steady-state ATP level

To test if altered mtDNA and mtRNA levels were associated with altered mitochondrial energy production, we measured ATP levels *in vivo* using a well-validated [20,43] transgenic strain expressing a luciferase gene. ATP levels were similar in control and UVC-exposed nematodes until ~24 h after the UVC exposure, despite a ~50% drop in the 3 h after the nematodes were plated on food plates (Figure 7). As observed previously using traditional methods for ATP analysis [44], ATP levels increased significantly during larval development. The UVC treatment resulted in a ~50% decrease in ATP levels at 24, 36, and

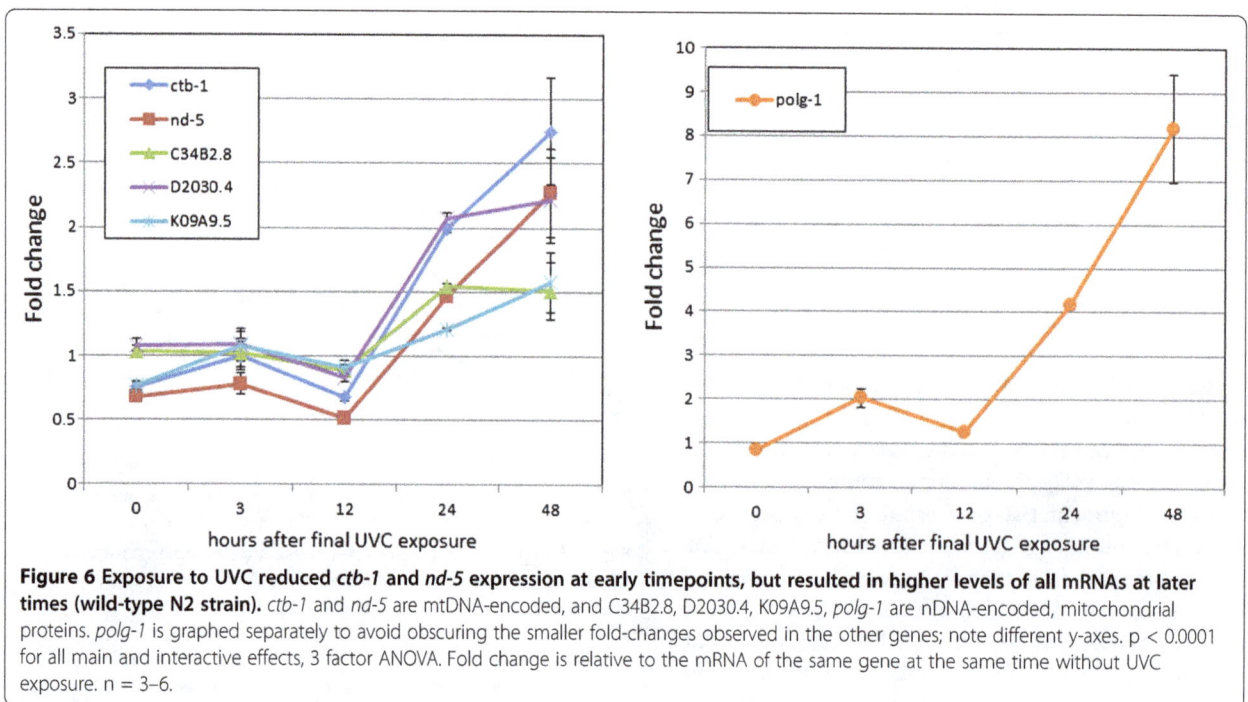

Figure 6 Exposure to UVC reduced *ctb-1* and *nd-5* expression at early timepoints, but resulted in higher levels of all mRNAs at later times (wild-type N2 strain). *ctb-1* and *nd-5* are mtDNA-encoded, and C34B2.8, D2030.4, K09A9.5, *polg-1* are nDNA-encoded, mitochondrial proteins. *polg-1* is graphed separately to avoid obscuring the smaller fold-changes observed in the other genes; note different y-axes. p < 0.0001 for all main and interactive effects, 3 factor ANOVA. Fold change is relative to the mRNA of the same gene at the same time without UVC exposure. n = 3–6.

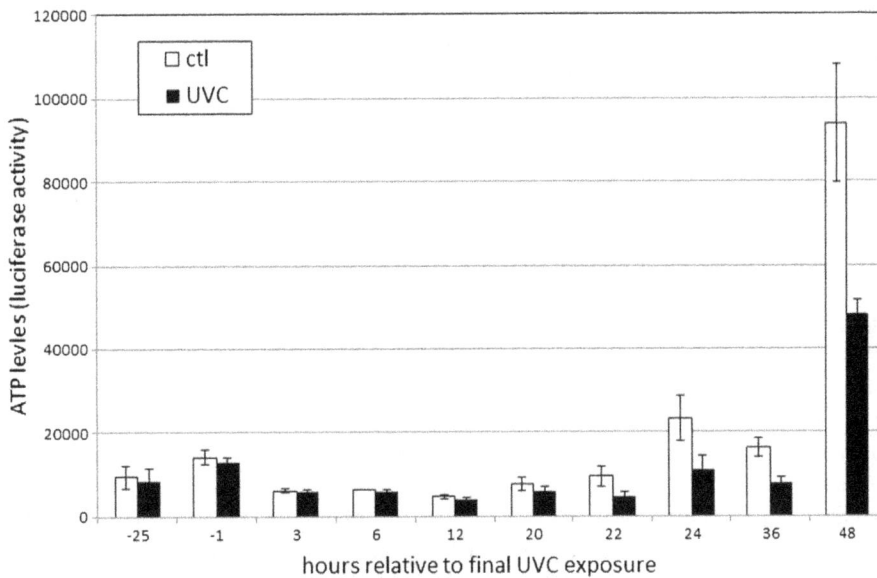

Figure 7 Exposure to UVC reduced ATP levels at later larval stages in developing *C. elegans*. The main effects of UVC and time were significant (p = 0.003 and p < 0.0001 respectively), but their interaction was not, precluding comparisons at specific timepoints. n = 5–7 separate experiments; 5 separate measurements per experiment were pooled for each "n".

48 h post-exposure, when ATP levels were rising significantly (Figure 7) (p = 0.003 and p < 0.0001 for main effects of UVC and time).

UVC exposure resulted in decreased oxygen consumption
Since ATP can also be produced anaerobically and is a function of both production and use, steady-state ATP levels are an indirect readout of oxidative phosphorylation

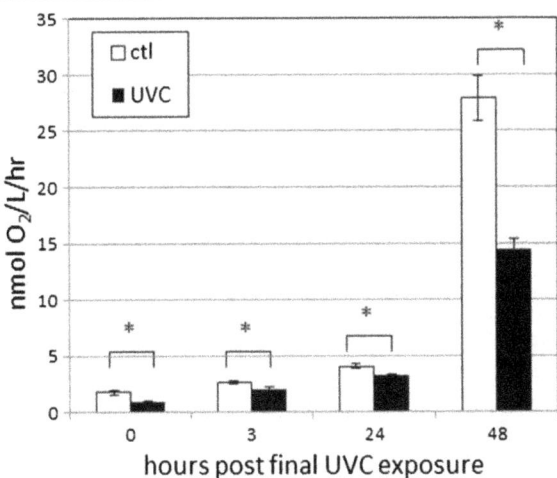

Figure 8 Exposure to UVC reduced oxygen consumption in larval *C. elegans*. n = 4–6 in 3 experiments. The effects of time and UVC and their interactions were all significant at p < 0.0001 (ANOVA); all FPLSD comparisons for the effect of UVC at individual timepoints were significant at p ≤ 0.001 (indicated by asterisks).

function. Therefore, to complement the ATP data, we also measured oxygen consumption in PE255 nematodes. Oxygen consumption, unlike ATP levels, did not drop between 0 and 3 h post-exposure (Figure 8), suggesting that the drop in ATP after addition of food resulted from a higher flux of ATP rather than an overall decrease in energy production. Consistent with previous research [44], we observed a strong increase in oxygen consumption during larval development. The UVC exposure resulted in a statistically significant (p ≤ 0.001, FPLSD) decrease in oxygen consumption at all timepoints. However, the degree of decrease varied (p < 0.0001 for time x treatment interaction, ANOVA): ~50% decrease at 0 and 48 h post-exposure, but ~20% at 3 and 24 h (Figure 8).

Discussion
Previous work has demonstrated that mtDNA damage generated by exposure to alkylating and oxidative agents can cause mitochondrial dysfunction in a cell culture system [14]. However, such damage is generally repairable in mtDNA [3,45]. In contrast, UVC-induced DNA damage is not repaired in mtDNA in *C. elegans* [19], although it can be slowly removed [15]. Here, we report on the effect of a serial UVC exposure, which results in highly persistent mtDNA damage, on genome-level transcription and mitochondrial function.

The strong overall effect of time on our transcriptomic profiles is not surprising, since the transcriptomic response to starvation in L1s is established within 6 h, and the response to food addition is established even more quickly (by 3 h) due to RNA polymerase II accumulation in the promoters of growth-related genes [46]. However, we were surprised not to observe a strong mitochondria-related transcriptomic response to serial UVC alone or in combination with the mtDNA intercalator EtBr. At the timepoints examined, the transcriptomic response to persistent mtDNA damage (from the UVC) and inhibition of mtDNA replication (from the EtBr) was mild and not very different than EtBr alone. Taken together, these results suggest that *C. elegans* lacks a way to specifically identify and respond transcriptionally to mtDNA damage, that this response is inactive at that time in development, or that any such response is very limited.

Although the transcriptomic response to EtBr by itself was quite robust, it did not include genes that are obviously related to mtDNA maintenance. Rather, the response was dominated by induction of "xenobiotic metabolism" (including cellular efflux pumps) as well as nuclear hormone receptor genes. The category of "xenobiotic metabolism," however, should be treated with caution since the actual substrate specificity of the corresponding enzymes has generally not been tested. Nonetheless, the degree of induction is remarkable, and adds to the growing literature on the ability of this nematode to transcriptionally modulate the metabolic response to xenobiotics [47-49].

UVC, EtBr, and the combination acted to inhibit development-related transcriptomic changes associated with food addition, and also altered the mRNA levels for genes involved in energy metabolism both during starvation and after food addition. This is consistent with the induction of glycolysis genes in human cells depleted of mtDNA [50]. It is also consistent with our other results that showed decreased ATP levels, oxygen consumption, and mtDNA copy number, since all of these typically increase during development. We note that we measured ATP levels and oxygen consumption only in PE255 nematodes, and the difference in UVC-induced mRNA levels indicates a need for caution in extrapolating results between PE255 and N2 nematodes. However, the developmental patterns that we observed were similar to those previously published for N2 nematodes, suggesting that overall mitochondrial function is likely similar in N2 and PE255 nematodes.

It is interesting that the observed decreases in mitochondrial function were not associated with a decrease in nDNA copy number. This suggests that development itself, as measured by cell division (which occurs according to an invariant pattern in *C. elegans*), was not significantly hindered. This conclusion is also supported by our previous observation of only a very slight delay in development at this dose of serial UVC [15]. This is surprising given the documented ability of mitochondrial dysfunction to inhibit larval development in *C. elegans* [9,51,52]. We propose two possibilities to explain this:

first, as suggested by previous work, that the developmental delay results not so much from mitochondrial dysfunction *per se*, but rather from a signaling event that presumably was not activated at this level of damage [52,53]; second, that the threshold of mitochondrial dysfunction required to hinder development was not reached. These hypotheses, as well as an exploration of effects in adults, are important areas of future research.

We hypothesized that since the DNA damage was repaired in nDNA but not mtDNA, transcription of ETC components would be imbalanced, resulting in mitochondrial dysfunction. While the decreases in mRNA levels that we observed at early times were not enormous (maximally 50%), we note that in human cells, mtRNA represents between 5% and 30% of total cellular RNA [54], suggesting that production of high levels is important. However, there was no induction of *hsp-6* and *hsp-60*, which respond to imbalance of ETC proteins [55]. This suggests the possibility of retrograde signaling that permits the organism to maintain an appropriate balance of ETC proteins. Similarly, there was not a strong transcriptomic signature indicative of oxidative stress (e.g., induction of *gst-4* or *gcs-1*: [56,57]), as might be expected if there were significant ETC dysfunction [58]. The lack of induction of these and other common general stress-response pathways also suggests that, although UVC is not entirely specific for nucleic acids, damage to other cellular macromolecules was not widespread. Overall, the relatively mild response to persistent mtDNA damage suggests that *C. elegans* has a significant ability to maintain mitochondrial function despite such damage, as we recently observed is true for primary human fibroblasts [59].

The significant induction in *polg-1* and ETC mRNAs at 24 and 48 h post-exposure may also explain in part the nematodes' ability to recover from damage, and to begin replenishing the mtDNA population by 48 h. It may be that *polg-1* was not induced at early timepoints because of the relatively low dependence on mitochondrial function exhibited by *C. elegans* at those developmental stages. That insensitivity has been previously demonstrated by studies showing that mitochondrial dysfunction results in developmental arrest at the L3 or L4 stage, not earlier [9,51,52], and that *C. elegans* lacking both copies of *polg-1* are able to survive to late larval stages and even in some cases early adulthood [28]. Similarly, the induction of ETC genes supports an adaptive response, and is consistent with the ability to tolerate and transcriptionally compensate for mtDNA depletion previously observed in HeLa cells [60].

A fuller understanding of the basic biology of mtDNA maintenance in *C. elegans* will help elucidate a more complete understanding of the replicative and transcriptional response to such damage in this organism. Mitochondrial biogenesis is an important response to mitochondrial stress or dysfunction in mammalian cells [61], and our mRNA induction data supports such a response in *C. elegans*. However, mitochondrial biogenesis *per se* has not been described in *C. elegans*. In addition, although there are many similarities with mammalian mtDNA, there are also differences. For example, TFAM has not been found in *C. elegans*—perhaps because if present, it may not have a transcriptional role, as appears to be the case in yeast [62]. It is also interesting that in *C. elegans* there are apparently no genes on the light strand, raising questions about how transcription and replication are coupled in this species, since light strand transcription is the mechanism for priming mtDNA replication in humans [63,64].

Conclusions

In summary, our results support the hypothesis that early life exposure to persistent mtDNA damage can lead to later life mitochondrial dysfunction. However, they also highlight the ability to compensate for or respond to such damage *in vivo*. Some of this capacity is likely the result of the ability to clear such damage via mitochondrial dynamics and autophagy [15]. An important direction of future research will be to investigate how deficiencies in those processes—which are observed in the human population—will affect the response to such damage.

Additional files

Additional file 1: Figure 1. The *C. elegans* mitochondrial genome, produced with Organellar GenomeDraw (Lohse et al., 2007). The blue arrow indicates the direction of transcription (Okimoto et al., 1992). mRNA levels of the two genes highlighted in purple were measured using RT-PCR. **Figure 2.** Exposure to EtBr (5 μg/mL) did not result in measureable DNA damage (measured 1 h after the third UVC exposure) in either genome, nor did it exacerbate UVC-induced DNA damage in either genome (p > 0.05 for main effect of EtBr and interaction term, 2 factor ANOVA). The exposures did not result in a marked change in mtDNA:nDNA ratio (bottom panel); time (p = 0.50), treatment (p = 0.91) and the interaction term (p = 0.89) were all statistically insignificant. Therefore, we could not make direct within-time comparisons by FPLSD. n = 4-8 per bar. **Figure 3.** Time and EtBr were the major drivers of differential gene expression by ANOVA and PCA. Even at the least stringent p-value, where 748 differentially expressed genes are expected to be identified by chance, no genes were differentially regulated in response to UVC in a way that was modulated by EtBr or EtBr and time. In the PCA (three views of same plot), the x-axis (component 1) explains 52% of variability, the y-axis 21%, and the z-axis 14%. Blue indicates -45 h, red -25 h, maroon -1 h, and grey 3 h. Diamonds indicate control samples, circles UVC, squares EtBr, and triangles UVC + EtBr. Analyses performed with GeneSpring. **Figure 4.** At 3 h, the combination treatment led to additional effects compared to EtBr alone. Development is the most-altered gene ontology; differences were also observed in transcription, protein catabolism, and organellar organization. Blue indicates higher expression in the combination than in EtBr alone. **Figure 5.** Some autophagy genes were induced by EtBr and UVC at later timepoints (top panel; *lgg-2* highlighted). No changes were observed in fusion or fission genes (bottom panel; *eat-3* highlighted). Red-blue scale coloration is based on comparison to mRNA levels in control samples at -45 h. Normalized intensity values are on a binary log scale (i.e. "1" indicates a 2-fold change, "2" a 4- fold change, ETC). n = 4-6. **Figure 6.** Many

cytochrome P450 genes were upregulated by exposure to ethidium bromide; shown are genes upregulated by EtBr and fitting the GO term "monooxygenase activity." The genes shown are *cyp-35B3* (highlighted in green), *cyp-13A7*, *cyp-35A5*, *cyp-35B1*, *cyp- 33C3*, *cyp-33C6*, *cyp-33C7*, *cyp-33D3*, *cyp-35B2*, *cyp-35A1*, *cyp-33C5*, and *cyp-33C4*. Red-blue scale coloration is based on comparison to mRNA levels in control samples at -45 h. Normalized intensity values are on a binary log scale (i.e. "1" indicates a 2-fold change, "2" a 4-fold change, ETC). n = 4-6. **Figure 7.** There is little change in expression of known DNA repair genes (from Boyd et al., 2010) either with time or treatment, with the exception of *pme-4* (highlighted). Red-blue scale coloration is based on comparison to mRNA levels in control samples at -45 h. Normalized intensity values are on a binary log scale (i.e. "1" indicates a 2-fold change, "2" a 4-fold change, ETC). n = 4-6. **Figure 8.** Effect of exposure to UVC, EtBr or both on mRNA levels for mtDNA-encoded (*ctb-1*, *nd-5*) and nDNA-encoded (C34B2.8, D2030.4, K09A9.5, *polg-1*) mitochondrial proteins. The legend is the same for all graphs. p < 0.05 for main effects of time, treatment, and genome, and genome x time interactions. Fold change is relative to the mRNA of the same gene at the same time without UVC exposure. n = 5-7 (samples derived from microarray experiment exposures, including additional samples not used for microarray). **Figure 9.** Effects of exposure to UVC in the PE255 strain. *polg-1* is graphed separately for consistency with Figure 6. *ctb-1* and *nd-5* are mtDNA-encoded, and C34B2.8, D2030.4, K09A9.5, *polg-1* are nDNA-encoded, mitochondrial proteins. The effect of UVC and gene (p = 0.016 and p < 0.0001 respectively) were significant, as was the interaction of UVC with gene (p = 0.003). No other main or interactive effects were significant (p > 0.05, 3 factor ANOVA). Comparisons at specific times could not be made due to the lack of significant interactions involving time. Gene-by-gene comparisons (across time) by FPLSD indicated that *polg-1* behaved differently than all other genes (p ≤ 0.003), and *nd-5* was distinct from K09A9.5 (p = 0.02). Fold change is relative to the mRNA of the same gene at the same time without UVC exposure n = 3-6.

Additional file 2: This file contains the "Union4" interactome described in the text (Methods section), containing 14334 nodes and 346484 edges. It is in the Cytoscape-compatible .sif file format.

Additional file 3: This file contains differentially expressed transcripts (defined as fold-change >1.2, p < 0.05 based on Rosetta Resolver analysis) for all pairwise treatment comparisons at the 3 h timepoint.

Competing interests
The authors declare that they have no competing interests.

Authors' contributions
MCKL, JPR, ITR, ASB, and AQJ carried out measurements of mtDNA damage, mtDNA and nDNA copy number, mRNA levels by RT-PCR, oxygen consumption, and ATP levels. AJB and TLC carried out microarray experiments. MCKL, JPR and JNM participated in study design and coordination; MCKL and JNM drafted the manuscript. All authors read and approved the final manuscript.

Acknowledgements
We thank Marni Falk for primer information, Alexandra Trifunovic for a plasmid-based mtDNA copy number standard curve, and Bernard Lemire for advice regarding oxygen consumption measurement. We thank Margaret Gustafson, Shawn Ahmed, and Jonathan Freedman for their advice and assistance in this study. This work was funded by NIEHS and NINDS (1P30 ES011961, 1R01-ES017540, and 1R21 NS065468 to JNM), the Society of Toxicology (Colgate-Palmolive Awards for Student Research Training in Alternative Methods to MCKL); American Foundation of Aging Research (GlaxoSmithKline Foundation Award to MCKL).

References
1. Schmidt CW: **Mito-conundrum unraveling environmental effects on mitochondria.** *Environ Heal Perspect* 2010, **118:**A292–A297.

2. Shaughnessy DT, Worth L, Lawler CP, McAllister KA, Longley MJ, Copeland WC: **Meeting report: Identification of biomarkers for early detection of mitochondrial dysfunction.** *Mitochondrion* 2010, 10:579–581.

3. Larsen NB, Rasmussen M, Rasmussen LJ: **Nuclear and mitochondrial DNA repair: similar pathways?** *Mitochondrion* 2005, 5:89–108.

4. Cohen BH: **Pharmacologic effects on mitochondrial function.** *Dev Disabil Res Rev* 2010, 16:189–199.

5. Gomez C, Bandez MJ, Navarro A: **Pesticides and impairment of mitochondrial function in relation with the parkinsonian syndrome.** *Front Biosci* 2007, 12:1079–1093.

6. Benhammou V, Tardieu M, Warszawski J, Rustin P, Blanche S: **Clinical mitochondrial dysfunction in uninfected children born to HIV-infected mothers following perinatal exposure to nucleoside analogues.** *Environ Mol Mutagen* 2007, 48:173–178.

7. Tsang WY, Lemire BD: **The role of mitochondria in the life of the nematode, *Caenorhabditis elegans*.** *Biochim Biophys Acta* 2003, 1638:91–105.

8. Breton S, Stewart DT, Hoeh WR: **Characterization of a mitochondrial ORF from the gender-associated mtDNAs of *Mytilus* spp. (Bivalvia: Mytilidae): Identification of the "missing" ATPase 8 gene.** *Mar Genom* 2010, 3:11–18.

9. Tsang WY, Lemire BD: **Mitochondrial genome content is regulated during nematode development.** *Biochem Biophys Res Commun* 2002, 291:8–16.

10. Braeckman BP, Houthoofd K, Vanfleteren JR: **Intermediary metabolism.** *WormBook* 2009,

11. May-Panloup P, Chretien MF, Malthiery Y, Reynier P: **Mitochondrial DNA in the oocyte and the developing embryo.** *Curr Top Dev Biol* 2007, 77:51–83.

12. Shoubridge EA: **Mitochondrial DNA segregation in the developing embryo.** *Hum Reprod* 2000, 15(Suppl 2):229–234.

13. Leung MC-K, Williams PL, Benedetto A, Au C, Helmke KJ, Aschner M, Meyer JN: ***Caenorhabditis elegans*: an emerging model in biomedical and environmental toxicology.** *Toxicol Sci* 2008, 106:5–28.

14. Furda AM, Marrangoni AM, Lokshin A, Van Houten B: **Oxidants and not alkylating agents induce rapid mtDNA loss and mitochondrial dysfunction.** *DNA Repair (Amst)* 2012, 11:684–692.

15. Bess AS, Crocker TL, Ryde IT, Meyer JN: **Mitochondrial dynamics and autophagy aid in removal of persistent mitochondrial DNA damage in *Caenorhabditis elegans*.** *Nucleic Acids Res* 2012, 40:7916–7931.

16. Kasiviswanathan R, Gustafson MA, Copeland WC, Meyer JN: **Human mitochondrial DNA polymerase gamma exhibits potential for bypass and mutagenesis at UV-induced cyclobutane thymine dimers.** *J Biol Chem* 2012, 287:9222–9229.

17. Cline SD: **Mitochondrial DNA damage and its consequences for mitochondrial gene expression.** *Biochim Biophys Acta* 2012, 1819:979–991.

18. Lewis JA, Fleming JT: **Basic Culture Methods.** In *Caenorhabditis elegans: Modern Biological Analysis of an Organism.* Edited by Epstein HF, Shakes DC. San Digo, CA: Academic Press; 1995:3–29.

19. Meyer JN, Boyd WA, Azzam GA, Haugen AC, Freedman JH, Van Houten B: **Decline of nucleotide excision repair capacity in aging *Caenorhabditis elegans*.** *Genome Biol* 2007, 8:R70.

20. Lagido C, Pettitt J, Flett A, Glover LA: **Bridging the phenotypic gap: real-time assessment of mitochondrial function and metabolism of the nematode *Caenorhabditis elegans*.** *BMC Physiol* 2008, 8:7.

21. Simonis N, Rual JF, Carvunis AR, Tasan M, Lemmens I, Hirozane-Kishikawa T, Hao T, Sahalie JM, Venkatesan K, Gebreab F, *et al:* **Empirically controlled mapping of the *Caenorhabditis elegans* protein-protein interactome network.** *Nat Methods* 2009, 6:47–54.

22. Alfarano C, Andrade CE, Anthony K, Bahroos N, Bajec M, Bantoft K, Betel D, Bobechko B, Boutilier K, Burgess E, *et al:* **The biomolecular interaction network database and related tools 2005 update.** *Nucleic Acids Res* 2005, 33:D418–424.

23. Zhong W, Sternberg PW: **Genome-wide prediction of C. elegans genetic interactions.** *Science* 2006, 311:1481–1484.

24. Lee I, Lehner B, Crombie C, Wong W, Fraser AG, Marcotte EM: **A single gene network accurately predicts phenotypic effects of gene perturbation in *Caenorhabditis elegans*.** *Nat Genet* 2008, 40:181–188.

25. Alexeyenko A, Sonnhammer EL: **Global networks of functional coupling in eukaryotes from comprehensive data integration.** *Genome Res* 2009, 19:1107–1116.

26. Ideker T, Ozier O, Schwikowski B, Siegel AF: **Discovering regulatory and signalling circuits in molecular interaction networks.** *Bioinformatics* 2002, 18(Suppl 1):S233–240.

27. Maere S, Heymans K, Kuiper M: **BiNGO: a Cytoscape plugin to assess overrepresentation of gene ontology categories in biological networks.** *Bioinformatics* 2005, 21:3448–3449.

28. Bratic I, Hench J, Henriksson J, Antebi A, Burglin TR, Trifunovic A: **Mitochondrial DNA level, but not active replicase, is essential for *Caenorhabditis elegans* development.** *Nucleic Acids Res* 2009, 37:1817–1828.

29. Rozen S, Skaletsky H: **Primer3 on the WWW for general users and for biologist programmers.** *Methods Mol Biol* 2000, 132:365–386.

30. Kodoyianni V, Maine EM, Kimble J: **Molecular basis of loss-of-function mutations in the glp-1 gene of *Caenorhabitis elegans*.** *Mol Biol Cell* 1992, 3:1199–1213.

31. Sulston J: **Cell Lineage.** In *The Nematode Caenorhabditis elegans.* Edited by Wood WB. Cold Spring Harbor, NY: Cold Spring Harbor Laboratory Press; 1988:123–155.

32. Golden TR, Beckman KB, Lee AH, Dudek N, Hubbard A, Samper E, Melov S: **Dramatic age-related changes in nuclear and genome copy number in the nematode *Caenorhabditis elegans*.** *Aging Cell* 2007, 6:179–188.

33. Emmons SW: **The Genome.** In *The Nematode Caenorhabditis elegans.* Edited by Wood WB. Cold Spring Harbor, NY: Cold Spring Harbor Laboratory Press; 1988:47–79.

34. Boyd WA, Crocker TL, Rodriguez AM, Leung MC, Lehmann DW, Freedman JH, Van Houten B, Meyer JN: **Nucleotide excision repair genes are expressed at low levels and are not detectably inducible in *Caenorhabditis elegans* somatic tissues, but their function is required for normal adult life after UVC exposure.** *Mutat Res* 2010, 683:57–67.

35. Hunter S, Jung D, Di Giulio R, Meyer J: **The QPCR assay for analysis of mitochondrial DNA damage, repair, and relative copy number.** *Methods* 2010, 51:444–451.

36. Hoogewijs D, Houthoofd K, Matthijssens F, Vandesompele J, Vanfleteren JR: **Selection and validation of a set of reliable reference genes for quantitative sod gene expression analysis in C. elegans.** *BMC Mol Biol* 2008, 9:9.

37. McLaggan D, Amezaga MR, Petra E, Frost A, Duff EI, Rhind SM, Fowler PA, Glover LA, Lagido C: **Impact of sublethal levels of environmental pollutants found in sewage sluge on a novel *Caenorhabditis elegans* model biosensor.** *PLoS One* 2012, 7(10):e46503.

38. Grad LI, Sayles LC, Lemire BD: **Isolation and functional analysis of mitochondria from the nematode Caenorhabditis elegans.** *Methods Mol Biol* 2007, 372:51–66.

39. Gaines G, Attardi G: **Intercalating drugs and low temperatures inhibit synthesis and processing of ribosomal RNA in isolated human mitochondria.** *J Mol Biol* 1984, 172:451–466.

40. Hall DB, Kelley SO, Barton JK: **Long-range and short-range oxidative damage to DNA: photoinduced damage to guanines in ethidium-DNA assemblies.** *Biochemistry* 1998, 37:15933–15940.

41. Kurbanyan K, Nguyen KL, To P, Rivas EV, Lueras AM, Kosinski C, Steryo M, Gonzalez A, Mah DA, Stemp ED: **DNA-protein cross-linking via guanine oxidation: dependence upon protein and photosensitizer.** *Biochemistry* 2003, 42:10269–10281.

42. Ichishita R, Tanaka K, Sugiura Y, Sayano T, Mihara K, Oka T: **An RNAi screen for mitochondrial proteins required to maintain the morphology of the organelle in *Caenorhabditis elegans*.** *J Biochem* 2008, 143:449–454.

43. Lagido C, McLaggan D, Flett A, Pettitt J, Glover LA: **Rapid sublethal toxicity assessment using bioluminescent *Caenorhabditis elegans*, a novel whole-animal metabolic biosensor.** *Toxicol Sci* 2009, 109:88–95.

44. Houthoofd K, Braeckman BP, Lenaerts I, Brys K, De Vreese A, Van Eygen S, Vanfleteren JR: **Ageing is reversed, and metabolism is reset to young levels in recovering dauer larvae of C. elegans.** *Exp Gerontol* 2002, 37:1015–1021.

45. Hunter SE, Gustafson MA, Margillo KM, Lee SA, Ryde IT, Meyer JN: **In vivo repair of alkylating and oxidative DNA damage in the mitochondrial and nuclear genomes of wild-type and glycosylase-deficient *Caenorhabditis elegans*.** *DNA Repair (Amst)* 2012, 11:857–863.

46. Baugh LR, Demodena J, Sternberg PW: **RNA Pol II accumulates at promoters of growth genes during developmental arrest.** *Science* 2009, 324:92–94.

47. Menzel R, Bogaert T, Achazi R: **A systematic gene expression screen of *Caenorhabditis elegans* cytochrome P450 genes reveals CYP35 as strongly xenobiotic inducible.** *Arch Biochem Biophys* 2001, 395:158–168.

48. Menzel R, Rodel M, Kulas J, Steinberg CE: **CYP35: xenobiotically induced gene expression in the nematode *Caenorhabditis elegans*.** *Arch Biochem Biophys* 2005, 438:93–102.

49. Lindblom TH, Dodd AK: **Xenobiotic detoxification in the nematode *Caenorhabditis elegans*.** *J Exp Zool* 2006, 305:720–730.

50. Behan A, Doyle S, Farrell M: Adaptive responses to mitochondrial dysfunction in the rho degrees Namalwa cell. *Mitochondrion* 2005, **5**:173–193.

51. Tsang WY, Sayles LC, Grad LI, Pilgrim DB, Lemire BD: Mitochondrial respiratory chain deficiency in *Caenorhabditis elegans* results in developmental arrest and increased life span. *J Biol Chem* 2001, **276**:32240–32246.

52. Ventura N, Rea SL, Schiavi A, Torgovnick A, Testi R, Johnson TE: p53/CEP-1 increases or decreases lifespan, depending on level of mitochondrial bioenergetic stress. *Aging Cell* 2009, **8**:380–393.

53. Torgovnick A, Schiavi A, Testi R, Ventura N: A role for p53 in mitochondrial stress response control of longevity in C. elegans. *Exp Gerontol* 2010, **45**:550–557.

54. Mercer TR, Neph S, Dinger ME, Crawford J, Smith MA, Shearwood AM, Haugen E, Bracken CP, Rackham O, Stamatoyannopoulos JA, *et al*: The human mitochondrial transcriptome. *Cell* 2011, **146**:645–658.

55. Durieux J, Wolff S, Dillin A: The cell-non-autonomous nature of electron transport chain-mediated longevity. *Cell* 2011, **144**:79–91.

56. An JH, Blackwell TK: SKN-1 links C. elegans mesendodermal specification to a conserved oxidative stress response. *Genes Dev* 2003, **17**:1882–1893.

57. Kahn NW, Rea SL, Moyle S, Kell A, Johnson TE: Proteasomal dysfunction activates the transcription factor SKN-1 and produces a selective oxidative-stress response in *Caenorhabditis elegans*. *Biochem J* 2008, **409**:205–213.

58. Dingley S, Polyak E, Lightfoot R, Ostrovsky J, Rao M, Greco T, Ischiropoulos H, Falk MJ: Mitochondrial respiratory chain dysfunction variably increases oxidant stress in *Caenorhabditis elegans*. *Mitochondrion* 2010, **10**:125–136.

59. Bess AS, Ryde IT, Hinton DE, Meyer JN: UVC-induced mitochondrial degradation via autophagy correlates with mtDNA damage removal in primary human fibroblasts. *J Biochem Mol Toxicol*. 2013, **27**:28–41.

60. Piechota J, Szczesny R, Wolanin K, Chlebowski A, Bartnik E: Nuclear and mitochondrial genome responses in HeLa cells treated with inhibitors of mitochondrial DNA expression. *Acta Biochim Pol* 2006, **53**:485–495.

61. Scarpulla RC: Nucleus-encoded regulators of mitochondrial function: Integration of respiratory chain expression, nutrient sensing and metabolic stress. *Biochim Biophys Acta* 2012, **1819**:1088–1097.

62. Shutt TE, Lodeiro MF, Cotney J, Cameron CE, Shadel GS: Core human mitochondrial transcription apparatus is a regulated two-component system in vitro. *Proc Natl Acad Sci USA* 2010, **107**:12133–12138.

63. Chang DD, Clayton DA: Priming of human mitochondrial DNA replication occurs at the light-strand promoter. *Proc Natl Acad Sci USA* 1985, **82**:351–355.

64. Kasiviswanathan R, Collins TR, Copeland WC: The interface of transcription and DNA replication in the mitochondria. *Biochim Biophys Acta* 2012, **1819**:970–978.

17

Maternal cadmium, iron and zinc levels, DNA methylation and birth weight

Adriana C. Vidal[1], Viktoriya Semenova[2,3], Thomas Darrah[4], Avner Vengosh[5], Zhiqing Huang[6], Katherine King[7,11], Monica D. Nye[6,8], Rebecca Fry[9], David Skaar[2], Rachel Maguire[2], Amy Murtha[10], Joellen Schildkraut[11], Susan Murphy[6] and Cathrine Hoyo[2]*

Abstract

Background: Cadmium (Cd) is a ubiquitous and environmentally persistent toxic metal that has been implicated in neurotoxicity, carcinogenesis and obesity and essential metals including zinc (Zn) and iron (Fe) may alter these outcomes. However mechanisms underlying these relationships remain limited.

Methods: We examined whether maternal Cd levels during early pregnancy were associated with offspring DNA methylation at regulatory sequences of genomically imprinted genes and weight at birth, and whether Fe and Zn altered these associations. Cd, Fe and Zn were measured in maternal blood of 319 women ≤12 weeks gestation. Offspring umbilical cord blood leukocyte DNA methylation at regulatory differentially methylated regions (DMRs) of 8 imprinted genes was measured using bisulfite pyrosequencing. Regression models were used to examine the relationships among Cd, Fe, Zn, and DMR methylation and birth weight.

Results: Elevated maternal blood Cd levels were associated with lower birth weight ($p = 0.03$). Higher maternal blood Cd levels were also associated with lower offspring methylation at the *PEG3* DMR in females ($\beta = 0.55$, se $= 0.17$, $p = 0.05$), and at the *MEG3* DMR in males ($\beta = 0.72$, se $= 0.3$, $p = 0.08$), however the latter association was not statistically significant. Associations between Cd and *PEG3* and *PLAGL1* DNA methylation were stronger in infants born to women with low concentrations of Fe ($p < 0.05$).

Conclusions: Our data suggest the association between pre-natal Cd and offspring DNA methylation at regulatory sequences of imprinted genes may be sex- and gene-specific. Essential metals such as Zn may mitigate DNA methylation response to Cd exposure. Larger studies are required.

Keywords: Cadmium, Zinc, Genomic imprinting, Epigenetics, Pediatrics, Obesity

Background

Cadmium (Cd) is a naturally occurring toxic group IIb transition metal that is ubiquitous in the earth's crust. Increased anthropogenic utilization of Cd in the last several decades has led to increased human exposure at high doses; exposure vectors are wide ranging, including waste and emissions from mining, smelting, industrial activities, sewage sludge, tobacco smoking and fruit and vegetables contaminated by the use of phosphate fertilizers in agriculture [1]. Cd is a nephrotoxin, neurotoxicant, osteotoxicant, and carcinogen [2]. Cellular effects include apoptosis, DNA fragmentation and chromatin structural changes. Cd exposure has also been implicated in the etiology of fetal growth restriction [1, 3–5].

Zinc (Zn), and iron (Fe) are essential metals found in wheat, seeds, beans, seafood, and red meats as well as dietary supplements, and over-the-counter drugs [6]. Because Zn and Fe are co-factor for numerous enzymes involved in nucleic acid synthesis and repair, they play a significant role in growth, development, and cellular functions [7, 8]. Animal and cross-sectional human data suggest that at moderate levels, Zn and Fe may mitigate Cd effects via trans-metallation processes; however empirical data remain limited in human.

In vitro and *in vivo* studies demonstrated that exposure to Cd modifies DNA methylation patterns [9–12],

* Correspondence: choyo@ncsu.edu
2Department of Biological Sciences, Center for Human Health and the Environment, North Carolina State University, Raleigh, NC 27695, USA
Full list of author information is available at the end of the article

although specific targets remain largely unknown. In humans, epigenetic targets for Cd exposure identified from unbiased approaches lack specificity, and the malleability of these epigenetic marks remains unknown. Moreover, although the timing of exposure during the life course is critical in determining severity of effects following exposure, human data is primarily from cross-sectional studies and reports in adults.

Parental allele-specific differentially methylated regions (DMRs) of imprinted genes are established in the gametes and in the early embryo, and are generally stable in tissues from all germ layers. Perturbations in the establishment or maintenance of these DMRs during early embryogenesis can result in systemic variability that may be detected in nearly any tissue [13, 14]. Aberrant methylation at some imprint regulatory regions has been associated with lower birth weight [15].

In the present analysis, we examine the association between levels of Zn, Fe and Cd in pregnant women and DNA methylation at imprinted regulatory DMRs in umbilical cord blood shown to be important in fetal growth and development or associated with other toxic metals including the *H19* DMR regulating the *IGF2/H19* domain, the *MEG3* DMR regulating the *MEG3* domain, the *SGCE/PEG10* DMR positioned between *Epsilon Sarcoglycan and Paternally Expressed Gene 10*, the *NNAT, MEST and PEG*. We hypothesized Cd exposure in utero alters offspring DNA methylation levels in the DMRs regulating genomically imprinted *NNAT, MEST, PEG3, PLAGL1, PEG10, IGF2, H19*, and *MEG3* DMRs and that maternal Zn and Fe levels alter these associations.

Methods

Study participants

Study participants were pregnant women who were enrolled as part of the Newborn Epigenetic STudy (NEST), a prospective cohort study of women and their offspring with the overarching goal of investigating the effects of *in utero* exposures on epigenetic profiles and phenotypes in children. Between 2009 and 2011, pregnant women were recruited from five prenatal clinics and obstetric care facilities at Duke University and Durham Regional Hospitals. Details of participant accrual have been previously described [16, 17]. Eligibility criteria were age 18 years or older, pregnant and intending to use one of two participating obstetric facilities in Durham County for delivery. Excluded were women who planned to relinquish custody of the index child, move states in the subsequent 3 years, or had an established HIV infection. In the 18-month period between April, 2009 and 2011, 2,548 women were approached and 1,700 consented (66.7 % response rate). The present analyses are limited to the first 319 infant-mother pairs for whom maternal

Zn, Fe and Cd blood levels and infant DNA methylation were measured. Maternal race, smoking status, BMI before pregnancy, parity, delivery route, and education were comparable in the 319 infant-mother pairs included in this study and the remainder of the cohort (p > 0.05). The study protocol was approved by the Institutional Review Boards of Duke and North Carolina State Universities.

Data and specimen collection

Participants completed a self-administered questionnaire at the time of enrollment that included social and demographic characteristics, reproductive history, lifestyle factors, and anthropometric measurements. At study enrollment, maternal peripheral blood samples were collected; the mean gestational age at maternal blood draw was 12 weeks. Infant cord blood specimens were collected at birth. The leukocyte-containing buffy coat was isolated following centrifugation at $3500 \times g$ for 20 min at 4 °C. Aliquots were prepared and stored at -80 °C.

DNA methylation analysis

Genomic DNA from buffy coat from umbilical cord blood specimens was extracted using PureGene reagents (Qiagen; Valencia, CA) and treated with sodium bisulfite using the Zymo EZ DNA Methylation Kit (Zymo Research, Irvine, CA). Bisulfite treatment modifies the DNA by converting unmethylated cytosines to uracils but leaves methylated cytosines unchanged. Pyrosequencing was performed using a Qiagen Pyromark Q96 MD Pyrosequencer. Primers and PCR conditions have been previously described [18, 19]. The percent methylation for each CG dinucleotide was calculated using PyroQ CpG Software (Qiagen). The percent methylation was analyzed at multiple CpG sites for nine imprinted gene DMRs, including the maternally methylated *NNAT, MEST, PEG3, PLAGL1, PEG10* DMRs and the paternally methylated *IGF2, H19*, and *MEG3* DMRs.

Measurement of Cd, Fe and Zn

Maternal Zn, Fe and Cd blood levels were measured in whole blood as nanograms per gram (ng/g; 1000 ng/g = 1025 ng/µl) using well-established solution-based ICP-MS methods [20–23]. Frozen maternal blood samples were equilibrated at room temperature, homogenized with a GlobalSpec laboratory slow shaker (GlobalSpec, East Greenbrush, NY) and ~0.2 mL aliquots were pipetted into a trace-metal-clean test tube and verified gravimetrically to ±0.001 mg using a calibrated mass balance. Samples were then spiked with internal standards consisting of known quantities (10 and 1 ng/g, respectively) of indium (In) and bismuth (Bi) (obtained from SCP Science), used to correct for instrumental drift. The solutions were then diluted using water purified to 18.2 MΩ/cm resistance (by a Milli-Q water purification system, Millipore, Bedford, Mass., USA) and acidified using ultra-pure 12.4 mol/L hydrochloric acid to result in a final concentration of 2 % hydrochloric acid (by volume). All standards, including aliquots of the certified NIST 955c, and procedural blanks were prepared by the same process.

Zn, Fe and Cd concentrations were measured using a Perkin Elmer DRC II (Dynamic Reaction Cell) axial field ICP-MS at the University of Massachusetts-Boston [20–23]. To clean sample lines and reduce memory effects, sample lines were sequentially washed with 18.2 MΩ cm resistance (by a Milli-Q water purification system, Millipore, Bedford, Mass., USA) water for 90 s and a 2 % nitric acid solution for 120 s between analyses. Procedural blanks were analyzed within each block of 10 samples, to monitor and correct for instrumental and procedural backgrounds. Calibration standards used to determine Zn and Cd in blood included aliquots of 18.2 MΩ cm resistance H_2O, NIST 955c SRM, and NIST 955c SRM spiked with known quantities of each metal in a linear range from 0.025 to 10 ng/g. Standards were prepared from 1000 mg/L single element standards obtained from SCP Science, USA. Method detection limits were calculated according to the two-step approach using the $t_{99}S_{LLMV}$ method (USEPA, 1993) at 99 % CI (t = 3.71). The MDLs for Zn and Cd yielded values of 278 and 83 pg/g parts per trillion, respectively. Limits of detection (LOD) and limits of quantification (LOQ) according to Long and Winefordner (1983) were less than ~43 pg/g and 129 pg/g for Zn, respectively and less than ~17 pg/g and 51 pg/g for Cd, respectively.

Measurement of folate
Maternal whole blood samples were sent to Craft Technologies (Wilson, NC, USA) for measurement of erythrocyte folate using a commercial kit, ID-Vit Folic acid (Immundiagnostic-ALPCO; Salem, NH, Ref KIF005) which uses the folate dependent strain *Lactobacillus rhamnosus* (taxon id 47715) in a 96 well format.

Statistical analyses
Covariates considered for confounded were race/ethnicity (White, African American, Hispanic, and other), and parity (nulliparous and multiparous), physical activity (≥3 days per week, yes/no), and maternal smoking (yes, no, and quit during pregnancy). Maternal Zn, Fe and Cd blood levels were natural log transformed to achieve a normal distribution. Since at moderate levels, Zn and Fe have been shown to interact with Cd and to mitigate cellular, epigenetic and phenotypic effects in vivo and in vitro [9, 11, 24, 25], we explored these potential effects

by categorizing Zn and Fe into high (top tertile) and low (bottom two tertiles) levels. We then modeled blood Cd on DMR methylation restricted to those with high and low levels of Fe or Zn. Factors evaluated for confounding were maternal age at delivery (less than 30 years, 30–39 years, and older than 40 years), the mother's educational achievement (high school graduate/less and college/beyond), household income (less than $24,999, $25,000–$49,999, $50,000–$100,000, and more than $100,000 per year), and BMI (kg/m^2, normal <25, overweight 25–30, obese 30–35, and extremely obese >35) calculated from self-reported maternal weight before pregnancy at last menstrual period and measured height at the study visit. Pre-pregnancy weight was verified with the hospital medical charts. The accuracy of retrospectively capturing weight was evaluated by abstracting weight from medical records of 237 cohort members who visited a Duke clinic within 6 months of their first prenatal visit for the pregnancy that made them eligible for the study, including a subset of 43 had visited within three months of their first prenatal clinic visit. The correlation between periconceptional self-reported and nurse-measured weight was 0.95 in the 237 and 0.98 in the 43 participants, ($p <$ 0.0001). Parturition data examined included gestational age (preterm <258 days and term >259 days), delivery route (vaginal and C-Section) and birth weight (in grams). Given that maternal erythrocyte folate levels can affect DNA methylation, we used measurements of folate using methods previously described [15] based on a published protocol [26]. Since childhood obesity may vary by ethnicity/race, pre-pregnancy obesity, and sex, we also explored the potential for effect modification of the associations between Cd and DNA methylations and obesity in early childhood in African Americans, Hispanics and Whites. Final models were adjusted for maternal race, maternal smoking status, erythrocyte folate levels, parity, prenatal physical activity, infant sex and maternal pre-pregnancy BMI. All statistical analyses were conducted in Stata Version 13.0 (Stata Corp, 2013) using the xtmixed function, and findings were replicated in SAS. These analyses were repeated using logistic regression models where DNA methylation was dichotomized at the 4th quartile, and weight at birth and age one year were categorized at <2500, 2500–4000 and >4000 g and <85th, 85-< 95th, and >95th percentile, respectively, and findings were comparable.

Results
Cd and socio-demographic characteristics
Maternal Cd levels did not vary by maternal age, pre-pregnancy obesity, gestational age at delivery, or by sex and birth weight of offspring. However, Cd levels were somewhat higher among Hispanic and African American women compared to White women ($p = 0.03$) (Table 1).

Cd blood concentrations were also higher among smoking mothers compared to nonsmoking mothers ($p = 0.01$), and were higher in women who delivered vaginally, compared to C-section deliveries ($p = 0.02$). These factors were accounted for in multivariable analysis.

Maternal Cd exposure and newborn DMR methylation

We evaluated the association between maternal Cd levels and DNA methylation at 9 differentially methylated regions of genomically imprinted genes in the offspring. We found a significant association between maternal Cd concentrations and altered methylation at the DMR regulating

Table 1 Distribution of maternal blood cadmium concentrations (ng/g) ($n = 319$)

Characteristic	Number	Mean	SD	p-value
Child Gender				0.73
Male	164	4.43	(6.66)	
Female	155	4.65	(5.53)	
Gestation Time				0.12
Preterm (<37 weeks)	39	3.07	(4.70)	
Normal(≥37 weeks)	280	4.74	(6.28)	
Birth Weight				0.61
Low Birth Weight (<2500)	31	4.67	(5.93)	
Normal Birth Weight(2500- < 4600)	281	4.58	(6.22)	
High Birth Weight (>4600)	5	1.84	(1.40)	
Maternal Age				0.35
Less than 30	187	4.93	(6.24)	
30-39	125	3.96	(6.08)	
40+	7	4.28	(2.94)	
Maternal Race				0.03
African American	111	4.71	(4.65)	
White	95	3.13	(5.07)	
Hispanic	101	5.44	(7.63)	
Other	12	6.48	(9.51)	
Maternal BMI				0.48
Less than 18.5	9	5.39	(7.46)	
18.5 to less than 25	111	4.20	(5.83)	
25 to less than 30	78	4.88	(5.90)	
30 to less than 35	39	2.95	(3.55)	
35+	29	3.87	(4.25)	
Maternal Smoking Status				0.01
Smoking Prior to Pregnancy	39	2.56	(3.13)	
Smoking During Pregnancy	46	6.44	(4.79)	
Never Smoke	225	4.42	(6.59)	
Delivery Route				0.02
Vaginal	198	5.16	(6.72)	
Cesarean section	120	3.50	(4.88)	

PEG3 ($\beta = 0.36$, se = 0.17 $p = 0.03$). We also found associations of borderline significance between maternal Cd concentrations and altered methylation at the DMRs regulating *MEG3* ($\beta = 0.44$, se = 0.30, $p = 0.14$), and *NNAT* ($\beta = 0.54$, se = 0.32, $p = 0.09$) (Table 2).

Associations may be specific to females at the *PEG3* ($\beta = 0.55$, $p = 0.05$) but not in males ($\beta = 0.09$, $p = 0.61$); whereas associations with the *MEG3* ($\beta = 0.72$, se = 0.41, $p = 0.08$), and *MEST* (beta = 0.47, se = 0.29, $p = 0.10$) DMRs may be specific to males and less evident in females. No evidence for sex-specific association at other DMRs was found.

Despite higher levels of Cd in Hispanics, restricting these analyses by self-reported ethnicity/race and further adjusting for sex of offspring revealed other consistent associations between Cd exposure and regulatory DMR methylation (data not shown).

Maternal Fe and Zn abundance in associations between Cd and DNA methylation at regulatory sequences of genomically imprinted genes

We also explored the extent to which maternal Zn and Fe altered the pattern of the associations observed between maternal Cd and offspring DNA methylation at the *MEG3*, *PLAGL1* and *PEG3*, by repeating the refined models, restricted to women and children with high concentrations of Zn or Fe (top tertile), and again among those with low levels (bottom two tertiles) (Fig. 1). We observed that higher Cd levels were associated with lower *PLAGL1* DMR methylation levels in women with lower Zn and Fe levels (Fig. 1a); the cross-product term for the interaction between Zn and Cd was $p = 0.04$, and that for Cd and Fe was ($p = 0.37$). We also found that higher *PEG3* DMR methylation levels were associated with higher Cd concentrations, but this association appeared limited to women with Zn levels in the top tertile ($p < 0.05$) (Fig. 1b). The cross-product term for the interaction between Cd and Zn was $p = 0.01$. This positive association between elevated Cd levels and higher

Table 2 Regression coefficients, standard errors and p-values for the association between maternal blood cadmium exposure and offspring DNA methylation at DMRs imprinted genes

DMRs	All β, SE, P-value	Males β, SE, P-value	Females β, SE, p-value
IGF2/H19	−0.02, 0.18, 0.91	0.06, 0.25, 0.80	−0.20, 0.25, 0.42
MEG3	0.44, 0.30, 0.14	0.72, 0.41, 0.08	0.37, 0.42, 0.38
MEST	0.05, 0.22, 0.83	0.47, 0.29, 0.10	−0.34, 0.34, 0.31
NNAT	0.54, 0.32, 0.09	0.61, 0.45, 0.17	0.41, 0.48, 0.39
PEG3	0.36, 0.17, 0.03	0.09, 0.17, 0.61	0.55, 0.28, 0.05
SGCE/PEG10	0.01, 0.19, 0.98	−0.23, 0.26, 0.36	0.38, 0.28, 0.18
PLAGL1	−0.20, 0.34, 0.56	−0.42, 0.50, 0.40	−0.17, 0.48, 0.72

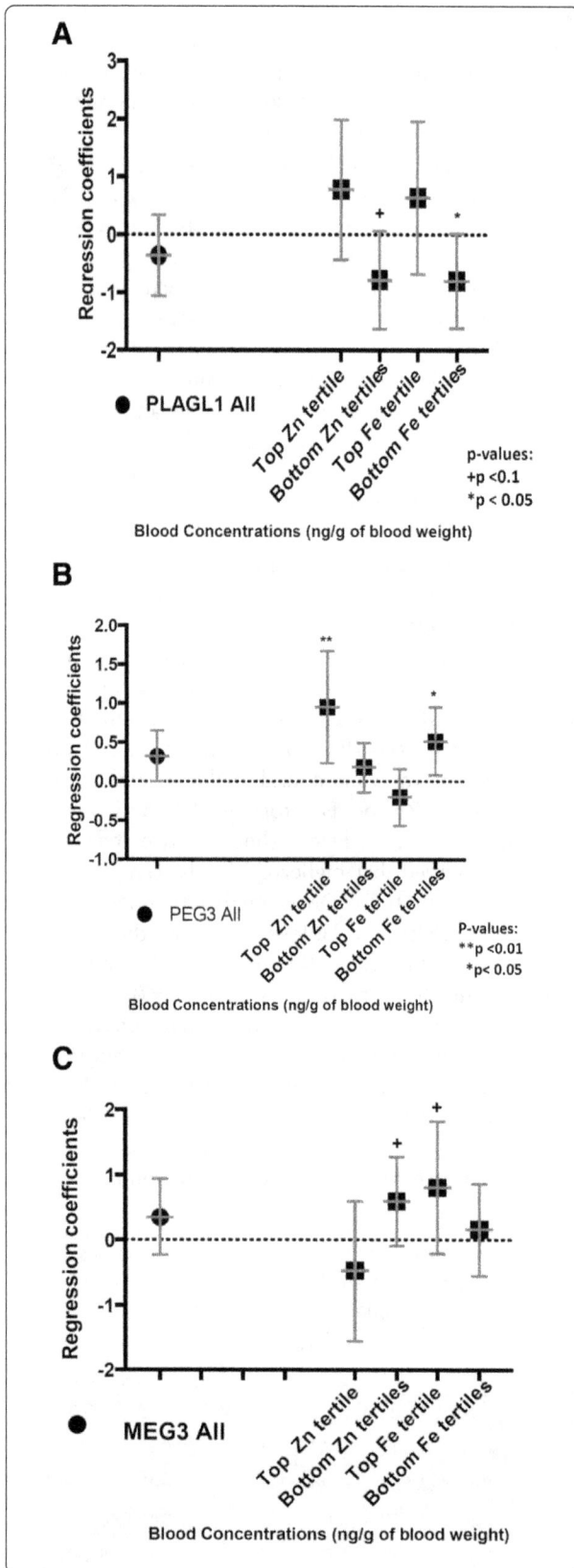

Fig. 1 Regression coefficients for the associations between maternal Cd and DNA methylation at newborns imprinted genes. **a**. Infants born to women with high blood Cd concentrations but with lower Zn and Fe levels, had lower DNA methylation at the *PLAGL1* DMR. **b**. Maternal higher Zn and Cd concentrations were associated with higher methylation at the *PEG3* DMR in newborns. **c**. No associations were observed for *MEG3*

PEG3 methylation was similar in women with high and low Fe levels (Fig. 1b); the cross-product term for the interaction between Fe and Cd was $p = 0.45$. We also found no evidence that the association between Cd levels and *MEG3* DMR methylation varied by Fe and Zn nutrient abundance (Fig. 1c).

Cd levels and birth weight

As Cd placental sequestration has been associated with fetal growth restriction; consequently, we also evaluated whether maternal Cd levels were associated with birth weight (Table 3). We found that higher maternal Cd concentrations in blood were associated with lower birth weight ($\beta = -51.89$, se = 24.20, $p = 0.03$).

Discussion

While the known effects of Cd include replacement of essential protein cofactors, protein disruption/misfolding, generation of oxidative stress, and endocrine disruption, epigenetic mechanisms are emerging as a dynamic

Table 3 Associations between maternal cadmium levels and birth weight

| | Adjusted associations of Log Cd and birth weight (n = 276) | | |
	β	se	p
Maternal			
Log Cd	−51.89	24.20	0.03
[a]Race/Ethnicity			
NH Black	−237.73	70.38	0.00
Hispanic	−164.34	72.27	0.02
NH Other	−222.72	134.09	0.10
Smoking			
Smoking during pregnancy	−173.52	106.27	0.10
Quit during pregnancy	−12.21	85.77	0.89
Pre-Pregnancy BMI	13.68	3.99	0.00
Prenatal physical Activity	5.23	64.31	0.94
Periconceptional antibiotic use	−94.61	60.38	0.12
Offspring			
Female	−107.72	52.19	0.04
Gestational Age at Delivery	26.48	2.19	0.00
Constant	−3996.97	633.10	0.00

Characteristics mutually adjusted
[a]Referents are non-Hispanic whites

mechanistic framework for how the environment interacts with the genome to influence low birth weight and cardio metabolic risk in later life. However, regions of the human epigenome targeted by these ubiquitous toxic metals are still unknown. Moreover, there is limited empirical longitudinal human data on the role of essential metals such as Zn and Fe, previously shown to be antagonists to Cd absorption in animal models [24, 25]. We conducted an analysis to determine whether maternal Cd concentrations, are associated with birth weight, DNA methylation alterations at multiple DMRs regulating genomically imprinted genes after accounting for maternal race/ethnicity, antibiotic use, physical activity, parity, cigarette smoking and sex. We also evaluated the extent to which the abundance of the essential minerals, Zn and Fe modify this association.

Our key finding was that elevated Cd levels were significantly associated with higher DNA methylation at the DMR regulating *PEG3*; these associations varied by Zn or Fe circulating levels. We also found that higher maternal Cd levels were associated with lower birth weight. Our data support that early Cd exposure is gene-specific as DNA methylation of several other DMRs evaluated in newborns were not associated with prenatal levels of Cd. DNA methylation at these regulatory DMRs are established in gametogenesis and embryogenesis and may be vulnerable to availability/abundance of circulating essential metals, including Fe and Zn. DNA methylation marks here examined have previously been associated with fetal development. If these findings are replicated in a larger study and from a wider scope of regulatory regions, our findings suggest that nutritional manipulation during vulnerable periods in life could alter disease course, in Cd-exposed populations. Moreover, if these epigenetic marks are confirmed to be stable in humans, these regions could be developed as markers of periconceptional Cd exposure, for potential use in risk assessment.

Our data suggest that Cd concentrations during early pregnancy are associated with lower levels of newborn's DNA methylation at the DMR regulating *PEG3*, and less consistently at *IGF2/H19* and *MEG3* and none with *PLAGL1* imprinted domains. *PEG3* is a paternally expressed imprinted gene, maps to chromosome 19q13.43 and encodes a zinc finger protein with a tumor suppressor function that plays a role in facilitating p53/c-*myc*-mediated apoptosis. *PEG3* also plays a critical role in brain development where it is mainly expressed in the mesencephalon and the pituitary gland [27]. Shifts in DNA methylation at the *PEG3* DMR have been shown to alter social and maternal nurturing behaviors in mice [27, 28] and to be associated with human cancer [19], presumably caused by a decrease in *PEG3* transcription [29, 30]. In support, a long term follow-up study, lower

PEG3 DMR methylation was recently associated with exposure to lead, a +2 toxic metal that tends to co-occur with Cd (Li et al., in press). Lower DNA methylation levels at the same *PEG3* DMR in males and *IGF2/H19* DMR in females have been associated with exposure to another environmentally abundant neurotoxin, lead, during the neonatal period (Li et al., in press).

While we know of no other study that has examined Cd exposure in relation to epigenetic dysregulation specifically targeting genomically imprinted genes, our findings that Cd exposure *in utero* is associated with DNA methylation differences is consistent with *in vitro* and *ex-vivo* systems studies showing that Cd is an effective inhibitor of DNA methyltransferase. Specifically, Cd initially induces DNA hypomethylation, although prolonged Cd exposure results in DNA hypermethylation and enhanced DNA methyltransferase activity [9]. In humans, gene-specific studies based on known gene function have shown DNA methylation alterations in response to Cd exposure [31, 32]; however, few have been conducted at birth to reflect the periconceptional environment [12]. Using the unbiased Illumina Human-Methylation450 BeadChip, maternal cigarette smoking, a common source of fetal Cd exposure, has been associated with altered DNA methylation at multiple CpG sites including 11 imprinted genes such as *AHRR*, *GFI1*, *IGF2* and *CYP1A1* in cord blood leukocyte DNA [33, 34]. In studies with small sample sizes [12, 35], *in utero* Cd exposure specifically was associated with CpG methylation differences in umbilical cord blood leukocyte DNA at multiple CpG sites mapping to genes involved in xenobiotic metabolism and inflammation [12], some of which may be sex-specific [36, 37]. Female-specific effects of Cd exposure have previously been reported in relation to birth weight, hypothesized to be due to lower iron in females that is associated with increased Cd intestinal absorption [38]. Therefore, while findings from these gene-specific and genome-scale studies do not include regions regulating *PLAGL1*, *MEG3* and *PEG3* examined here, together they support that *in utero* Cd exposure alters the epigenome.

Our findings that the association among maternal Cd and CpG methylation vary by Zn and Fe concentrations are consistent with the toxicity of these essential metals when present in excess, and reduced intestinal absorption reported in animal models. Both Zn and Fe have been shown to mitigate cellular, epigenetic and phenotypic effects *in vivo* and *in vitro* [9, 11, 23, 24, 39]. Mechanisms by which Fe or Zn may decrease harmful effects of Cd exposure remain unknown, although are an active topic of investigation. Studies suggest that marginal intakes of Zn, Fe, and Ca cause the accumulation of Cd in the duodenum, which results in a greater rate of Cd absorption and a greater accumulation in the internal organs [24, 25], which may influence fetal development and epigenetic dysregulation. However, these associations may also depend on other essential elements as well as age and sex. Cd may compete with essential metals for binding to transporter molecules. Indeed, Fe deficiency has been shown to upregulate Fe transporters and subsequently, increased Cd in duodenal mucosa [40, 41]. Deficiencies or excesses of these essential metals can contribute to epigenetic alterations and/or other mechanisms to influence phenotypes such as birth weight and childhood obesity [42], associations that may vary by race/ethnicity as our present results suggest. Zn and Fe are essential co-factor for many enzymes that epigenetically modify DNA and histones, and maternal Zn excess or deficiencies may program offspring growth trajectories by altering epigenetic modifications of DNA and histones [39, 43, 44] at labile loci. Together, our findings corroborate animal and *in vitro* data [9, 24, 25].

A strength of our study is its longitudinal design in early life, as few studies examine Cd exposure before birth. Because Cd and Zn measurements were made in erythrocytes at gestational age <12 weeks, and many heavy metals bind to erythrocytes (a 120 day lifespan), metal concentrations examined here likely represent those of the periconceptional environment. As nutrient concentrations vary by ethnicity (NHANES), another strength is the multiethnic composition of the cohort, enabling examination of the effects of Cd and Zn on the four major ethnic group in the US: Whites, Blacks, Hispanics and Asians. However, given race/ethnic heterogeneity, we cannot exclude the possibility that our inability to find statistically significant associations between altered methylation at other DMRs in response to Cd exposure could be due, in part, to our limited statistical power in race-specific analyses. While statistical power was adequate for overall analyses, we are underpowered for examining higher-order interaction by race. Also, we examined only eight DMRs of more than 65 genes currently known to be imprinted in humans, these 65 genes themselves represent only 1-5 % of the human genome [45]. Analysis of the methylation status of a wider spectrum of the epigenome will be required to clarify the spectrum of genes and pathways that contribute to the association between maternal Cd and DNA methylation alterations in newborns. Despite these limitations, our data suggest that maternal exposure to Cd is associated with aberrant DNA methylation at multiple regions previously associated with preterm birth [46], fetal growth restriction and neurodevelopmental disorders, as previously reported in other geographic regions [36, 47]. With replication, *PLAGL1* and *PEG3* could be considered among epigenetic regions perturbed by Cd exposure early *in utero*.

Conclusions

Although epigenetic mechanisms have been proposed to link early Cd exposure to human health, human data are still limited, as epigenetic targets that may influence human health are still unknown. We present data consistent with the hypothesis that maternal Cd exposure in early pregnancy alters DNA methylation at multiple DMRs in offspring with sex and possibly race/ethnic-specific effects, and that Zn may mitigate these effects. We also contribute data suggesting that early Cd exposure is associated with lower birth weight. As our data were too limited for mediation analyses, larger studies are required to confirm these findings and to determine the role of other imprinted and non-imprinted genes in the associations between Cd, Fe and Zn exposure in epigenetic alterations with known methylation profiles, and low birth weight, a consistent risk factor for childhood obesity and other chronic diseases. Such efforts would contribute data to nutritional policy related to these ubiquitous toxic metals.

Abbreviations
Cd: Cadmium; Fe: Iron; Zn: Zinc; DMR: Differentially methylated region.

Competing interests
The authors declare that they have no competing interests.

Authors' contributions
ZH and DS performed the experiments. SM, AM and CH supervised the data collection and experimental work. RM managed the data. SV, TD, AV, ACV and RF contributed in the analysis and interpretation of the data. SV, ACV, and CH were involved in drafting the manuscript. TD, AV, KK, MN, AM, and JS, critically revised the manuscript for important intellectual content. CH conceived of the study, and participated in its design and coordination. All authors read and approved the final manuscript.

Acknowledgments
This work was supported by National Institutes of Health grants ES016772 and ES005948 and greatly benefited from funding by the National Children's Study Placental Consortium (NCS Formative Research Project LOI2-BIO-18) to THD (NIH: NO1-HD-5-3422) and an ORISE Fellowship to KK. This work does not represent the official view of the US EPA. We thank Carole Grenier, Erin Erginer, Allison Barratt, Cara Davis, and Alissa White for excellent technical support.

Author details
[1]Department of Surgery, Division of Urology, Cedars-Sinai Medical Center, Los Angeles, CA 90048, USA. [2]Department of Biological Sciences, Center for Human Health and the Environment, North Carolina State University, Raleigh, NC 27695, USA. [3]Department of Public Health, Brody School of Medicine, East Carolina University, Greenville, NC 27834, USA. [4]Division of Water, Climate, and the Environment, School of Earth Sciences, The Ohio State University, Columbus, OH 43210, USA. [5]Nicholas School of the Environment, Duke University, Research Drive, Durham, NC 27710, USA. [6]Division of Gynecologic Oncology, Department of Obstetrics and Gynecology, Duke University School of Medicine, Research Drive, Durham, NC 27710, USA. [7]Environmental Public Health Division, U.S. Environmental Protection Agency, Chapel Hill, NC 27599, USA. [8]University of North Carolina at Chapel Hill, Lineberger Comprehensive Cancer Center, 450 West Drive, Chapel Hill, NC 27599, USA. [9]Department of Environmental Sciences and Engineering, Gillings School of Global Public Health, UNC-Chapel Hill, Chapel Hill, NC 27599, USA. [10]Division of Maternal Fetal Medicine, Department of Obstetrics and Gynecology, Duke University School of Medicine, Erwin Drive, Durham, NC 27710, USA. [11]Department of Community and Family Medicine and Duke

Cancer Institute, Duke University School of Medicine, Erwin Drive, Durham, NC 27710, USA.

References

1. Cadmium [http://toxtown.nlm.nih.gov/text_version/chemicals.php?id=63]
2. Registry: http://www.atsdr.cdc.gov/. 2011.
3. Hou L, Zhang X, Wang D, Baccarelli A. Environmental chemical exposures and human epigenetics. Int J Epidemiol. 2012;41(1):79–105.
4. Menai M, Heude B, Slama R, Forhan A, Sahuquillo J, Charles MA, et al. Association between maternal blood cadmium during pregnancy and birth weight and the risk of fetal growth restriction: the EDEN mother-child cohort study. Reprod Toxicol. 2012;34(4):622–7.
5. Scott ME, Shvetsov YB, Thompson PJ, Hernandez BY, Zhu X, Wilkens LR, et al. Cervical cytokines and clearance of incident human papillomavirus infection: Hawaii HPV cohort study. Int J Cancer. 2013;133(5):1187–96.
6. Zinc: Fact Sheet for Health Professionals [http://ods.od.nih.gov/factsheets/Zinc-HealthProfessional/].
7. Matovic V, Buha A, Bulat Z, Dukic-Cosic D. Cadmium toxicity revisited: focus on oxidative stress induction and interactions with zinc and magnesium. Arh Hig Rada Toksikol. 2011;62(1):65–76.
8. Rogalska J, Brzoska MM, Roszczenko A, Moniuszko-Jakoniuk J. Enhanced zinc consumption prevents cadmium-induced alterations in lipid metabolism in male rats. Chem Biol Interact. 2009;177(2):142–52.
9. Takiguchi M, Achanzar WE, Qu W, Li G, Waalkes MP. Effects of cadmium on DNA-(Cytosine-5) methyltransferase activity and DNA methylation status during cadmium-induced cellular transformation. Exp Cell Res. 2003;286(2):355–65.
10. Reichard JF, Schnekenburger M, Puga A. Long term low-dose arsenic exposure induces loss of DNA methylation. Biochem Biophys Res Commun. 2007;352(1):188–92.
11. Jiang G, Xu L, Song S, Zhu C, Wu Q, Zhang L, et al. Effects of long-term low-dose cadmium exposure on genomic DNA methylation in human embryo lung fibroblast cells. Toxicology. 2008;244(1):49–55.
12. Sanders AP, Smeester L, Rojas D, Debussycher T, Wu MC, Wright FA, et al. Cadmium exposure and the epigenome: Exposure-associated patterns of DNA methylation in leukocytes from mother-baby pairs. Epigenetics. 2014;9(2):212–21.
13. Woodfine K, Huddleston JE, Murrell A. Quantitative analysis of DNA methylation at all human imprinted regions reveals preservation of epigenetic stability in adult somatic tissue. Epigenetics Chromatin. 2011;4(1):1.
14. Hoyo C, Murphy SK, Jirtle RL. Imprint regulatory elements as epigenetic biosensors of exposure in epidemiological studies. J Epidemiol Community Health. 2009;63(9):683–4.
15. Hoyo C, Daltveit AK, Iversen E, Benjamin-Neelon SE, Fuemmeler B, Schildkraut J, et al. Erythrocyte folate concentrations, CpG methylation at genomically imprinted domains, and birth weight in a multiethnic newborn cohort. Epigenetics. 2014;9(8):1120–30.
16. Liu Y, Murphy SK, Murtha AP, Fuemmeler BF, Schildkraut J, Huang Z, et al. Depression in pregnancy, infant birth weight and DNA methylation of imprint regulatory elements. Epigenetics. 2012;7(7):735–46.
17. Vidal AC, Murphy SK, Murtha AP, Schildkraut JM, Soubry A, Huang Z, et al. Associations between antibiotic exposure during pregnancy, birth weight and aberrant methylation at imprinted genes among offspring. Int J Obes (Lond). 2013;37(7):907–13.
18. Murphy SK, Huang Z, Hoyo C. Differentially methylated regions of imprinted genes in prenatal, perinatal and postnatal human tissues. PLoS One. 2012;7(7), e40924.
19. Nye MD, Hoyo C, Huang Z, Vidal AC, Wang F, Overcash F, et al. Associations between methylation of paternally expressed gene 3 (PEG3), cervical intraepithelial neoplasia and invasive cervical cancer. PLoS One. 2013;8(2), e56325.
20. Darrah TH, Prutsman-Pfeiffer JJ, Poreda RJ, Ellen Campbell M, Hauschka PV, Hannigan RE. Incorporation of excess gadolinium into human bone from medical contrast agents. Metallomics. 2009;1(6):479–88.
21. DeLoid G, Cohen JM, Darrah T, Derk R, Rojanasakul L, Pyrgiotakis G, et al. Estimating the effective density of engineered nanomaterials for in vitro dosimetry. Nat Commun. 2014;5:3514.
22. McLaughlin MP, Darrah TH, Holland PL. Palladium(II) and platinum(II) bind strongly to an engineered blue copper protein. Inorg Chem. 2011;50(22):11294–6.
23. Sprauten M, Darrah TH, Peterson DR, Campbell ME, Hannigan RE, Cvancarova M, et al. Impact of long-term serum platinum concentrations on neuro- and ototoxicity in Cisplatin-treated survivors of testicular cancer. J Clin Oncol. 2012;30(3):300–7.
24. Reeves PG, Chaney RL. Marginal nutritional status of zinc, iron, and calcium increases cadmium retention in the duodenum and other organs of rats fed rice-based diets. Environ Res. 2004;96(3):311–22.
25. Brzoska MM, Moniuszko-Jakoniuk J. Interactions between cadmium and zinc in the organism. Food Chem Toxicol. 2001;39(10):967–80.
26. Piyathilake CJ, Robinson CB, Cornwell P. A practical approach to red blood cell folate analysis. Anal Chem Insights. 2007;2:107–10.
27. Li L, Keverne EB, Aparicio SA, Ishino F, Barton SC, Surani MA. Regulation of maternal behavior and offspring growth by paternally expressed Peg3. Science. 1999;284(5412):330–3.
28. Chiavegatto S, Sauce B, Ambar G, Cheverud JM, Peripato AC. Hypothalamic expression of Peg3 gene is associated with maternal care differences between SM/J and LG/J mouse strains. Brain Behav. 2012;2(4):365–76.
29. Deng Y, Wu X. Peg3/Pw1 promotes p53-mediated apoptosis by inducing Bax translocation from cytosol to mitochondria. Proc Natl Acad Sci U S A. 2000;97(22):12050–5.
30. Johnson MD, Wu X, Aithmitti N, Morrison RS. Peg3/Pw1 is a mediator between p53 and Bax in DNA damage-induced neuronal death. J Biol Chem. 2002;277(25):23000–7.
31. Arita A, Shamy MY, Chervona Y, Clancy HA, Sun H, Hall MN, et al. The effect of exposure to carcinogenic metals on histone tail modifications and gene expression in human subjects. J Trace Elem Med Biol. 2012;26(2–3):174–8.
32. Hossain MB, Vahter M, Concha G, Broberg K. Low-level environmental cadmium exposure is associated with DNA hypomethylation in Argentinean women. Environ Health Perspect. 2012;120(6):879–84.
33. Joubert BR, Haberg SE, Nilsen RM, Wang X, Vollset SE, Murphy SK, et al. 450 K epigenome-wide scan identifies differential DNA methylation in newborns related to maternal smoking during pregnancy. Environ Health Perspect. 2012;120(10):1425–31.
34. Murphy SK, Adigun A, Huang Z, Overcash F, Wang F, Jirtle RL, et al. Gender-specific methylation differences in relation to prenatal exposure to cigarette smoke. Gene. 2012;494(1):36–43.
35. Smeester L, Yosim AE, Nye MD, Hoyo C, Murphy SK, Fry RC. Imprinted genes and the environment: links to the toxic metals arsenic, cadmium, lead and mercury. Genes (Basel). 2014;5(2):477–96.
36. Kippler M, Engstrom K, Mlakar SJ, Bottai M, Ahmed S, Hossain MB, et al. Sex-specific effects of early life cadmium exposure on DNA methylation and implications for birth weight. Epigenetics. 2013;8(5):494–503.
37. Kippler M, Tofail F, Hamadani JD, Gardner RM, Grantham-McGregor SM, Bottai M, et al. Early-life cadmium exposure and child development in 5-year-old girls and boys: a cohort study in rural Bangladesh. Environ Health Perspect. 2012;120(10):1462–8.
38. Akesson A, Berglund M, Schutz A, Bjellerup P, Bremme K, Vahter M. Cadmium exposure in pregnancy and lactation in relation to iron status. Am J Public Health. 2002;92(2):284–7.
39. Maret W, Sandstead HH. Possible roles of zinc nutriture in the fetal origins of disease. Exp Gerontol. 2008;43(5):378–81.
40. Min KS, Iwata N, Tetsutikawahara N, Onosaka S, Tanaka K. Effect of hemolytic and iron-deficiency anemia on intestinal absorption and tissue accumulation of cadmium. Toxicol Lett. 2008;179(1):48–52.
41. Flanagan PR, McLellan JS, Haist J, Cherian G, Chamberlain MJ, Valberg LS. Increased dietary cadmium absorption in mice and human subjects with iron deficiency. Gastroenterology. 1978;74(5 Pt 1):841–6.
42. Yang QY, Liang JF, Rogers CJ, Zhao JX, Zhu MJ, Du M. Maternal obesity induces epigenetic modifications to facilitate Zfp423 expression and enhance adipogenic differentiation in fetal mice. Diabetes. 2013;62(11):3727–35.
43. Fatemi M, Hermann A, Pradhan S, Jeltsch A. The activity of the murine DNA methyltransferase Dnmt1 is controlled by interaction of the catalytic domain with the N-terminal part of the enzyme leading to an allosteric activation of the enzyme after binding to methylated DNA. J Mol Biol. 2001;309(5):1189–99.
44. Somoza JR, Skene RJ, Katz BA, Mol C, Ho JD, Jennings AJ, et al. Structural snapshots of human HDAC8 provide insights into the class I histone deacetylases. Structure. 2004;12(7):1325–34.

45. Luedi PP, Dietrich FS, Weidman JR, Bosko JM, Jirtle RL, Hartemink AJ. Computational and experimental identification of novel human imprinted genes. Genome Res. 2007;17(12):1723–30.

46. Liu Y, Hoyo C, Murphy S, Huang Z, Overcash F, Thompson J, et al. DNA methylation at imprint regulatory regions in preterm birth and infection. Am J Obstet Gynecol. 2013;208(5):e391–7. 395.

47. Kippler M1, Tofail F, Gardner R, Rahman A, Hamadani JD, Bottai M, et al. Maternal cadmium exposure during pregnancy and size at birth: a prospective cohort study. Environ Health Perspect. 2012;120(2):284–9.

18

Antinociceptive tolerance to NSAIDs microinjected into dorsal hippocampus

Gulnazi Gurtskaia, Nana Tsiklauri, Ivliane Nozadze, Marina Nebieridze and Merab G Tsagareli[*]

Abstract

Background: Pain is characterized as a complex experience, dependent not only on the regulation of nociceptive sensory systems, but also on the activation of mechanisms that control emotional processes in limbic brain areas such as the amygdala and the hippocampus. Several lines of investigations have shown that in some brain areas, particularly the midbrain periaqueductal gray matter, rostral ventro-medial medulla, central nucleus of amygdala and nucleus raphe magnus, microinjections of non-steroidal anti-inflammatory drugs (NSAIDs) induce antinociception with distinct development of tolerance. The present study was designed to examine whether microinjection of NSAIDs, clodifen, ketorolac and xefocam into the dorsal hippocampus (DH) leads to the development of antinociceptive tolerance in male rats.

Methods: The experiments were carried out on experimental and control (with saline) white male rats. Animals were implanted with a guide cannula in the DH and tested for antinociception following microinjection of NSAIDs into the DH in the tail-flick (TF) and hot plate (HP) tests. Repeated measures of analysis of variance with post-hoc Tukey-Kramer multiple comparison tests were used for statistical evaluations.

Results: We found that microinjection of these NSAIDs into the DH induces antinociception as revealed by a latency increase in the TF and HP tests compared to controls treated with saline into the DH. Subsequent tests on days 2 and 3, however, showed that the antinociceptive effect of NSAIDs progressively decreased, suggesting tolerance developed to this effect of NSAIDs. Both pretreatment and post-treatment with the opioid antagonist naloxone into the DH significantly reduced the antinociceptive effect of NSAIDs in both pain models.

Conclusions: Our results indicate that microinjection of NSAIDs into the DH induces antinociception which is mediated via the opioid system and exhibits tolerance.

Keywords: Antinociception, Endogenous opioids, Hot plate test, Non-opioid tolerance, NSAIDs, Tail-flick reflex

Background

Emotional distress is an intrinsic and the most undesirable feature of painful states. Pain is characterized as a complex experience, dependent not only on the regulation of nociceptive sensory systems, but also on the activation of mechanisms that control emotional processes in limbic brain areas such as the amygdala and the hippocampus [1]. The involvement of the hippocampal formation (HF) in nociception has been suggested in several studies [2-4]. Just recently, some abnormalities in hippocampal functioning with persistent pain have been shown [5]. Particularly, mice with spared nerve injury (SNI) neuropathic pain were unable to extinguish contextual fear and showed increased anxiety-like behavior. Additionally, mice with SNI compared with sham animals exhibited hippocampal reduced extracellular signal-regulated kinase expression and phosphorylation, decreased neurogenesis, and altered short-term synaptic plasticity [5].

Furthermore, morphine microinjections in the dorsal hippocampus (DH) produced antinociceptive effects in the formalin-induced orofacial pain model in rats [6]. Recent evidence suggests the participation of cholinergic, opioidergic and GABA-ergic systems of the DH in the modulation of nociception in guinea pigs [2]. Moreover, opioid peptides are important modulators of information processing in the hippocampus. When activated, opioid

* Correspondence: tsagareli@biphysiol.ge
Dept of Neurophysiology, Ivane Beritashvili Center for Experimental Biomedicine, Gotua Street 14, Tbilisi 0160, Georgia

receptors play a key role in central pain modulation mechanisms, and the HF is a structure that expresses significant densities of this kind of receptors [7,8]. In addition, the hippocampus is anatomically connected to components of the pain neuromatrix, including the amygdala and the descending pain pathway with the periaqueductal gray (PAG) – the rostral ventromedial (RVM) region of medulla [9]. However, specific neural substrates and circuitry mediating opioid-induced hippocampal antinociception are unknown.

We have recently shown that in the PAG, the central nucleus of amygdala (CeA), and the nucleus raphe magnus (NRM), microinjection of non-steroidal anti-inflammatory drugs (NSAIDs) induces antinociception with some effects of tolerance and cross-tolerance to morphine [10-14]. These findings strongly support the suggestion of endogenous opioid involvement in NSAIDs antinociception and tolerance in the descending pain-control system [15-19]. However, involvement of NSAIDs antinociception in the HF is still a matter of controversy. For example, indomethacin did not protect against significant pain-induced down-regulation of neurokinin-1 (NK-1) and brain derived-neurotropic factor (BDNF) receptor genes in the hippocampus, suggesting that although analgesic drug treatment reduces nociceptive sensory activation in the spinal cord, it is insufficient to prevent the impact of pain on the hippocampus [20].

In this study, we have examined whether microinjection of the widely used NSAIDs diclofenac, ketorolac, and xefocam into the DH induces antinociception and whether this action is mediated via the endogenous opioid system.

Methods
Animals
The experiments were carried out on male Wistar rats, 200-250 g in body weight, bred at Beritashvili Center for Experimental Biomedicine. The experimental protocol was approved by the local Bioethic Committee of the Center. Every effort was made to minimize both the number of animals used and their suffering. Guidelines of the International Association for the Study of Pain regarding animal experimentation were followed throughout [21].

Surgical procedures
Under anesthesia with thiopental (55 mg/kg, i.p. "Kievmed", Ukraine), a 12 mm-long stainless steel guide cannula (Small Parts, Inc, USA) was stereotaxically implanted into the DH bilaterally (AP:-4.3; L:±2.5; H:2.8) according to the coordinates in the atlas of Paxinos and Watson [22] siting the tip 2 mm above the DH. Guides were anchored to the cranium by dental cement. The guide cannula was plugged with a stainless steel stylet. Thereafter, the rats were handled every day for 3 days for 15 min. During this

time, the stylet was removed and 14 mm-long stainless steel microinjection cannula was inserted into the guide cannula to reach the DH, but no drug was injected. This helped to habituate the rats to the injection procedure and to reduce artifacts arising from mechanical manipulation during the test days. Five days after surgery a microinjection cannula, attached to a 50-μl Hamilton syringe (Hamilton, Inc, USA), was introduced through the guide cannula, and the drug was microinjected while the rat was gently restrained.

Drugs
Clodifen (diclofenac sodium, 75 μg/0.5 μl, RotexMedica, Germany), ketorolac (ketorolac tromethamine, 90 μg/0.5 μl, Zee Drugs, India) or xefocam (lornoxicam, 12 μg/0.5 μl, Nycomed, Austria) were injected through the microinjection cannula; the guide cannula was then plugged with a stainless steel stylet. Saline was injected in the same volume (0.5 μl, GalichPharm, Ukraine) and manner in a separate group of rats for controls. Solutions were microinjected in about 10 seconds.

Behavioral testing
Twenty minutes post microinjection, i.e. 10-min before the peak of the drugs' effect is normally reached, animals were tested for antinociception using the tail-flick (TF) and hot plate (HP) tests. For the TF test, the distal part of the tail was stimulated with a light beam and the latency measured until the tail was reflexively flicked away from the beam (IITC #33, IITC Life Science, Inc., Woodland Hills, CA, USA). For the HP test, the rat was placed on a 55°C hot plate and the latency to the first hindpaw licking or jumping was measured (IITC #39). The cut-off time was 20 s for both TF and HP latencies. Each rat was tested with both tail flick (TF) and hot plate (HP) in the same session. A similar procedure was followed for the repeated microinjection of clodifen, ketorolac, xefocam or saline for four consecutive days.

In control experiments, saline microinjections into the DH was followed by a non-selective opioid receptor antagonist naloxone (0.5 μl, GalichPharm, Ukraine) and tested for TF and HP latencies for the three consecutive days.

In the second set of experiments, twenty minutes after NSAIDs administration we tested on whether posttreatment with a non-selective opioid receptor antagonist naloxone in the DH diminishes NSAID-induced antinociception on the 1st, 2nd and 3rd experimental days. In the third set of experiments, rats pretreated with the same dose of naloxone in the DH were followed by TF and HP tests. 10 min after rats were treated with NSAIDs in the same dose as in the first and second set of experiments and were then tested again. Different animal groups were used for experiments 1, 2 and 3. The number of rats in each group was five or six.

Histology

At the end of each set of experiments, the microinjection sites were marked with 2 μl of saturated solution of Pontamine Sky Blue (Sigma Chemical, Co.) and the animal was euthanized with an overdose of ester. After fixation by immersion in 10% formalin, the brain was sectioned and counterstained with Cresyl Violet. The microinjection sites were histologically verified and plotted according to Paxinos and Watson (1997) stereotaxic atlas coordinates [22]. Representative microinjection sites are shown in Figure 1.

Statistical analysis

All data are presented as mean±S.E.M. Repeated measures of analysis of variance (ANOVA) with *post-hoc* Tukey-Kramer multiple comparison test were used for statistical comparisons between treated and saline groups, and treated and naloxone groups, respectively. The Kolmogorov–Smirnov test was applied to verify normality. The statistical software utilized was InStat 3.05 (GraphPad Software, USA). Statistical significance between vehicle control and treated groups, and naloxone and treated groups of rats was acknowledged if $P < 0.05$.

Results

We found that microinjection of NSAIDs into the DH produced antinociception as revealed by a latency increase in TF and HP compared to the baseline control of intact rats and a control group with saline microinjected into the same site as well. The TF latency significantly increased for clodifen [ANOVA: $F(4, 16) = 20.189$, $P < 0.0001$], ketorolac [ANOVA: $F(4,20) = 22.314$, $P < 0.0001$], and xefocam [ANOVA: $F(4,16) = 32.42$, $P < 0.0001$]. We found similar significant differences in the HP latencies for clodifen [ANOVA: $F(4,16) = 21.53$, $P < 0.0001$], for ketorolac [ANOVA: $F(4,20) = 17.764$, $P < 0.0001$], and for xefocam [ANOVA: $F(4,16) = 39.463$, $P < 0.0001$], respectively. Subsequent NSAIDs microinjections caused progressively less antinociception, so by day 4 there was no effect, similar to

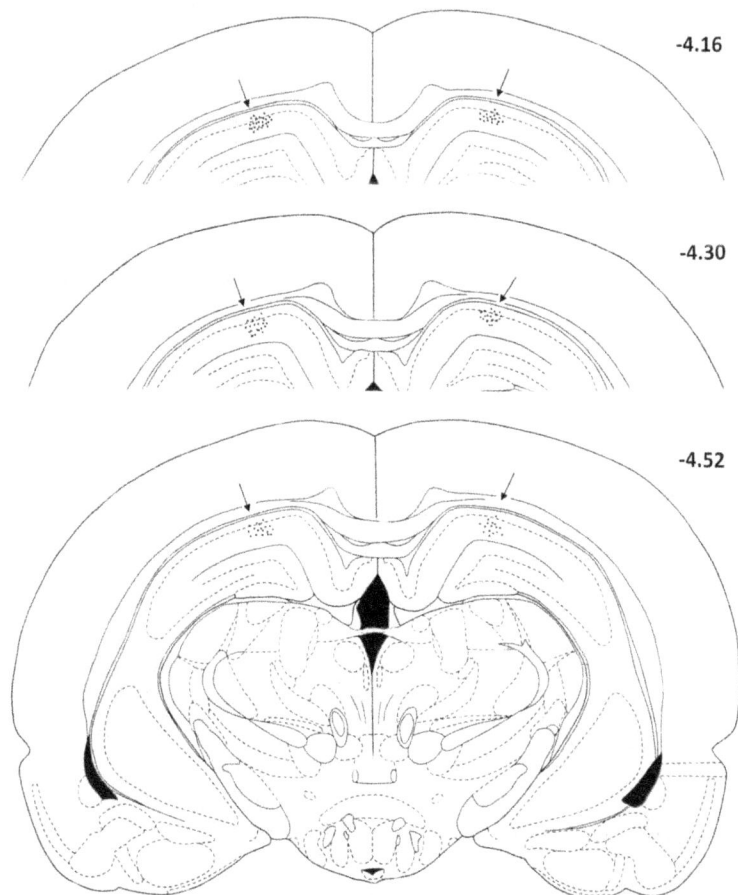

Figure 1 Serial coronal sections of the rat brain showing placement of microinjections bilaterally in the DH (black arrows). The numbers to the right of sections represent millimeters relative to bregma, adapted from the Paxinos and Watson (1997) stereotaxic atlas [22].

saline microinjections for both the TF and the HP tests (Figure 2).

Control testing with saline microinjections into the DH followed by a non-selective opioid receptor antagonist naloxone statistically did not change the latency to respond in the TF [ANOVA: $F_{(5,24)} = 0.8914$, $P = 0.5024$, not significant] and HP [ANOVA: $F_{(5,24)} = 0.1463$, $P = 0.9792$, not significant] tests respectively for the first, second and third days ($P > 0.05$) (Figure 3A, B).

In the second set of experiments, we tested if post-treatment with the non-selective opioid receptor antagonist naloxone in the DH diminishes NSAID-induced antinociception at the first, second and third experimental days. Twenty minutes after NSAID administration, microinjection of naloxone in the DH significantly decreased antinociceptive effects of these drugs at the first day in the TF for clodifen [ANOVA: $F_{(5,20)} = 26.906$,

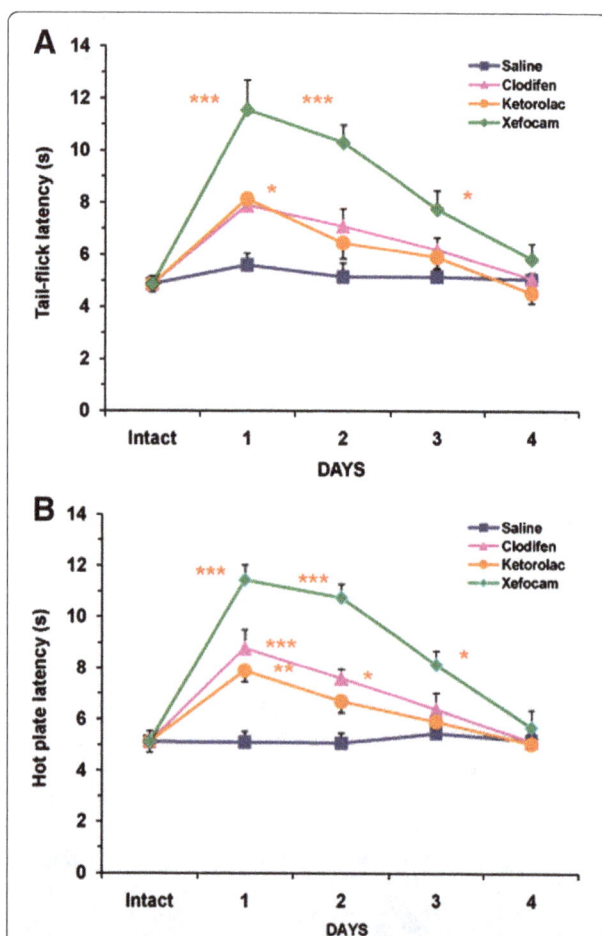

Figure 3 Control experiments of post-treatment with naloxone after microinjection of saline into the DH does not significantly change TF (A) and HP (B) latencies either for the first or second and third days ($P > 0.05$). Number of rats $N = 5$/group.

Figure 2 Microinjections of NSAIDs into the DH for four consecutive days result in a progressive decrease in TF (A) and HP (B) latencies as compared to vehicle saline control. The number of rats in the control group $N = 16$/group, in the treated groups for clodifen $N = 5$/group, for ketorolac $N = 6$/group, and for xefocam $N = 5$/group, respectively. *- $P < 0.05$, **- $P < 0.01$, ***- $P < 0.001$.

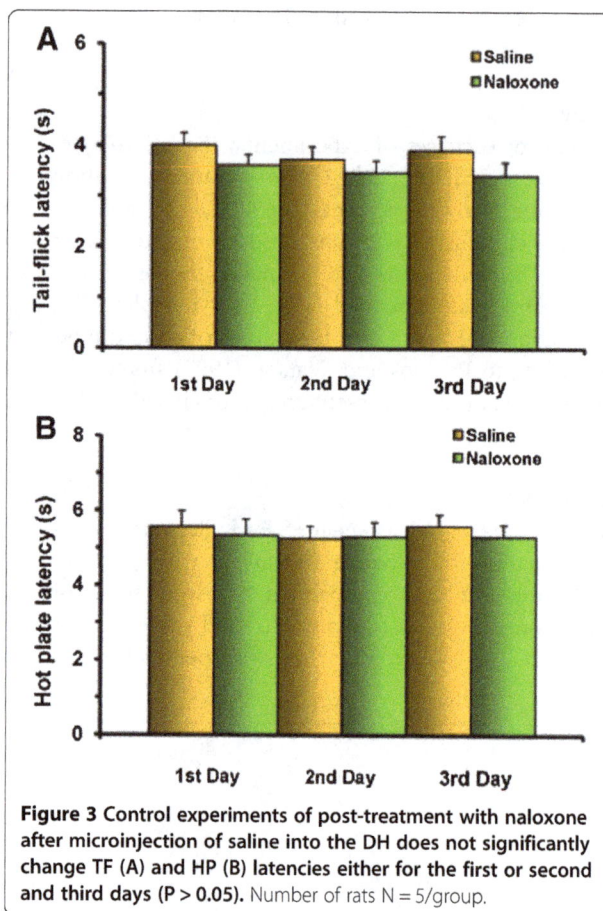

$P < 0.0001$], ($t = 13.161$, $P < 0.001$) (Figure 4A), for ketorolac [ANOVA: $F_{(5,20)} = 24.701$, $P < 0.0001$], ($t = 10.691$, $P < 0.001$) (Figure 4B), and for xefocam [ANOVA: $F_{(5,20)} = 22.412$, $P < 0.0001$], ($t = 9.745$, $P < 0.001$) (Figure 4C). At the second and third experimental days, naloxone showed generally trend effects (Figure 4), except for xefocam at the second experimental day where the difference between xefocam and naloxone injected groups is significant ($P < 0.05$) (Figure 4C).

The same effects we discovered in the HP test for clodifen [ANOVA: $F_{(5,20)} = 11.341$, $P < 0.0001$], ($t = 6.679$, $P < 0.01$) (Figure 4D), for ketorolac [ANOVA: $F_{(5,20)} = 33.093$, $P < 0.0001$], ($t = 12.141$, $P < 0.001$) (Figure 4E), and for xefocam [ANOVA: $F_{(5,20)} = 35.494$, $P < 0.0001$], ($t = 13.068$, $P < 0.001$) (Figure 4F, C). At the second and third experimental days, naloxone showed generally trend effects (Figure 4), except for ketorolac in the second experimental day where the difference between ketorolac and naloxone injected groups is significant ($P < 0.01$) (Figure 4E).

In the third set of experiments, we tested if pretreatment with naloxone prevents antinociception induced by NSAID microinjected into the DH. Pretreatment with

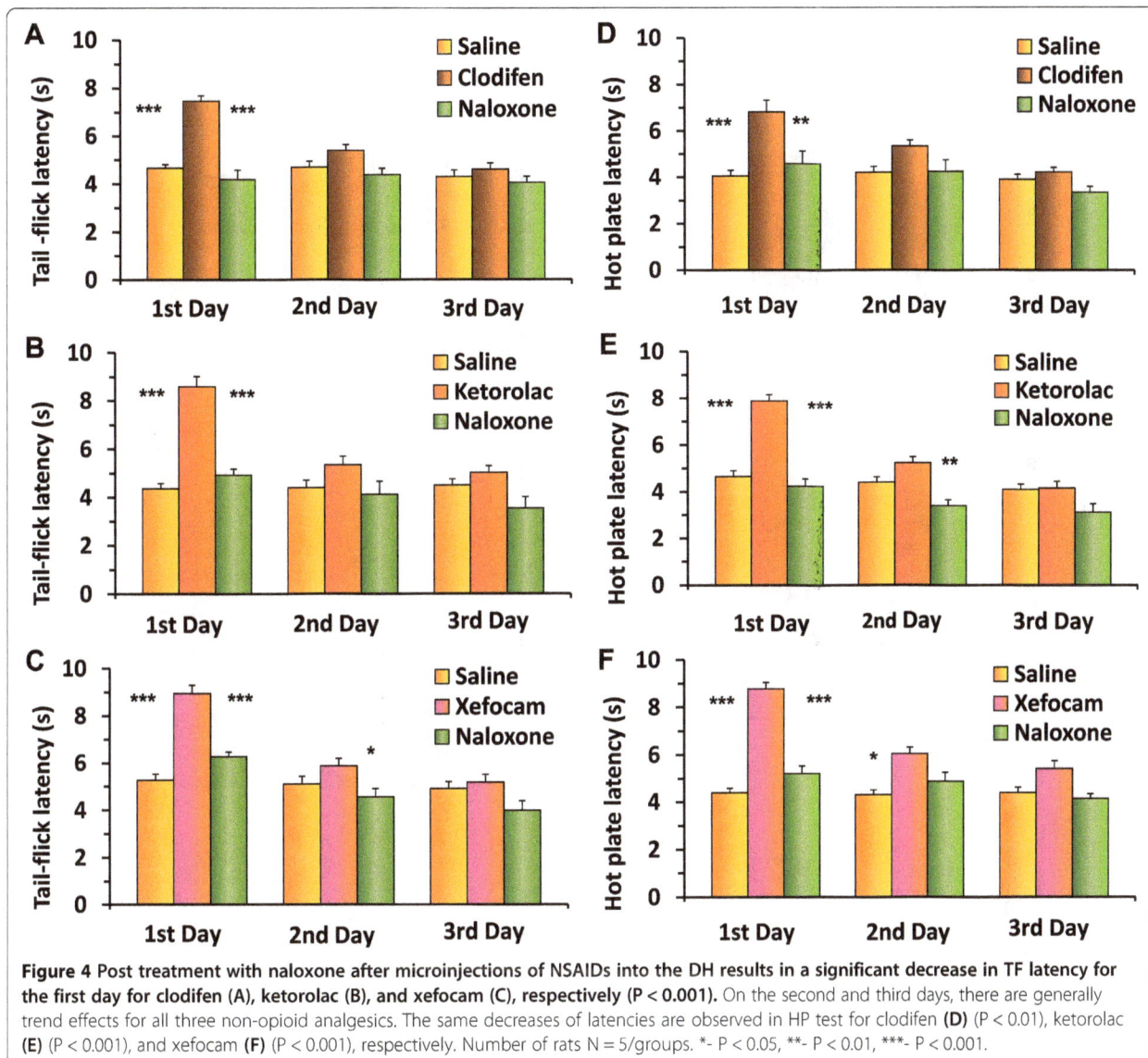

Figure 4 Post treatment with naloxone after microinjections of NSAIDs into the DH results in a significant decrease in TF latency for the first day for clodifen (A), ketorolac (B), and xefocam (C), respectively (P < 0.001). On the second and third days, there are generally trend effects for all three non-opioid analgesics. The same decreases of latencies are observed in HP test for clodifen **(D)** (P < 0.01), ketorolac **(E)** (P < 0.001), and xefocam **(F)** (P < 0.001), respectively. Number of rats N = 5/groups. *- P < 0.05, **- P < 0.01, ***- P < 0.001.

naloxone completely prevented the analgesic effects of clodifen (Figure 5A), ketorolac (Figure 5B), and xefocam (Figure 5C) in the TF test. The differences between NSAIDs injected and naloxone injected groups are not significant (Figure 5). The same results are in the HP test for clodifen (Figure 6A), ketorolac (Figure 6B), and xefocam (Figure 6C), respectively.

Discussion

The present results demonstrate that microinjections of the NSAIDs, clodifen, ketorolac and xefocam into the DH induce antinociception. This confirms our and other colleagues previous results with systemic, intraperitoneal administration of NSAIDs [23,24], and results using microinjection of the same NSAIDs into the PAG [15,16]. In the other experiments in rats, responses of spinal dorsal horn wide-dynamic range neurons to mechanical noxious

stimulation of a hindpaw were strongly inhibited by intravenous dipyrone (metamizol) [25].

Importantly, repeated microinjections of NSAIDs into the DH resulted in a progressive decrease in antinociceptive effectiveness, i.e. induced tolerance similar to that observed with intra-PAG, CeA and NRM injections [11,12,14-17], and reminiscent of the effect of opiates. For example, it has recently been shown that repeated intrathecal injections of a selective delta opioid receptor (DOPR) agonists deltorphin II or morphine induce tolerance effects on antihyperalgesic and antinociceptive responses in rodents [26].

A major involvement of opioidergic mechanisms in tolerance to the analgesic effect of NSAIDs is unusual, because traditionally the cellular and molecular actions of opioids were thought to differ from those of non-opioid analgesics. However, one interesting aspect of NSAIDs administration, namely tolerance, emphasizes their similarity to opioid

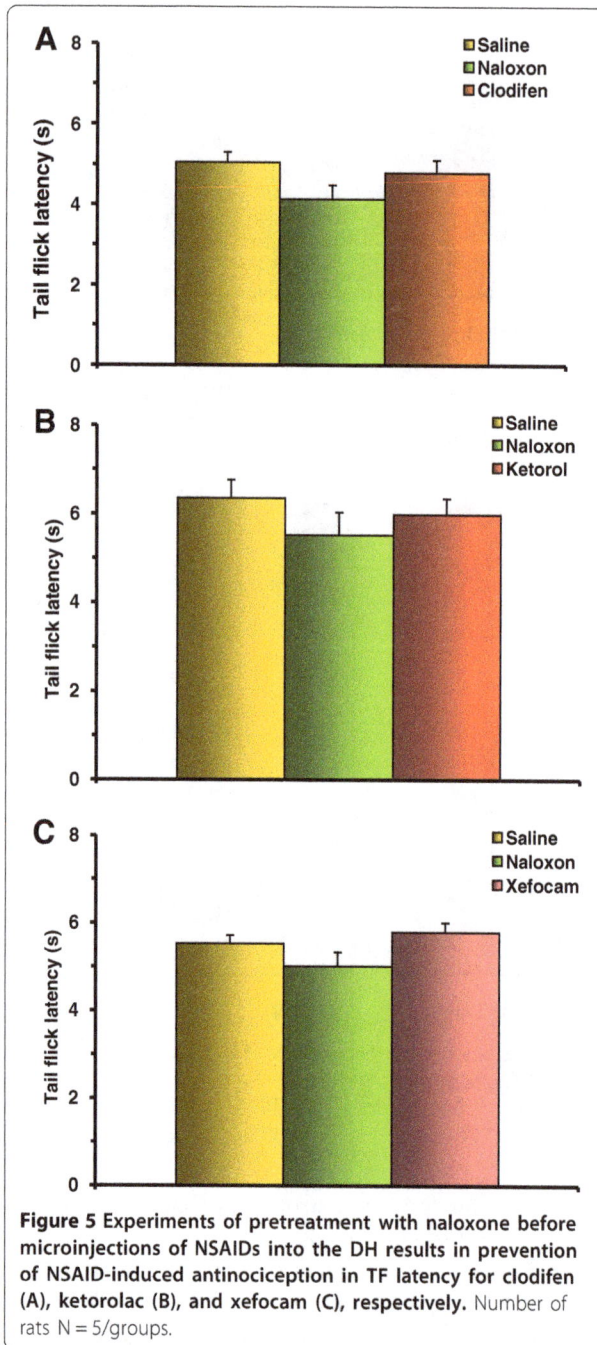

Figure 5 Experiments of pretreatment with naloxone before microinjections of NSAIDs into the DH results in prevention of NSAID-induced antinociception in TF latency for clodifen (A), ketorolac (B), and xefocam (C), respectively. Number of rats N = 5/groups.

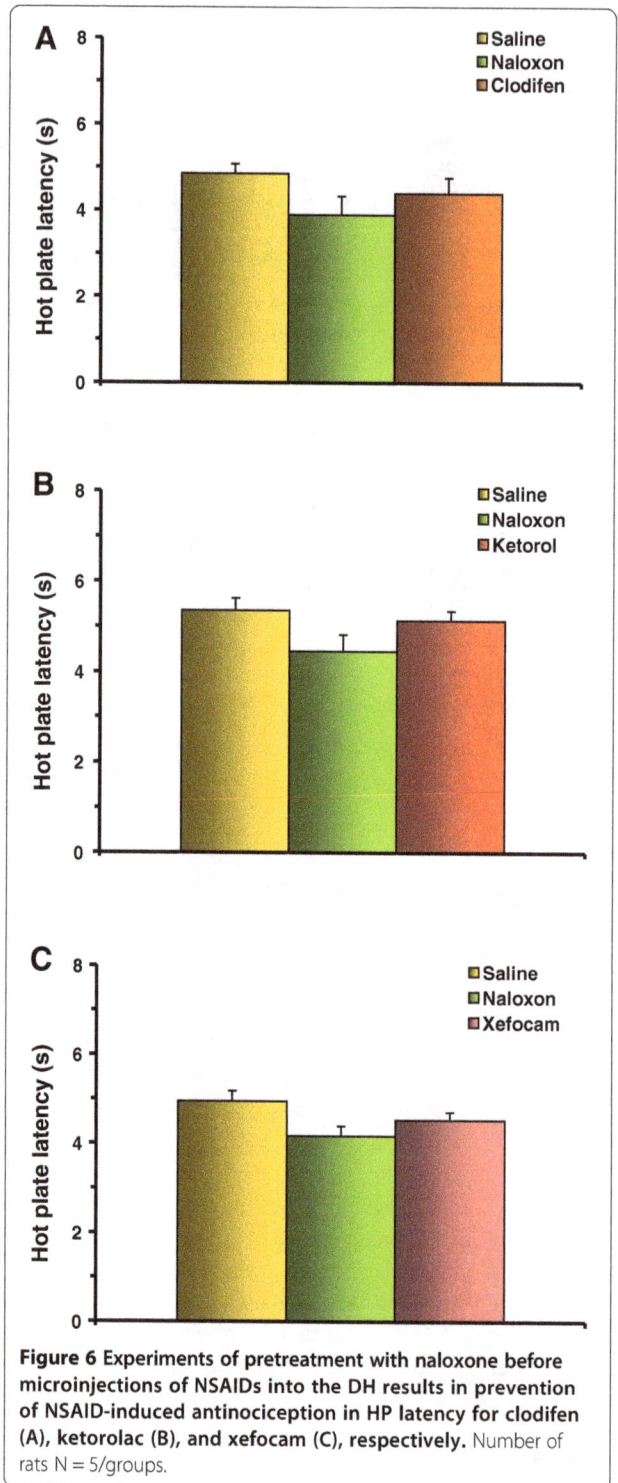

Figure 6 Experiments of pretreatment with naloxone before microinjections of NSAIDs into the DH results in prevention of NSAID-induced antinociception in HP latency for clodifen (A), ketorolac (B), and xefocam (C), respectively. Number of rats N = 5/groups.

analgesics. Indeed, microinjection of metamizol into PAG [13,15,16,18], or into CeA [11,18], progressively led to a loss of their antinociceptive effects, i.e. produced tolerance. Furthermore, tolerance to metamizol was accompanied by cross-tolerance to morphine as if opioid analgesics had been repeatedly administered [16,17].

The mechanism producing tolerance to NSAIDs can be due to the participation of endogenous opioids [19,27,28]. Herein we clearly showed that a non-selective opioid receptor antagonist naloxone significantly diminishes

NSAIDs-induced antinociception on the first day, and on the second and third days shows trend effects. Our findings affirm the results of other investigators that microinjection of dipyrone and aspirin, and systemic dipyrone are abolished by systemically injected and/or microinjections of the opioid antagonists, naloxone, and CTOP (D-phe-Cys-Tyr-D-trp-Orn-thr-Pen-thr-NH2) [15,23,25,27]. The latter is a cyclic analog of the neuropeptide somatostatin and is known to block the analgesic effect of morphine [15]. Moreover, endogenous opioids are involved in the potentiation of analgesia observed with the combination of morphine plus dipyrone (metamizol). The release of endogenous opioids by dipyrone could enhance exogenous opiate effects, explaining the need for more naloxone to counteract the antinociception produced by morphine plus dipyrone [27].

The mechanisms whereby NSAIDs, in general, engage endogenous opioids are not completely understood. There is a proposed model for the PAG where γ-amino-butyric acid (GABA) containing synapses act as the plausible site where NSAIDs could converge with endogenous opioids. The PAG output neurons that drive antinociception via downstream relays, like the RVM, is tonically inhibited by local GABA-ergic synapses [19,28]. Endogenous opioids reduce presynaptic release of GABA in the PAG. Furthermore, activation of μ-opioid receptors in the PAG brings about an elevation of the intracellular concentration of arachidonic acid metabolites. One of the pathways leads to the formation of hepoxilins, which increase potassium conductance. This in turn hyperpolarizes the presynaptic GABA-ergic terminals and decreases GABA release [29]. Disinhibition of PAG output neurons would thus drive antinociception in the downstream loop of the PAG–RVM–spinal dorsal horn [30,31]. For this pathway to function, however, an activation of μ-opioid receptors seems to be necessary, because naloxone or CTOP blocks the effect of PAG-microinjected metamizol or aspirin [15,23].

As stated above, the action of either opioid or non-opioid analgesics in the PAG leads to an excitation of PAG output neurons and this causes an activation of RVM off-cells and an inhibition of RVM on-cells, thus leading to antinociception (analgesia). When tolerance develops, PAG microinjections of morphine [32], or metamizol [15], are no longer capable of affecting RVM neurons and inducing analgesia. These results show further neuronal relationships between opioid and non-opioid analgesics as regards the descending pain-control and modulation system [19,30]. In addition, metamizol probably can act via endocannabinoids in the downstream PAG-RVM axis reducing inflammation pain in rats [33].

There is evidence that GABAergic mediation of opioid effects is a widespread phenomenon and occurs throughout most of CNS. A co-localization between hippocampal μ-opioid receptors and GABA-ergic interneurons in CA1, CA3 and dentate gyrus has been shown in rats [34]. The localization of μ-opioid receptors on GABA-ergic neurons suggests that these receptors, when activated, can directly control the hippocampal GABA-ergic neurons' activity [34,35]. Several studies have shown that activation of the

opioid receptors can lead to the inhibition of interneuron activity resulting in diminished GABA release and the disinhibition of hippocampal pyramidal neurons [36-38].

Our results support the hypothesis that modulation of nociceptive response in the DH could occur in a manner similar to that proposed for the PAG [9,19,28,39]. It is therefore likely that in this study the antinociception observed after microinjection of NSAIDs into the DH occurs through the inhibition of tonically active GABA-ergic interneurons. In addition, involvement of the downstream PAG-RVM axis mechanism is also possible.

Conclusions

In conclusion, our data showed for the first time that repeated microinjections of NSAIDs into the DH induce antinociception that is opioid mediated. These findings confirmed previous studies indicating that the antinociceptive action of NSAIDs may be mediated via the endogenous opioid system, as it is blocked by naloxone and exhibits tolerance.

Competing interests
There is no conflict of interest in the present work.

Authors' contributions
GG, NT, and IN equally contributed to data collection. MN carried out histological control. MGT designed conception, finally analyzed the data and drafted the manuscript. All authors read, contributed to and approved the final manuscript.

Acknowledgement
This work was supported by the Georgian National Science Foundation.

References
1. Craig KD: Emotions and psychobiology. In *Wall and Mellzack's Textbook of Pain*. 5th edition. Edited by McMahon SB, Koltzenburg M. London: Elsevier; 2006:231–240.
2. Favaroni Mendes LA, Menescal-de-Oliveira L: Role of cholinergic, opioidergic and GABA-ergic neuro-transmission of the dorsal hippocampus in the modulation of nociception in guinea pigs. *Life Sci* 2008, 83:644–650.
3. Liu MG, Chen J: Roles of the hippocampal formation in pain information processing. *Neurosci Bull* 2009, 25:237–266.
4. McKenna JE, Melzack R: Analgesia produced microinjection in dentate gyrus. *Pain* 1992, 49:105–112.
5. Mutso AA, Radzicki D, Baliki MN, Huang L, Banisadr G, Centeno MV, Radulovic J, Martina M, Miller RJ, Apkarian AV: Abnormalities in hippocampal functioning with persistent pain. *J Neurosci* 2012, 32:5747–5756.
6. Erfanparast A, Tamaddonfard E, Farshid AA, Khalilzadeh E: Antinociceptive effect of morphine microinjections into the dorsal hippocampus in the formalin-induced orofacial pain in rats. *Veter Res Forum* 2010, 1:83–89.
7. Drake CT, Patterson TA, Simmons ML, Chavkin C, Milner TA: k-opioid receptor-like immune-reactivity in guinea pig brain: ultrastructural localization in presynaptic terminals in hippocampal formation. *J Comp Neurol* 1996, 370:377–395.
8. McLean S, Rothman RB, Jacobson AE, Rice KC, Herkenham M: Distribution of opiate receptor subtypes and enkephalin and dynorphin immunoreactivity in the hippocampus of squirrel, guinea pig, rat, and hamster. *J Comp Neurol* 1987, 255:497–510.
9. Fields HL, Basbaum AI, Heinricher MM: Central nervous system mechanisms of pain modulation. In *Wall and Mellzack's Textbook of Pain*. 5th edition. Edited by McMahon SB, Koltzenburg M. London: Elsevier; 2006:125–143.

10. Tsagareli MG, Tsiklauri ND, Gurtskaia GP, Nozadze IR, Kandelaki RA, Abzianidze EV: Tolerance effects induced by NSAIDs micro-injections into the central nucleus of the amygdala in rats. *Neurophysiology* 2009, **41**:404–408.

11. Tsagareli MG, Tsiklauri N, Gurtskaia G, Nozadze I, Abzianidze E: The central nucleus of amygdala is involved in tolerance to the antinociceptive effect of NSAIDs. *Health* 2010, **2**:64–68.

12. Tsagareli MG, Nozadze I, Tsiklauri N, Gurtskaia G: Tolerance to non-opioid analgesics is opioid sensitive in the nucleus raphe magnus. *Front Neurosci* 2011, **5**:92.

13. Tsiklauri N, Nozadze I, Gurtskaia G, Abzianidze E, Tsagareli M: Tolerance induced by non-opioid analgesic microinjections into rat's periaqueductal gray and nucleus raphe. *Georgian Med News* 2010, **180**:47–55.

14. Tsiklauri ND, Nozadze IR, Gurtskaia GP, Tsagareli MG: Opioid sensitivity of analgesia induced by microinjections of non-steroidal anti-inflammatory drugs into the *nucleus raphe magnus*. *Neurophysiology* 2011, **43**:213–216.

15. Tortorici V, Aponte Y, Acevedo H, Nogueira L, Vanegas H: Tolerance to non-opioid analgesics in PAG involves unresponsiveness of medullary pain-modulating neurons in male rats. *Eur J Neurosci* 2009, **29**:1188–1196.

16. Tortorici V, Vanegas H: Opioid tolerance induced by metamizol (dipyrone) microinjections into the periaqueductal gray of rats. *Eur J Neurosci* 2000, **12**:4074–4080.

17. Tsagareli MG, Tsiklauri N: *Behavioral Study of 'Non-Opioid Tolerance'.* New York: Nova Biomedical Publishers, Inc.; 2012.

18. Tsagareli MG, Tsiklauri N, Nozadze I, Gurtskaia G: Tolerance effects of NSAIDs microinjected into central amygdala, periaqueductal grey, and nucleus raphe: possible cellular mechanism. *Neural Regen Res* 2012, **7**:1029–1039.

19. Vanegas H, Vazquez E, Tortorici V: NSAIDs, opioids, cannabinoids and the control of pain by the central nervous system. *Pharmaceuticals* 2010, **3**:1335–1347.

20. Duric V, McCarson KE: Effects of analgesic or antidepressant drugs on pain- or stress-evoked hippocampal and spinal neurokinin-1receptor and brain-derived neurotrophic factor gene expression in the rat. *J Pharmacol Exp Therapeutics* 2006, **319**:1235–1243.

21. Zimmermann M: Ethical guidelines for investigations of experimental pain in conscious animals. *Pain* 1983, **16**:109–110.

22. Paxinos G, Watson C: *The Rat Brain in Stereotaxic Coordinates.* San Diego: Academic Press; 1997.

23. Pernia-Andrade AJ, Tortorici V, Venegas H: Induction of opioid tolerance by lysine acetyl-salicylate in rats. *Pain* 2004, **111**:191–200.

24. Tsiklauri N, Viatchenko-Karpinski V, Voitenko N, Tsagareli MG: Non-opioid tolerance in juvenile and adult rats. *Eur J Pharmacol* 2010, **629**:68–72.

25. Vazquez E, Hernandez N, Escobar W, Vanegas H: Antinociception induced by intravenous dipyrone (metamizol) upon dorsal horn neurons: Involvement of endogenous opioids at the periaqueductal gray matter, the nucleus raphe magnus, and the spinal cord in rats. *Brain Res* 2005, **1048**:211–217.

26. Beaudry H, Proteau-Gagné A, Li S, Dory Y, Chavkin C, Gendron L: Differential noxious and motor tolerance of chronic delta opioid receptor agonists in rodents. *Neurosci* 2009, **61**:381–391.

27. Hernandez-Delgadillo GP, Cruz SL: Endogenous opioids are involved in morphine and dipyrone analgesic potentiation in the tail flick test in rats. *Eur J Pharmacol* 2006, **546**:54–59.

28. Heinricher MM, Ingram SL: The brainstem and nociceptive modulation. In *Science of Pain*. Edited by Basbaum AI, Bushnell MC. San Diego: Elsevier; 2009:593–626.

29. Vaughan CW: Enhancement of opioid inhibition of GABAergic synaptic transmission by cyclo-oxygenase inhibitors in rat periaqueductal grey neurons. *British J Pharmacol* 1998, **123**:1479–1481.

30. Wessendorf MW, Vaughan CW, Vanegas H: Rethinking the PAG and RVM: supraspinal modulation of nociception by opioids and nonopioids. In *11th World Congress Pain*. Edited by Flor H, Kalso E, Dostrovsky JO. Seattle: IASP Press; 2006:311–320.

31. Morgan MM, Kelsey L, Whittier A, Deborah M, Hegarty A, Sue AA: Periaqueductal gray neurons project to spinally projecting GABAergic neurons in the rostral ventromedial medulla. *Pain* 2008, **140**:376–386.

32. Tortorici V, Morgan MM, Vanegas H: Tolerance to repeated microinjection of morphine into the periaqueductal gray is associated with changes in the behavior of off- and on-cells in the rostral ventromedial medulla of rats. *Pain* 2001, **89**:237–244.

33. Escobar W, Ramirez K, Avila C, Limongi R, Vanegas H, Vazquez E: Metamizol, a non-opioid analgesic, acts via endocannabinoids in the PAG-RVM axis during inflammation in rats. *Eur J Pain* 2012, **16**:676–689.

34. Kalyuzhny AE, Wessendorf MW: Relationship of mu- and delta-opioid receptors to GABAergic neurons in the central nervous system, including antinociceptive brainstem circuits. *J Comp Neurol* 1998, **392**:528–547.

35. Kalyuzhny AE, Wessendorf MW: CNS GABA neurons express the mu-opioid receptor: immunocytochemical studies. *NeuroReport* 1997, **8**:3367–3372.

36. Svoboda KR, Lupica CR: Opioid inhibition of hippocampal interneurons via modulation of potassium and hyperpolarization-activated cation currents. *J Neurosci* 1998, **18**:7084–7098.

37. Cohen GA, Doze VA, Madison DV: Opioid inhibition of GABA release from presynaptic terminals of rat hippocampal interneurons. *Neuron* 1992, **2**:325–335.

38. Lupica CR, Proctor WR, Dunwiddie TV: Dissociation of mu and delta opioid receptor-mediated reductions in evoked and spontaneous synaptic inhibition in the rat hippocampus in vitro. *Brain Res* 1992, **593**:226–238.

39. Heinricher MM, Tavares I, Leith JL, Lumb BM: Descending control of nociception: specificity, recruitment and plasticity. *Brain Res Rev* 2009, **60**:214–225.

19

Influence of external calcium and thapsigargin on the uptake of polystyrene beads by the macrophage-like cell lines U937 and MH-S

Ebru Diler[1]*, Marion Schwarz[1], Ruth Nickels[2], Michael D Menger[2], Christoph Beisswenger[3], Carola Meier[1] and Thomas Tschernig[1]

Abstract

Background: Macrophages are equipped with several receptors for the recognition of foreign particles and pathogens. Upon binding to these receptors, particles become internalized. An interaction of particles with macrophage surface receptors is accompanied by an increase in cytosolic calcium concentration. This calcium is provided by intracellular stores and also by an influx of external calcium upon activation of the calcium channels. Nevertheless, the role of calcium in phagocytosis remains controversial. Some researchers postulate the necessity of calcium in Fc-receptor-mediated phagocytosis and a calcium-independent phagocytosis of complement opsonized particles. Others refute the need for calcium in Fc-receptor-mediated phagocytosis by macrophages.

Methods: In this study, the influence of external calcium concentrations and thapsigargin on the phagocytosis of polystyrene latex beads by the macrophage-like cell lines MH-S (murine) and differentiated U937 (human) was analyzed. The phagocytosis efficiency was determined by flow cytometry and was evaluated statistically by ANOVA test and Dunett's significance test, or ANOVA and Bonferroni's Multiple Comparison.

Results: Acquired data revealed an external calcium-independent way of internalization of non-functionalized polystyrene latex beads at free calcium concentrations ranging from 0 mM to 3 mM. The phagocytosis efficiency of the cells is not significantly decreased by a complete lack of external calcium. Furthermore, the presence of thapsigargin, known to lead to an increase of cytosolic calcium levels, did not have a significant enhancing influence on bead uptake by MH-S cells and only an enhancing effect on bead uptake by macrophage-like U937 cells at an external calcium concentration of 4 mM.

Conclusion: The calcium-independent phagocytosis process and the decrease of phagocytosis efficiency in the presence of complement receptor inhibitor staurosporine lead to the assumption that besides other calcium independent receptors, complement receptors are also involved in the uptake of polystyrene beads. The comparison of the phagocytosis efficiencies of both cell types in bivalent cation-free HBSS buffer and in cell medium, leads to the conclusion that it is more likely that other media ingredients such as magnesium are of greater importance for phagocytosis of non-functionalized polystyrene beads than calcium.

Keywords: Phagocytosis, Particle clearance, Macrophages, Calcium

* Correspondence: ebru.diler@uks.eu
[1]Institute of Anatomy, Saarland University, Kirrberger Str. 100, 66424 Homburg, Saar, Germany
Full list of author information is available at the end of the article

Background

The important role of macrophages in host defense against infection is known since Elie Metchnikoffs description of phagocytosis and the proposal that stimulation of phagocytes is essential for immunity [1]. Macrophages are also involved in clearance of cellular debris resulting from apoptosis or necrosis [2-4]. The recognition of endogenous danger signals resulting from cell necrosis and the stimulation of macrophages by cellular debris makes macrophages one of the frontline danger sensors [5]. In general, macrophages mediate host defense, wound healing and immune regulation. Besides phagocytosis of microorganisms and erythrocytes [6], macrophages also can uptake percoll and particles, such as polystyrene beads by endocytosis, which enables the investigation of cellular and molecular mechanisms of phagocytosis [7]. This is the most important mechanism for the clearance of particles and fibers in the lung. Furthermore, particle clearance by macrophages enables targeted drug delivery to macrophages, thereby minimizing the side effects of drugs caused by systemic application. Surface functionalization of beads can maximize particle uptake e.g. by Fc-receptor-mediated uptake [8] and provides a more directed delivery to the cells. Biodegradable nanoparticles, functionalized with mannose for targeted and enhanced uptake by macrophages, which bear reactive oxygen species detoxifying catalase, were demonstrated to be scavenged by macrophages [9].

Survival of macrophages depends - to a significant extent - on Ca^{2+} influx [10]. Furthermore, Ca^{2+} is demonstrated to be essential for the efficient killing of internalized pathogens by macrophages. The inhibition of macrophage Ca^{2+} signaling by infection with *M. tuberculosis* retards the maturation of the phagolysosomes, leading to the intracellular survival of the pathogen [11]. The intracellular Ca^{2+} concentration, whether maintained by internal or external Ca^{2+} sources, was also revealed to be essential for Fc-receptor-mediated phagocytosis [12]. Incubation of some cell types with the tumor promoter thapsigargin was demonstrated to increase intracellular Ca^{2+} levels by inhibiting Ca^{2+} reuptake from the cytosol by sarco-endoplasmic reticulum ATPases [13,14].

Since data on the systemic influence of calcium on the phagocytosis efficiency of polystyrene beads by macrophages was not determined so far, the aim of this study was to analyze the influence of external Ca^{2+} concentration and thapsigargin concentration on macrophage reference cell lines. The beads were neither opsonized with complement nor functionalized with immunoglobulins. The two different cell lines - the murine alveolar macrophage cell line MH-S [15] and the activated human lymphoma cell-line U937 [16] - were used as reference cell lines. The phagocytosis efficiency was evaluated by the uptake of fluorescence dye-labeled polystyrene beads. The data revealed an external calcium-independent ingestion of polystyrene beads at physiological calcium concentrations. The phagocytosis efficiency was only slightly enhanced by a high external calcium level of 4 mM in MH-S cells, if thapsigargin was not present. Activated U937 cells showed only a significant increase in phagocytosis at an external calcium level of 4 mM if 10 nM thapsigargin was present. This cell type was not influenced by external calcium levels, if thapsigargin was not present in cell medium. Furthermore, thapsigargin did not elevate the phagocytosis efficiency in standard cell culture medium RPMI1640 with 10% FCS, FCS-free RPMI1640 and in calcium free HBSS buffer.

Understanding the mechanisms of bead uptake by macrophages is essential for the therapeutic nano- and microparticle delivery to macrophages as a potential approach for targeted drug delivery [17].

Results

Influence of thapsigargin concentration and medium composition on phagocytosis

The influence of the thapsigargin concentration on the phagocytosis of the fluorescent beads by differentiated (activated) U937 and MH-S cells was analyzed in RPMI1640 medium supplemented with 10% FCS. An initial number of 5×10^5 cells were incubated with increasing concentrations of thapsigargin prior to the incubation with 1×10^7 beads. A number of 1×10^4 cells were analyzed by flow cytometry for increased fluorescence intensity caused by the uptake of particles. The graph in Figure 1 shows that a thapsigargin concentration in the range of 10 nM to 1 μM did not significantly influence the phagocytosis by U937 cells and MH-S cells (Figure 1).

The effect of 10 nM thapsigargin on the phagocytosis efficiency of differentiated U937 cells was investigated in RPMI1640 medium with 10% FCS (Figure 2A) in RPMI1640 medium without FCS (Figure 2B) and in external Ca^{2+}-free, Mg^{2+}-free and FCS-free HBSS buffer. No significant influence of 10 nM thapsigargin was determined on the phagocytosis efficiency of differentiated U937 cells in all three medium compositions (Figure 2). On the other hand, the comparison of the phagocytosis efficiencies in different media showed significant differences for phagocytosis of the beads by differentiated U937 cells. Figure 3 shows that the lowest phagocytosis efficiency was achieved in Ca^{2+}-free and Mg^{2+}-free HBSS buffer, followed by the value achieved in RPMI1640 medium without FCS. The highest phagocytosis rate was achieved in FCS-containing RPMI1640 medium.

The concentration of 10 nM thapsigargin did not influence the phagocytosis efficiency of MH-S cells for the beads significantly in any of the medium compositions

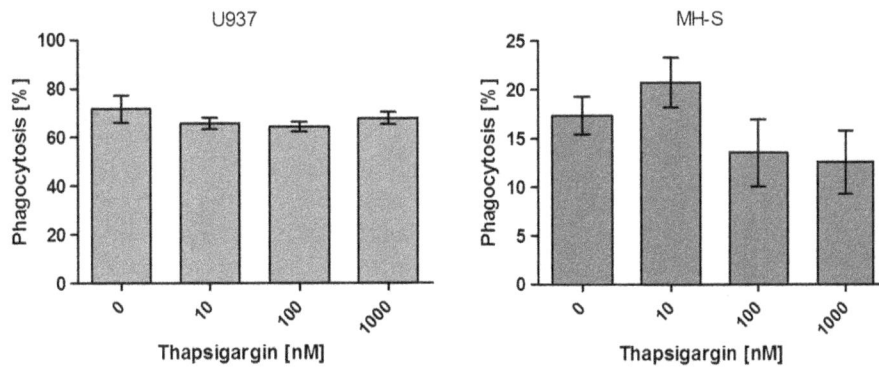

Figure 1 Influence of thapsigargin concentrations from 10 nM to 1 µM on the number of phagocytic cells. Phagocytosis efficiency was determined by FACS analysis.

used to determine the phagocytosis efficiency in this study (Figure 4). However, in contrast to the differentiated U937 cells, the phagocytosis efficiency of MH-S cells in HBSS buffer did not significantly differ from the phagocytosis efficiency in FCS-free RPMI1640 medium. In FCS-containing RPMI1640 medium, the MH-S cells showed a significantly higher phagocytosis efficiency than in HBSS buffer or in FCS-free RPMI1640 medium (Figure 5).

Influence of increasing external calcium ion concentrations on phagocytosis

To determine the effect of external calcium on the phagocytosis efficiency of macrophages, the reference cell lines MH-S and differentiated U937, were incubated in Ca^{2+}-free, Mg^{2+}-free and FCS-free HBSS buffer for one hour. Subsequently, gradually increasing concentrations of calcium chloride were added to the medium and the cells were incubated for an additional hour prior to incubation with 1×10^7 beads at 37°C. To determine the influence of thapsigargin, the same phagocytosis assays were also performed in the presence of 10 nM thapsigargin.

Figure 6 shows that external calcium did not significantly influenced the phagocytosis of beads by differentiated U937

in the range of 1 mM to 4 mM. In contrast, the presence of 10 nM thapsigargin led to a significant increase in the phagocytosis efficiency at a calcium level of 4 mM.

To exclude a decrease in the phagocytosis efficiency due to the lack of Mg^{2+} or FCS, RPMI1640 medium containing 10% FCS was incubated with 1 mM EGTA, which was demonstrated to be effective in chelating the total free Ca^{2+} in FCS-containing RPMI1640 medium (personal communication with Dr. Eva Schwarz, Saarland University Medical Center, Germany). Subsequently, increasing concentrations of $CaCl_2$ were added to 1 mM EGTA containing RPMI1640 + 10% FCS medium. The EGTA-calcium complex was not removed, but as determined by the software maxchelator, the present EGTA chelates not more than 1 mM of the added external Ca^{2+} (http://maxchelator.stanford.edu/webmaxc/webmaxcE.htm). Figure 7 shows that the addition of 1, 2, and 4 mM external Ca^{2+} to 1 mM EGTA-containing medium did not enhance the phagocytosis efficiency of differentiated U937 cells for the polystyrene beads significantly. According to the calculations made by maxchelator, these external calcium values correspond to 0 mM, 1 mM, and 3 mM free calcium. These values also do not differ significantly from

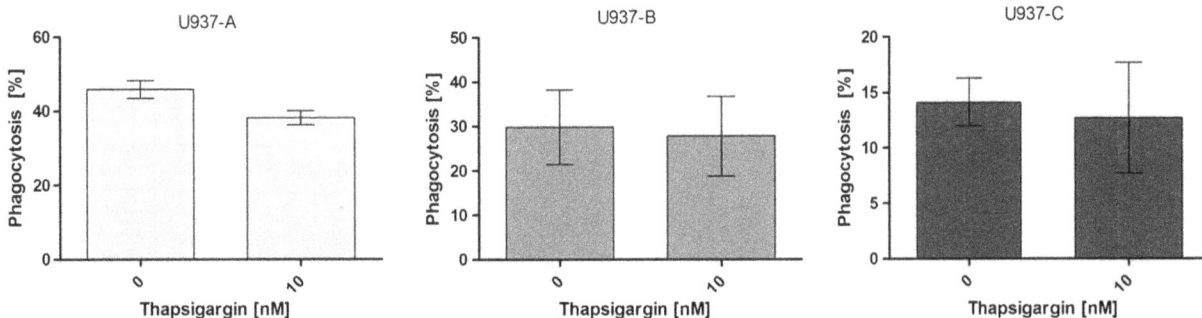

Figure 2 The influence of thapsigargin on phagocytosis by differentiated U937 cells in RPMI1640 medium with 10% FCS (A), in RPMI1640 medium without FCS (B) and in HBSS buffer (C). No significant influence by thapsigargin was determined in any medium composition.

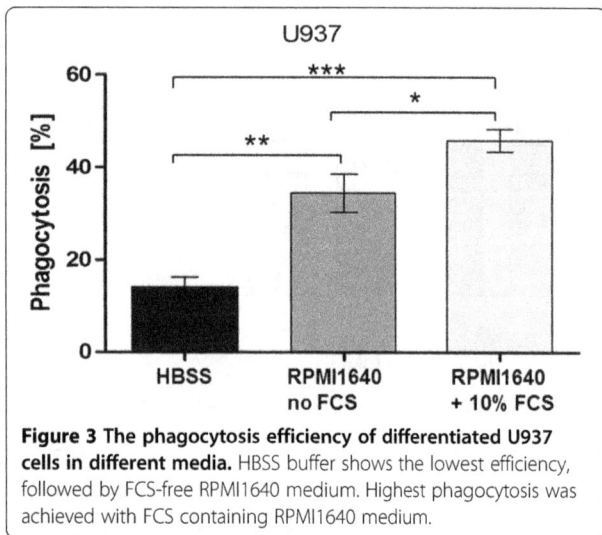

Figure 3 The phagocytosis efficiency of differentiated U937 cells in different media. HBSS buffer shows the lowest efficiency, followed by FCS-free RPMI1640 medium. Highest phagocytosis was achieved with FCS containing RPMI1640 medium.

the phagocytosis efficiency og U937 cells in chelator-free RPMI1640 + 10%FCS. A significant increase in phagocytosis was achieved only by the addition of 5 mM Ca^{2+} to the EGTA containing medium.

The phagocytosis efficiency of MH-S cells were not significantly affected in HBSS buffer that contains a free Ca^{2+}-concentration of 0, 0.5 mM, 1 mM and 2 mM. A significant increase in the uptake of beads by MH-S cells could be determined at a free external calcium level of with 4 mM. The presence of 10 nM thapsigargin did not significantly influence the phagocytosis efficiency. The cells showed rather a decreased uptake of the beads in 0.5 mM and 1 mM calcium containing buffer with 10 nM thapsigargin (Figure 8).

Cytotoxicity of the medium supplements and the uptake of beads

To determine the cytotoxic effects of the media, medium supplements (thapsigargin and calcium ions) and the phagocytosis of the polystyrene beads on the differentiated U937 and MH-S cells, a toxicity assay that correlates the release of cytosolic LDH, caused by cell lysis, to

the cytotoxicity of the reactants was used. A number of 1.5×10^4 cells were used for each assay condition. The maximal level of cell lysis was determined by incubating the cells with lysis buffer leading to the lysis of 100% of the cells. These values served then as reference values for the determination of the percental cytotoxicity of RPMI1640 medium, RPMI1640 medium with 10% FCS, HBSS buffer, HBSS buffer with 5 mM Ca^{2+}, HBSS buffer with 10 nM and 1 μM thapsigargin (Th). The cytotoxicity was determined for each condition in the presence and the absence of beads. The cell to beads ratio used in this assay was 1:20, according to the ratio used in the assays.

The results of the toxicity assay for both reference cell lines can be seen in Figure 9. In general, the spontaneous lysis activity of the cells in media is less than 10% and the uptake of beads did not further increase the LDH activity, hence the phagocytosis of the beads was not cytotoxic per se. The addition of 10 nM and 1 μM thapsigargin had a greater cytotoxic effect on the MH-S cells (up to 25.5%) whereas the U937 cells remained unaffected by 10 nM thapsigargin and were only slightly affected by 1 μM thapsigargin (10% cytotoxicity). In contrast, the presence of 5 mM Ca^{2+} in HBSS buffer caused a higher cell lysis of U937 cells of up to 46%. The addition of 5 mM calcium to HBSS buffer caused the lysis of up to 29% MH-S cells.

Determination of the adherence of beads to the cells

To verify that data obtained from the phagocytosis assays reflect the bead internalization by the cells and not only their adherence to the cells the assays were performed under two conditions that inhibit phagocytosis. However, the adherence of the beads to cells is not inhibited by these methods.

First, the cells were incubated with beads at 4°C. It was previously shown that incubation of macrophages at this temperature was not lethal and did not influence the ligand binding to cells. In contrary, the ingestion of the target by the phagocytic cells is inhibited at this

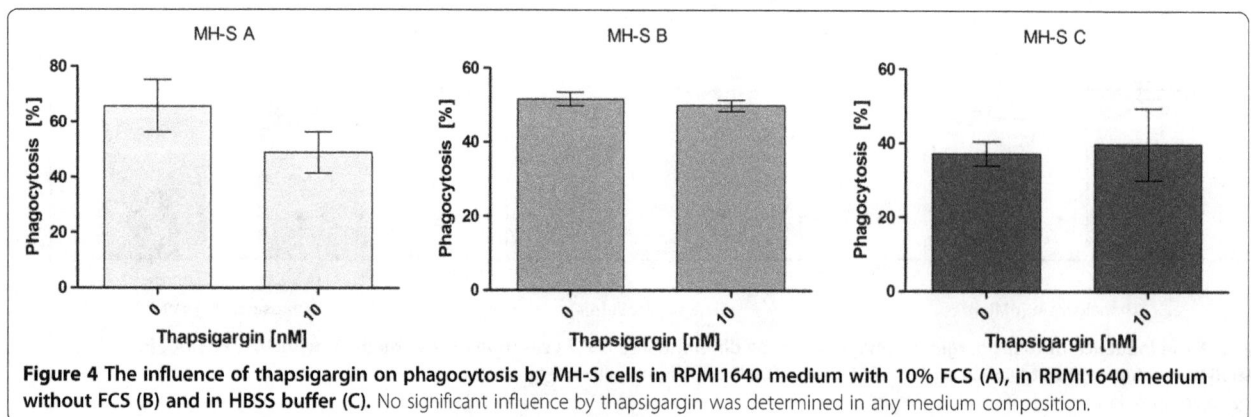

Figure 4 The influence of thapsigargin on phagocytosis by MH-S cells in RPMI1640 medium with 10% FCS (A), in RPMI1640 medium without FCS (B) and in HBSS buffer (C). No significant influence by thapsigargin was determined in any medium composition.

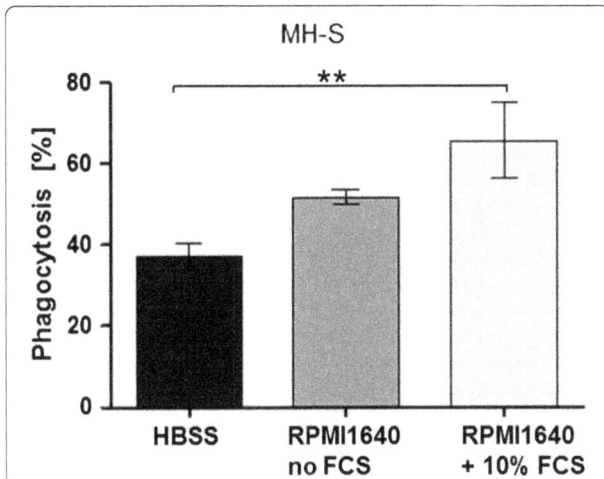

Figure 5 The phagocytosis efficiency of MH-S cells in different media. HBSS buffer shows the lowest efficiency, followed by FCS-free RPMI1640 medium. Highest phagocytosis was achieved with FCS containing RPMI1640 medium.

temperature [18]. Our data revealed that at 4°C, a significantly lower number of both type of cells were fluorescent due to bead adherence (Figure 10). This value for cells that adhered to beads (2.8% of MH-S cells and 0.9% of differentiated U937 cells) is lower than significant differences in assay conditions, where phagocytosis is performed at 37°C.

The second method for inhibiting the phagocytosis of beads was the use of three phagocytosis inhibitors: cytochalasin D (Cyto D: 5 µg ml^{-1} and 15 µg ml^{-1}), nocodazole (Noc: 3 µg ml^{-1}) and staurosporine (Stau: 10 µM). Additionally, a mixture of Cyto D and Noc or a mixture of Cyto D, Noc and Stau were added to the cells. The assay was performed at 37°C and the cells were incubated with the beads for 2 hours. Figure 10 shows that each inhibitor by its own caused a significant decrease in the phagocytosis of the beads but a residual phagocytosis still remained. Adding 15 µg ml^{-1} of Cyto D or a mixture of Noc and Cyto D caused a decrease in the

percentage of fluorescent MH-S cells down to 0.96% and 1.3% compared to a phygocytosis efficiency of 17.13% at inhibitor-free conditions. These values were much higher for differentiated U937 cells (6.2% and 4.4%) but both cell types were strongly inhibited in their ability of ingesting beads by the simultaneous presence of all of the three inhibitors (MH-S: 0.7%, U937: 1%). These values were comparable to the results obtained from the phagocytosis assays performed at 4°C (Figure 10).

Both methods showed that the percentage of cells showing fluorescence due to bead adherence is much lesser than significant differences achieved in phagocytosis efficiencies due to different conditions. Therefore, adherence of beads did not falsify the results.

Discussion and conclusion

Macrophages and neutrophils are professional phagocytosis cells of the innate immune system. The uptake of large particles (>0.5 µm) occurs in an actin-dependent manner. It has been demonstrated that many cells, such as bladder and thyroid epithelial cells, also accomplish phagocytosis [19] but professional phagocytes, like macrophages, possess phagocytic receptors that increase the target particle range and the phagocytosis rate [20]. The mechanisms underlying phagocytosis by macrophages are complex and provide important tools for the essential role of the cells in the uptake and degradation of infectious agents, senescent cells, particles, tissue remodeling, immune response and inflammation [21].

Macrophages are equipped with receptors for Fc-mediated, complement-mediated and pathogenic conserved motifs-mediated phagocytosis [21]. Although ligand binding to all of these receptors promotes phagocytosis, the effects of receptor signaling differ. Whereas FcR-mediated phagocytosis results in the production and secretion of proinflammatory mediators like arachidionic acid and reactive oxygen species, complement receptor (CR)-mediated phagocytosis does not cause the release of these mediators [22,23]. Interaction of ligands with phagocytic receptors for

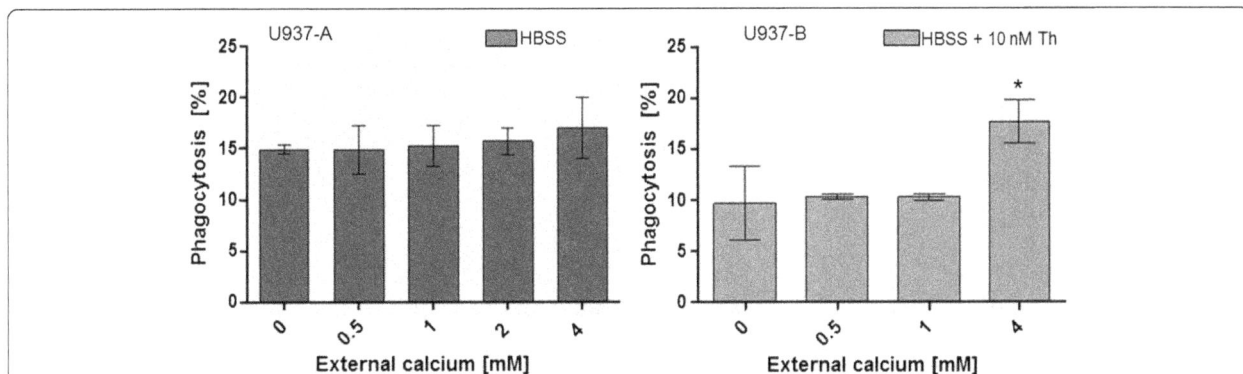

Figure 6 The phagocytosis efficiency of U937 cells dependent on external calcium ion concentrations in HBSS buffer without thapsigargin (dark grey bars) and with 10 nM thapsigargin (light grey bars). Th: thapsigargin. Statistical significance is marked by asterisks.

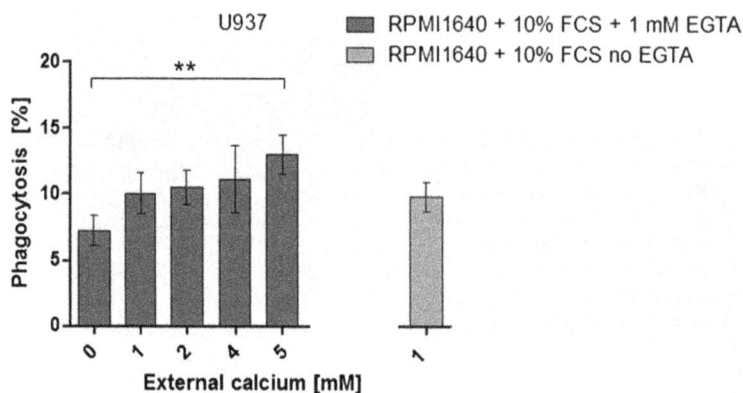

Figure 7 The phagocytosis of beads by U937 cells in RPMI 1640 + 10% FCS with 1 mM EGTA and gradually increasing levels of external calcium ions (dark grey bars) compared to phagocytosis of cells incubated in EGTA free RPMI 1640 + 10% FCS with 1 mM Ca^{2+} (light grey bar). Statistical significance is marked by an asterisk.

immunoglobulins (FcγR) and for complement proteins induces the activation of phospholipase C and phospholipase D, which in turn leads to the formation of Ca^{2+} mobilizing second messengers. This, on the other hand, is involved in the activation of store-operated calcium entry (SOCE) channels in the plasma membrane, resulting in a Ca^{2+} flux from the extracellular medium. It is generally accepted that an increase in cytosolic Ca^{2+} is an early signal that accompanies phagocytic ingestion, but the elevation of cytososlic Ca^{2+} is required for the promotion of an efficient ingestion of foreign particles by some, but not all, receptors. In 1985 Lew et al. showed that antibody/FcR generated phagocytosis relies on an increase of cytosolic Ca^{2+} concentration upon receptor activation, whereas activation of the complement receptor C3b/bi generates a Ca^{2+}-independent phagocytosis mechanism in human neutrophils. They determined a decrease in Fc-receptor-mediated phagocytosis after increasing the intracellular Ca^{2+}-buffering capacity of quin2, which was more pronounced in the absence of extracellular calcium. In contrast, a decrease in complement-mediated phagocytosis of yeast cells was not observed despite increasing the intracellular Ca^{2+} buffering by quin2 [24]. Nevertheless, the

question of the necessity of Ca^{2+} for the phagocytosis of foreign particles is controversial [25]. Some studies in murine macrophages verified a decrease of phagocytic ingestion of IgG opsonized or non-opsonized latex beads due to Ca^{2+} chelation [26-28], whereas others reported effective phagocytosis of IgG opsonized red blood cells at low cytosolic Ca^{2+} levels [29-31].

In this study, the influence of external calcium levels and thapsigargin concentrations were investigated with regard to the phagocytosis efficiency for non-IgG functionalized, fluorescence-labeled polystyrene beads. The phagocytosis assays were applied on two different reference cell lines: the murine alveolar macrophage derived MH-S [15] and human lymphoma monocyte like cell line U937 [16], which were differentiated to adherent, phagocytosis-exhibiting macrophage-like cells by PMA, previous to performing phagocytosis assays.

The data acquired from thapsigargin containing assay set-ups, external Ca^{2+} free conditions, and a stepwise increase in external Ca^{2+} concentrations revealed that external calcium concentrations of 1 mM and 2 mM did not influence the uptake of non-functionalized beads by differentiated U937 cells and MH-S cells in HBSS buffer.

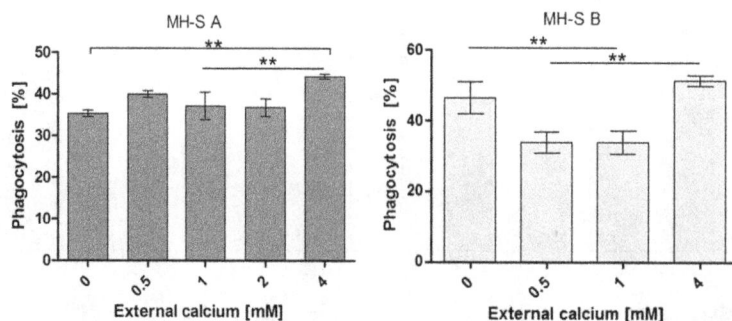

Figure 8 The phagocytosis efficiency of MH-S cells dependent on external calcium ion concentrations in HBSS buffer without thapsigargin (dark grey bars) and with 10 nM thapsigargin (light grey bars). Statistical significance is marked by asterisks.

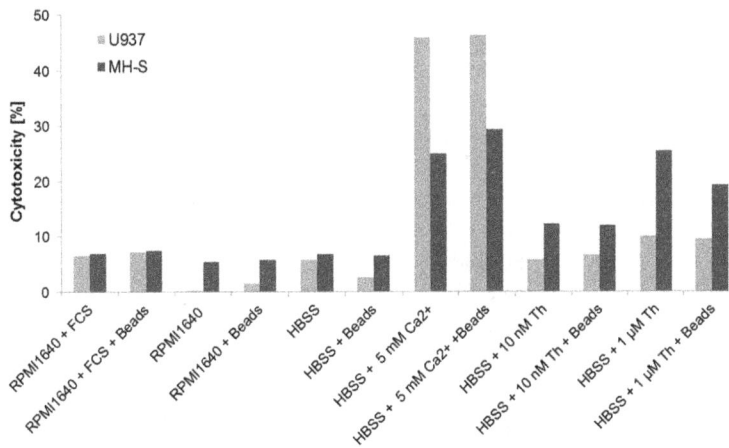

Figure 9 The cytotoxic effect of medium composition, supplements and bead internalization on MH-S cells (dark grey bars) and differentiated U937 cells (light grey bars). The cytotoxicity is determined by the activity of LHD, which is released from lysed cells. A number of 1.5×10^4 cells that were completely lysed by lysis buffer served as reference.

Furthermore, neither the presence nor the absence of thapsigargin also affected the phagocytosis efficiency of these cells at physiological calcium levels. The phagocytosis efficiency of differentiated U937 cells was not even affected in their phagocytosis efficiency at an external calcium level of 4 mM. This situation changed if 10 nM thapsigargin was present in HBSS buffer. Whereas external free calcium concentrations of 1 mM and 2 mM were still ineffective in increasing the phagocytosis efficiency of differentiated U937 cells, the presence of

thapsigargin enhanced phagocytosis efficiency from 9.6% to 17.7% at an external calcium concentration of 4 mM. The cytotoxicity assay showed that the increased calcium levels in HBSS buffer caused a high level of cell death of up to 46%, which was probably caused either by high osmotic pressure or by an increase in intracellular calcium levels, known to cause the death of cells [32]. To exclude decreased phagocytosis efficiency due to the lack of FCS or Mg^{2+}, phagocytosis assays with differentiated U937 cells were performed in 1 m EGTA containing

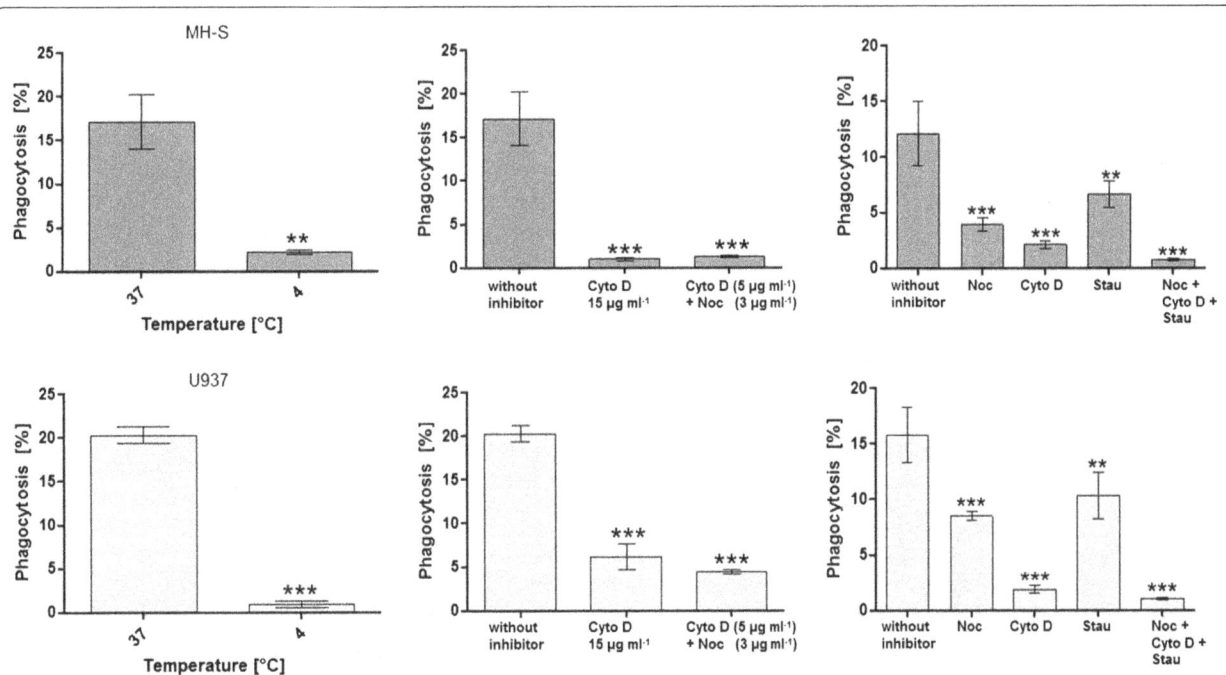

Figure 10 Comparison of the percentage of fluorescent cells under phagocytosis inhibiting conditions (4°C and inhibitors) with phagocytosis efficiency under non-inhibitory conditions.

RPMI1640 + 10% FCS medium. This concentration of EGTA was shown to be effective in chelating the complete free calcium of the FCS containing medium (personal communication with Dr. Eva Schwarz, Saarland University). The phagocytosis efficiency of differentiated U937 cells in this medium did not show a significant difference to the phagocytosis efficiency in EGTA-free RPMI1640 + 10% FCS medium. Further increase of external calcium only showed significant enhancement in phagocytosis efficiency at a calcium concentration of 5 mM, which according to the maxchelator software, corresponds to 4 mM free calcium. But, the amount of free calcium in FCS is not known, and probably the calcium level is much higher than 4 mM. This data also provided a hint to the insignificant role of physiological calcium levels on phagocytosis.

MH-S cells showed some differences in phagocytosis efficiency at an external calcium concentration of 4 mM. In the absence of thapsigargin, the presence of 4 mM external free calcium in HBSS buffer increased the phagocytosis efficiency of MH-S cells significantly from 35% to 44%, whereas in the presence of 10 nM thapsigargin, no enhancement of the phagocytosis efficiency of MH-S cells was determined. Nevertheless, neither cell line showed any differences in their phagocytosis efficiency in the range of free external calcium at the range of 0 mM to 2 mM in HBSS buffer. We can conclude that, at physiological free calcium levels, which, according to free calcium measurements of the sera of healthy individuals, is at the range of 1.175 mM – 1.375 mM [33], the efficiency of phagocytosis of beads by MH-S cells and differentiated U937 cells is not affected by calcium.

It was previously demonstrated that the tumor promoter thapsigargin increases intracellular free Ca^{2+}-levels by inhibiting the Ca^{2+} reuptake from the cytosol into the ER-lumen by sarco-endoplasmic reticulum ATPases [13,14]. In this study, experimental set-ups with increasing thapsigargin concentrations in RPMI1640 + 10% FCS revealed that the phagocytosis behavior of differentiated U937 cells and MH-S cells is not affected by the presence of thapsigargin, even at concentrations of 1 μM. As mentioned, a concentration of 10 nM thapsigargin was only effective in enhancing the phagocytosis efficiency of U937 cells in HBSS buffer with 4 mM calcium, but not at lower extracellular calcium levels. According to the cytotoxicity assay, differentiated U937 cells seem to be resistant to the presence of thapsigargin even at high concentrations. MH-S cells, on the other hand, were highly sensitive to the presence of thapsigargin, leading to a cell lysis of up to 25.5%.

The uptake of beads by differentiated U937 cells in Ca^{2+}-free, Mg^{2+}-free HBSS buffer was low, compared to the phagocytosis efficiency in FCS-free RPMI 1640 medium, which, according to the manufacturer, contains 1 mM free Ca^{2+}. However, after verifying that this

external Ca^{2+} concentration does not have an increasing effect on phagocytosis efficiency, it can be concluded that other supplements such as magnesium, which is also not present in HBSS, could have a more pronounced influence on the phagocytosis efficiency of these cells. In fact, the suppression of phagocytosis caused by lowered extracellular levels of magnesium was previously demonstrated in rat alveolar macrophages [34,35].

All of the data acquired in this study indicate that the uptake of non-functionalized polystyrene beads with a size of 1 μm by MH-S cells and by differentiated U937 cells does not depend on external calcium at physiological levels or on the addition of thapsigargin. The beads used in this study, were not opsonized with antibodies or with complement proteins but the latter type of opsonization cannot be excluded in phagocytosis assays performed in FCS-containing medium. As mentioned above, complement-mediated phagocytosis was demonstrated to be Ca^{2+} independent in human neutrophils [24]. Therefore, a complement-mediated, Ca^{2+}- independent phagocytosis of polystyrene beads is a possible way of bead uptake by the reference macrophage-like cell lines used. This conclusion is further supported by the results obtained from phagocytosis studies performed in the presence of staurosporine. The uptake of beads by both cell types was significantly reduced when the complement receptor inhibitor staurosporine was added to the medium. Therefore, the calcium- independent phagocytosis process and the influence of staurosporine on bead uptake reveal a possible complement receptor-dependent way of polystyrene bead entry. However, taking into account that staurosporine did not completely inhibit the bead uptake, interaction of beads with other receptors could also cause the uptake of beads in an Ca^{2+}-independent manner.

In conclusion, a comparison of the particle uptake by differentiated U937 cells and MH-S cells in Ca^{2+}-containing HBSS with that in FCS-free RPMI 1640 medium indicated that other PRMI1640 ingredients, for example magnesium ions, could be more necessary for an efficient phagocytosis than free external calcium ions. Experiments to reveal the influence of external magnesium are in preparation and should shed some light onto the mechanisms involved in the uptake of polystyrene beads by macrophage-like U937 cells and MH-S cells.

Methods

Cells

The murine alveolar macrophages cell line MH-S was obtained from Sigma-Aldrich (Germany). These cells were grown in RPMI 1640 medium (Lonza, Germany) containing 10% heat inactivated fetal bovine serum (PAA, Germany), 100 Units ml^{-1} penicillin, 100 μg ml^{-1}

streptomycin (both antibiotics from PAA, Germany) and 50 μM β- mercaptoethanol (gibco life technologies, Darmstadt, Germany) at 37°C in a humidified atmosphere with 5% CO_2. To detach the cells from culture flasks a few milliliters of a mixture of 500 μg ml^{-1} trypsin with 220 μg ml^{-1} EDTA were added to the adherent cells, which were then incubated at 37°C for fifteen minutes. Cells were then collected by centrifugation and resuspended in medium. Then 0.5×10^6 or 1×10^6 cells were disseminated on 12 well-plates (Greiner Bio-One, Frickenhausen, Germany). After 15 hours the cells were used for the phagocytosis assay.

The monocyte-like human lymphoma U937 cell line was cultivated in RPMI 1640 medium with 10% fetal bovine serum, 100 Units ml^{-1} penicillin and 100 μg ml^{-1} streptomycin. For differentiation into adherent macrophage-like cells capable of phagocytosis, cells were incubated with 50 ng ml^{-1} phorbol 12-myristate 13-acetate (PMA) (Sigma Aldrich) for 20 hours, washed with medium once, and then incubated in medium for 48 hours at 37°C in a humidified atmosphere with 5% CO_2. Subsequently the cells were used for the phagocytosis assay.

Phagocytosis of fluorescent beads

Fluoresbrite® Yellow Green Microspheres (Polysciences GmbH, Eppenheim, Germany) with a size of 1 μm were used for phagocytosis assays. 0.5×10^6 or 1×10^6 cells were incubated with 1×10^7 or 2×10^7 beads (20× excess of beads), respectively, for 2 hours.

To determine the thapsigargin influence on the efficiency of phagocytosis, 5×10^5 cells were incubated with 100 nM, 400 nM, 1 μM, and 10 μM thapsigargin for 1 h previous to phagocytosis. Then, 1×10^7 beads were added to the cells and incubated for 2 hours.

External Ca^{2+} influence was determined by using Ca^{2+} free and Mg^{2+} free Hank's Balanced Salt Solution (HBSS). After growth of the cells in RPMI 1640 with 10% FCS, the medium was removed, the cells were washed with phosphate-buffered saline (PBS) and then incubated in HBSS buffer with a stepwise increase in the concentration of $CaCl_2$ rising from 0.5 - 5 mM $CaCl_2$ with or without 10 nM thapsigargin for one hour previous to bead addition. The phagocytosis efficiency was analyzed by flow cytometry.

To decrease the level of free Ca^{2+} in RPMI 1640 medium containing 10% FCS, the medium was incubated with sterile filtered 1 mM ethylenglycol tetraacetic acid (EGTA). A number of 5×10^5 cells per well were incubated in EGTA containing medium for 20 minutes and then increasing concentrations of $CaCl_2$ from 0.5 mM to 5 mM were added stepwise to the cells. After an incubation period of 30 minutes, 1×10^7 beads with a size of 1 μm were added and the cells incubated with beads for 2 hours in a humidified

incubator at 37°C with 5% CO_2. Subsequently, the bead-containing medium was removed and cells were washed with PBS prior to trypsinization. The cells were fixed with 4% paraformaldehyde solution in PBS pH 7.4 and stored at 4°C for several days until analysis by flow cytometry.

Flow cytometric analysis of phagocytosis efficiency

The phagocytosis efficiencies were determined by using a BD FACScan™ flow cytometer (Becton- Dickinson, Heidelberg, Germany). Point plotting of the events measured in the fluorescence channel (ordinate) versus total events measured in the forward scatter channel (abscissa) revealed the number of cells that internalized fluorescent beads. MH-S cells and differentiated U937 cells that were not incubated with fluorescent beads were used to determine the auto fluorescence and to define the dot plot panel sizes. The phagocytosis efficiency of cells was defined as the percentage of cells that internalized beads with reference to the total cells analyzed by flow cytometry. The number of cells analyzed was between 2×10^3 and 1×10^4. The number of beads internalized by each cell was not considered in the determination of the efficiency of phagocytosis.

LDH cytotoxicity assay

To determine the cytotoxic effects of different media compositions (RPMI1640, RPMI1640 + 10%FCS and HBSS) and supplements (5 mM Ca^{2+}, 10 nM thapsigargin, and 1 μM thapsigargin), the Pierce™ LDH Cytotoxicity Assay Kit from Thermo Scientific (Schwerte, Germany) was used. To determine cytotoxic effect of internalization of polystyrene beads, the assay was performed in the absence and also in the presence of beads (beads to cell ratio: 20:1). The assay was performed according to the manufacturer's instructions for chemical compound mediated cytotoxicity. Fluorescence of media compositions and LDH activity in FCS was determined in a cell-free manner and subtracted from sample results. However, in contrast to the instructions, spontaneous LDH activity was not subtracted from the sample results, because, besides toxic effect of calcium, thapsigargin and uptake of beads, the aim was also to determine the lytic effect of media compositions per se.

Determination of adhesion of beads to the cells

The portion of bead adherence to the macrophage-like cells was determined by incubating cells and beads to a ratio of 1:20 in RPMI1640 + 10% FCS medium at 4°C. After two hours of incubation, the cells were washed with ice-cold PBS and then trypsinized. After fixation, 1×10^4 cells were analyzed by flow cytometer (FACSCalibur, Becton-Dickinson, Heidelberg, Germany). The second method for determining adherence of beads to the macrophage-like cells used was the addition of phagocytosis inhibitors to the cell medium previous to phagocytosis. For this purposes, the cells were incubated in RPMI1640 + 10% FCS medium with cytochalasin D (5 µg ml^{-1} or 15 µg ml^{-1}), nocodazole (3 µg ml^{-1}) or staurosporin (10 µM). Furthermore, a mixture of cytochalasin D (5 µg ml^{-1}) and nocodazole or a mixture of cytochalasin D (5 µg ml^{-1}), nocodazole (3 µg ml^{-1}) and staurosporine (10 µM) were added to the medium. The cells were incubated in inhibitor containing medium for two hours at 37°C. Subsequently the polystyrene beads were added and phagocytosis was accomplished for two hours at 37°C. A number of 1×10^4 cells were analyzed by flow cytometer.

Statistics

Calculations, graphical illustration of data and statistical analysis were accomplished with GraphPad Prism (GraphPad Software Inc., La Jolla, USA). Data are presented as mean ± standard deviation. The significance in mean value differences (P < 0.05) were determined by t-test and analysis of variance (ANOVA) with the post-hoc analysis of Dunnett's or Bonferroni's Multiple Comparison Test and labeled with asterisks.

Abbreviations

ATPase: Adenylpyrophosphatase, Adenosine Triphosphatase; CR: Complement receptor; Cyto D: Cytochalasine D; EDTA: Ethylenediaminetetraacetic acid; EGTA: Ethylene glycol tetraacetic acid; ER: Endoplasmic reticulum; FCS: Fetal calf serum; HBSS: Hank's Balanced Salt Solution; MH-S: Murine alveolar macrophage cell line; Noc: Nocodazole; PBS: Phosphate buffered saline; PMA: Phorbol-12-myristat-13-acetat; Stau: Staurosporine; U937: Human monocyte like cell line.

Competing interests

The authors declare that they have no competing interests.

Authors' contributions

ED and TT conceived the study and conducted the experiments. MS and RN were responsible for the cell culture, performed the phagocytosis assays, flow cytometry and data analysis. CB, MM and CM participated in the study design and were involved in the interpretation of the results as well as in the drafting of the manuscript. ED participated in all parts of the study and wrote the manuscript. All authors read and approved the final manuscript.

Acknowledgment

The authors are thankful to Ann-Mary Soether for proofreading and to Andreas Kamyschnikow for technical help.

Author details

[1]Institute of Anatomy, Saarland University, Kirrberger Str. 100, 66424 Homburg, Saar, Germany. [2]Institute for Clinical & Experimental Surgery, Saarland University, Homburg, Saar, Germany. [3]Department of Internal Medicine V-Pulmonology, Allergology, Respiratory Intensive Care Medicine, Saarland University Hospital, Homburg, Saar, Germany.

References

1. Nathan C: Metchnikoff's Legacy in 2008. Nat Immunol 2008, 9(7):695–698.
2. Erwig L, Henson P: Clearance of apoptotic cells by phagocytes. Cell Death Differ 2007, 15(2):243–250.
3. Erwig L-P, Henson PM: Immunological consequences of apoptotic cell phagocytosis. Am J Pathol 2007, 171(1):2–8.
4. Zhang X, Mosser DM: Macrophage activation by endogenous danger signals. J Pathol 2008, 214(2):161–178.
5. Kono H, Rock KL: How dying cells alert the immune system to danger. Nat Rev Immunol 2008, 8(4):279–289.
6. Stossel TP: How Do Phagocytes Eat? Ann Intern Med 1978, 89(3):398–402.
7. Pratten MK, Lloyd JB: Pinocytosis and phagocytosis: the effect of size of a particulate substrate on its mode of capture by rat peritoneal macrophages cultured in vitro. Biochim Biophys Acta Gen Subj 1986, 881(3):307–313.
8. Pacheco P, White D, Sulchek T: Effects of microparticle size and Fc density on macrophage phagocytosis. PLoS One 2013, 8(4):e60989.
9. Saraf A, Dasani A, Soni A: Targeted delivery of catalase to macrophages by using surface modification of biodegradable nanoparticle. IJPSR, 4(8):2221–2229.
10. Tano J-Y, Vazquez G: Requirement for non-regulated, constitutive calcium influx in macrophage survival signaling. Biochem Biophys Res Commun 2011, 407(2):432–437.
11. Malik ZA, Denning GM, Kusner DJ: Inhibition of Ca2+ signaling by Mycobacterium tuberculosisis associated with reduced phagosome-lysosome fusion and increased survival within human macrophages. J Exp Med 2000, 191(2):287–302.
12. Young J, Ko SS, Cohn ZA: The increase in intracellular free calcium associated with IgG gamma 2b/gamma 1 Fc receptor-ligand interactions: role in phagocytosis. Proc Natl Acad Sci 1984, 81(17):5430–5434.
13. Thastrup O, Cullen PJ, Drøbak B, Hanley MR, Dawson AP: Thapsigargin, a tumor promoter, discharges intracellular Ca2+ stores by specific inhibition of the endoplasmic reticulum Ca2 (+)-ATPase. Proc Natl Acad Sci 1990, 87(7):2466–2470.
14. Treiman M, Caspersen C, Christensen SB: A tool coming of age: thapsigargin as an inhibitor of sarco-endoplasmic reticulum Ca < sup > 2 + </sup > – ATPases. Trends Pharmacol Sci 1998, 19(4):131–135.
15. Larrick JW, Fischer D, Anderson S, Koren H: Characterization of a human macrophage-like cell line stimulated in vitro: a model of macrophage functions. J Immunol 1980, 125(1):6–12.
16. Sundström C, Nilsson K: Establishment and characterization of a human histiocytic lymphoma cell line (U-937). Int J Cancer 1976, 17(5):565–577.
17. Kumar M: Nano and microparticles as controlled drug delivery devices. J Pharm Pharm Sci 2000, 3(2):234–258.
18. Griffin FM, Griffin J, Leider JE, Silverstein S: Studies on the mechanism of phagocytosis I. Requirements for circumferential attachment of particle-bound ligands to specific receptors on the macrophage plasma membrane. J Exp Med 1975, 142(5):1263–1282.
19. Rabinovitch M: Professional and non-professional phagocytes: an introduction. Trends Cell Biol 1995, 5(3):85–87.
20. Indik ZK, Park J-G, Hunter S, Schreiber A: The molecular dissection of Fc gamma receptor mediated phagocytosis. Blood 1995, 86(12):4389–4399.
21. Aderem A, Underhill DM: Mechanisms of phagocytosis in macrophages. Annu Rev Immunol 1999, 17(1):593–623.
22. Aderem A, Wright S, Silverstein S, Cohn Z: Ligated complement receptors do not activate the arachidonic acid cascade in resident peritoneal macrophages. J Exp Med 1985, 161(3):617–622.
23. Wright SD, Silverstein S: Receptors for C3b and C3bi promote phagocytosis but not the release of toxic oxygen from human phagocytes. J Exp Med 1983, 158(6):2016–2023.
24. Lew DP, Andersson T, Hed J, Di Virgilio F, Pozzan T, Stendahl O: Ca2 + –dependent and Ca2 + –independent phagocytosis in human neutrophils. Nature 1985, 315(6019):509–511.
25. Nunes P, Demaurex N: The role of calcium signaling in phagocytosis. J Leukoc Biol 2010, 88(1):57–68.
26. Hishikawa T, Cheung JY, Yelamarty RV, Knutson DW: Calcium transients during Fc receptor-mediated and nonspecific phagocytosis by murine peritoneal macrophages. J Cell biol 1991, 115(1):59–66.
27. Ichinose M, Asai M, Sawada M: β-endorphin enhances phagocytosis of latex particles in mouse peritoneal macrophages. Scand J Immunol 1995, 42(3):311–316.
28. Ichinose M, Asai M, Sawada M: Enhancement of phagocytosis by dynorphin A in mouse peritoneal macrophages. J Neuroimmunol 1995, 60(1):37–43.
29. McNeil P, Swanson J, Wright S, Silverstein S, Taylor D: Fc-receptor-mediated phagocytosis occurs in macrophages without an increase in average [Ca++] i. J Cell biol 1986, 102(5):1586–1592.

30. Di Virgilio F, Meyer BC, Greenberg S, Silverstein SC: **Fc receptor-mediated phagocytosis occurs in macrophages at exceedingly low cytosolic Ca2+ levels.** *J Cell biol* 1988, **106**(3):657–666.

31. Greenberg S, El Khoury J, Di Virgilio F, Kaplan EM, Silverstein SC: **Ca (2+)-independent F-actin assembly and disassembly during Fc receptor-mediated phagocytosis in mouse macrophages.** *J Cell biol* 1991, **113**(4):757–767.

32. Yue C, Soboloff J, Gamero AM: **Control of type I interferon-induced cell death by Orai1-mediated calcium entry in T cells.** *J Biol Chem* 2012, **287**(5):3207–3216.

33. Ladenson JH, Bowers GN: **Free calcium in serum. I. Determination with the Ion-specific electrode, and factors affecting the results.** *Clin Chem* 1973, **19**(6):565–574.

34. Ishiguro S, Miyamoto A, Tokushima T, Ueda A, Nishio A: **Low extracellular Mg2+ concentrations suppress phagocytosis in vitro by alveolar macrophages from rats.** *Magnes Res* 2000, **13**(1):11–18.

35. Nishio A, Kikuchi K, Ueda A, Miyamoto A, Ishiguro S, Rayssiguier Y, Mazur A, Durlach J: *Phagocytosis by Alveolar Macrophages During Dietary Magnesium Deficiency in Adult Rats,* Advances in Magnesium Research: Nutrition and Health. 2001:297–300.

20

A Phase 1 dose-ranging study examining the effects of a superabsorbent polymer (CLP) on fluid, sodium and potassium excretion in healthy subjects

Lee W Henderson[1], Howard C Dittrich[1], Alan Strickland[2], Thomas M Blok[3], Richard Newman[4], Thomas Oliphant[5] and Detlef Albrecht[1*]

Abstract

Background: CLP is an orally administered, non-absorbed, superabsorbent polymer being developed to increase fecal excretion of sodium, potassium and water in patients with heart failure and end-stage renal disease. This study was conducted to evaluate the safety of CLP, and to explore dose-related effects on fecal weight, fecal and urine sodium and potassium excretion, and serum electrolyte concentrations.

Methods: This Phase 1, open-label, dose-escalation study included 25 healthy volunteers, who were administered CLP orally immediately prior to four daily meals for 9 days at doses of 7.5, 15.0, and 25.0 g/day (n = 5/group). An additional dose group received 15.0 g/day CLP under fasting conditions, and an untreated cohort (n = 5) served as control. Twenty-four-hour fecal and urinary output was collected daily. Samples were weighed, and sodium, potassium, and other ion content in stool and urine were measured for each treatment group. Effects on serum cation concentrations, other standard laboratory values, and adverse events were also determined.

Results: At doses below 25.0 g/day, CLP was well tolerated, with a low frequency of self-limiting gastrointestinal adverse events. CLP increased fecal weight and fecal sodium and potassium content in a dose-related manner. Concomitant dose-related decreases in urinary sodium and potassium were observed. All serum ion concentrations remained within normal limits.

Conclusions: In this study, oral CLP removed water, sodium and potassium from the body via the gastrointestinal tract in a dose related fashion. CLP could become useful for patients with fluid overload and compromised kidney function in conditions such as congestive heart failure, salt sensitive hypertension, chronic kidney disease and end stage renal disease.

Trial registration: NCT01944007

Keywords: Superabsorbent polymer, Dose ranging, Pharmacodynamics, Gastrointestinal fluid removal, Gastrointestinal sodium removal

* Correspondence: dalbrecht@sorbent.com
[1]Sorbent Therapeutics Inc, 710 Lakeway Drive, Suite 290, Sunnyvale, CA 94085, USA
Full list of author information is available at the end of the article

Background

Fluid overload and sodium retention are central components in the pathophysiology of heart failure, with up to 90% of hospitalizations in heart failure caused by symptoms and signs of fluid overload [1,2]. There is also growing evidence that hypervolemia *per se* is independently associated with mortality [3,4]. Concomitant renal dysfunction (chronic kidney disease; CKD) has a strong association with poor outcomes in heart failure patients [5,6]. Diuretics are the cornerstone of acute and chronic heart failure therapy, but concerns have been raised about the safety and therapeutic efficacy of high dose diuretic therapy [2,7-9], diuretic resistance in the presence of declining renal function and undesired serum electrolyte effects [10,11]. The use of cationic exchange resins for removal of excess sodium and water via the gastrointestinal tract from edematous patients was under considerable study in the late 1940s and early 1950s [12]. These products failed to achieve a significant therapeutic presence, in large measure due to the high dosage required (up to 150 g/day), problems in taking the large amounts of unpalatable resins, significant abdominal side effects and the advent of loop diuretics. Recently, interest in the use of the gastrointestinal tract to remove fluid and/or ions using polymers of enhanced efficacy and improved tolerability has been renewed [13,14].

New treatment options for fluid and ion management are a significant medical need [2]. CLP (Cross Linked Polyelectrolyte) is a novel, non-absorbed, superabsorbent polymer that, given orally, absorbs water, sodium and potassium in the gastrointestinal tract with eventual elimination in the feces. The clinical effects of CLP in patients with congestive heart failure and impaired kidney function were recently reported in a Phase 2, double-blind, placebo-controlled study. Patients administered 15 g/day CLP lost significantly more weight, had a higher proportion of improvement in New York Heart Association (NYHA) class and showed a trend for improvement in both the six minute walk test and the Kansas City Cardiomyopathy Questionnaire compared to patients receiving placebo [13]. This exploratory Phase 1 study was done before the Phase 2 study and the purpose was to evaluate the safety of CLP, and to explore the dose-related effects on fecal weight, and urine and fecal sodium and potassium excretion.

Methods

The study was conducted in accordance with International Conference on Harmonisation Good Clinical Practice guidelines and other applicable regulatory requirements and laws. The study protocol was reviewed and approved by the IntegReview Ethical Review Board, Austin, Texas. All subjects provided written informed consent prior to study participation. Trial registration number: NCT01944007.

Healthy volunteers at least 18 years of age considered to be in good general health (no renal, cardiac, hepatic or other major organ dysfunction) and with no prior history of major gastrointestinal surgery, conditions affecting motility, or dyspepsia requiring treatment within the previous 6 months were recruited by the Clinical Pharmacology Research Unit at the Jasper Clinic, Kalamazoo, Michigan.

This Phase 1, open-label, dose-escalation study recruited 25 healthy volunteers who were randomized into five groups (n = 5/group): a) Control (untreated), b) 7.5 g CLP/day, c) 15.0 g CLP/day, d) 15.0 g CLP/day (fasted) and e) 25.0 g CLP/day. CLP was administered orally in size 00 hydroxypropylmethylcellulose capsules immediately prior to meals (breakfast, lunch, dinner, and snack) in 4 doses divided equally for 9 days, except in the 15.0 g/day fasted group who received the medication 1 hour prior to meals to evaluate the effects of CLP on an empty stomach. With the exception of administration of study medication, untreated control subjects were exposed to the same conditions and procedures as CLP subjects. All subjects were given identical, standardized meals that were controlled for the amount of calories, level of sodium (~5000 mg per day ±100 mg), fiber content (10-15 g per day), fat content, and approximate recommended Dietary Reference Intakes. The study subjects were requested to consume all of their meals. Clinic staff monitored and recorded complete ingestion of the meals served during the study. All fluid intake was recorded.

Subjects were admitted to the research unit on Day -1 (baseline); CLP was administered on Days 1 through 9, and subjects were discharged on Day 10.

Fecal and urine samples for each 24-hour period were collected daily during the treatment period and were weighed and analyzed for sodium, potassium, magnesium, calcium, and phosphorus. Daily samples were pooled for analysis. Analyses of ion content in feces were performed by inductively coupled plasma-optical emission spectroscopy (ICP-OES) at Galbraith Labs Inc. (Knoxville, Tennessee). Urine samples and safety laboratories were analyzed at Bronson Methodist Hospital Laboratory (Kalamazoo, Michigan), using standard clinical automated chemistry techniques.

Safety assessments included daily monitoring of adverse events, vital signs and serum chemistries. Hematology, urinalysis, and 12-lead electrocardiogram (ECG) were measured at baseline and prior to discharge. All blood samples were drawn in the fasting stage before breakfast.

Endpoints

Endpoints to evaluate the pharmacologic activity of CLP included stool weight, fecal content of sodium, potassium, calcium, magnesium and phosphorus, and urine content of sodium, potassium, calcium, magnesium and phosphorus. Safety and tolerability evaluations were based on frequency and severity of adverse events, clinical safety labs and vital signs.

Statistical analysis

Fecal ion content, fecal weight, urine ion content and serum ion concentration data were summarized for each CLP dose group and the control group using descriptive statistics for an empirically determined steady state period (Days 5-9). The steady state period is illustrated for stool weight for the 15 g/day fed group in Figure 1. Due to the exploratory nature of the study and the small sample size, no formal confirmatory statistical analysis was performed.

For these descriptive statistical analyses, data collected during the steady-state period were analyzed as the daily average of values measured on Days 5-9. Least squares mean profiles and empirical standard errors for each CLP dose group versus control were estimated via generalized estimating equations in accordance with a 2-group repeated measures analysis of variance (RM-ANOVA) assuming compound symmetry. The least squares means and corresponding 95% confidence intervals from the RM-ANOVA were then used to depict expected cumulative (Days 5-9) mean values for each pairing of CLP versus control. The incidence of treatment-emergent adverse events for each group was determined. Hematology, serum chemistry and quantitative urinalysis analytes were summarized by treatment group using descriptive statistics; qualitative urinalysis analytes were summarized by treatment group. Descriptive statistics were performed on vital signs data for each treatment group. ECG data were

summarized for each treatment group as normal or abnormal; abnormal findings were categorized further with regard to clinical significance.

Results

Subjects ranged in age from 22 to 68 years (mean, 38.0 years). Approximately half of the subjects (56%) were male, and dose groups were not balanced with regard to gender: the control group comprised only females, and all but the 15.0 g/day fed group, which included 2 males and 3 females, had a male to female ratio of 4:1. The sample was predominantly Caucasian (84% of subjects).

Fecal weight

Mean fecal weight was higher in all CLP groups compared to the control group during study Days 5-9. Mean fecal weight values increased in a dose-related manner and were similar in the fed and fasted 15.0 g/day CLP groups (Figure 2).

Fecal ion content

Mean fecal sodium and potassium content were higher in all CLP groups compared to the control group (Figure 3), and increased in a dose-related manner. Mean fecal magnesium and calcium content were similar across treatment groups and fecal phosphorus was lower than the control group at 15.0 g/day. No differences between fed and fasted state were noted for fecal content of any of the ions.

Urine ion content

Mean urine sodium and potassium were lower in all CLP groups than the control group, with values in CLP groups showing an inverse relationship to dose (Figure 4).

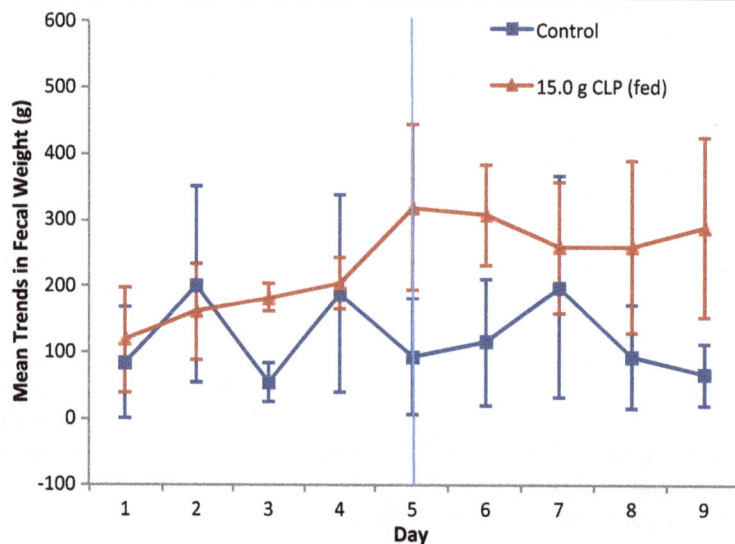

Figure 1 Daily fecal weight following 15.0 g/day CLP for 9 days under fed conditions. Values are means ± 95% confidence intervals. Blue line indicates start of steady state.

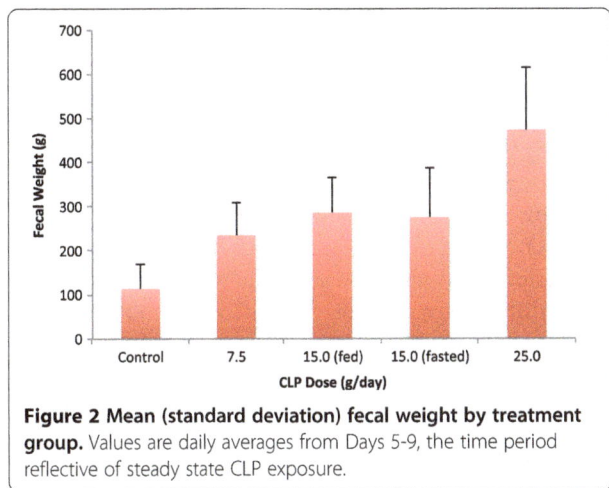

Figure 2 Mean (standard deviation) fecal weight by treatment group. Values are daily averages from Days 5-9, the time period reflective of steady state CLP exposure.

Treatment groups were similar with respect to urine calcium and magnesium, whereas there was an increase in urine phosphorus content at higher doses. There were no noteworthy differences in mean urine cation content values under fed versus fasting conditions.

Serum ion concentrations

There were no clinically meaningful changes in mean serum ion concentrations during the study. A dose dependent drop in serum potassium resulted in a borderline low serum potassium level in the 25.0 g/day CLP group (Table 1).

Safety

Adverse events

No serious adverse events were reported. At doses below 25.0 g/day, CLP was well tolerated. Two subjects in the 25.0 g/day group discontinued CLP dosing on Day 4 due to gastrointestinal adverse events: one due to repeated episodes of moderately severe vomiting, and the other due to abdominal distension, nausea and abdominal pain. Events for both subjects resolved completely without medical treatment prior to discharge on Day 9, five days after termination of dosing. The most frequently reported adverse events were gastrointestinal in nature and appeared to be dose related. However, gastrointestinal adverse events were also reported for 4 of 5 subjects in the control group. The most common gastrointestinal event was nausea. Diarrhea was reported for 1 subject each in the 25.0 g/day CLP and control groups, and no constipation was reported for any of the subjects on CLP, but it was reported for 2 subjects in the control group. All adverse events were mild to moderate in severity, tended to be transient, and resolved without pharmacologic intervention.

Hematology, clinical chemistries, and other safety assessments

No clinically significant changes in mean hematology values were observed in any treatment group. With the exception of the serum carbon dioxide concentration (CO_2), there were no noteworthy changes in mean clinical chemistry values. As shown in Figure 5, serum CO_2 decreased as the dose of the acidic CLP polymer increased, and in the 25.0 g/day CLP group, fell below the

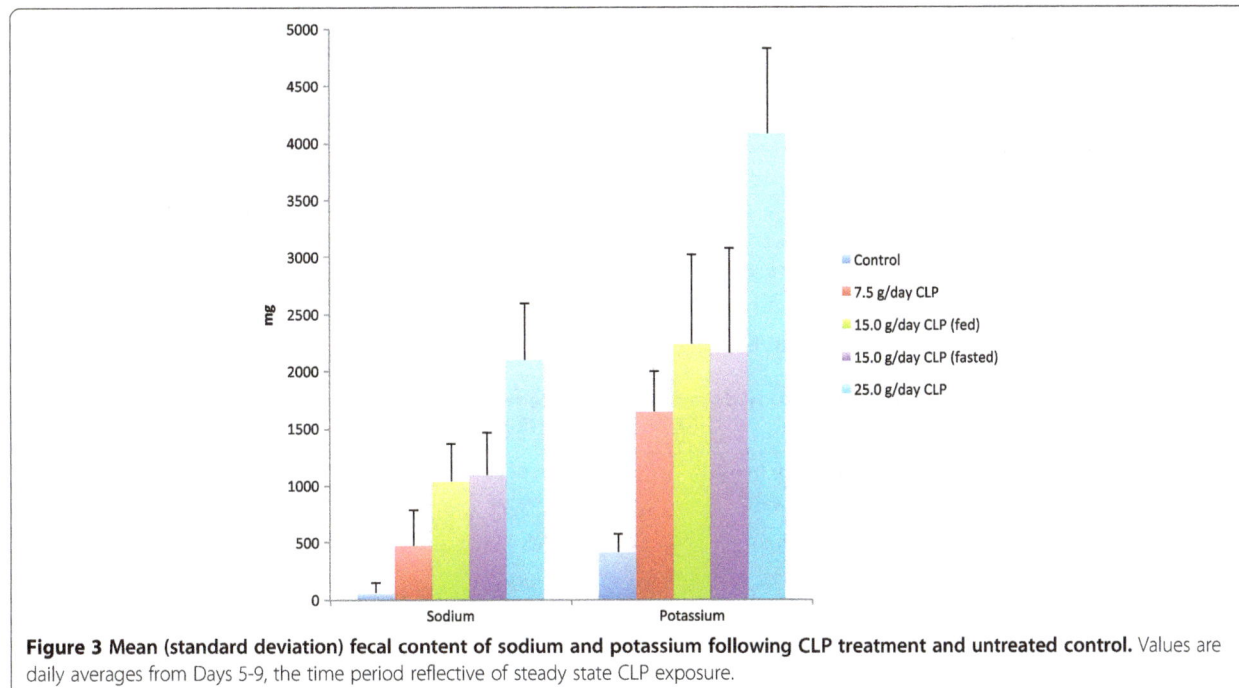

Figure 3 Mean (standard deviation) fecal content of sodium and potassium following CLP treatment and untreated control. Values are daily averages from Days 5-9, the time period reflective of steady state CLP exposure.

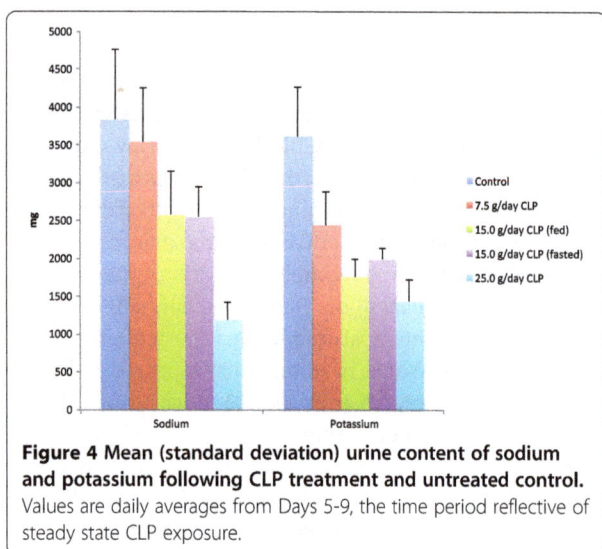

Figure 4 Mean (standard deviation) urine content of sodium and potassium following CLP treatment and untreated control. Values are daily averages from Days 5-9, the time period reflective of steady state CLP exposure.

lower limit of normal on Day 4, and remained decreased until the end of dosing on Day 9. No clinically significant changes in urinalysis were observed, and there were no noteworthy changes in vital signs or ECGs.

Discussion

This Phase 1 study was conducted to evaluate the tolerability and effects of three different doses of CLP, a novel, non-absorbed superabsorbent polymer, on fecal weight and fecal and urine ion content. No serious adverse events occurred in the 25 subjects studied. At CLP doses below 25.0 g/day, there was a low incidence of self-resolving, mild adverse events. The 25.0 g/day dose immediately prior to meals caused more gastrointestinal adverse events, which resulted in 2 subjects discontinuing the study medication. There was no clinically meaningful difference between groups who received 15.0 g/day CLP under fasting and fed states on any endpoint. Fecal weight, sodium and potassium in the stool were increased relative to control in a dose-related fashion, with a 15.0 g dose removing approximately 3.0 mEq of sodium and 3.4 mEq of potassium per gram of polymer. Serum potassium and serum sodium concentrations were within the normal range for

all subjects, with the 25.0 g/day CLP group showing a borderline low potassium level. Serum CO_2 decreased as the dose of CLP increased; however, only for the 25.0 g/day CLP group did the serum CO_2 fall below the normal range (23-32 mmol/L).

While there were small changes in fecal phosphorus content, this was considered clinically inconsequential. The reduction in urine sodium and potassium is considered to reflect a normal homeostatic compensation of the kidney for the loss of these cations in the stool [15].

Previous studies with cation exchange resins in the treatment of patients with heart failure and fluid overload demonstrated removal of sodium and potassium via the gastrointestinal route [12]. However, these products failed to achieve a significant therapeutic presence for fluid management, due to the high doses required (up to 150 g/day), problems in taking the large amounts of unpalatable resins, significant abdominal side effects and the advent of loop diuretics. The much higher cation binding capacity of CLP may offer the opportunity to remove up to 1.0 g of sodium with a lower dose of drug, improving efficiency and gastrointestinal tolerability. Moreover, the superabsorbent water binding capacity of CLP allows for direct fluid removal via the fecal route without causing diarrhea.

Removal of sodium and fluid in the feces may prove beneficial in patients with kidney failure and fluid overload, as well as in those with heart failure and CKD where the effectiveness of diuretics is limited and diuretic resistance is an increasing problem [2,7-9]. High dietary sodium intake has been implicated in target organ damage in kidney and heart cells via increases in blood pressure and oxidative stress, reduction of arterial elasticity and fibrotic cell remodeling [16]. Dietary sodium restriction is recommended in the management of hypertension, heart failure and CKD [16-18]. Studies have shown the beneficial effects of dietary sodium reduction to lower blood pressure and reduce deaths from heart attack and stroke [19,20]. In patients with salt sensitive treatment resistant hypertension, systolic blood pressure reductions of over 20 mmHg have been reported after dietary sodium restriction [21]. Sodium reduction also lowered proteinuria in chronic kidney disease patients [22]. However, dietary sodium

Table 1 Mean serum ion concentrations during study days 5-9 by treatment group

	CLP Dose (g/day)				Control (n = 5)
	7.5 (n = 5)	15.0 (Fed) (n = 4)	15.0 (Fasted) (n = 5)	25.0 (n = 5)	
Sodium (mmol/L)	141.1 (1.4)	138.5 (1.8)	141.0 (2.6)	137.4 (1.6)	139.4 (1.6)
Potassium (mmol/L)	4.6 (0.3)	4.3 (0.3)	4.3 (0.4)	3.7 (0.2)	4.8 (0.5)
Magnesium (mmoL/L)	0.8 (0.0)	0.8 (0.0)	0.8 (0.0)	0.7 (0.0)	0.9 (0.0)
Calcium (mmol/L)	2.4 (0.0)	2.3 (0.1)	2.4 (0.1)	2.3 (0.1)	2.4 (0.1)
Phosphorus (mmol/L)	1.5 (0.2)	1.4 (0.1)	1.3 (0.1)	1.2 (0.1)	1.6 (0.2)

Values are the mean (standard deviation) of daily averages from Days 5-9.

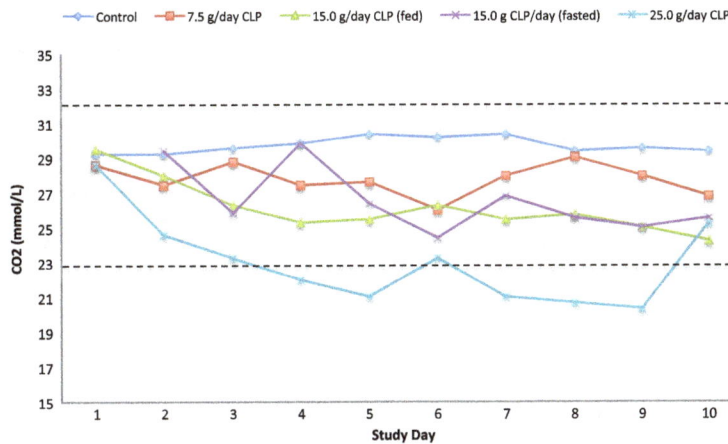

Figure 5 Mean serum carbon dioxide (CO$_2$) concentration for each treatment group by study day. Dashed lines represent the normal range (23-32 mmol/L).

restriction is difficult to achieve and a 15.0 g/day dose of CLP could remove a clinically meaningful amount of sodium from the systemic circulation [23].

The fecal removal of up to 2.0 g potassium from the body may have desirable benefits for patients at risk for hyperkalemia such as CKD or heart failure patients, especially patients with a glomerular filtration rate of ≤ 60 mL/min who have a higher risk for the occurrence of hyperkalemia [24]. Kayexelate (polystyrene sulfonate), the only approved potassium removing agent, has significant tolerability and safety concerns which would render it inadequate to treat hyperkalemia on a chronic use basis [25,26]. Recently, a study with RLY5016 has demonstrated that hyperkalemia may be prevented with a potassium binding oral polymer [14]. However, in a previously reported Phase 2, double-blind, placebo-controlled study in heart failure patients, no differences were observed between CLP and placebo in serum potassium concentrations. This may have been the result of the concomitant administration of an aldosterone antagonist, which alters serum potassium balance [13].

The main weakness of this study is that the small number of study subjects in each group does not permit formal statistical analysis of differences between groups. A strength of the study is the rigor with which subjects were selected and monitored as inpatients in a metabolic study unit with strict control of total dietary caloric, ion and fluid intake and collection of urine and fecal samples for the duration of the study.

Conclusions

In this study of healthy volunteers, CLP increased fecal weight and fecal sodium and potassium content in a dose-related manner, and doses below 25.0 g/day were well tolerated, with infrequent, self-limiting gastrointestinal adverse events. CLP may represent a new therapeutic tool for the removal of fluid, sodium and potassium via

the gastrointestinal tract in patients with fluid and sodium overload in conditions such as congestive heart failure, salt sensitive hypertension, CKD and end stage renal disease.

Competing interests
This study was sponsored by Sorbent Therapeutics Inc., Sunnyvale, CA, USA. All authors have completed the Unified Competing Interest form at http://www.icmje.org/coi_disclosure.pdf (http://www.icmje.org/coi_disclosure.pdf) (available on request from the corresponding author) and declare the following: LWH, HCD and DA are employees of Sorbent Therapeutics Inc., Sunnyvale, CA, USA. DA is a stockholder of Relypsa Inc. AS and RN are paid expert advisors engaged by Sorbent Therapeutics, Inc. to support the design, conduct and analysis of this study. TMB is an employee of the Jasper Clinic's Clinical Research Unit, Kalamazoo, MI, which was engaged by Sorbent Therapeutics, Inc. to conduct this study. TO is an employee of Innovative Analytics, Kalamazoo, MI, which was engaged by Sorbent Therapeutics, Inc. to conduct the data management and statistical analysis for this study. None of the authors received payments for their contributions to the manuscript.

Authors' contributions
All authors contributed significantly to the study design (LWH, TMB, AS, RN) and conduct (TMB, TO), data analysis (TO) and interpretation (LWH, AS, RN, HCD, DA). They were involved in the drafting and revising of the manuscript and gave full approval for the final version to be published.

Acknowledgments
For their contributions in the conduct, analysis and reporting of this study, the authors would like to thank Jolene Shorr and Linda De Young, PhD, for editorial assistance, Karen Tindall, BS, and Sandra Mann, BA MT, of Innovative Analytics (Kalamazoo, MI) for data management support, Kay Bentley, BS, of Innovative Analytics (Kalamazoo, MI) for programming support, and finally, Barbara Gullotti, BSN, RN, the Lead Study Nurse, Nabil Ghazal, BS, the Project Manager and Julia Jenkins, RD, the Dietician at Jasper Clinic's Clinical Research Unit (Kalamazoo, MI).

Author details
[1]Sorbent Therapeutics Inc, 710 Lakeway Drive, Suite 290, Sunnyvale, CA 94085, USA. [2]Alan Strickland Consulting, 101 Waterlily, Lake Jackson, TX 77566, USA. [3]Jasper Clinic's Clinical Research Unit, 526 Jasper Street, Kalamazoo, MI 49007, USA. [4]RnD Services, LLC, 635 Bent Creek Ridge, Deerfield, IL 60015, USA. [5]Innovative Analytics, 161 East Michigan Ave, Kalamazoo, MI 49007, USA.

References

1. Adams KF Jr, Fonarow GC, Emerman CL, LeJemtel TH, Costanzo MR, Abraham WT, Berkowitz RL, Galvao M, Horton DP, ADHERE Scientific Advisory Committee and Investigators: Characteristics and outcomes of patients hospitalized for heart failure in the United States: rationale, design, and preliminary observations from the first 100,000 cases in the Acute Decompensated Heart Failure National Registry (ADHERE). *Am Heart J* 2005, 149(2):209–216.

2. Brandimarte F, Mureddu GF, Boccanelli A, Cacciatore G, Brandimarte C, Fedele F, Gheorghiade M: Diuretic therapy in heart failure: current controversies and new approaches for fluid removal. *J Cardiovasc Med* 2010, 11(8):563–570.

3. Drazner MH, Rame JE, Stevenson LW, Dries DL: Prognostic importance of elevated jugular vein pressure and third heart sound in patients with heart failure. *N Engl J Med* 2001, 345(8):574–581.

4. Costanzo MR, Guglin ME, Saltzberg MT, Jessup ML, Bart BA, Teerlink JR, Jaski BE, Fang JC, Feller ED, Haas GJ, Anderson AS, Schollmeyer MP, Sobotka PA, UNLOAD Trial Investigators: Ultrafiltration versus intravenous diuretics for patients hospitalized for acute decompensated heart failure. *J Am Coll Cardiol* 2007, 49:675–683. Erratum, *J Am Coll Cardiol* 2007, 49:1136.

5. Cowie MR, Komajda M, Murray-Thomas T, Underwood J, Ticho B: Prevalence and impact of worsening renal function in patients hospitalized with decompensated heart failure: results of the prospective outcomes study in heart failure (POSH). *Eur Heart J* 2006, 27:1216–1222.

6. Heywood JT, Fonarow GC, Costanzo MR, Mathur VS, Wigneswaran JR, Wynne J: High prevalence of renal dysfunction and its impact on outcome in 118,465 patients hospitalized with acute decompensated heart failure: a report from the ADHERE database. *J Card Fail* 2007, 13(6):422–430.

7. Ahmed A, Husain A, Love TE, Gambassi G, Dell'Italia LJ, Francis GS, Gheorghiade M, Allman RM, Meleth S, Bourge RC: Heart failure, chronic diuretic use, and increase in mortality and hospitalization: an observational study using propensity score methods. *Eur Heart J* 2006, 27(12):1431–1439.

8. Domanski M, Tian X, Haigney M, Pitt B: Diuretic use, progressive heart failure, and death in patients in the DIG study. *J Card Fail* 2006, 12(5):327–332.

9. Eshaghian S, Horwich TB, Fonarow GC: Relation of loop diuretic dose to mortality in advanced heart failure. *Am J Cardiol* 2006, 97(12):1759–1764.

10. Cotter G, Dittrich HC, Weatherley BD, Bloomfield DM, O'Connor CM, Metra M, Massie BM, Protect Steering Committee, Investigators, and Coordinators: The PROTECT pilot study: a randomized, placebo-controlled, dose-finding study of the adenosine A1 receptor antagonist rolofylline in patients with acute heart failure and renal impairment. *J Card Fail* 2008, 14(8):631–640. Epub 2008 Sep 14.

11. Stanton BA, Kaissling B: Adaptation of distal tubule and collecting duct to increased Na delivery. II. Na + and K + transport. *Am J Physiol* 1988, 255:F1269–F1275.

12. Dock W, Frank NR: Cation exchangers: their use and hazards as aids in managing edema. *Am Heart J* 1950, 40:638–645.

13. Costanzo MR, Heywood JT, Massie BM, Iwashita J, Henderson L, Mamatsashvilli M, Sisakian H, Hayrapetyan H, Sager P, van Veldhuisen DJ, Albrecht D: A double-blind, randomized, parallel, placebo-controlled study examining the effect of cross-linked polyelectrolyte in heart failure patients with chronic kidney disease. *Eur J Heart Fail* 2012, 14(8):922–930.

14. Pitt B, Anker SD, Bushinsky DA, Kitzman DW, Zannad F, Huang I-Z on behalf of the PEARL-HF investigators: Evaluation of the efficacy and safety of RLY5016, a polymeric potassium binder, in a double-blind, placebo-controlled study in patients with chronic heart failure (the PEARL-HF) trial. *Eur Heart J* 2011, 32(7):820–828.

15. Linz D, Wirth K, Linz W, Heuer HOO, Frick W, Hofmeister A, Heinelt U, Arndt P, Schwahn U, Boehm M, Ruetten H: Antihypertensive and laxative effects by pharmacological inhibition of sodium-proton-exchanger subtype 3-mediated sodium absorption in the gut. *Hypertension* 2012, 60:1560–1567.

16. Appel LJ, Frohlich ED, Hall JE, Pearson TA, Sacco RL, Seals DR, Sacks FM, Smith SC, Vafiadis DK, Van Horn LV: The importance of population-wide sodium reduction as a means to prevent cardiovascular disease and stroke. *Circulation* 2011, 123:1138–1143.

17. Whelton PK, Appel LJ, Sacco RL, Anderson CAM, Antman EM, Campbell N, Dunbar SB, Frohlich ED, Hall JE, Jessup M, Labarthe DR, MacGregor DA, Sacks FM, Stamler J, Vafiadis DK, Van Horn LV: Sodium, blood pressure, and cardiovascular disease: further evidence supporting the American Heart Association Sodium Reduction Recommendations. *Circulation* 2012. 10.1161/CIR.0b013e318279acbf.

18. Hunt SA, Abraham WT, Chin MH, Feldman AM, Francis GS, Ganiats TG, Jessup M, Konstam MA, Mancini DM, Michl K, Oates JA, Rahko PS, Silver MA, Stevenson LW, Yancy CW: 2009 focused update incorporated into the ACC/AHA 2005 Guidelines for the Diagnosis and Management of Heart Failure in Adults: a report of the American College of Cardiology Foundation/American Heart Association Task Force on Practice Guidelines: developed in collaboration with the International Society for Heart and Lung Transplantation. *Circulation* 2009, 119(14):e391–e479.

19. Sacks FM, Svetkey JP, Vollmer WM, Appel LJ, Bray GA, Harsha D, Obarzanek E, Conlin PR, Miller ER, Simons-Morton DG, Karanja N, Lin PH: Effects on blood pressure of reduced dietary sodium and the Dietary Approaches to Stop Hypertension (DASH) diet. DASH-Sodium Collaborative Research Group. *N Engl J Med* 2001, 334(1):3–10.

20. Cook NR, Cutler JA, Obarzanek E, Buring JE, Rexrode KM, Kumanyika SK, Appel LJ, Whelton PK: Long term effects of dietary sodium reduction on cardiovascular disease outcomes: observational follow-up of the Trials of Hypertension Prevention (TOHP). *BMJ* 2007, 334:885–888.

21. Pimenta E, Gaddam KK, Oparil S, Aban I, Husain S, Dell'Italia LJ, Calhoun DA: Effects of dietary sodium reduction on blood pressure in subjects with resistant hypertension: results from a randomized trial. *Hypertension* 2009, 54:475–481.

22. Slagman MCJ, Waanders F, Hemmelder MH, Woittiez AJ, Janssen WMT, Lambers Heerspink HJ, Navis G, Laverman GD: Moderate dietary sodium restriction added to angiotensin converting enzyme inhibition compared with dual blockade in lowering proteinuria and blood pressure: randomized controlled trial. *BMJ* 2011, 343:d4366. 10.1136/bmj.d4366.

23. Centers for Disease Control and Prevention: Usual sodium intakes compared with current dietary guidelines — United States, 2005–2008. *MMWR* 2011, 60:1413–1417.

24. Pitt B, Bakris G, Ruilope LM, DiCarlo L, Mukherjee R, EPHESUS Investigators: Serum potassium and clinical outcomes in the Eplerenone Post-Acute Myocardial Infarction Heart Failure Efficacy and Survival Study (EPHESUS). *Circulation* 2008, 118(16):1643–1650.

25. Sterns RH, Rojas M, Bernstein P, Chennupati S: Ion-exchange resins for treatment of hyperkalemia: are they safe and effective? *J Am Soc Nephrol* 2010, 21:733–735.

26. Watson M, Abbott KC, Yuan CM: Damned if you do, damned if you don't: potassium binding resins in hyperkalemia. *Clin J Am Soc Nephrol* 2010, 5:1723–1726.

21

Pharmacokinetics and safety issues of an accidental overdose of 2,000,000 IU of vitamin D$_3$ in two nursing home patients: a case report

Jody van den Ouweland[1*], Hanneke Fleuren[2], Miranda Drabbe[3] and Hans Vollaard[2]

Abstract

Background: Administration of intermittent high doses of vitamin D$_3$ is increasingly used as a strategy for rapid normalization of low 25-hydroxyvitamin D (25(OH)D) blood concentrations in patients with vitamin D deficiency. Here, we describe the pharmacokinetics of an accidental single oral overdose of 2,000,000 IU of vitamin D$_3$ in two elderly nursing home patients and discuss safety issues.

Case presentation: Two patients, a Caucasian 90-year old man and a 95-year old woman, were monitored from 1 h up to 3 months after intake for clinical as well as biochemical signs of vitamin D intoxication. Blood vitamin D$_3$ concentrations showed a prompt increase with the highest peak area already hours after the dose, followed by a rapid decrease to undetectable levels after day 14. Peak blood 25(OH)D$_3$ concentrations were observed 8 days after intake (527 and 422 nmol/L, respectively (ref: 50–200 nmol/L)). Remarkably, plasma calcium levels increased only slightly up to 2.68 and 2.73 mmol/L, respectively (ref: 2.20–2.65 mmol/L) between 1 and 14 days after intake, whereas phosphate and creatinine levels remained within the reference range. No adverse clinical symptoms were noted.

Conclusion: A single massive oral dose of 2,000,000 IU of vitamin D$_3$ does not cause clinically apparent toxicity requiring hospitalization, with only slightly elevated plasma calcium levels in the first 2 weeks. Toxicity in the long term cannot be excluded as annual doses of 500,000 IU of vitamin D$_3$ for several years have shown an increase in the risk of fractures. This means that plasma calcium levels may not be a sensitive measure of vitamin D toxicity in the long term in the case of a single high overdose. To prevent a similar error in the future, the use of multiple-dose bottles need to be replaced by smaller single-unit dose formulations.

Keywords: Vitamin D, Intoxication, Single high dose

Background

Vitamin D deficiency is a highly prevalent condition, present in approximately 30–50% of the general population [1], and may be as high as 100% in institutionalized elderly patients [2,3]. Vitamin D supplementation is increasingly advised, but compliance with daily dosing regimens is low [4]. Because serum 25-hydroxyvitamin D$_3$ (25(OH)D$_3$), the functional indicator of vitamin D status, has a long half-life of about 2 months [5], there is great interest in intermittent dosing for patient convenience and long-term adherence. Administration of 100,000 IU of cholecalciferol (vitamin D$_3$) every 4 months for 5 years showed a 22% reduction in the risk of osteoporotic fractures [6], similar to studies using a daily dose of 800 IU [7]. On the contrary, rapid increases in serum 25(OH)D from intermittent high doses of 500,000 IU of vitamin D$_3$ once a year for 3–5 years in older women, have been shown to increase the risk of falls and fractures by 26% compared with the use of a placebo [8]. In clinical studies using high-dose regimens of up to 600,000 IU of vitamin D$_3$, there has been surprisingly little concern for vitamin D toxicity. Plasma calcium and urinary calcium excretion both are recognized markers of vitamin D toxicity [5]. In the few clinical studies that have analyzed plasma calcium levels and/or urinary calcium excretion within a month after dosing, calcium levels were found to be unchanged or only slightly elevated within the reference range following a loading dose of 300,000 IU [9], 500,000 IU [10], 540,000 IU [11], or 600,000 IU [12,13].

* Correspondence: j.v.d.ouweland@cwz.nl
[1]Department of Clinical Chemistry, Canisius Wilhelmina Hospital, Weg door Jonkerbos 100, 6532 SZ Nijmegen, The Netherlands
Full list of author information is available at the end of the article

Here, we describe the pharmacokinetics of an accidental overdosing by 2,000,000 IU vitamin D_3 in two elderly nursing home patients and discuss safety issues from single massive oral doses of vitamin D_3.

Case presentation

In Waelwick, a nursing home near Nijmegen, all residents receive osteoporosis prophylaxis with oral vitamin D_3 doses of 100,000 IU three times a year as a lyophilized solution (2 mL vitamin D_3 aquosum FNA, 50,000 IU/mL). Two nursing home patients each received an accidental single overdose of 2,000,000 IU vitamin D from a whole bottle of a concentrated vitamin D_3 solution (40 mL vitamin D_3 aquosum FNA 50,000 IU/mL). The pharmacy department was surprised by the order for 25 new bottles immediately after the dose, as the two 40-mL bottles would have

lasted for half of a year of treatment for the patients at the ward. It then became clear that an overdose had been given. For safety reasons, we immediately started biochemical and clinical monitoring of both patients. Plasma calcium, phosphate, creatinine, and 25(OH)D levels were measured from 1 h after dosing up to 106 days (case 1) and 71 days (case 2) (Figure 1, Table 1). Vitamin D_3 was measured at time points 1 h, 0.5, 1, 2, 8, and 14 days after dosing (Figure 1). Because of the nature of this study, baseline concentrations (prior to dosing) were lacking. Unfortunately, we lacked the opportunity for measuring 1,25-dihydroxyvitamin D and 24,25-dihydroxyvitamin D (because of limited availability of plasma material), parathyroid hormone (PTH) and bone turnover markers (lack of the appropriate blood containers or pre-analytical conditions), and urinary calcium excretion (lack of urine collection).

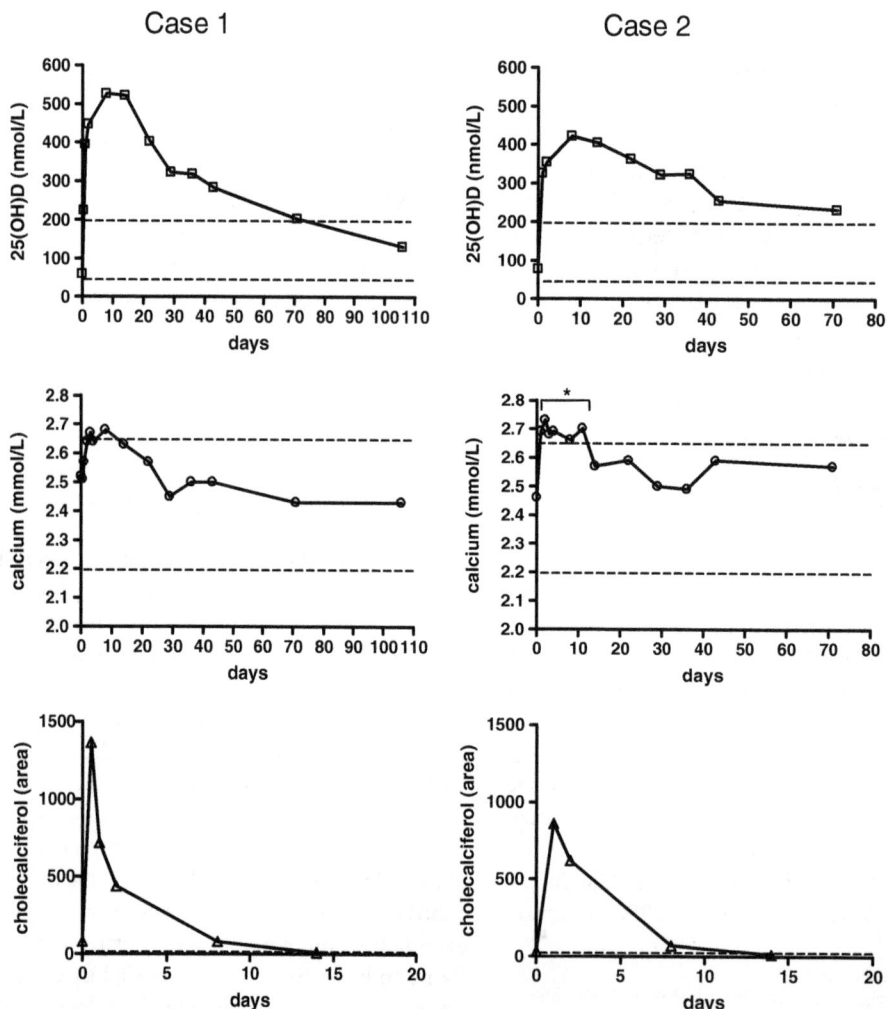

Figure 1 Time course of plasma calcidiol and calcium concentrations, as well as semi-quantitative measurements of plasma vitamin D_3 (cholecalciferol), after a single oral dose of 2,000,000 IU of vitamin D to two nursing home residents. The asterisk indicates the individual calcium measurements that show a biologically significant difference from baseline concentrations. Note the time-scale differences between the vitamin D_3 (cholecalciferol) and the upper plots.

Table 1 Biochemical values from single high-dose vitamin D3 administration in two cases

		Reference range	1 h	5.5 h	1d	2d	3d	4d	8d	11d	14d	22d	29d	36d	43d	60d	71d	106d
Case 1	Calcidiol (nmol/L)	50-200	59	**224**	**395**	**448**			**527**		**522**	**403**	**323**	**318**	**283**		**203**	131
	Calcium (mmol/L)	2.20-2.65	2.52	2.51	2.57	2.64	**2.67**	2.64	**2.68**		2.63	2.57	2.45	2.5	2.5		2.43	2.43
	Phosphate (mmol/L)	0.80-1.40	1.08	1.09	1.05	1.30	1.13	1.14	1.37		1.32	1.01	1.00	0.98	0.97			0.96
	Creatinine (µmol/L)	60-110	64	65	66	68	69	73	69		77	75	71	69	63	66	75	65
Case 2	Calcidiol (nmol/L)	50-200	77		**326**	**354**			**422**		**405**	**363**	**322**	**324**	**255**		**233**	
	Calcium (mmol/L)	2.20-2.65	2.46		**2.69**	**2.73**	**2.68**	**2.69**	**2.66**	**2.70**	2.57	2.59	2.50	2.49	2.59		2.57	
	Phosphate (mmol/L)	0.80-1.40	0.91		1.20	1.06	1.12	1.05	1.13	1.02	1.07	0.82	0.82	0.89	0.87		**0.79**	
	Creatinine (µmol/L)	50-90	**45**		51	**44**	55	54	52	52	**49**	52	**41**	50	54		**45**	

Values outside the reference range are indicated in bold. h, hours; d, days. Conversion factors: calcidiol (mg/dL = 0.4 × mmol/L), calcium (mg/dL = 4 × mmol/L), phosphate (mg/dL = 3.1 × mmol/L), creatinine (mg/dL = 0.01 × µmol/L).

Measurements of plasma 25(OH)D concentrations, as well as semi-quantitative measurement of vitamin D_3 (monitoring peak area), were performed using liquid chromatography-tandem mass spectrometry as previously described [14]. Plasma calcium, phosphate, and creatinine levels were measured on a routine clinical chemistry analyzer (Modular; Roche Diagnostics, Mannheim, Germany). Changes of biological significance were calculated from reference change (RCV, at a 95% confidence interval) according to the formula RCV = $Z \times 2^{1/2}$ $(CV_a^2 + CV_a^2)^{1/2}$ [15], where Z = 1.96 (i.e., the Z-score for 95% confidence), CV_a = analytical variation, and CV_i = intra-individual variation. For calcium, CV_a and CV_i were 1.5% and 1.9%, respectively [16].

Case 1 was a 90-year-old man of Caucasian origin, with normal kidney function (estimated glomerular filtration rate by Modification of Diet in Renal Disease (MDRD) equation >60 mL/min), and an absence of significant pathology. He did not report any clinical signs or symptoms of vitamin D toxicity. His plasma calcium was 2.52 mmol/L 1 h after dosing and showed a non-significant increase from day 1 to day 8, with a maximum of 2.68 mmol/L at day 8. After 8 days, plasma calcium levels fell to within the reference range (2.2–2.65 mmol/L) (Figure 1). At first measurement, 1 h after gift, vitamin D3 was already detected. The vitamin D_3 peak area showed a prompt increase with the highest peak area already at the second measurement, 5.5 h after dosing, followed by a rapid decrease to undetectable levels at day 14. Plasma 25(OH)D_3 concentrations also were already markedly increased 5.5 h after dosing, but rose more slowly than vitamin D_3, reaching a maximum of 527 nmol/L at day 8. Over the following 3-month period, 25(OH)D_3 concentrations decreased by 50% over an approximately 50-day period. At the end of the 106-day follow-up period, the patient's 25(OH)D_3 concentration was 113 nmol/L and fell within the laboratory reference range (50–200 nmol/L). Plasma phosphate and creatinine levels showed a modest increase within the reference range (Table 1).

Case 2 relates to a 95-year-old woman of Caucasian origin, with normal kidney function (MDRD >60 mL/min) and an absence of significant pathology. She did not report any clinical signs or symptoms of vitamin D toxicity. Her plasma calcium was 2.46 mmol/L 1 h after dosing and showed a biologically significant increase from day 1 to day 11 with a maximum of 2.73 mmol/L at the second day. After 11 days, plasma calcium levels dropped to within the reference range of 2.2–2.65 mmol/L (Figure 1). Vitamin D_3 peak area was highest at the first measurement opportunity, being 1-day post-dose, followed by a rapid decrease to undetectable levels after day 14. Plasma 25(OH)D_3 concentrations also were already markedly increased 1 day after dosing, but rose more slowly than vitamin D_3, reaching a maximum of 422 nmol/L at day 8. At the end of the 71-day follow-up period, the 25(OH)D_3 concentration was 233 nmol/L, with an approximate 50% decrease from the highest level being still above the upper normal limit of 200 nmol/L. Plasma phosphate and creatinine levels both showed a modest increase within the reference range (Table 1).

Discussion

Pharmacokinetic studies in human volunteers given a single large oral dose of 100,000 IU of vitamin D_3 indicate that serum vitamin D_3 and 25(OH)D_3 levels peak on days 1 and 7, respectively [17,18]. The vitamin D_3 concentrations fell rapidly, being close to baseline by day 7, with a much slower fall of the 25(OH)D_3 concentrations. Plasma calcium levels did not rise at any time, and no subject experienced hypercalcemia at any of the measured time points [17]. The pharmacokinetic profiles of our two cases resembled those from the 100,000 IU study and emphasize the importance of measuring 25(OH)D and calcium concentrations over the first 14 days for identifying the maximum blood concentrations. The half-life of the plasma 25(OH)D levels of about 50 days in case 1 is comparable to a half-life of about 2 months as described previously [5]. The relatively normal 25(OH)D_3 concentrations in our nursing home residents (59 nmol/L in case 1 and 77 nmol/L in case

2) at the first measurement (1 h post-dosing) can be explained as the result of previous osteoporosis prophylaxis treatments with 100,000 IU of oral vitamin D_3. However, we cannot exclude the possibility that the plasma 25(OH)D concentrations were already increased 1 h after the high dose of vitamin D_3, implicating that the baseline 25(OH)D values in both cases actually may have been lower.

The toxicity of vitamin D in daily administration has been studied extensively. The present view is that hypercalcemia is the hazard criterion for vitamin D [19]. Thus, vitamin D toxicity is supposed to be inseparable from hypercalcemia. Hypercalcemia does not occur with daily doses up to 40,000 IU of vitamin D_3 and serum levels of 25(OH)D_3 up to 500 nmol/L, well above naturally occurring levels of 25(OH)D_3 [20]. Most patients with an overdose of vitamin D_3 are not seen by a physician until they are admitted to the emergency department with clinical signs of intoxication, such as life-threatening dehydration, after a prolonged period of oral intake of high-dose vitamin D, either from contaminated food components [21,22] or supplements with errors in manufacturing and/or labeling [23,24].

Much less is known about the toxicity of vitamin D_3 following a single high oral dose of vitamin D_3. In studies using 300,000 IU [9], 540,000 IU [11], and 600,000 IU [12,13] of oral vitamin D_3, no adverse effects were noted and plasma calcium levels or urinary calcium excretion did not change, or only slightly increased for a short period of time, with all cases remaining within the physiological range. In contrast to these reassuring data, Sanders et al. [8] found a significant increase in the risk of falls (+15%) and fractures (+26%) in a randomized controlled trial with an annual dose of 500,000 IU vitamin D_3 for 3–5 years in older women compared with placebo. Falls and fractures occurred especially within the first 3 months following the annual dose of vitamin D_3. In that study, plasma calcium levels and urinary calcium excretion were not measured; however, bearing in mind the former data, it is unlikely that hypercalcemia occurred in the study. These unexpected findings led Rossini et al. [13,25] to investigate dose-dependent short-term effects on bone turnover markers of a single bolus of vitamin D_3. A single dose of 600,000 IU of vitamin D_3 increased serum C-terminal telopeptide of type 1 collagen and cross-linked N-telopeptide of type 1 collagen significantly at day 1, attained a peak increment greater than 50% at day 3, and subsequently decreased almost back to baseline values at day 90, without statistically significant changes in plasma calcium [13]. Their results indicate that the use of oral megadoses greater than 100,000 IU of vitamin D may be counterproductive and that the safety issues surrounding vitamin D dosing should not be limited to early markers of vitamin D toxicity as plasma hypercalcemia or increased

urinary calcium excretion [13,25]. A possible explanation is the fact that the level of 1,25 dihydroxy-vitamin D is regulated much stronger in the endocrine system than in the autocrine system of vitamin D [5]. If the plasma level of calcidiol (the substrate of the autocrine vitamin D system) increases sharply after a loading dose that deviates too much from the maximum physiological daily dose with sunlight (20,000 IU), this might result in toxic intracellular calcitriol levels in the autocrine vitamin D system without toxic circulating calcitriol levels in the endocrine system of vitamin D and without hypercalcemia. If that is the case, we need other markers than hypercalcemia to prove vitamin D toxicity in the autocrine system, such as bone turnover markers [13]. In any case, more studies are needed to evaluate potential adverse effects of high-dose vitamin D treatment on bone metabolism in relation to fracture risk and risk of falls.

The present study displays some limitations. We lacked the opportunity for studying other relevant parameters in the risk assessment for vitamin D_3, such as measurement of urinary calcium excretion and plasma levels of 1,25-dihydroxyvitamin D, 24,25-dihydroxyvitamin D, PTH, and bone turnover markers. Because of the nature of this study, baseline concentrations (prior to dosing) of biochemical parameters such as plasma vitamin D_3, 25(OH)D, and calcium were lacking.

Conclusion

In our two patients, the massive single overdose of 2,000,000 IU of vitamin D_3 did not result in immediate clinical and biochemical toxicity requiring hospitalization, with only slightly elevated plasma calcium levels in the first 2 weeks. However, toxicity in the long term cannot be excluded as an annual dose of 500,000 IU of vitamin D_3 for several years has shown an increased risk of fractures. This may implicate that markers other than plasma calcium measurement, such as bone turnover markers, are needed to assess the safety of high doses of vitamin D in the long term. Clearly, the safety of high-dose vitamin D supplementation warrants further study. To prevent a similar error in the future, the use of multiple-dose bottles were replaced by smaller single-unit dose formulations of 25.000 IU/mL. In general, we believe that available formulations of vitamin D_3 should not exceed 100,000 IU, as long as the safety of high doses of vitamin D in the long term has not been established.

Consent

Written informed consent for publication of their clinical details was obtained from the relatives of both patients. A copy of the written consent is available for review by the Editor of this journal.

Abbreviations
25(OH)D: 25-hydroxyvitamin D; CV_a: analytical variation; CV_i: intra-individual variation; RCV: reference change value.

Competing interests
The authors declare that they have no competing interests.

Authors' contributions
MD was the treating physician of the patients reported. JvdO carried out the biochemical measurements, evaluated the test results and drafted the manuscript. HF and HV evaluated the test results and helped to draft the manuscript. All authors read and approved the final version of the manuscript.

Acknowledgments
The authors declare that they have no acknowledgments and/or sources of funding.

Author details
[1]Department of Clinical Chemistry, Canisius Wilhelmina Hospital, Weg door Jonkerbos 100, 6532 SZ Nijmegen, The Netherlands. [2]Department of Clinical Pharmacy, Canisius-Wilhelmina Hospital, Nijmegen, The Netherlands. [3]Nursing Home Waelwick, Ewijk Beuningen, The Netherlands.

References
1. Holick MF: Vitamin D: evolutionary, physiological and health perspectives. *Curr Drug Targets* 2011, **12**:4–18.
2. Lips P: Vitamin D deficiency and secondary hyperparathyroidism in the elderly: consequences for bone loss and fractures and therapeutic implications. *Endocr Rev* 2001, **22**:477–501.
3. Pilz S, Dobnig H, Tomaschitz A, Kienreich K, Meinitzer A, Friedl C, Wagner D, Piswanger-Sölkner C, März W, Fahrleitner-Pammer A: Low 25-hydroxyvitamin D is associated with increased mortality in female nursing home residents. *J Clin Endocrinol Metab* 2012, **97**:E653–E657.
4. Bischoff-Ferrari HA: How to select the dose of vitamin D in the management of osteoporosis. *Osteoporosis Int* 2007, **18**:401–407.
5. Vieth R: The Pharmacology of Vitamin D. In *Chapter 57 in Feldman, Pike and Adams*. 3, volume IIth edition. Edited by Vitamin D. London, UK: Academic; 2011.
6. Trivedi DP, Dolf R, Khaw KT: Effect of four monthly oral vitamin D3 (cholecalciferol) supplementation on fractures and mortality in men and women living in the community: randomised double blind controlled trial. *BMJ* 2003, **326**:469–475.
7. Dawson-Hughes B, Heaney RP, Holick MF, Lips P, Meunier PJ, Vieth R: Estimates of optimal vitamin D status. *Osteoporosis Int* 2005, **16**:713–716.
8. Sanders KM, Stuart AL, Williamson EJ, Simpson JA, Kotowicz MA, Young D, Nicholson GC: Annual high-dose oral vitamin D and falls and fractures in older women. A randomized controlled trial. *JAMA* 2010, **303**:1815–1822.
9. Romagnoli E, Mascia ML, Cipriani C, Fassino V, Mazzei F, D'Erasmo E, Carnevale V, Scillitani A, Minisola S: Short and long-term variations in serum calciotropic hormones after a single very large dose of ergocalciferol (vitamin D2) or cholecalciferol (vitamin D3) in the elderly. *J Clin Endocrinol Metab* 2008, **93**:3015–3020.
10. Bacon CJ, Gamble GD, Horne AM, Scott MA, Reid IR: High-dose oral vitamin D3 supplementation in the elderly. *Osteoporos Int* 2009, **20**:1407–1415.
11. Amrein K, Sourij H, Wagner G, Holl A, Pieber TR, Smolle KH, Stojakovic T, Schnedl C, Dobnig H: Short term effects of high dose oral vitamin D3 in critically ill vitamin D deficient patients: a randomized, double blind, placebo controlled pilot study. *Crit Care* 2011, **15**:R104.
12. Cipriani C, Romagnoli E, Scillatani A, Chiodini I, Clerico R, Carnevale V, Mascia ML, Battista C, Viti R, Pileri M, Eller-Vainicher C, Minisola S: Effect of a single oral dose of 600,000 IU of cholecalciferol in serum calciotropic hormones in young subjects with vitamin D deficiency: A prospective intervention study. *J Clin Endocrinol Metab* 2010, **95**:4771–4777.
13. Rossini M, Gatti D, Viapiana O, Fracassi E, Idolazzi L, Zanoni S, Adami S: Short term effects on bone turnover markers of a single high dose of oral vitamin D3. *J Clin Endocrinol Metab* 2012, **97**:E622–E626.
14. van den Ouweland JM, Beijers AM, Demacker PN, van Daal H: Measurement of 25-OH-vitamin D in human serum using liquid chromatography tandem-mass spectrometry with comparison to radioimmunoassay and automated immunoassay. *J Chromatogr B Analyt Technol Biomed Life Sci* 2010, **878**:1163–1168.
15. Fraser CG: *Biological Variation: From Principles to Practice*. Washington: AACC press; 2001:67–70.
16. Ricós C, Iglesias N, García-Lario JV, Simón M, Cava F, Hernández A, Perich C, Minchinela J, Alvarez V, Doménech MV, Jiménez CV, Biosca C, Tena R: Within-subject biological variation in disease: collated data and clinical consequences. *Ann Clin Biochem* 2007, **44**:343–352.
17. Ilahi M, Armas LA, Heaney RP: Pharmacokinetics of a single, large dose of cholecalciferol. *Am J Clin Nutr* 2008, **87**:688–691.
18. Heaney RP, Armas LA, Shary JR, Bell NH, Binkley N, Hollis BW: 25-Hydroxylation of vitamin D3: relation to circulating vitamin D3 under various input conditions. *Am J Clin Nutr* 2008, **87**:1738–1742.
19. Vieth R: Vitamin D toxicity, policy, and science. *J Bone Miner Res* 2007, **22**(Suppl 2):V64–V68.
20. Vieth R: Vitamin D supplementation, 25-hydroxyvitamin D concentrations and safety. *Am J Clin Nutr* 1999, **69**:842–856.
21. Vieth R, Pinto TR, Reen BS, Wong MM: Vitamin D poisoning by table sugar. *Lancet* 2002, **359**:672.
22. Down PF, Polak A, Regan RJ: A family with massive acute vitamin D intoxication. *Postgrad Med J* 1979, **55**:897–902.
23. Araki T, Holick MF, Alfonso BD, Charlap E, Romero CM, Rizk D, Newman LG: Vitamin D intoxication with severe hypercalcemia due to manufacturing and labeling errors of two dietary supplements made in the United States. *J Clin Endocrinol Metab* 2011, **96**:3603–3608.
24. Lowe H, Cusano NE, Binkley N, Blaner WS, Bilezikian JP: Vitamin D toxicity due to a commonly available "over the counter" remedy from the Dominican Republic. *J Clin Endocrinol Metab* 2011, **96**:291–295.
25. Rossini M, Adami S, Viapiana O, Fracassi E, Idolazzi L, Povine MR, Gatti D: Dose-dependent short-term effects of single high doses of oral vitamin D3 on bone turnover markers. *Calcif Tissue Int* 2012, **91**:365–369.

22

Medication errors related to transdermal opioid patches: lessons from a regional incident reporting system

Henrik Lövborg[1,2*], Mikael Holmlund[1] and Staffan Hägg[1]

Abstract

Objective: A few cases of adverse reactions linked to erroneous use of transdermal opioid patches have been reported in the literature. The aim of this study was to describe and characterize medication errors (MEs) associated with use of transdermal fentanyl and buprenorphine.

Methods: All events concerning transdermal opioid patches reported between 2004 and 2011 to a regional incident reporting system and assessed as MEs were scrutinized and characterized. MEs were defined as "a failure in the treatment process that leads to, or has the potential to lead to, harm to the patient".

Results: In the study 151 MEs were identified. The three most common error types were wrong administration time 67 (44%), wrong dose 34 (23%), and omission of dose 20 (13%). Of all MEs, 118 (78%) occurred in the administration stage of the medication process. Harm was reported in 26 (17%) of the included cases, of which 2 (1%) were regarded as serious harm (nausea/vomiting and respiratory depression). Pain was the most common adverse reaction reported.

Conclusions: Of the reported MEs related to transdermal fentanyl and buprenorphine, most occurred during administration. Improved routines to ascertain correct and timely administration and educational interventions to reduce MEs for these drugs are warranted.

Keywords: Transdermal patch, Opioids, Fentanyl, Buprenorphine, Medication errors, Incident reporting system

Background

The usage of transdermal patches which allows continuous and prolonged delivery of medications is increasing. Less frequent dosing, lower peak plasma drug concentration compared with other types of administration forms and avoidance of first-passage metabolism are some reported benefits suggesting that this administration form may have increased compliance, effectiveness and safety compared to oral administration [1,2]. In addition, patches offer the potential to deliver medications that would otherwise require injections. Moreover, future advances in the technology will probably increase the utilization of drug patches further.

Sporadic case reports indicate however specific problems related with this drug form, such as incorrect use of multiple patches [3,4], ingestion of used or unused patches [5] and skin reaction [6]. Since potent drugs linked to serious adverse reactions are administered through transdermal patches, medication errors may lead to serious adverse health consequences. The American Food and Drug Administration (FDA) states that opioids poses the highest risk of harm and death, among approved transdermal patches, because of their risk to cause respiratory depression [7] and has, along with other organizations, issued warnings regarding unsafe use of these patches [8,9]. There are also previous reports of serious and fatal cases due to erroneous administration of multiple patches of rivastigmine, an anticholinergic drug used to treat dementia [4,10]. Prevalence and characteristics of medications errors related to transdermal opioid patches has not

* Correspondence: Henrik.Lovborg@lio.se
[1]Department of Clinical Pharmacology and Department of Medical and Health Sciences, Linköping University, Linköping, Sweden
[2]Clinical Pharmacology, University Hospital, S-581 85 Linköping, Sweden

been systematically compiled and presented in the scientific literature and such information is needed to develop effective preventive measures. This study was therefore undertaken to describe and characterize medication errors regarding transdermal opioid patches, containing fentanyl and buprenorphine, submitted to a regional incident reporting system.

Method
Data source
Reports on medication errors were identified in a web-based incident reporting system for the healthcare organization within the County Council of Östergötland, Southeastern Sweden. Permission to access the data was obtained from the patient safety department of the County Council. Ethical review was not required for this study, based on national legislation [11]. The database did not contain information that was directly or indirectly identifying individual subjects. The catchment area in this study comprised 431 075 persons (2011). All are encouraged to report all types of incidents and risks. Incident and risk were defined by the county council as "an unexpected event or observation that leads to or has the potential to lead to harm to a patient, relative or family member, employee, equipment, or organization". In this study all events concerning transdermal opioid patches reported between 2004 and 2011 were scrutinized. The data included free text description of the incident, reporting clinic, and date of the incident.

Cases
For incident reports to be included in this study they had to be classified as MEs according to the definition "a failure in the treatment process that leads to or has the potential to lead to harm to patients" [12], and concern transdermal opioid patches with fentanyl or buprenorphine as active ingredients (e.g. fentanyl in Durogesic and Matrifen or buprenorphine in Norspan). "Pain relief patch" is a commonly used term for these patches among healthcare employees and MEs described with this term have accordingly been included. To reliably identify reports when searching the database, the key terms used included the words *patch, fentanyl, buprenorphine, transdermal, Norspan, Durogesic, Matrifen* and a number of misspellings of these terms. Patches with e.g. lidocaine for local anesthetic use were excluded.

Classification
During ME classification substance, drug brand name, harm, reactions, and error type have been determined. Serious harm was classified in accordance with the WHO definition of a serious adverse event or reaction, i.e. a reaction that results in death, requires inpatient hospitalization or prolongation if existing hospitalization,

results in persistent disability/incapacity, or is life threatening [13]. The MedDRA (Medical Dictionary for Regulatory Activities) terminology was used describe the type of adverse reactions reported [14]. In some reports more than one incident was described. In this case incidents considered to causally relate to the first one in the medication process was not included. Also sequentially repeated incidents of the same type in a single report were classified as a single incident. 60 proposed error types, as previously described [15] were used to categorize the MEs (Table 1), based on the free text description of the case. Reports were anonymized and were not traceable back to medical records. Therefore no thorough root cause analysis was possible to perform. Due to lack of information in some incident reports the error type "unclassifiable" was added, and to further analyze our results sub-error types were created for "wrong time" and "wrong dose". The authors collectively developed the inclusion and exclusion criteria and data extraction. Inclusion of and extraction of data was performed by MH and HL by consensus.

Results
During the study period a total of 102 270 incident reports were submitted. Selection of opioid patch related MEs are shown in Figure 1. Of all incident reports 13,3% (n = 13 617) concerned medications. Of these, 279 contained at least one of the key terms and were reviewed. Of the reviewed incident reports 149 were selected for this study in accordance with the inclusion criteria. In two incident reports more than one ME was found which resulted in two additional MEs and a total of 151 MEs were included in the analysis. Of the MEs, 66% (n = 100) concerned fentanyl, 28% (n = 42) unknown substance, and 6% (n = 9) buprenorphine. Of the included MEs 48% (n = 73) were reported during 2010 and 2011.

In total, 11 different types of MEs were identified. Some error types may however be found in several stages of the medication process while others are stage specific (Table 1). Administration errors were most commonly reported, and the most frequently occurring error in this category was administration at the wrong time (n = 67). In the prescribing stage wrong transcription errors were most common (n = 9), and in the dispensing stage wrong dose (n = 4), shown in Table 2.

MEs in the prescribing stage were often due to incorrect use of electronic systems for prescribing or electronic medical records. In the dispensing stage slips and lapses occurred as causes, and in the administration step lack of compliance with routines, e.g. scheduling visits to outpatients to change patch, was a common cause. The two most frequent error types reported, wrong time and wrong dose, were further analyzed by the addition of subtypes. Wrong time MEs were divided into late (92%, n = 62), early (3% n = 2) and unknown (5%, n = 3).

Table 1 Categories of error types used in this study [15]

Prescribing		Dispensing	Administration and monitoring
Decision making	**Communication**		
- Allergy	- Allergy information	- Ambiguous information on label	- Contamination
			- Incompatibility errors
- Calculation error	- Decimal place error	- Incompatibility errors	- Extra dose
- Interaction drug and disease	- Ambiguous drug name	- Contamination	- Lack of control of patient identity
		- Expired drug	
- Interaction between drug and laboratory test	- Ambiguous drug prescription	- Omission of dose	- Omission of dose
- Drug to drug interaction	- P.r.n. prescription without a maximum limit	- Omission of documentation of drug dispensing	- Lack of documentation of the drug administration
- Extra drug	- P.r.n. prescription without a minimum dose interval	- Omission of control of the drug prescription	- Lack of control of agreement between administered drug and prescribed drug
- Omission of a drug prescription			
- Wrong concentration	- Omission of indication for treatment including p.r.n. prescriptions	- Substitution error	- Unordered drug
- Wrong drug form		- Unordered drug	- Wrong dose
- Wrong dose		- Unordered electrolyte	- Wrong patient
- Wrong dosing interval		- Wrong concentration	- Wrong dosing interval
- Wrong drug			
	- Illegible handwriting	- Wrong drug form	- Wrong rate
- Wrong route of administration	- Omission of rate of infusion	- Wrong dose	- Wrong route of administration
- Wrong duration of treatment	- Discrepancy between dose intervals	- Extra dose	- Wrong technique
- Wrong strength/unit		- Wrong strength per unit	- Wrong time
- Omission of ordering laboratory tests	- Discrepancy between indication of dose	- Wrong dilution fluid	- Omission of documentation of side-effects of the drug treatment
	- Wrong transcription		

The error types are listed from left to right in the order of the medication process.

As evident from the short descriptions in the reports scheduling of visits and assigning personnel to the task of changing patches were the most common cause of late administration.

Of the 34 MEs with wrong dose, 13 were cases of too high dose, 10 were cases of too low dose, and 4 with unspecified wrong dose. Of the cases with too high dose, 7 were cases where the old patch were not removed before a new patch was applied.

Harm was reported for 17% (n = 26) of the MEs as shown in Table 3. In two cases there were reports of serious harm. In the first case a patient who ingested a fentanyl patch is described. This patient experienced a respiratory depression and during intubation for respiratory care the patch was discovered in the pharynx. The second case concerns a patient who received a higher dose than prescribed. At admittance to hospital health care personnel found two sets of patches of the prescribed dose on the patient, who was experiencing nausea, vomiting, and pain. The observed adverse reactions (in some cases more than one reaction per ME) were pain (n = 16), withdrawal syndrome (n = 4),

fatigue (n = 3), anxiety (n = 2), discomfort (n = 1), dizziness (n = 1), respiratory depression (n = 1), nausea/vomiting (n = 1), tremor (n = 1) and confusional state (n = 1).

Discussion

This is, to our knowledge, the first systematic study assessing and categorizing medication errors concerning transdermal opioid patches. A considerable proportion, 54%, of the MEs assessed in this study constitutes of wrong time - late and omission of doses. The difference between these two error types was the time of discovery; incidents discovered before the next administration were categorized as wrong time – late and incidents discovered at the next scheduled administration or later were categorized as omission of dose. These errors often appeared to be caused by unsatisfactory planning and inadequate patch changing routines. As for all error types, we were unable to perform a full root cause analysis to fully explain what occurred prior to the errors of late administration. It is also important to note that incidents and errors are often consequences of failures in the

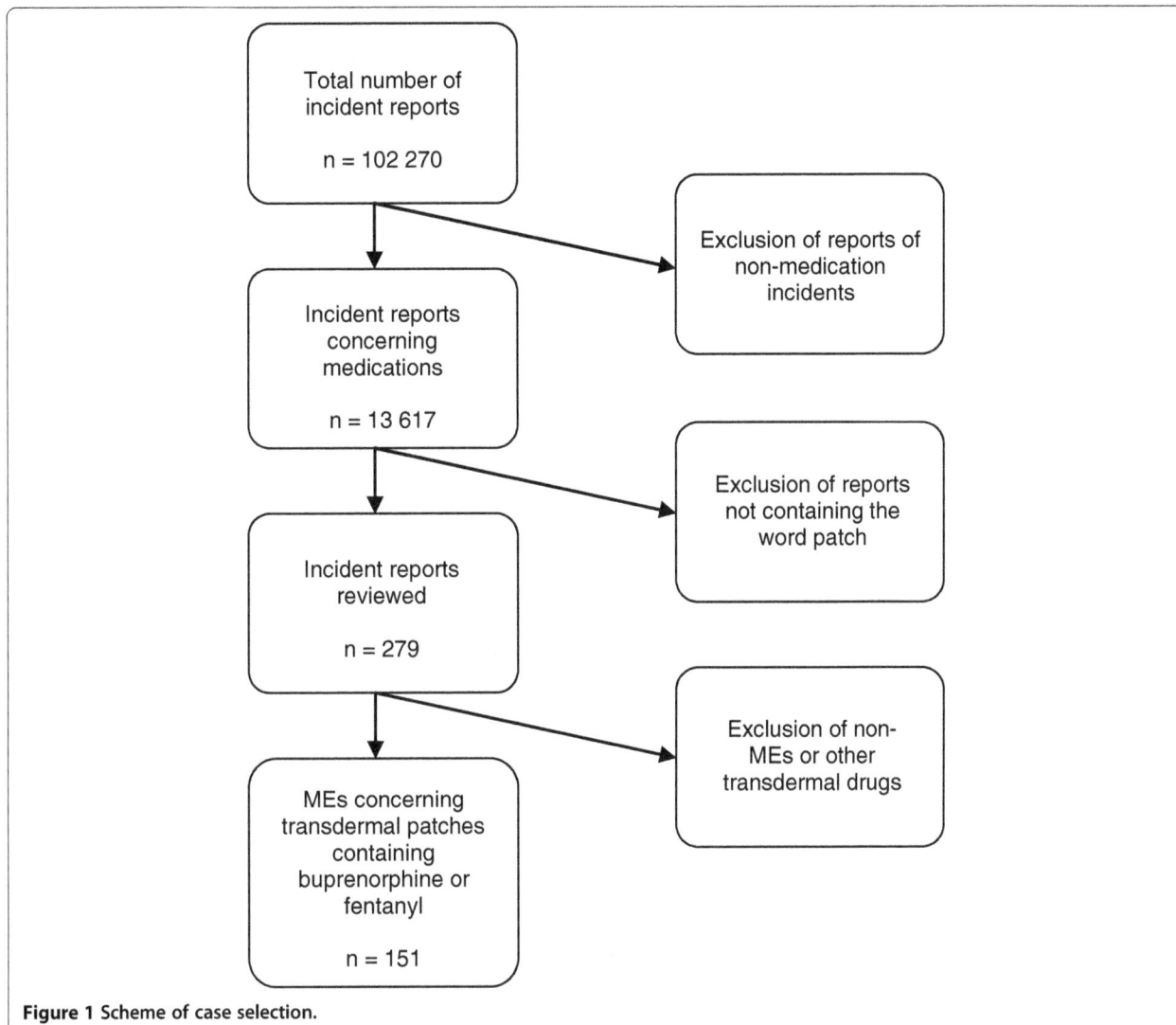

Figure 1 Scheme of case selection.

system rather than solely the act of the individual [16], information that was not available in this dataset on a case by case basis.

Wrong dose constituted 23% of the reported MEs, a diverse error type that was further divided into several subtypes. Analyzing wrong dose – high as well as wrong dose – low, we found that difficulties in handling doses consisting of more than one patch, often with different strengths, sometimes caused problems. Studies have shown that the amount of drug present in used fentanyl patches may be high, in some cases up to 60% of the initial amount [17,18]. As well as potential risk of causing an overdose this could enhance other risks associated with fentanyl use, such as the risk for ADRs. Due to these facts we have considered forgetting to remove old patches when applying a new ones as potentially harmful and this is an important dosage form specific ME. Constituting 21% of the reports of wrong doses, the risks with forgetting old patches on patients may not be

considered negligible. Educating healthcare personnel in transdermal opioid pain management and the importance of carefully checking patient for old patches before applying new ones would likely reduce the risk of overdosing.

Of all prescribing MEs, 74% were categorized as wrong transcription or omission of a drug prescription. Mutual for these two error types is that there seemed to be issues concerning electronic prescribing systems and knowledge about how to use it properly. There were also cases where a prescription was noted in the medical record but not transcribed into a separate system for ordering multi-dose packaging. Knowledge about routines related to documenting drug related information in the journal appeared to be another issue. At the same time it is important to note that these systems are likely to reduce mediation errors relating to prescriptions [19,20].

In our study we also found one case of ingestion of a fentanyl patch, which ended up causing the patient

Table 2 Error types found in the different stages of the medication process

Error type	Prescribing	Dispensing	Administration	Unknown[†]	Total (%)
Wrong time	0	1	66		67(44)
Wrong dose	4	4	25	1	34(23)
Omission of dose	0	2	18		20(13)
Wrong transcription	9	0	0		9(6)
Unclassifiable*	0	0	0	6	6(4)
Omission of a drug prescription	5	0	0		5(3)
Lack of documentation of the drug administration	0	0	2		2(1)
Wrong dosing interval	0	0	2		2(1)
Wrong technique	0	0	3		3(2)
Ambiguous drug prescription	1	0	0		1(1)
Lack of control of agreement between administered drug and prescribed drug	0	0	1		1(1)
Wrong route of administration	0	0	1		1(1)
SUM (%)	19(112)	7(5)	8(78)	7(5)	151 (100)

*MEs with no suitable error type [†]Data didn't provide enough information to determine in what stage in the medication process the ME occurred.

serious harm. A multicenter case series concerning whole fentanyl patch ingestion reports hospital admittance in about 78% of the cases with serious adverse reactions like coma, respiratory depression and tachycardia [5]. Patient education regarding the serious risks that this type of misuse can cause could possibly increase the safety in using these types of drugs, with the exception of intentional misuse. The second case of serious harm in our study was categorized as wrong dose – high; a patient who was treated with a relatively high dose, 250 µg, was discovered to have two sets of patches of the prescribed dose on his body at the same time. This most likely contributed to his symptoms that caused admission. Both accidental and voluntary misuse of fentanyl patches causing fatal and nonfatal intoxications are described in the literature [17,21].

The third most commonly reported error type, omission of dose, had the highest proportion of harm (40%). Most common reaction in this category was, as expected, that the patients suffered from pain breakthrough and withdrawal symptoms. Omission of dose, as well as late doses, was often related to inadequate routines for scheduling and performing change of patch.

Interestingly several studies states that using transdermal patches may increase compliance [22,23], but an American study reviewing 644 medication errors with opioids found a higher rate of omission errors with fentanyl patches then with other opioids in different dosage forms, 36% and 12% respectively [1,23,24]. This is in line with our data where reports on omission of doses were relatively common.

The three most commonly reported error types i.e. wrong time, wrong dose, and omission of dose, constitute 80% of all MEs included in this study. Of these 90% occurred in the administration phase of the medication

process. We suspected that this uneven distribution of MEs in the medication process partly could be explained by which profession that had predominantly reported the cases included in this study. However this data was not accessible for the years 2004 and 2005, but for the remaining years nurses were submitting the vast majority of the reports (not shown). This may have influenced in what phase of the medication process and what type of errors that were reported. We also suspect that we have an underestimation of MEs in the dispensing stage since neither hospital nor community pharmacies were reporting MEs to the database used in this study.

There are some limitations of this study that needs to be taken into consideration when interpreting the results. Even though reporting incidents to the database used in this study is mandatory for the employees in the county council, underreporting is substantial. It has been estimated that at most 10% of all incidents in our region are reported (personal communication patient safety officer). It is also likely that certain categories of healthcare personnel are more prone to report particular error

Table 3 Patient harm by error type

Error type	No harm	Harm	
		Nonserious	Serious
Omission of dose: n = 20	12	8	0
Wrong time: n = 67	59	8	0
Wrong dose: n = 34	27	6	1
Wrong transcription: n = 9	8	1	0
Wrong technique: n = 3	2	1	0
Wrong route of administration: n = 1	0	0	1
Remaining error types	17	0	0
SUM: n = 151	125	24	2

types, making it challenging to draw conclusion of how common these errors are in the clinical setting. However, the lack of published data on specific problems relating to transdermally delivered drugs warrants this kind of study to capture signals and patterns on MEs with these drugs. In the analysis of MEs we did not have access to medical records therefore some clinical information about the incident, the measures taken and the outcome for the patient was not available. We were not able to check medical record or interview personnel and patients. Doing so would have yielded a deeper understanding of the causes of the errors performed. However, that was neither possible using this data source, nor the scope of this study. Another limitation was the fact that the time of discovery could not always be assessed. Incidents where omission of dose could not be accurately determined were categorized as wrong time-late. As most of the patients had healthcare personnel administering the fentanyl or buprenorphine patches, we only came across very few cases where the patients were self-administrating, a setting with a potentially different pattern of MEs. Furthermore, it is essential to know that ME is a term that is quite imprecisely used in the literature and there are numerous definitions [15,25]. This makes studies in this field difficult to compare. Inclusion of cases considered a ME according to our definition, is to some extent subjective. To reduce the risk of misclassification, only cases where the assessors reached a consensus, were included.

Conclusions

Using an incident reporting system we were able to describe and characterize medication errors related to transdermal fentanyl and buprenorphine. The vast majority of the reported errors occurred during administration. Improved routines to ascertain correct and timely administration of these drugs and educational interventions focusing on this stage of the medication process are suggested.

Competing interests
The authors declare that they have no competing interests.

Authors' contributions
HL and MH carried out the data retrieval and analysis and drafted the manuscript. SH and HL participated in the design of the study and interpretation of the data. All authors read and approved the final manuscript.

Acknowledgement
The authors would like to thank the County Council of Östergötland for providing data and Ingela Jakobsson for assistance with data handling. Research and preparation of manuscript funded by the County Council of Östergötland.

References
1. Durand C, Alhammad A, Willett KC: Practical considerations for optimal transdermal drug delivery. Am J Health Syst Pharm 2012, 69:116–124.
2. Wohlrab J, Kreft B, Tamke B: Skin tolerability of transdermal patches. Expert Opin Drug Deliv 2011, 8:939–948.
3. Fentanyl patches: preventable overdose. Prescrire Int 2010, 19:22–25.
4. Lövborg H, Jönsson AK, Hägg S: A fatal outcome after unintentional overdosing of rivastigmine patches. Curr Drug Saf 2012, 7:30–32.
5. Mrvos R, Feuchter AC, Katz KD, Duback-Morris LF, Brooks DE, Krenzelok EP: Whole fentanyl patch ingestion: a multi-center case series. J Emerg Med 2012, 42:549–552.
6. Sindali K, Sherry K, Sen S, Dheansa B: Life-threatening coma and full-thickness sunburn in a patient treated with transdermal fentanyl patches: a case report. J Med Case Reports 2012, 6:220.
7. Lee M, Phillips J: Transdermal patches: high risk for error? Drug Topics 2002, 54–55.
8. Fentanyl Transdermal System (marketed as Duragesic) Information. [http://www.fda.gov/drugs/drugsafety/postmarketdrugsafetyinformationfor patientsandproviders/ucm114961.htm]
9. Grissinger M, Gaunt MJ: Reducing patient harm with the use of fentanyl transdermal system. Consult Pharm 2009, 24:864–872.
10. Hoffman RS, Manini AF, Russell-Haders AL, Felberbaum M, Mercurio-Zappala M: Use of pralidoxime without atropine in rivastigmine (carbamate) toxicity. Hum Exp Toxicol 2009, 28:599–602.
11. The act concerning the ethical review of research involving humans. Swedish Code of Statutes 2003, 460.
12. Ferner RE, Aronson JK: Clarification of terminology in medication errors: definitions and classification. Drug Saf 2006, 29:1011–1022.
13. World Health Organisation Collaborating Centre for International Drug Monitoring: adverse reaction terminology. [http://www.who-umc.org]
14. MedDRA - Medical Dictionary for Regulatory Activities. [http://www.meddra.org/]
15. Lisby M, Nielsen LP, Brock B, Mainz J: How should medication errors be defined? Development and test of a definition. Scand J Public Health 2012, 40:203–210.
16. Reason J: Human error: models and management. BMJ 2000, 320:768–770.
17. Kornick CA, Santiago-Palma J, Moryl N, Payne R, Obbens EAMT: Benefit-risk assessment of transdermal fentanyl for the treatment of chronic pain. Drug Saf 2003, 26:951–973.
18. Kress HG, Boss H, Delvin T, Lahu G, Lophaven S, Marx M, Skorjanec S, Wagner T: Transdermal fentanyl matrix patches Matrifen and Durogesic DTrans are bioequivalent. Eur J Pharm Biopharm 2010, 75:225–231.
19. Jozefczyk KG, Kennedy WK, Lin MJ, Achatz J, Glass MD, Eidam WS, Melroy MJ: Computerized prescriber order entry and opportunities for medication errors: comparison to tradition paper-based order entry. J Pharm Pract 2013, 26:434–437.
20. Villamanan E, Larrubia Y, Ruano M, Velez M, Armada E, Herrero A, Alvarez-Sala R: Potential medication errors associated with computer prescriber order entry. Int J Clin Pharm 2013, 35:577–583.
21. Kim HK, Smiddy M, Hoffman RS, Nelson LS: Buprenorphine may not be as safe as you think: a pediatric fatality from unintentional exposure. Pediatrics 2012, 130:e1700–e1703.
22. Clemens KE, Klaschik E: Clinical experience with transdermal and orally administered opioids in palliative care patients–a retrospective study. Jpn J Clin Oncol 2007, 37:302–309.
23. Dy SM, Shore AD, Hicks RW, Morlock LL: Medication errors with opioids: results from a national reporting system. J Opioid Manage 2007, 3:189–194.
24. Tanner T, Marks R: Delivering drugs by the transdermal route: review and comment. Skin Res Tech 2008, 14:249–260.
25. Pintor-Mármol A, Baena M: Terms used in patient safety related to medication: a literature review. Pharmacoepidemiol Drug Saf 2012, 21:799–809.

23

Effect of novobiocin on the viability of human gingival fibroblasts (HGF-1)

Anna K Szkaradkiewicz[1], Tomasz M Karpiński[2*] and Andrzej Szkaradkiewicz[2]

Abstract

Background: Novobiocin is a coumarin antibiotic, which affects also eukaryotic cells inhibiting activity of Heat shock protein 90 (Hsp90). The Hsp90 represents a molecular chaperone critical for stabilization and activation of many proteins, particularly oncoproteins that drive cancer progression. Currently, Hsp90 inhibitors focus a significant attention since they form a potentially new class of drugs in therapy of cancer. However, in the process of tumorigenesis a significant role is played also by the microenvironment of the tumour, and, in particular, by cancer-associated fibroblasts (CAFs). This study aimed at examination of the effect played by novobiocin on viability of human gingival fibroblasts (HGF-1).

Methods: The studies were conducted using 24 h cultures of human gingival fibroblasts – HGF-1 (CRL-2014) in Chamber Slides, in presence of 0.1, 0.5, 1.0, 2.5 or 5.0 mM novobiocin. Cell viability was evaluated using fluorescence test, ATP assay and LDH release.

Results: Viability of HGF-1 was drastically reduced after 5 hour treatment with novobiocin in concentrations of 1 mM or higher. In turn, the percentage of LDH-releasing cells after 5 h did not differ from control value although it significantly increased after 10 h incubation with 1 mM and continued to increase till the 20th hour.

Conclusions: The obtained data indicate that novobiocin may induce death of human gingival fibroblasts. Therefore, application of the Hsp90 inhibitor in neoplastic therapy seems controversial: on one hand novobiocin reduces tumour-associated CAFs but, on the other, it may induce a significant destruction of periodontium.

Keywords: Novobiocin, Hsp90, Human gingival fibroblasts, Viability, Cell death

Introduction

Novobiocin represents a coumarin antibiotic produced by *Streptomyces spheroides* and *Streptomyces niveus* strains and manifesting activity against Gram-positive bacteria [1]. The antibiotic exerts mainly bacteriostatic activity, inhibiting function of ATP-dependent gyrase [2,3]. In addition, in recent years novobiocin was found to act also on eukaryotic cells, blocking chaperone activity of 90 kDa heat shock proteins (Hsp90) through competitive binding to the Hsp90 C-terminal ATP binding site [4,5]. Due to inhibition of Hsp90, many oncoproteins linked to all six hallmarks of cancer progression (angiogenesis, immortalization, metastasis, impaired apoptosis, insensitivity to antigrowth signals and autocrine growth) undergo degradation in cancer cells [6]. Currently, inhibitors of Hsp90

are thought to represent promising agents, providing a new class of drugs in cancer therapy. In parallel, recent studies indicate that the microenvironment of the tumour and activated fibroblasts in particular play a significant role in the process of tumourigenesis [7-9]. These cancer-associated fibroblasts (CAFs) may promote both tumour growth and progression [9,10]. In parallel, it has already been recognised that some oncological drugs may induce periodontium destruction, resulting in a permanent architectural defect [11,12]. Gingival fibroblasts represent the prevailing periodontal tissue cells while their injury during cancer therapy may determine pathology in periodontium. Nevertheless, data on effects of novobiocin on human fibroblasts still remain unavailable.

Taking the above into consideration, present investigations aimed at analysis of novobiocin effect on viability of human gingival fibroblasts (HGF-1).

* Correspondence: tkarpin@interia.pl
[2]Department of Medical Microbiology, University of Medical Sciences, Wieniawskiego 3, str., 61-712 Poznań, Poland
Full list of author information is available at the end of the article

Materials and Methods

Cell cultures

Gingival fibroblasts HGF-1 (CRL-2014, ATCC) were cultured in T-25 culture vessels (Nunc), in an incubators at the temperature of 37°C, in atmosphere of 5% CO_2. Culture medium consisted of DMEM (ATCC) enriched with 10% FBS (Sigma-Aldrich).

Fluorescence viability assay

Viability assays in gingival fibroblasts, HGF-1 employed the fluorescence test of Live/Dead Viability/Cytotoxicity Kit (Invitrogen, USA). The test allows to distinguish viable cells (stained with green-fluorescent calcein-AM) from dead cells (stained with red-fluorescent ethidium homodimer-1). In the studies novobiocin (Sigma-Aldrich) was used. The culture medium consisted of DMEM (ATCC) enriched with 10% FBS (Sigma-Aldrich). The studies took advantage of 24 h cultures of gingival fibroblasts, HGF-1, which following incubation were subjected to triple rinsing. The tests in triple repetitions were conducted in culture Lab-Tek Chamber Slides (Nunc) in presence of culture medium alone - control (0.5×10^6 cells of HGF-1) and in presence of novobiocin (in concentrations of 0.1, 0.5, 1, 2.5 or 5 mM/L/0.5×10^6 HGF-1 cells). The samples were incubated for 20 h at 37°C in presence of 5% CO_2. In addition, the samples were incubated with 1 mM/L novobiocin for 5 and 10 h. Following the incubation the cells were rinsed with culture medium and their cell viability was assayed. The readout took advantage of the fluorescence microscope, Nikon Eclipse E200 (magnif. of 1000×).

ATP assay

ATP content of HGF-1 gingival fibroblasts was evaluated using a luminescence test (CellTiter-Glo Luminescent Cell Viability Assay, Promega). The culture medium consisted of DMEM (ATCC), enriched with 10% FBS (Sigma-Aldrich). In the studies 24 h cultures of HGF-1 gingival fibroblasts were used, which following incubation were subjected to triple rinsing. The studies, in three repetitions, were conducted in culture medium alone – the control (10^5 HGF-1 cells) and in presence of novobiocin (0.1, 0.5, 1, 2.5 or 5 mM/L/10^5 HGF-1 cells). The prepared cells were incubated for 20 h at the temperature of 37°C in presence of 5% CO_2. Subsequently, they were rinsed with culture medium and subjected to the test evaluating ATP content. The results were read out using a luminometer (GloMax, Promega). In presence of ATP a light is emitted which is read out in relative light units (RLU). Intensity of the emitted light quants is directly related to quantity of ATP present in the test. Viability of fibroblasts was calculated as a percentage of light intensity (RLU) emitted from experimental samples to intensity emitted from control samples, which was set as representing 100% viability.

LDH release

The tests of LDH release were conducted using CytoTox 96 Non-Radioactive Cytotoxicity Assay kits (Promega, Madison). In the studies 24 h cultures of HGF-1 gingival fibroblasts were used which, following incubation were rinsed three times. The studies were performed in medium alone – the control (10^5 HGF-1 cells) and in presence of novobiocin (0.1, 0.5, 1, 2.5 or 5 mM/L/10^5 HGF-1 cells). The tubes were centrifuged at 500 rpm for 4 min at the temperature of 20°C. The prepared cells were incubated for 20 h at the temperature of 37°C in presence of 5% CO_2. In addition the samples with novobiocin at the concentration of 1 mM/L were incubated for 5 and 10 hours. The studies were conducted as specified by the producer. The results were read out as absorbance at 492 nm. The percentage of cytotoxicity was calculated as a quotient of absorbance reflecting LDH release in experimental samples to absorbance value reflecting LDH release in samples with maximum lysis.

Statistical methods

Results obtained in the studies were subjected to analysis using the STATISTICA 8 software for Windows operational system. Comparative analysis of ATP levels and studies on LDH release employed the unifactorial analysis of variance (one-way ANOVA) with the Tukey-Kramer's test. Comparative analysis of gingival fibroblast viability took advantage of the non-parametric Mann-Whitney's test and the Kruskal-Wallis'es test. A difference was considered significant when $p < 0.05$.

Results

In the studies percentage of viable HGF-1 fibroblasts in control samples using the fluorescence test ranged between 94 and 99% (97.6 ± 2.32%), while in ATP assay the average value in the control samples was taken as 100%. In neither of the tests a significant difference could be detected between viability in control samples and viability of fibroblasts incubated with novobiocin at concentrations of 0.1 mM or 0.5 mM. However, gingival fibroblast viability was markedly reduced ($p < 0.0001$) following application of novobiocin at the concentration of 1 mM. No significant differences in fibroblast viability were detected in samples treated with 1 mM, 2.5 mM or 5 mM novobiocin (Figures 1 and 2).

In control samples the percentage of LDH-releasing cells ranged between 1 and 3.5% (2.8 ± 1.76%). No significant difference could be detected between LDH levels in the control samples and LDH levels in samples incubated with novobiocin at the concentrations of 0.1 mM or 0.5 mM. Levels of LDH were markedly increased

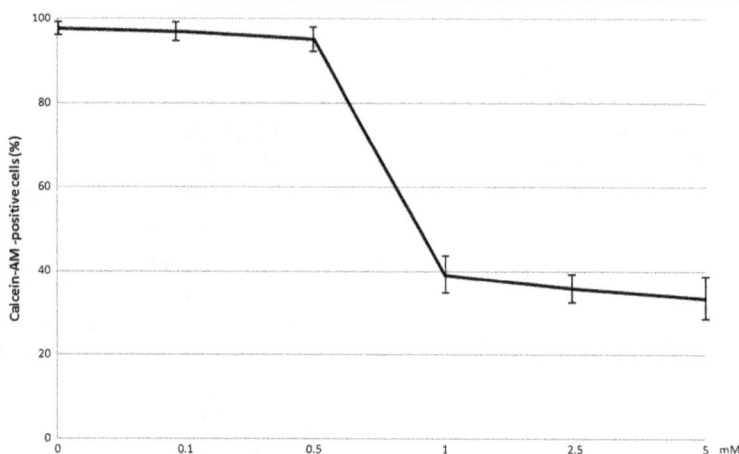

Figure 1 Viability of gingival fibroblasts (fluorescence test) after 20 h incubation with examined novobiocin concentrations. The studies were conducted in triple repetitions. The obtained results represent mean values ± SD (denoted in bars).

($p < 0.0001$) in fibroblast cultures subjected to novobiocin action at the concentration of 1 mM. No significant alterations were noted in LDH levels in samples incubated with 1 mM, 2.5 mM or 5 mM novobiocin (Figure 3).

Viability of HGF-1 fibroblasts treated with novobiocin at the concentration of 1 mM obtained in fluorescence test and that obtained in LDH release tests differed between each other: in fluorescence test viability of HGF-1 underwent a significant reduction already after 5 h and it did not change in consecutive time points of testing, in turn in LDH release assays the viability decreased significantly after 10 h culture and continued to increase till the 20th hour (Figure 4).

Discussion

The Hsp90 plays essential roles in the folding, maturation and activity of many proteins that are involved in signal transduction and transcriptional regulation [5]. The

proteins which are known to interact with Hsp90 include glucocorticoid receptors [13], Akt/Protein kinase B and Raf-1 [14], the tumor suppressor protein TP53 [15] and NOS family members [16]. The anti-cancer effects induced by novobiocin and its analogues through Hsp90 inhibition have already been well described [4,5]. Therefore, Hsp90 chemical inhibitors may find application in oncological therapy [17,18]. Moreover, application of Hsp90 inhibitors is considered in treatment of certain infectious diseases, because in eukaryotic cells Hsp90 is essential for the replication of obligatory intracellular parasites [19,20]. In recent years, development of neoplastic process has been found to be contributed by CAFs present in tumour stroma [9,10]. In parallel, fibroblasts represent prevailing connective tissue cells which provide integrity to its structure.

In this study we have examined for the first time effect of novobiocin on viability of human gingival fibroblasts

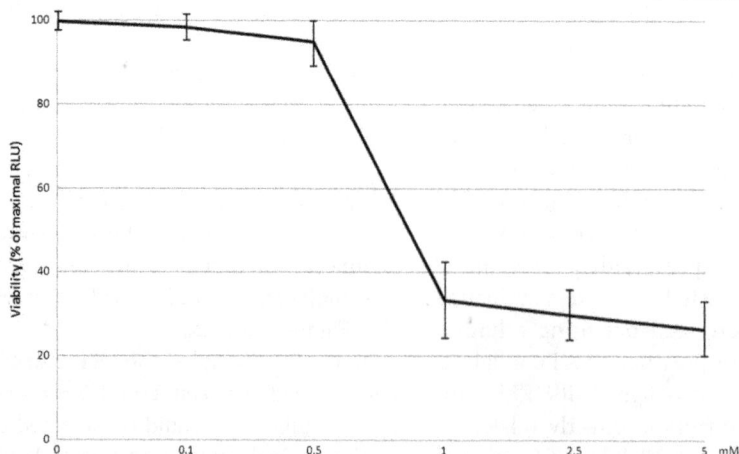

Figure 2 Viability of gingival fibroblasts (ATP assay) after 20 h incubation with examined novobiocin concentrations. The studies were conducted in triple repetitions. The obtained results represent mean values ± SD (denoted in bars).

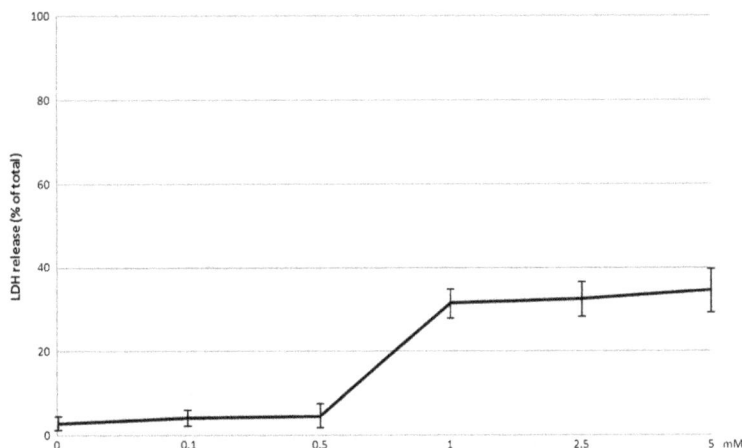

Figure 3 Release of LDH in 20 h culture of gingival fibroblasts with the examined novobiocin concentrations. The studies were conducted in triple repetitions. The obtained results represent mean values ± SD (denoted in bars).

(HGF-1), which are the dominant periodontal tissue cells [21,22]. Using a fluorescent test and ATP assay we have shown that novobiocin in doses of 0.1 and 0.5 mM failed to alter cell viability. Nevertheless, 0.5 mM novobiocin has insignificantly decreased viability of fibroblasts using ATP assay. The test represents the most sensitive assay of cell viability [23], which may explain differences in the obtained results. Using both tests we have demonstrated a significant decrease in HGF-1 viability following their 20 h incubation with 1 mM novobiocin. Percentage of viable fibroblasts following their 20 h incubation with 1.0, 2.5 and 5.0 mM novobiocin has amounted to 20-38% and it has not been dependent on the dose of novobiocin. In an earlier study by Calamia et al. [24], a significant reduction was noted in viability of human chondrocytes also in presence of 1 mM novobiocin. Results of Shelton et al. [25] contrast with those of ours. The authors demonstrated that novobiocin in concentration of 0.252 mM

markedly inhibited proliferation of Jurkat T-lymphocytes, significantly reducing their viability. In turn, novobiocin at the dose of 0.4353 mM significantly reduced proliferation of K562 human erythroleukaemic cells [26]. However, the data pertain leukaemic cells, which as neoplastic cells may be particularly sensitive to Hsp90 inhibitors. The suggestion has been supported by reports showing that Hsp90 in cancer cells has a higher affinity for Hsp90 inhibition drugs than the Hsp90 in normal cells [27].

The demonstrated by us novobiocin-mediated decreased viability of fibroblasts seems to result from induction of an apoptotic response. The suggestion, in turn, corresponds with the data indicating that novobiocin and its derivatives may induce cell death along the apoptosis pathway [24,26,28]. In our study we have conducted also fibroblast viability tests following 5, 10 and 20 h treatment with 1 mM novobiocin, using for the purpose the fluorescence test and LDH assay. It has been already

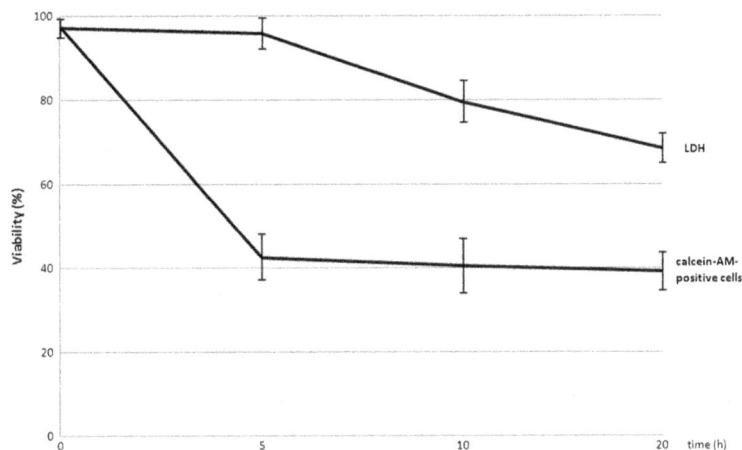

Figure 4 Viability of gingival fibroblasts (fluorescence test and LDH test) in culture with 1 mM novobiocin after 5 h, 10 h and 20 h incubation. The studies were conducted in triple repetitions. The obtained results represent mean values ± SD (denoted in bars).

well established that stable cytoplasmic enzyme lactate dehydrogenase (LDH) is released from necrotic cells and, therefore, the use of LDH assay establishes cell death by necrosis [23]. After 5 h incubation of fibroblasts with 1 mM novobiocin, the percentage of viable cells in fluorescence test has been significantly reduced and has shown no statistical alterations in consecutive time points of testing. In turn, LDH release upon 1 mM novobiocin treatment has been significantly higher after 10 h than in corresponding control and increased further till 20 h. The results remain in contrast to the detected decrease in fibroblast viability already after 5 h exposure, using fluorescence test and ATP assay. This may indicate that LDH assay represents a test less sensitive than the remaining two tests applied in the study, in accordance to the earlier observation of Weyermann et al. [23]. However, on the other hand it also seems probable that novobiocin in concentration of at least 1 mM induces fibroblast apoptosis, leading after 10 hour incubation to post-apoptotic lysis of the fibroblasts. The phenomenon of post-apoptotic lysis has already been well described and referred to the post-apoptotic change as secondary necrosis [29,30].

Conclusion

Data presented in this study indicate that novobiocin may induce death of human gingival fibroblasts. Therefore, application of this Hsp90 inhibitor drug in neoplastic therapy seems controversial: novobiocin on one hand reduces tumour-associated CAFs and, on the other, its application may lead to a severe destruction of periodontium.

Competing interests
The authors declare no competing interests.

Authors' contributions
AKS and TMK: study conception and design, participation in performation of the experimental studies and data analysis, drafting of the manuscript; AS: coordination and help in interpretation of the study results. All authors read and approved the final manuscript.

Acknowledgements
The studies were financed by the Poznań University of Medical Sciences research project No. 502-14-02209324-08456.

Author details
[1]Department of Conservative Dentistry and Periodontology, University of Medical Sciences, Bukowska 70, str., 60-812, Poznań, Poland. [2]Department of Medical Microbiology, University of Medical Sciences, Wieniawskiego 3, str., 61-712 Poznań, Poland.

References
1. Limson BM, Romansky MJ: Novobiocin, a new antibiotic; laboratory and clinical evaluation of thirty patients with bacterial pneumonia. *Antibiotic Med Clin Ther* 1956, 2:277–281.
2. Gellert M, O'Dea MH, Itoh T, Tomizawa J: Novobiocin and coumermycin inhibit DNA supercoiling catalysed by DNA gyrase. *Proc Natl Acad Sci U S A* 1976, 73:4474–4478.
3. Sugino A, Higgins NP, Brown PO, Peebles CL, Cozzarelli NR: Energy coupling in DNA gyrase and the mechanism of action of novobiocin. *Proc Natl Acad Sci U S A* 1978, 75:4838–4842.
4. Marcu MG, Chadli A, Bouhouche I, Catelli M, Neckers L: The heat shock protein 90 antagonist novobiocin interacts with a previously unrecognized ATP-binding domain in the carboxyl terminus of the chaperone. *J Biol Chem* 2000, 275(47):37181–37186.
5. Donnelly A, Blagg BSJ: Novobiocin and additional inhibitors of the Hsp90 C-terminal nucleotide-binding pocket. *Curr Med Chem* 2008, 15(26):2702–2717.
6. Piper PW, Millson SH: Spotlight on the microbes that produce heat shock protein 90-targeting antibiotics. *Open Biol* 2012, 2(12):120138.
7. Lorusso G, Ruegg C: The tumor microenvironment and its contribution to tumor evolution toward metastasis. *Histochem Cell Biol* 2008, 130:1091–1103.
8. Räsänen K, Vaheri A: Activation of fibroblasts in cancer stroma. *Exp Cell Res* 2010, 316:2713–2722.
9. Cirri P, Chiarugi P: Cancer-associated-fibroblasts and tumour cells: a diabolic liaison driving cancer progression. *Cancer Metastasis Rev* 2012, 31:195–208.
10. Polanska UM, Orimo A: Carcinoma-associated fibroblasts: non-neoplastic tumour-promoting mesenchymal cells. *J Cell Physiol* 2013, 228:1651–1657.
11. Wright WE: Periodontium destruction associated with oncology therapy. Five case reports. *J Periodontol* 1987, 58(8):559–563.
12. Epstein JB, Thariat J, Bensadoun RJ, Barasch A, Murphy BA, Kolnick L, Popplewell L, Maghami E: Oral complications of cancer and cancer therapy: from cancer treatment to survivorship. *CA Cancer J Clin* 2012, 62(6):400–422.
13. Bresnick EH, Dalman FC, Sanchez ER, Pratt WB: Evidence that the 90-kDa heat shock protein is necessary for the steroid binding conformation of the L cell glucocorticoid receptor. *J Biol Chem* 1989, 264(9):4992–4997.
14. Jia W, Yu C, Rahmani M, Krystal G, Sausville EA, Dent P, Grant S: Synergistic antileukemic interactions between 17-AAG and UCN-01 involve interruption of RAF/MEK – and AKT – related pathways. *Blood* 2003, 102:1284–1832.
15. Blagosklonny MV, Toretsky J, Bohen S, Neckers L: Mutant conformation of p53 translated in vitro or in vivo requires functional HSP90. *Proc Natl Acad Sci U S A* 1996, 93(16):8379–8383.
16. Kone BC: Protein-protein interactions controlling nitric oxide synthases. *Acta Physiol Scand* 2000, 168(1):27–31.
17. Gao Z, Garcia-Echeverri C, Jensen MR: Hsp90 inhibitors: clinical development and future opportunities in oncology therapy. *Curr Opin Drug Discov Devel* 2010, 13(2):193–202.
18. Geller R, Vignuzzi M, Andino R, Frydman J: Evolutionary constraints onchaperone – mediated folding provide an antiviral approach refractory to development of drug resistance. *Genes Dev* 2007, 21:195–205.
19. Isaacs JS, Xu W, Neckers L: Heat shock protein 90 as a molecular target for cancer therapeutics. *Cancer Cell* 2003, 3:213–217.
20. Shahinas D, Liang M, Datti A, Pillai DR: A repurposing strategy identifies novel synergistic inhibitors of Plasmodium falciparum heat shock protein 90. *J Med Chem* 2010, 53:3552–3557.
21. Koka S, Reinhardt RA: Periodontal pathogen-related stimulation indicates unique phenotype of primary cultured human fibroblasts from gingiva and periodontal ligament: implications for oral health disease. *J Prosthet Dent* 1997, 77:191–196.
22. Ara T, Kurata K, Hirai K, Uchihashi T, Uematsu T, Imamura Y, Furusawa K, Kurihara S, Wang PL: Human gingival fibroblasts are critical in sustaining inflammation in periodontal disease. *J Periodontal Res* 2009, 44:21–27.
23. Weyermann J, Lochmann D, Zimmer A: A practical note on the use of cytotoxicity assays. *Int J Pharm* 2005, 288:369–376.
24. Calamia V, De Andrés MG, Oreiro N, Ruiz-Romero C, Blanco FJ: Hsp90 inhibition modulates nitric oxide production and nitric oxide-induced apoptosis in human chondrocytes. *BMC Musculoskelet Disord* 2011, 12:237.
25. Shelton SN, Shawgo ME, Matthews SB, Lu Y, Donnelly AC, Szabla K, Tanol M, Vielhauer GA, Rajewski RA, Matts RL, Blagg BSJ, Robertson JD: KU135, a novel novobiocin-derived C-terminal inhibitor of the 90-kDa heat shock protein, exerts potent antiproliferative effects in human leukemic cells. *Mol Pharmacol* 2009, 76(6):1314–1322.
26. Wu LX, Xu JH, Zhang KZ, Lin Q, Huang XW, Wen CX, Chen YZ: Disruption of the Bcr-Abl/Hsp90 protein complex: a possible mechanism to inhibit Bcr-Abl-positive human leukemic blasts by novobiocin. *Leukemia* 2008, 22:1402–1409.

27. Kamal A, Thao L, Sensintaffar J, Zhang L, Boehm MF, Fritz LC, Burrows FJ: **A high-affinity conformation of Hsp90 confers tumour selectivity on Hsp90 inhibitors.** *Nature* 2003, **425**:407–410.

28. Le Bras G, Radanyi C, Peyrat JF, Brion JD, Alami M, Marsaud V, Stella B, Renoir JM: **New novobiocin analogues as antiproliferative agents in breast cancer cells and potential inhibitors of heat shock protein 90.** *J Med Chem* 2007, **50**(24):6189–6200.

29. Schwab BL, Guerini D, Didszun C, Bano D, Ferrando-May E, Fava E, Tam J, Xu D, Xanthoudakis S, Nicholson DW, Carafoli E, Nicotera P: **Cleavage of plasma membrane calcium pumps by caspases: a link between apoptosis and necrosis.** *Cell Death Differ* 2002, **9**:818–831.

30. Skulachev VP: **Bioenergetic aspects of apoptosis, necrosis and mitoptosis.** *Apoptosis* 2006, **11**:473–485.

24

Assessment of pharmacokinetic changes of meropenem during therapy in septic critically ill patients

João Goncalves-Pereira[1,2*], Nuno Elvas Silva[3], André Mateus[3], Catarina Pinho[3] and Pedro Povoa[1,2]

Abstract

Background: Meropenem is a carbapenem antibiotic commonly used in critically ill patients to treat severe infections. The available pharmacokinetic (PK) data has been mostly obtained from healthy volunteers as well as from clinical studies addressing selected populations, often excluding the elderly and also patients with renal failure. Our aim was to study PK of meropenem in a broader population of septic critically ill patients.

Methods: We characterized the PK of meropenem in 15 critically ill patients during the first 36 hrs of therapy. Aditionally, whenever possible, we collected a second set of late plasma samples after 5 days of therapy to evaluate PK intra-patient variability and its correlation with clinical course.
Patients received meropenem (1 g every 8 hrs IV). Drug plasma profiles were determined by high-performance liquid chromatography. The PK of meropenem was characterized and compared with clinical parameters.

Results: Fifteen septic critically ill patients (8 male, median age 73 yrs) were included. The geometric mean of the volume of distribution at the steady state (V_{ss})/weight was 0.20 (0.15-0.27) L/kg. No correlation of V_{ss}/weight with severity or comorbidity scores was found. However the Sequential Organ Failure Assessment score correlated with the V_{ss}/weight of the peripheral compartment ($r^2 = 0.55$, p = 0.021). The median meropenem clearance (Cl) was 73.3 (45–120) mL/min correlated with the creatinine (Cr) Cl ($r^2 = 0.35$, p = 0.033).
After 5 days (N = 7) although V_{ss} remained stable, a decrease in the proportion of the peripheral compartment (V_{ss2}) was found, from 61.3 (42.5-88.5)% to 51.7 (36.6-73.1)%. No drug accumulation was noted.

Conclusions: In this cohort of septic, unselected, critically ill patients, large meropenem PK heterogeneity was noted, although neither underdosing nor accumulation was found. However, Cr Cl correlated to meropenem Cl and the V_{ss2} decreased with patient's improvement.

Keywords: Meropenem, β-lactam antibiotics, Pharmacokinetics, Intensive care unit

Background

Meropenem is a carbapenem antibiotic with a broad antibacterial spectrum, commonly used in critically ill patients to treat severe infections. Its dose and schedule are based on pharmacokinetic (PK) data mostly obtained from healthy volunteers, as well as from clinical studies [1]. However in critically ill patients, seldom evaluated, this drug often presents different PK behaviour, and conventional dosing may fail to provide adequate antibiotic concentrations [2-4] due to both fluid shifts and therapeutic interventions. Moreover elderly patients and patients with renal failure are commonly excluded from PK studies and, therefore, it may be even more difficult to generalize the results.

Some populations, especially those with augmented renal clearance seem to be at special risk of sub-therapeutic drug concentration. Therapeutic drug monitoring has been proposed to minimize dosage inadequacy, reducing the occurrence of sub-therapeutic concentrations or drug accumulation [5]. Our purpose was to characterize the concentration time profile of meropenem in a broad

* Correspondence: joaogpster@gmail.com
[1]Polyvalent Intensive Care Unit, São Francisco Xavier Hospital, CHLO, Lisbon, Portugal, Estrada do Forte do Alto do Duque, Lisboa 1449-005, Portugal
[2]CEDOC, Faculty of Medical Sciences, New University of Lisbon, Lisbon, Portugal, Campo dos Mártires da Pátria, 130, Lisboa 1169-056, Portugal
Full list of author information is available at the end of the article

population of critically ill infected patients in the early stages of infection treatment, to determine if the recommended dose resulted in adequate plasma concentrations, according to the minimal inhibitory concentration (MIC) of susceptible bacteria. We also intended to characterize PK late profile, after at least 5 days of therapy, in particular volume of distribution at steady state (V_{ss}) and clearance (Cl), to unveil changes on drug PK behaviour during patient clinical course, and consequently the need for a dosage adjustment during therapy [6].

Methods

The study was approved by the Ethics Committee of the Centro Hospitalar de Lisboa Ocidental. All patients or their legal representatives provided written informed consent.

Infected critically ill patients requiring intravenous meropenem (by decision of the attending physician), admitted to the intensive care unit (ICU) between May of 2009 and May of 2010, were recruited, irrespectively of comorbidities or of renal function. Only patients receiving renal replacement therapy were excluded.

All patients received 1000 mg of meropenem every 8 hrs by an intravenous central line infusion during 30 minutes. The exact duration of the infusion was registered for accurate PK calculations. The line was flushed after meropenem infusion to ensure administration of the entire vial of the drug.

Collected data (Table 1) included Simplified Acute Physiology Score (SAPS) II score [7], Sequential Organ

Failure Assessment (SOFA) [8] score on the day of sample collection, Charlson comorbidity score [9], measured creatinine (Cr) Cl (in 4 hrs urine samples).

Sampling

Sampling was performed within the first 36 hrs after starting antibiotic therapy (early samples) and repeated, whenever possible, in the 5th or 6th day of therapy (late samples). Five mL blood samples were collected into heparin-lithium test tubes immediately before the beginning of infusion and after 15, 30, 45, 60, 90, 120, 180, 360 and 480 min of the start of antibiotic infusion, which covers the times of expected peak and trough drug concentrations. The exact time of collection of the sample was registered. Blood samples were immediately centrifuged at 3000 rpm (roughly 1000*g) and at 4°C, during 10 min. Two mL of plasma aliquots were separated into polypropylene tubes containing an equal volume of 3-(N-morpholino) propanesulfonic acid (MOPS) as stabilizing solution. The mixture was immediately frozen at -40°C before being transferred into -80°C (within 48 hrs), where were kept pending analysis. Drug quantifications were made within 3 months as of collection.

Analytical determinations

The concentration of meropenem in plasma was determined by high-performance liquid chromatography (HPLC). Separation was performed at 35°C using a XTerra® MS C18 cartridge (Waters, inc.) equipped

Table 1 Demographic and clinical data

Patient	Gender	Age (years)	Weight (kg)	MV	Cr Cl (mL/min)	Infection focus	Vasop	Surgery	Charlson	SAPS II	SOFA
1	M	73	77	No	76.7	Lung	Yes	No	4	26	4
2	F	58	55	Yes	25.0	Lung	No	No	3	44	5
3	F	77	65	No	66.7	Intra-abdominal	No	Yes	9	48	4
4	M	79	78	No	23.3	Intra-abdominal	No	Yes	6	38	2
5	F	78	85	Yes	81.7	Bacteremia	No	No	9	47	4
6	M	73	78	Yes	65.0	Unknown	Yes	Yes	5	43	8
7	F	76	80	Yes	43.3	Intra-abdominal	Yes	Yes	3	72	8
8	M	53	60	No	15.0	Skin/Soft tissue	Yes	No	6	34	6
9	F	71	90	Yes	NA	Intra-abdominal	No	Yes	6	37	3
10	M	41	80	Yes	116.7	Intra-abdominal	No	No	1	35	5
11	M	51	70	Yes	41.7	Lung	Yes	No	4	50	9
12	F	90	75	Yes	NA	Central nervous system	No	Yes	6	58	6
13	M	34	63	Yes	95.0	Lung	No	No	0	32	2
14	M	67	80	Yes	226.7	Lung	No	No	3	47	4
15	F	76	100	No	51.7	Intra-abdominal	No	Yes	3	47	2
Median [IQR]		73 [21]	78 [12.5]		65.0 (40)				4 [3]	44 [11.5]	4 [2.5]

Surgery was considered when was performed in the last 24 h before patients' admission to the Intensive Care Unit. M- Male; F-Female; MV – Invasive mechanical ventilation; Cr Cl – Creatinine Clearance; Vasop – Vasopressors; Charlson – Charlson comorbidity score; SAPS II – Simplified acute physiology score II; SOFA – Sequential organ failure assessment score; IQR – Interquartile range; NA-Not available.

with a Symmetry® C18 guard column (Waters, inc.). The UV detection was performed at 300 nm.

At the time of analysis, samples were thawed at room temperature. One mL of plasma sample spiked with ertapenem (as internal standard) was loaded into the cartridge. The cartridges were washed two times with 1 mL of phosphate buffer and eluted with 1 mL of acetonitrile. The eluted solutions were evaporated under vacuum, at room temperature. The residue was dissolved in 60 µL of pure water and injected into the HPLC system.

The mobile phase consisted of a mixture of 92% phosphate buffer (pH 7.4) and 8% acetonitrile pumped at 1 mL/min. The autosampler temperature was kept at 4°C and the injection volume was 5 to 25 µL.

This method showed to be linear over a range of 0.35-100 mg/L of meropenem concentration with a correlation coefficient always >0.998. Intra-assay accuracy ranged from –5.5% to –1.8% and precision was less than 3.9%. Inter-assay accuracy ranged from –8.1% to –1.4% and precision was less than 4.8%. The lower limit of quantification was 0.35 mg/L.

The method has also showed to be sensitive and specific in plasma samples obtained from intensive care patients not receiving meropenem, but a large number of other drugs commonly used in critically ill patients (including sedatives, vasopressors and other antibiotics).

Pharmacokinetics

Data were analyzed by WinNonlin 5.0.1 software (Pharsight Corp., Mountain View, California). A two-compartment model with zero order input and first order elimination was fitted into meropenem plasma profiles, using the least squares method. The model is considered to be well adjusted, with a mean r^2 of 0.95 (ranging from 0.77 to 1.00) – Figure 1. The following PK parameters were calculated: elimination half-life ($t_{1/2}$), volume of distribution at steady state associated to the central (V_{ss1}) and to the peripheral (V_{ss2}) compartments, area-under-the concentration-time curve (AUC) and total serum meropenem Cl.

We also measured trough concentrations to assess the possibility of drug accumulation.

The relationship between both meropenem Cl and Vd on one hand, and clinical relevant characteristics on the other hand, especially Cr Cl, SOFA score and Charlson comorbidity score, were assessed. A second set of late samples were collected whenever possible. We evaluated the differences between early and late meropenem PK to evaluate its relationship with patients' improvement.

Finally we evaluated ability of conventional dose of meropenem to achieve a time over minimal inhibitory concentration (T > MIC) of 100%, assuming a MIC of 2 mg/L (the European Committee on Antimicrobial Susceptibility Testing (EUCAST) for *Pseudomonas aeruginosa*).

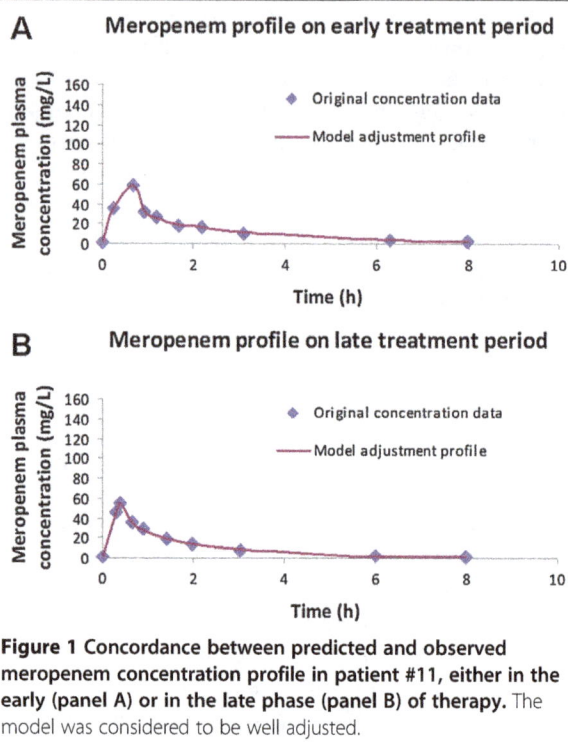

Figure 1 Concordance between predicted and observed meropenem concentration profile in patient #11, either in the early (panel A) or in the late phase (panel B) of therapy. The model was considered to be well adjusted.

Statistical analysis

Descriptive statistical analysis was performed. Continuous variables were expressed as median [interquartile range]. The PK parameters were expressed as geometric mean (95% confidence interval of the mean) to account for the log distribution of the data.

Correlations between severity and comorbidity scores with either V_{ss} or V_{ss2} and between Cr Cl and meropenem Cl were assessed using the Spearman rank correlation test and paired samples were assessed by the Wilcoxon signed rank test according to the data non normal distribution.

Data were analyzed using PASW Statistics v.18.0 (SPSS, Chicago, IL). All statistics were two-tailed, and significance level was defined as $p < 0.05$.

Results

Early meropenem pharmacokinetics

Fifteen critically ill patients (eight male, median age 73 [21] yrs) were included in the study. Their clinical and demographic data are presented in Table 1.

Despite their old age, their clinical severity was relatively low with a median SOFA score of 4 and a SAPS II score of 44. Ten patients were receiving invasive mechanical ventilation and five were on vasopressors at the time of the first meropenem measurement. Seven patients were submitted to an abdominal surgery before enrolment. One patient died still in the ICU.

Individual and geometric mean of PK parameters measured at the first 36 hrs of antibiotic therapy are shown in Table 2. The geometric mean of V_{ss}, normalized to patients' weight, at the early stage of treatment was 0.20 (0.15-0.27) L/kg. No significant correlation of V_{ss}/weight was found with either SOFA score ($r^2 = 0.25$, p = 0.068), SAPS II ($r^2 < 0.01$, p = 1.0) or Charlson comorbidity score ($r^2 = 0.06$, p = 0.389). However the SOFA score was correlated with the V_{ss2}/weight ($r^2 = 0.55$, p = 0.002). Meropenem Cl geometric mean was 73.3 (45–120) mL/min, which was significantly correlated with the measured Cr Cl ($r^2 = 0.35$, p = 0.033).

Fourteen (93%) patients had meropenem concentrations at 8 hrs above the European Committee on Antimicrobial Susceptibility Testing (EUCAST) for *Pseudomonas aeruginosa* (2 mg/L) and therefore had a T > MIC of 100%. Only one had a trough concentration below that threshold (Table 2). Six patients had a trough concentration higher than 8 mg/L (4 times above the same threshold).

No adverse effects related to the antibiotic infusion were reported.

Evolution of meropenem pharmacokinetics

In seven patients a late set of samples were collected. Early discharge from the ICU (3 patients), de-escalation of the antibiotic therapy (3 patients), incomplete data (1 patient) and withdrawal of consent (1 patient) precluded the completion of a second PK profile in the 8 patients.

In this subset of patients, the V_{ss}/weight slightly decrease, from 0.25 (0.17-0.36) L/kg to 0.23 (0.1-0.53) L/kg from the early to the late set of measurements (Table 3). This difference was associated with a relative decrease of the weight of the V_{ss2}, roughly 10% in 5 days, from 61.3 (42.5-88.5)% to 51.7 (36.6-73.1)%. Significant interpatient variability was again noted.

In these 7 patients no accumulation of meropenem was found from the early to the late set of samples. However in 4 of them a trough concentration below 2 mg/dL was noted, probably related with the improvement in renal function. This translated in a lower T > MIC at this time point.

Discussion

In this study we evaluated the PK of meropenem in 15 septic critically ill patients. We found important heterogeneity of both Cl, which parallels Cr Cl, and of V_{ss}. Moreover, we noted a relative decrease of V_{ss2}, in parallel with patients' improvement (assessed by the SOFA score). Despite the variability of the PK parameters, only one of our 15 patients had a trough level lower than 1 mg/L in early samples and no significant meropenem accumulation between early and late samples were noted.

Table 2 Initial meropenem pharmacokinetic parameters

Patient N°	V_{ss}	V_{ss}/weight	V_{ss2}/V_{ss}	AUC	Cl	$T_{1/2}$	Peak	Trough	T > 2 mg/L	T > 4 mg/L	T > 8 mg/L
	L	L/Kg	%	L/mg.h	mL/min	h	mg/L	mg/L	100%	90%	70%
1	19.6	0.25	50.6%	157.1	106.7	2.9	63.3	3.0	100%	100%	100%
2	NA	NA	NA	264.7	63.3	1.5	NA	11.9	100%	100%	100%
3	13.6	0.21	56.3%	253.3	65	2.6	94.1	8.6	100%	100%	85%
4	13.6	0.17	78.4%	160.1	103.3	1.7	102.3	4.8	100%	85%	50%
5	13.4	0.16	51.8%	129.2	128.3	1.3	80.1	2.7	100%	90%	65%
6	32.7	0.42	93.7%	134.9	123.3	3.4	52.0	3.0	100%	100%	100%
7	18.6	0.23	73.6%	479.2	35	6.4	84.7	NA	100%	100%	100%
8	14.9	0.25	88.7%	465.9	35	5.0	91.3	NA	100%	100%	75%
9	6.7	0.07	90.4%	232.5	71.7	1.4	192.5	4.4	100%	75%	50%
10	13.0	0.16	58.4%	139.5	120	1.5	85.1	2.4	100%	75%	50%
11	20.9	0.30	68,6%	107.3	155	1.9	58.6	2.9	100%	100%	100%
12	13.6	0.18	79.2%	304.2	55	3.5	119.8	8.6	75%	50%	35%
13	17.1	0.27	34.9%	81.4	205	1.3	56.9	0.6	100%	100%	55%
14	22.5	0.28	53.1%	120.7	138.3	2.1	48.4	4.1	100%	100%	100%
15	13.0	0.13	68.6%	315.3	53.3	3.3	124.2	12.5	100%	90%	70%
Geometric mean	15.7	0.2	63.1%	190.2	73.3	2.3	85.9	3.8	100%	100%	100%
95% CI	12.7-19.4	0.15-0.27	52.7-75.5%	138.4-261.4	45-120	1.8-3.1	69.2-106.6	2.3-6.2			

V_{ss} – Volume of distribution at steady state; V_{ss2} - Volume of distribution at steady state (peripheral compartment); AUC – Area under the concentration-time curve; Cl – Meropenem clearance; $T_{1/2}$ – Half life; NA- Data not available; IQR – Interquartile range; 95% CI - 95% confidence interval of the mean; T > – Percentage of time that meropenem concentration was above 2, 4 and 8 mgL.

Table 3 Comparison of early and late clinical and pharmacokinetic parameters in the 7 patients who completed two pharmacokinetic assessments

	Early	Late	P-value*
Cr Cl (mL/min)	66.7 [31.7]	106.7 [46.7]	0.128
SOFA	6 [3.5]	3 [1]	0.042
V_{ss} (L)	18.5 (13.0-26.4)	17.3 (7.3-41.0)	0.866
V_{ss}/**Weight** (l/kg)	0.25 (0.17-0.36)	0.23 (0.1-0.53)	0.866
V_{ss2}/V_{ss} (%)	61.3 (42.5-88.5)	51.7 (36.6-73.1)	0.176
Cl (mL/min)	120 (75-188.3)	135 (73.3-228.3)	0.398
Trough (mg/L)	2.6 (1.1-6.4)	1.5 (0.4-5.9)	0.172

Cr Cl – Creatine Clearance; SOFA- Sequential organ failure assessment score; V_{ss} – Volume of distribuition at steady state; V_{ss2} – Volume of distribution at steady state of the peripheral compartment; Cl – Meropenem Clearance; Early – Parameters measured within the first 36 hrs of meropenem therapy; Late – Parameters measured after the 5th day of meropenem therapy. *Wilcoxon signed ranks test. Data presented as geometric mean (95% confidence interval of the mean) or median [IQR].

Similarly to our findings, the clinical studies addressing meropenem PK in septic patients have generally reported high V_{ss} and Cl, with large inter-patient variability, exceeding a twofold variation [10-12]. This variability of PK parameters in septic patients treated with meropenem was noted both in the same patient during infection treatment and between different patients [10].

The mean meropenem V_{ss} in patients with ventilator associated pneumonia has been reported to be as high as 0.47 L/kg [12] or as low as 0.11 L/kg [11]. In our study the geometric mean V_{ss} was 0.20 L/kg, which is in the range of the values reported in volunteers [1], although we noted large inter-patient variability (Table 2).

The β-lactam antibiotics are hydrophilic drugs usually eliminated by the kidney. In septic critically ill patients Cr Cl is commonly aumengted and this has been shown to occur in septic surgical or trauma patients [13] as well as in medical patients [14]. Moreover patients with normal plasma creatinine frequently have aumengted Cr Cl that may be unrecognized without direct measurement [15].

Meropenem Cl has been noted to be correlated, as in our study, with the Cr Cl [16] and increases in drug Cl may lead to underexposure and facilitate the emergence of resistance, especially when long antibiotic courses are used. Nevertheless the relationship with Cr Cl is not linear and changes in Cr Cl may not reliably predict variations in β-lactam PK [17]. In a study addressing 11 surgical patients no change in meropenem Cl was noted between the first and the fourth day of therapy, despite an increase of roughly 25% in Cr Cl [18], which was similar to our results. In the same cohort the authors again noted a decrease, although non significant, of meropenem mean V_{ss}, from 0.22 ± 0.06 to 0.17 ± 0.06 L/kg, accompanying clinical improvement [18]. In another study, addressing 25 critically ill patients (either from the ICU or from hemato-oncology) [19], the authors noted low

trough concentrations and T > MIC due to increased Cl and Vd. Again these differences were only partly explained by increased Cr Cl. Conversely, drug accumulation occurred in ICU subjects with decreased renal function and therapeutic drug monitoring (TDM) was advised [19].

Since β-lactam TDM is not widely available, population PK models have been proposed. Moreover the model was improved in one study [20] by the inclusion of amikacin TDM and correctly predicted Vd and Cl of 4 different β-lactam antibiotics. In another study of population PK [21] imipenem Cl was found to be correlated with patients' demographic characteristics (age, weight and height) as well as with Cr Cl.

In our study we were able to unveil a relative decrease of the V_{ss2} during treatment, which maybe consequence of the reversal of fluid shifts and decrease of the interstitial compartment fluid volume [22].

Changes in PK may lead either to sub-therapeutic concentrations or to drug accumulation. In a study, 25% of patients with severe sepsis or septic shock did not attained the intended target after the first dose of 1 g of meropenem; this was due to a large V_{ss} (0.43 [Interquartile range 0.43] L/kg) [23]. Also an increase in Cl and a lower T > MIC of β-lactam antibiotics, may follow the increase in Cr Cl, noted in several septic critically ill patient, and contributed to treatment failure [24]. Several of these studies excluded patients with the lower Cr Cl (either measured or estimated). On the contrary, we choose to include all critically ill septic patients in order to increase the external validity. However we aknowledge that this may also help to explain why we only found one patient with augmented renal [25] or meropenem Cl.

To overcome the altered PK of critically ill patients TDM has been proposed [5]. However, currently therapeutic target concentrations are poorly defined and β-lactam TDM is seldom available in most hospitals. Proposed targets of β-lactam antibiotics ranged between 40 to 60% of T > MIC [26] but a T > MIC as high as 100% [27] or 40% T > 4*MIC [23] has also been suggested. Acording to our findings, the use of TDM seems to be not usefull in an unselected population of critically ill septic patients. In fact, only one of our patients had a Cr Cl higher than normal, above 130 mL/min (Table 1). However that same patient was the only one who did not attained a T > MIC of 100%. Besides, we did not find evidence of either underdosing or drug accumulation between early and late measurements.

However we believe that this strategy may be usefull for selected patients at high risk of PK changes, particularly those with augmented renal clearance [28], although better definition of the target concentrations is probably needed.

Continuous infusion of β-lactam antibiotics has also been proposed to achieve an improved concentration profile and a T > MIC of 100% [29,30]. This strategy, despite its biological plausibility, has produced disapointing results so far. Two recent randomized prospective studies both unveiled a non-significant decrease in hospital mortality with continuous infusion of β-lactam antibiotics, despite higher microbiological response. The first one included 60 patients treated with piperacillin/tazobactam, meropenem or ticarcillin [31]. Hospital mortality was 10% in the continuous group versus 20% in the intermittent arm (p = 0.47). Another study included 240 patients treated with a high dose of meropenem (6 g/day), either by continuous or intermittent infusion [32]. Hospital mortality was 17.5% vs 23.3%, respectivelly (p = 0.34). Similarly, a meta-analysis of another 14 prospective studies [33] and a retrospective matched case–control study of piperacillin/tazobactam [34], again failed to show a survival benefit. It should be noted that, if changes in the Vd and high MIC are not considered, with continuous infusion concentration of the antibiotic might be always under the MIC.

Overall it seems that both these strategies, continuous infusion of β-lactam antibiotics and TDM, are probably helpful in the presence of bacteria with a high MIC or a high inoculum or in the presence of augmented renal clearance [35], especially in the early phases of therapy [36].

This study has some limitations namely it is single center and included a relativelly small number of patients. Beside we did not measured patients weight daily although we were not able to find a correlation between patients' fluid balance and Vd. Nevertheless it also had some strengths: only critically ill septic patients were included, different infection focus were studied and an evaluation of early as well as late PK parameters was performed.

In the present study we confirmed the PK adequacy of the commonly used dose of meropenem to treat an unselected population of septic critically ill patients not receiving renal replacement therapy. As a result we did not find any evidence that the generalized use of meropenem TDM would be useful or cost-effective. Identification of sub-groups of patients most likely to benefit from this pratice should be performed before the general use of TDM monitoring can be recommended.

Conclusions

In a population of septic critically ill patients meropenem PK was found to have important heterogeneity, especially Cl and V_{ss}. A decrease of V_{ss2} was noted to parallel patients' improvement in the second meropenem PK assessment. Trough levels were found to be above 2 mg/dL in almost all patients at early samples but only in half of patients in late samples.

Abbreviations
AUC: Area under the concentration time curve; Cl: Clearance; Cr: Creatinine; ICU: Intensive Care Unit; HPLC: High performance liquid chromatography; MIC: Minimum inhibitory concentration; PK: Pharmacokinetic; SAPS: Simplified acute physiology score; SOFA: Sequential organ failure assessment; T>MIC: Antibiotic concentration time over bacteria MIC; $t_{1/2}$: Half-life; TDM: Therapeutic drug monitoring; V_{ss}: Volume of distribution at steady state; V_{ss1}: Volume of distribution of the central compartment at steady state; V_{ss2}: Volume of distribution of the peripheral compartment at steady state.

Competing interest
J.G.P. has received honoraria and served as advisor of Pfizer, Astra-Zeneca, Gilead, Abbott, Wyeth-Lederle, Janssen-Cilag, Merck Sharp & Dohme P.P. has received honoraria and served as advisor of Astra Zeneca, Ely-Lilly, Gilead, Janssen-Cilag, Merck Sharp & Dohme, Novartis and Pfizer. All other authors had no competing interests to declare.

Authors' contributions
JGP conceived the study. JGP, NES and PP participated in the original design and in writing the original protocol. JGP and PP collected the samples and clinical data. NES, AM and CP developed the HPLC methodology, performed laboratory testing and pharmacokinetic modelling. All authors analysed data. JGP, NES and PP draft the manuscript. All authors have read and approved the final manuscript.

Financial support
Unrestricted research grant from Astra-Zeneca who also supplied purified meropenem for laboratory testing. Merck, Sharp and Dohme supplied purified ertapenem for laboratory testing.
The WinNonlin software was used under an academic license from Pharsight Corporation to the Faculty of Pharmacy, University of Lisbon, Lisbon, Portugal.

Author details
[1]Polyvalent Intensive Care Unit, São Francisco Xavier Hospital, CHLO, Lisbon, Portugal, Estrada do Forte do Alto do Duque, Lisboa 1449-005, Portugal. [2]CEDOC, Faculty of Medical Sciences, New University of Lisbon, Lisbon, Portugal, Campo dos Mártires da Pátria, 130, Lisboa 1169-056, Portugal. [3]Faculty of Pharmacy, University of Lisbon, Lisbon, Portugal, Av. Prof. Gama Pinto, Lisbon 1649-003, Portugal.

References
1. Zhanel GG, Wiebe R, Dilay L, Thomson K, Rubinstein E, Hoban DJ, Noreddin AM, Karlowsky JA: **Comparative review of the carbapenems.** *Drugs* 2007, 67:1027–1052.
2. Pea F, Viale P: **Bench-to-bedside review: appropriate antibiotic therapy in severe sepsis and septic shock–does the dose matter?** *Crit Care* 2009, 13:214.
3. Roberts JA, Lipman J: **Antibacterial dosing in intensive care: pharmacokinetics, degree of disease and pharmacodynamics of sepsis.** *Clin Pharmacokinet* 2006, 45:755–773.
4. Goncalves-Pereira J, Povoa P: **Antibiotics in critically ill patients: a systematic review of the pharmacokinetics of beta-lactams.** *Crit Care* 2011, 15:R206.
5. Sime FB, Roberts MS, Peake SL, Lipman J, Roberts JA: **Does beta-lactam pharmacokinetic variability in critically Ill patients justify therapeutic drug monitoring? a systematic review.** *Ann Intensive Care* 2012, 2:35.
6. Triginer C, Izquierdo I, Fernandez R, Rello J, Torrent J, Benito S, Net A: **Gentamicin volume of distribution in critically ill septic patients.** *Intensive Care Med* 1990, 16:303–306.
7. Le Gall JR, Lemeshow S, Saulnier F: **A new simplified acute physiology score (SAPS II) based on a European/North American multicenter study.** *JAMA* 1993, 270:2957–2963.
8. Vincent JL, Moreno R, Takala J, Willatts S, De Mendonca A, Bruining H, Reinhart CK, Suter PM, Thijs LG: **The SOFA (Sepsis-related organ failure assessment) score to describe organ dysfunction/failure: on behalf of the working group on sepsis-related problems of the European society of intensive care medicine.** *Intensive Care Med* 1996, 22:707–710.

9. Charlson ME, Pompei P, Ales KL, MacKenzie CR: A new method of classifying prognostic comorbidity in longitudinal studies: development and validation. *J Chronic Dis* 1987, **40**:373–383.

10. Roberts JA, Kirkpatrick CM, Roberts MS, Robertson TA, Dalley AJ, Lipman J: **Meropenem dosing in critically ill patients with sepsis and without renal dysfunction: intermittent bolus versus continuous administration? Monte Carlo dosing simulations and subcutaneous tissue distribution.** *J Antimicrob Chemother* 2009, **64**:142–150.

11. Jaruratanasirikul S, Sriwiriyajan S, Punyo J: **Comparison of the pharmacodynamics of meropenem in patients with ventilator-associated pneumonia following administration by 3-hour infusion or bolus injection.** *Antimicrob Agents Chemother* 2005, **49**:1337–1339.

12. de Stoppelaar F, Stolk L, van Tiel F, Beysens A, van der Geest S, de Leeuw P: Meropenem pharmacokinetics and pharmacodynamics in patients with ventilator-associated pneumonia. *J Antimicrob Chemother* 2000, **46**:150–151.

13. Fuster-Lluch O, Geronimo-Pardo M, Peyro-Garcia R, Lizan-Garcia M: Glomerular hyperfiltration and albuminuria in critically ill patients. *Anaesth Intensive Care* 2008, **36**:674–680.

14. Baptista JP, Udy AA, Sousa E, Pimentel J, Wang L, Roberts JA, Lipman J: **A comparison of estimates of glomerular filtration in critically ill patients with augmented renal clearance.** *Crit Care* 2011, **15**:R139.

15. Udy AA, Baptista JP, Lim NL, Joynt GM, Jarrett P, Wockner L, Boots RJ, Lipman J: **Augmented renal clearance in the ICU: results of a multicenter observational study of renal function in critically ill patients with normal plasma creatinine concentrations*.** *Crit Care Med* 2014, **42**:520–527.

16. Kitzes-Cohen R, Farin D, Piva G, De Myttenaere-Bursztein SA: **Pharmacokinetics and pharmacodynamics of meropenem in critically ill patients.** *Int J Antimicrob Agents* 2002, **19**:105–110.

17. Casu GS, Hites M, Jacobs F, Cotton F, Wolff F, Beumier M, De Backer D, Vincent JL, Taccone FS: **Can changes in renal function predict variations in beta-lactam concentrations in septic patients?** *Int J Antimicrob Agents* 2013, **42**:422–428.

18. Lovering AM, Vickery CJ, Watkin DS, Leaper D, McMullin CM, White LO, Reeves DS, MacGowan AP: **The pharmacokinetics of meropenem in surgical patients with moderate or severe infections.** *J Antimicrob Chemother* 1995, **36**:165–172.

19. Binder L, Schworer H, Hoppe S, Streit F, Neumann S, Beckmann A, Wachter R, Oellerich M, Walson PD: **Pharmacokinetics of meropenem in critically ill patients with severe infections.** *Ther Drug Monit* 2013, **35**:63–70.

20. Delattre IK, Musuamba FT, Verbeeck RK, Dugernier T, Spapen H, Laterre PF, Wittebole X, Cumps J, Taccone FS, Vincent JL, Jacobs F, Wallemacq PE: **Empirical models for dosage optimization of four beta-lactams in critically ill septic patients based on therapeutic drug monitoring of amikacin.** *Clin Biochem* 2010, **43**:589–598.

21. Sakka SG, Glauner AK, Bulitta JB, Kinzig-Schippers M, Pfister W, Drusano GL, Sorgel F: **Population pharmacokinetics and pharmacodynamics of continuous versus short-term infusion of imipenem-cilastatin in critically ill patients in a randomized, controlled trial.** *Antimicrob Agents Chemother* 2007, **51**:3304–3310.

22. Nduka OO, Parrillo JE: **The pathophysiology of septic shock.** *Crit Care Clin* 2009, **25**:677–702. vii.

23. Taccone FS, Laterre PF, Dugernier T, Spapen H, Delattre I, Witebolle X, De Backer D, Layeux B, Wallemacq P, Vincent JL, Jacobs F: **Insufficient beta-lactam concentrations in the early phase of severe sepsis and septic shock.** *Crit Care* 2010, **14**:R126.

24. Lipman J, Wallis SC, Boots RJ: **Cefepime versus cefpirome: the importance of creatinine clearance.** *Anesth Analg* 2003, **97**:1149–1154.

25. Carlier M, De Waele JJ: **Identifying patients at risk for augmented renal clearance in the ICU - limitations and challenges.** *Crit Care* 2013, **17**:130.

26. Andes D, Anon J, Jacobs MR, Craig WA: **Application of pharmacokinetics and pharmacodynamics to antimicrobial therapy of respiratory tract infections.** *Clin Lab Med* 2004, **24**:477–502.

27. McKinnon PS, Paladino JA, Schentag JJ: **Evaluation of area under the inhibitory curve (AUIC) and time above the minimum inhibitory concentration (T > MIC) as predictors of outcome for cefepime and ceftazidime in serious bacterial infections.** *Int J Antimicrob Agents* 2008, **31**:345–351.

28. Hayashi Y, Lipman J, Udy AA, Ng M, McWhinney B, Ungerer J, Lust K, Roberts JA: **Beta-Lactam therapeutic drug monitoring in the critically ill:** optimising drug exposure in patients with fluctuating renal function and hypoalbuminaemia. *Int J Antimicrob Agents* 2012, **41**:162–166.

29. Nicolau DP: **Pharmacodynamic optimization of beta-lactams in the patient care setting.** *Crit Care* 2008, **12**(4):S2.

30. Kasiakou SK, Sermaides GJ, Michalopoulos A, Soteriades ES, Falagas ME: **Continuous versus intermittent intravenous administration of antibiotics: a meta-analysis of randomised controlled trials.** *Lancet Infect Dis* 2005, **5**:581–589.

31. Dulhunty JM, Roberts JA, Davis JS, Webb SA, Bellomo R, Gomersall C, Shirwadkar C, Eastwood GM, Myburgh J, Paterson DL, Lipman J: **Continuous infusion of beta-lactam antibiotics in severe sepsis: a multicenter double-blind, randomized controlled trial.** *Clin Infect Dis* 2012, **56**:236–244.

32. Chytra I, Stepan M, Benes J, Pelnar P, Zidkova A, Bergerova T, Pradl R, Kasal E: **Clinical and microbiological efficacy of continuous versus intermittent application of meropenem in critically ill patients: a randomized open-label controlled trial.** *Crit Care* 2012, **16**:R113.

33. Roberts JA, Webb S, Paterson D, Ho KM, Lipman J: **A systematic review on clinical benefits of continuous administration of beta-lactam antibiotics.** *Crit Care Med* 2009, **37**:2071–2078.

34. Goncalves-Pereira J, Oliveira BS, Janeiro S, Estilita J, Monteiro C, Salgueiro A, Vieira A, Gouveia J, Paulino C, Bento L, Povoa P: **Continuous infusion of piperacillin/tazobactam in septic critically ill patients–a multicenter propensity matched analysis.** *PLoS One* 2012, **7**:e49845.

35. Carlier M, Carrette S, Roberts JA, Stove V, Verstraete AG, Hoste E, Decruyenaere J, Depuydt P, Lipman J, Wallis SC, De Weale JJ: **Meropenem and piperacillin/tazobactam prescribing in critically ill patients: does augmented renal clearance affect pharmacokinetic/pharmacodynamic target attainment when extended infusions are used?** *Crit Care* 2013, **17**:R84.

36. Goncalves-Pereira J, Paiva JA: **Dose modulation: a new concept of antibiotic therapy in the critically ill patient?** *J Crit Care* 2013, **28**:341–346.

Permissions

The contributors of this book come from diverse backgrounds, making this book a truly international effort. This book will bring forth new frontiers with its revolutionizing research information and detailed analysis of the nascent developments around the world.

We would like to thank all the contributing authors for lending their expertise to make the book truly unique. They have played a crucial role in the development of this book. Without their invaluable contributions this book wouldn't have been possible. They have made vital efforts to compile up to date information on the varied aspects of this subject to make this book a valuable addition to the collection of many professionals and students.

This book was conceptualized with the vision of imparting up-to-date information and advanced data in this field. To ensure the same, a matchless editorial board was set up. Every individual on the board went through rigorous rounds of assessment to prove their worth. After which they invested a large part of their time researching and compiling the most relevant data for our readers.

The editorial board has been involved in producing this book since its inception. They have spent rigorous hours researching and exploring the diverse topics which have resulted in the successful publishing of this book. They have passed on their knowledge of decades through this book. To expedite this challenging task, the publisher supported the team at every step. A small team of assistant editors was also appointed to further simplify the editing procedure and attain best results for the readers.

Apart from the editorial board, the designing team has also invested a significant amount of their time in understanding the subject and creating the most relevant covers. They scrutinized every image to scout for the most suitable representation of the subject and create an appropriate cover for the book.

The publishing team has been an ardent support to the editorial, designing and production team. Their endless efforts to recruit the best for this project, has resulted in the accomplishment of this book. They are a veteran in the field of academics and their pool of knowledge is as vast as their experience in printing. Their expertise and guidance has proved useful at every step. Their uncompromising quality standards have made this book an exceptional effort. Their encouragement from time to time has been an inspiration for everyone.

The publisher and the editorial board hope that this book will prove to be a valuable piece of knowledge for researchers, students, practitioners and scholars across the globe.

List of Contributors

Chung-Hang Leung
State Key Laboratory of Quality Research in Chinese Medicine, Institute of Chinese Medical Sciences, University of Macau, Macao, China

Daniel Shiu-Hin Chan
Department of Chemistry, Hong Kong Baptist University, Kowloon Tong, Hong Kong

Ying-Wei Li
Centre for Cancer and Inflammation Research, School of Chinese Medicine, Hong Kong Baptist University, Kowloon Tong, Hong Kong

Wang-Fun Fong
Centre for Cancer and Inflammation Research, School of Chinese Medicine, Hong Kong Baptist University, Kowloon Tong, Hong Kong

Dik-Lung Ma
Department of Chemistry, Hong Kong Baptist University, Kowloon Tong, Hong Kong

Anthony Cahn
Medicines Discovery and Development, Gunnels Wood Road, Stevenage Herts SG1 2NY, UK

Simon Hodgson
Medicines Discovery and Development, Gunnels Wood Road, Stevenage Herts SG1 2NY, UK

Robert Wilson
Medicines Discovery and Development, Gunnels Wood Road, Stevenage Herts SG1 2NY, UK

Jonathan Robertson
Medicines Discovery and Development, Gunnels Wood Road, Stevenage Herts SG1 2NY, UK

Joanna Watson
GlaxoSmithKline, Stockley Park West, Uxbridge, Middlesex UB11 1BT, UK

Misba Beerahee
Medicines Discovery and Development, Gunnels Wood Road, Stevenage Herts SG1 2NY, UK

Steve C Hughes
GlaxoSmithKline, Park Road, Ware SG12 0DP, UK

Graeme Young
GlaxoSmithKline, Park Road, Ware SG12 0DP, UK

Rebecca Graves
Medicines Discovery and Development, Gunnels Wood Road, Stevenage Herts SG1 2NY, UK

David Hall
Medicines Discovery and Development, Gunnels Wood Road, Stevenage Herts SG1 2NY, UK

Sjoerd van Marle
PRA International, Stationsweg 163, Zuidlaren 9741 GP, the Netherlands

Roberto Solari
Medicines Discovery and Development, Gunnels Wood Road, Stevenage Herts SG1 2NY, UK

David G Levitt
Department of Integrative Biology and Physiology, University of Minnesota, 6-125 Jackson Hall, 321 Church St. S. E, Minneapolis, MN 55455, USA

Ronald G Hall II
Department of Pharmacy Practice, Texas Tech University Health Sciences Center, School of Pharmacy, Dallas, USA
Department of Clinical Sciences, University of Texas Southwestern, Dallas, USA

Kathleen A Hazlewood
Department of Pharmacy Practice, Texas Tech University Health Sciences Center, School of Pharmacy, Dallas, USA
Current affiliation: University of Wyoming School of Pharmacy, Swedish Family Medicine Residency Program, Englewood, USA

Sara D Brouse
Department of Pharmacy Practice, Texas Tech University Health Sciences Center, School of Pharmacy, Dallas, USA
Current affiliation: University of Kentucky Healthcare, Lexington, USA

Christopher A Giuliano
Department of Pharmacy Practice, Texas Tech University Health Sciences Center, School of Pharmacy, Amarillo, USA

Krystal K Haase
Department of Pharmacy Practice, Texas Tech University Health Sciences Center, School of Pharmacy, Amarillo, USA

Chistopher R Frei
Division of Pharmacotherapy, University of Texas, Austin, USA

Nicolas A Forcade
Division of Pharmacotherapy, University of Texas, Austin, USA
Current affiliation: Mission Regional Medical Center, Mission, USA

Todd Bell
Department of Internal Medicine, Texas Tech University Health Sciences Center, School of Medicine, Amarillo, USA

Roger J Bedimo
Department of Internal Medicine, University of Texas Southwestern, Dallas, USA

Carlos A Alvarez
Department of Pharmacy Practice, Texas Tech University Health Sciences Center, School of Pharmacy, Dallas, USA
Department of Clinical Sciences, University of Texas Southwestern, Dallas, USA

Marie Parel
Hospices Civils de Lyon, Clinical Oncology Pharmacy Department, Pierre-Bénite, France

Florence Ranchon
Hospices Civils de Lyon, Clinical Oncology Pharmacy Department, Pierre-Bénite - Université Lyon 1, EMR 3738, Lyon, France

Audrey Nosbaum
Hospices Civils de Lyon, Allergy and Clinical Immunology Department, Pierre-Bénite, France

Benoit You
Oncologie Médicale, Centre d'Investigation des Thérapeutiques en Oncologie et Hématologie de Lyon (CITOHL), Centre Hospitalier Lyon-Sud, Hospices Civils de Lyon, Lyon - Université Lyon 1, EMR 3738, Lyon, France.

Nicolas Vantard
Hospices Civils de Lyon, Clinical Oncology Pharmacy Department, Pierre-Bénite, France

Vérane Schwiertz
Hospices Civils de Lyon, Clinical Oncology Pharmacy Department, Pierre-Bénite, France

Chloé Gourc
Hospices Civils de Lyon, Clinical Oncology Pharmacy Department, Pierre-Bénite, France

Noémie Gauthier
Hospices Civils de Lyon, Clinical Oncology Pharmacy Department, Pierre-Bénite, France

Marie-Gabrielle Guedat
Hospices Civils de Lyon, Clinical Oncology Pharmacy Department, Pierre-Bénite, France

Sophie He
Hospices Civils de Lyon, Clinical Oncology Pharmacy Department, Pierre-Bénite, France

Eléna Kiouris
Hospices Civils de Lyon, Clinical Oncology Pharmacy Department, Pierre-Bénite, France

Céline Alloux
Hospices Civils de Lyon, Clinical Oncology Pharmacy Department, Pierre-Bénite, France

Thierry Vial
Centre Régional de pharmacovigilance de Lyon, France

Véronique Trillet-Lenoir
Oncologie Médicale, Centre d'Investigation des Thérapeutiques en Oncologie et Hématologie de Lyon (CITOHL), CentreHospitalier Lyon-Sud, Hospices Civils de Lyon, Lyon - Université Lyon 1, EMR 3738, Lyon, France

Gilles Freyer
Oncologie Médicale, Centre d'Investigation des Thérapeutiques en Oncologie et Hématologie de Lyon (CITOHL), CentreHospitalier Lyon-Sud, Hospices Civils de Lyon, Lyon - Université Lyon 1, EMR 3738, Lyon, France

Frédéric Berard
Hospices Civils de Lyon, Allergy and Clinical Immunology Department, Pierre-Bénite, France

Catherine Rioufol
Hospices Civils de Lyon, Clinical Oncology Pharmacy Department, Pierre-Bénite - Université Lyon 1, EMR 3738, Lyon, France

R Preston Mason
Cardiovascular Division, Department of Medicine, Brigham and Women's Hospital, Harvard Medical School, 02115 Boston, MA, USA
Elucida Research LLC, 01915 Beverly, MA, USA

Robert F Jacob
Elucida Research LLC, 01915 Beverly, MA, USA

J Jose Corbalan
Department of Chemistry and Biochemistry, Ohio University, 45701 Athens, OH, USA

Damian Szczesny
Department of Chemistry and Biochemistry, Ohio University, 45701 Athens, OH, USA

Kinga Matysiak
Department of Chemistry and Biochemistry,Ohio University, 45701 Athens, OH, USA

Tadeusz Malinski
Department of Chemistry and Biochemistry,Ohio University, 45701 Athens, OH, USA

Elizabeth Brunner
Eli Lilly and Company, Lilly Corporate Center, Indianapolis, Indiana 46285, USA

Deborah M Falk
Eli Lilly and Company, Lilly Corporate Center, Indianapolis, Indiana 46285, USA

Meghan Jones
Eli Lilly and Company, Lilly Corporate Center, Indianapolis, Indiana 46285, USA

Debashish K Dey
Eli Lilly and Company, Lilly Corporate Center, Indianapolis, Indiana 46285, USA

Chetan Chinmaya Shatapathy
Eli Lilly and Company, Lilly Corporate Center, Indianapolis, Indiana 46285, USA

Shamol Saha
Department of Pharmacology & Experimental Therapeutics, Laboratory of Molecular Neurobiology, Boston University School of Medicine, Boston, MA 02118, USA

Yinghui Hu
Department of Pharmacology & Experimental Therapeutics, Laboratory of Translational Epilepsy, Boston University School of Medicine, 72 East Concord Street, Boston, MA 02118, USA

Stella C Martin
Department of Pharmacology & Experimental Therapeutics, Laboratory of Molecular Neurobiology, Boston University School of Medicine, Boston, MA 02118, USA

Sabita Bandyopadhyay
Department of Pharmacology & Experimental Therapeutics, Laboratory of Translational Epilepsy, Boston University School of Medicine, 72 East Concord Street, Boston, MA 02118, USA

Shelley J Russek
Department of Pharmacology & Experimental Therapeutics, Laboratory of Translational Epilepsy, Boston University School of Medicine, 72 East Concord Street, Boston, MA 02118, USA

David H Farb
Department of Pharmacology & Experimental Therapeutics, Laboratory of Molecular Neurobiology, Boston University School of Medicine, Boston, MA 02118, USA

Kyla H Thomas
School of Social and Community Medicine, University of Bristol, Canynge Hall 39 Whatley Road, Bristol BS8 2PS, UK.
Health and Wellbeing Division, Department for Children, Adults and Health, South Gloucestershire Council Badminton Road, Yate, Bristol, UK

Richard M Martin
School of Social and Community Medicine, University of Bristol, Canynge Hall 39 Whatley Road, Bristol BS8 2PS, UK

John Potokar
The Academic Unit of Psychiatry, University of Bristol, Bristol, UK

Munir Pirmohamed
Centre for Drug Safety Science, University of Liverpool, Liverpool, UK

David Gunnell
School of Social and Community Medicine, University of Bristol, Canynge Hall 39 Whatley Road, Bristol BS8 2PS, UK

Brian K Schilling
Department of Health and Sport Sciences, The University of Memphis, 161 Roane Fieldhouse, 38152 Memphis, TN, USA

Kelley G Hammond
Department of Health and Sport Sciences, The University of Memphis, 161 Roane Fieldhouse, 38152 Memphis, TN, USA

Richard J Bloomer
Department of Health and Sport Sciences, The University of Memphis, 161 Roane Fieldhouse, 38152 Memphis, TN, USA

Chaela S Presley
University of Tennessee Health Sciences Center, Memphis, TN, USA

Charles R Yates
University of Tennessee Health Sciences Center, Memphis, TN, USA

Lise Aagaard
Clinical Pharmacology, Institute of Public Health, Faculty of Health Sciences, University of Southern Denmark, J.B. Winsløws Vej 19, DK - 5000 Odense C, Denmark

Danish Pharmacovigilance Research Project (DANPREP), Copenhagen, Denmark

Ebba Holme Hansen
Section for Social and Clinical Pharmacy, Department of Pharmacy, Faculty of Health and Medical Sciences, University of Copenhagen, Copenhagen, Denmark
Danish Pharmacovigilance Research Project (DANPREP), Copenhagen, Denmark

Elisabeth Ersvaer
Institute of Clinical Science, University of Bergen, Bergen, Norway
Institute of Biomedical Laboratory Sciences, Bergen University College, Nygårdsgaten 112, P.O. Box 7030, N-5020 Bergen, Norway

Annette K Brenner
Institute of Clinical Science, University of Bergen, Bergen, Norway

Kristin Vetås
Institute of Clinical Science, University of Bergen, Bergen, Norway

Håkon Reikvam
Institute of Clinical Science, University of Bergen, Bergen, Norway

Øystein Bruserud
Institute of Clinical Science, University of Bergen, Bergen, Norway
Department of Medicine, Haukeland University Hospital, Bergen, Norway

Jennifer R Bellis
Research & Development, Alder Hey Children's NHS Foundation Trust, Liverpool, UK

Jamie J Kirkham
Department of Biostatistics, University of Liverpool, Liverpool, UK

Anthony J Nunn
Department of Women's & Child Health, University of Liverpool, Liverpool, UK

Munir Pirmohamed
Department of Molecular and Clinical Pharmacology, University of Liverpool, Liverpool, UK

Zhi-duo Hou
Department of Rheumatology, the First Affiliated Hospital of Shantou University Medical College, No.57 Chang Ping Road, Shantou 515041, Guangdong Province, China

Zheng-yu Xiao
Department of Rheumatology, the First Affiliated Hospital of Shantou University Medical College, No.57 Chang Ping Road, Shantou 515041, Guangdong Province, China

Yao Gong
Department of Rheumatology, the First Affiliated Hospital of Shantou University Medical College, No.57 Chang Ping Road, Shantou 515041, Guangdong Province, China

Yu-ping Zhang
Department of Rheumatology, the First Affiliated Hospital of Shantou University Medical College, No.57 Chang Ping Road, Shantou 515041, Guangdong Province, China

Qing Yu Zeng
Research Unit of Rheumatology, Shantou University Medical College, No.22 Xin Ling Road, Shantou 515041, Guangdong Province, China

Jose E Cancado
Division of Pulmonary, Allergy, Critical Care and Sleep Medicine, University of Miami School of Medicine, Miami, FL 33136, USA

Eliana S Mendes
Division of Pulmonary, Allergy, Critical Care and Sleep Medicine, University of Miami School of Medicine, Miami, FL 33136, USA

Johana Arana
Division of Pulmonary, Allergy, Critical Care and Sleep Medicine, University of Miami School of Medicine, Miami, FL 33136, USA

Gabor Horvath
Department of Pulmonology, Semmelweis University School of Medicine, Budapest, Hungary

Maria E Monzon
Division of Pulmonary, Allergy, Critical Care and Sleep Medicine, University of Miami School of Medicine, Miami, FL 33136, USA

Matthias Salathe
Division of Pulmonary, Allergy, Critical Care and Sleep Medicine, University of Miami School of Medicine, Miami, FL 33136, USA

Adam Wanner
Division of Pulmonary, Allergy, Critical Care and Sleep Medicine, University of Miami School of Medicine, Miami, FL 33136, USA

Maxwell CK Leung
Nicholas School of the Environment, Duke University, Durham, NC, USA
Integrated Toxicology and Environmental Health Program, Duke University, Durham, NC, USA

John P Rooney
Nicholas School of the Environment, Duke University, Durham, NC, USA
Integrated Toxicology and Environmental Health Program, Duke University, Durham, NC, USA

Ian T Ryde
Nicholas School of the Environment, Duke University, Durham, NC, USA

Autumn J Bernal
Integrated Toxicology and Environmental Health Program, Duke University, Durham, NC, USA

Amanda S Bess
Nicholas School of the Environment, Duke University, Durham, NC, USA
Integrated Toxicology and Environmental Health Program, Duke University, Durham, NC, USA

Tracey L Crocker
Nicholas School of the Environment, Duke University, Durham, NC, USA

Alex Q Ji
Nicholas School of the Environment, Duke University, Durham, NC, USA

Joel N Meyer
Nicholas School of the Environment, Duke University, Durham, NC, USA
Integrated Toxicology and Environmental Health Program, Duke University, Durham, NC, USA

Adriana C. Vidal
Department of Surgery, Division of Urology, Cedars-Sinai Medical Center, Los Angeles, CA 90048, USA

Viktoriya Semenova
Department of Biological Sciences, Center for Human Health and the Environment, North Carolina State University, Raleigh, NC 27695, USA
Department of Public Health, Brody School of Medicine, East Carolina University, Greenville, NC 27834, USA

Thomas Darrah
Division of Water, Climate, and the Environment, School of Earth Sciences, The Ohio State University, Columbus, OH 43210, USA

Avner Vengosh
Nicholas School of the Environment, Duke University, Research Drive, Durham, NC 27710, USA

Zhiqing Huang
Division of Gynecologic Oncology, Department of Obstetrics and Gynecology, Duke University School of Medicine, Research Drive, Durham, NC 27710, USA

Katherine King
Environmental Public Health Division, U.S. Environmental Protection Agency, Chapel Hill, NC 27599, USA
Department of Community and Family Medicine and Duke Cancer Institute, Duke University School of Medicine, Erwin Drive, Durham, NC 27710, USA

Monica D. Nye
Division of Gynecologic Oncology, Department of Obstetrics and Gynecology, Duke University School of Medicine, Research Drive, Durham, NC 27710, USA
University of North Carolina at Chapel Hill, Lineberger Comprehensive Cancer Center, 450 West Drive, Chapel Hill, NC 27599, USA

Rebecca Fry
Department of Environmental Sciences and Engineering, Gillings School of Global Public Health, UNC-Chapel Hill, Chapel Hill, NC 27599, USA

David Skaar
Department of Biological Sciences, Center for Human Health and the Environment, North Carolina State University, Raleigh, NC 27695, USA

Rachel Maguire
Department of Biological Sciences, Center for Human Health and the Environment, North Carolina State University, Raleigh, NC 27695, USA

Amy Murtha
Division of Maternal Fetal Medicine, Department of Obstetrics and Gynecology, Duke University School of Medicine, Erwin Drive, Durham, NC 27710, USA

Joellen Schildkraut
Department of Community and Family Medicine and Duke Cancer Institute, Duke University School of Medicine, Erwin Drive, Durham, NC 27710, USA

Susan Murphy
Division of Gynecologic Oncology, Department of Obstetrics and Gynecology, Duke University School of Medicine, Research Drive, Durham, NC 27710, USA

Cathrine Hoyo
Department of Biological Sciences, Center for Human Health and the Environment, North Carolina State University, Raleigh, NC 27695, USA

Gulnazi Gurtskaia
Dept of Neurophysiology, Ivane Beritashvili Center for Experimental Biomedicine, Gotua Street 14, Tbilisi 0160, Georgia

Nana Tsiklauri
Dept of Neurophysiology, Ivane Beritashvili Center for Experimental Biomedicine, Gotua Street 14, Tbilisi 0160, Georgia

Ivliane Nozadze
Dept of Neurophysiology, Ivane Beritashvili Center for Experimental Biomedicine, Gotua Street 14, Tbilisi 0160, Georgia

Marina Nebieridze
Dept of Neurophysiology, Ivane Beritashvili Center for Experimental Biomedicine, Gotua Street 14, Tbilisi 0160, Georgia

Merab G Tsagareli
Dept of Neurophysiology, Ivane Beritashvili Center for Experimental Biomedicine, Gotua Street 14, Tbilisi 0160, Georgia

Ebru Diler
Institute of Anatomy, Saarland University, Kirrberger Str. 100, 66424 Homburg, Saar, Germany

Marion Schwarz
Institute of Anatomy, Saarland University, Kirrberger Str. 100, 66424 Homburg, Saar, Germany

Ruth Nickels
Institute for Clinical & Experimental Surgery, Saarland University, Homburg, Saar, Germany

Michael D Menger
Institute for Clinical & Experimental Surgery, Saarland University, Homburg, Saar, Germany

Christoph Beisswenger
Department of Internal Medicine V-Pulmonology, Allergology, Respiratory Intensive Care Medicine, Saarland University Hospital, Homburg, Saar, Germany

Carola Meier
Institute of Anatomy, Saarland University, Kirrberger Str. 100, 66424 Homburg, Saar, Germany

Thomas Tschernig
Institute of Anatomy, Saarland University, Kirrberger Str. 100, 66424 Homburg, Saar, Germany

Lee W Henderson
Sorbent Therapeutics Inc, 710 Lakeway Drive, Suite 290, Sunnyvale, CA 94085, USA

Howard C Dittrich
Sorbent Therapeutics Inc, 710 Lakeway Drive, Suite 290, Sunnyvale, CA 94085, USA

Alan Strickland
Alan Strickland Consulting, 101 Waterlily, Lake Jackson, TX 77566, USA

Thomas M Blok
Jasper Clinic's Clinical Research Unit, 526 Jasper Street, Kalamazoo, MI 49007, USA

Richard Newman
RnD Services, LLC, 635 Bent Creek Ridge, Deerfield, IL 60015, USA

Thomas Oliphant
Innovative Analytics, 161 East Michigan Ave, Kalamazoo, MI 49007, USA

Detlef Albrecht
Sorbent Therapeutics Inc, 710 Lakeway Drive, Suite 290, Sunnyvale, CA 94085, USA

Jody van den Ouweland
Department of Clinical Chemistry, Canisius Wilhelmina Hospital, Weg door Jonkerbos 100, 6532 SZ Nijmegen, The Netherlands

Hanneke Fleuren
Department of Clinical Pharmacy, Canisius-Wilhelmina Hospital, Nijmegen, The Netherlands

Miranda Drabbe
Nursing Home Waelwick, Ewijk Beuningen, The Netherlands

Hans Vollaard
Department of Clinical Pharmacy, Canisius-Wilhelmina Hospital, Nijmegen, The Netherlands

Henrik Lövborg
Department of Clinical Pharmacology and Department of Medical and Health Sciences, Linköping University, Linköping, Sweden
Clinical Pharmacology, University Hospital, S-581 85 Linköping, Sweden

Mikael Holmlund
Department of Clinical Pharmacology and Department of Medical and Health Sciences, Linköping University, Linköping, Sweden

Staffan Hägg
Department of Clinical Pharmacology and Department of Medical and Health Sciences, Linköping University, Linköping, Sweden

Anna K Szkaradkiewicz
Department of Conservative Dentistry and Periodontology, University of Medical Sciences, Bukowska 70, str., 60-812, Poznań, Poland

Tomasz M Karpiński
Department of Medical Microbiology, University of Medical Sciences, Wieniawskiego 3, str., 61-712 Poznań, Poland

Andrzej Szkaradkiewicz
Department of Medical Microbiology, University of Medical Sciences, Wieniawskiego 3, str., 61-712 Poznań, Poland

João Goncalves-Pereira
Polyvalent Intensive Care Unit, São Francisco Xavier Hospital, CHLO, Lisbon, Portugal, Estrada do Forte do Alto do Duque, Lisboa 1449-005, Portugal
CEDOC, Faculty of Medical Sciences, New University of Lisbon, Lisbon, Portugal, Campo dos Mártires da Pátria, 130, Lisboa 1169-056, Portugal

Nuno Elvas Silva
Faculty of Pharmacy, University of Lisbon, Lisbon, Portugal, Av. Prof. Gama Pinto, Lisbon 1649-003, Portugal

André Mateus
Faculty of Pharmacy, University of Lisbon, Lisbon, Portugal, Av. Prof. Gama Pinto, Lisbon 1649-003, Portugal

Catarina Pinho
Faculty of Pharmacy, University of Lisbon, Lisbon, Portugal, Av. Prof. Gama Pinto, Lisbon 1649-003, Portugal

Pedro Povoa
Polyvalent Intensive Care Unit, São Francisco Xavier Hospital, CHLO, Lisbon, Portugal, Estrada do Forte do Alto do Duque, Lisboa 1449-005, Portugal
CEDOC, Faculty of Medical Sciences, New University of Lisbon, Lisbon, Portugal, Campo dos Mártires da Pátria, 130, Lisboa 1169-056, Portugal